RADIOLOGY 101

The Basics and Fundamentals of Imaging

FIFTH EDITION

RADIOLOGY 101
The Basics and Fundamentals of Imaging

FIFTH EDITION

Thomas A. Farrell, MB, BCh
Attending Radiologist
Evanston Northwestern Healthcare
University of Chicago School of Medicine
Chicago, Illinois

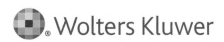

Philadelphia • Baltimore • New York • London
Buenos Aires • Hong Kong • Sydney • Tokyo

Acquisitions Editor: Sharon Zinner
Development Editor: Eric McDermott
Editorial Coordinator: John Larkin
Production Project Manager: Barton Dudlick
Design Coordinator: Holly McLaughlin
Manufacturing Coordinator: Beth Welsh
Prepress Vendor: TNQ Technologies

Fifth edition

9 8 7 6 5 4 3 2 1

Printed in China

Library of Congress Cataloging-in-Publication Data

ISBN-13: 978-1-4963-9298-5

Cataloging in Publication data available on request from publisher.

shop.lww.com

To my wife Laurie and daughters Niamh and Ciara.

Welcome to the fifth edition of *Radiology 101, the Basics and Fundamentals of Imaging.*

The labor(s) of love continue a full 2 decades after the publication of the first edition. While the practice of medicine and the specialty of radiology have changed a great deal since 1999, the basics and fundamentals are still as relevant and important as ever.

What has changed in this edition? You have seen the first change on the cover; Dr Wilbur Smith, one of the previous editors has hung up his lead apron after many years of service to the field of pediatric radiology. However, his legacy and that of the late Dr Bill Erkonen live on.

Radiology 101 is written for those seeking an understanding of imaging and for many readers it may be their introduction to the subject. By reading this book you should get an insight into the contribution made by imaging to the practice of medicine and that regardless of your experience or responsibilities in medicine, we hope your knowledge will be enhanced.

With each edition, we have strived to make the book relevant and readable. For the fifth edition, all chapters have been rewritten with expanded content in the chest, abdomen, and spine chapters, and we have added a new chapter on pelvic imaging, including obstetric ultrasound. We have deliberately kept our tables and lists of differential diagnoses short and our interesting cases to a minimum as there are plenty of bigger textbooks covering the various radiological subspecialties. Much of this book is concerned with ordering and interpretation of appropriate tests and the American College of Radiology Appropriateness Criteria© are widely referenced.

Whether you are "Rad oblivious" or "Rad curious," we urge you to seize the opportunity to become better acquainted with the specialty and all it has to offer. We strongly recommend volunteering for a radiology elective where you will witness firsthand many of the tests and thought processes described in this book. Better still, why not apply for a radiology residency—we are always looking for good people?

Thomas A. Farrell, MB, BCh

Contributing Authors

William J. Ankenbrandt, MD
Department of Radiology
NorthShore University HealthSystem
Clinical Associate Professor of Radiology
The University of Chicago Pritzker School of Medicine
Chicago, Illinois

Carolyn Donaldson, MD
Department of Radiology
NorthShore University HealthSystem
Clinical Assistant Professor of Radiology
The University of Chicago Pritzker School of Medicine
Chicago, Illinois

Laurie L. Fajardo, MD, MBA
Clinical Professor of Radiology
Department of Radiology
The University of Utah School of Medicine
Salt Lake City, Utah

Thomas A. Farrell, MB, BCh
Attending Radiologist
Evanston Northwestern Healthcare
University of Chicago School of Medicine
Chicago, Illinois

Nicholas Florence, MD
Resident Physician
Department of Radiology
University of Chicago
Chicago, Illinois

Bojan Petrovic, MD
Department of Radiology
NorthShore University HealthSystem
Clinical Assistant Professor
The University of Chicago Pritzker School of Medicine
Chicago, Illinois

Ethan A. Smith, MD
Clinical Assistant Professor
Department of Radiology
Cincinnati Children's Hospital
Cincinnati, Ohio

Wilbur L. Smith, MD
Former Professor and Chair
Department of Radiology
Wayne State University School of Medicine
Detroit Receiving Hospital
Detroit, Michigan

Christopher M. Straus, MD
Associate Professor
Department of Radiology
The University of Chicago Pritzker School of Medicine
Chicago, Illinois

Stephen Thomas, MD
Associate Professor
Department of Radiology
The University of Chicago Pritzker School of Medicine
Chicago, Illinois

Limin Yang, MD, PhD
Clinical Associate Professor
Department of Radiology
The University of Iowa
Iowa City, Iowa

Contents

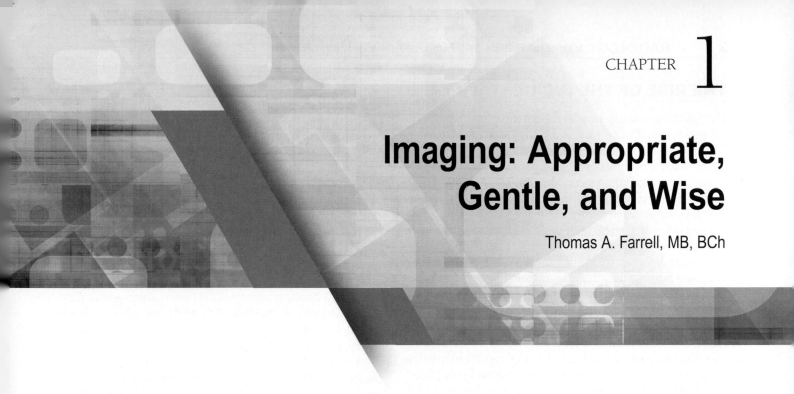

CHAPTER 1

Imaging: Appropriate, Gentle, and Wise

Thomas A. Farrell, MB, BCh

CHAPTER OUTLINE

More than a century has passed since Wilhelm Roentgen discovered X-rays, and in that time the impact of diagnostic imaging on patient care has been immeasurable. The innovation of techniques and technologies such as ultrasound, mammography CT, MRI, and positron emission tomography (PET) scanning have created a specialty central to the practice of medicine. However, this evolution has resulted in a significant increase in the population's cumulative exposure to ionizing radiation and the potential increase in cancer risk.

There has been a sevenfold increase in radiation exposure to the population of the United States from medical radiation since the early 1980s, with CT as the largest source of medical radiation exposure. The 2009 National Council on Radiation Protection and Measurements, Report No. 160—Ionizing Radiation Exposure of the Population of the United States—showed that medical exposure to patients is one of the largest sources of radiation exposure to Americans, nearly equaling the exposure from background sources. Although the United States has about 5% of the world's population, it accounts for 12% of all radiologic procedures and about half of all nuclear medicine procedures. It has been estimated that approximately 29,000 future cancers could be related to CT scans performed in the United States in 2007.

The United States spends twice as much on health care as any other high-income country in the world with heavy utilization of imaging technology as a contributory factor. In 2016, the United States spent 17.8% of its gross domestic product (GDP) on medical spending compared with other countries including Canada, the United Kingdom, Germany, Japan, and Sweden who spent between 9.6% and 12.4% of GDP on health care. Utilization of medical services in the United States was comparable to those of other nations—except in diagnostic imaging where 118 MRIs per 1,000 population was performed compared with a mean in all 11 countries of 82 per 1,000 population. Similarly, 245 CTs per 1,000 of the US population was performed compared with 151 per 1,000 population in other countries.

Reasons for this increase in utilization of diagnostic imaging are many and varied, including fear of litigation, the payment mechanisms and financial incentives in the US healthcare system, and self-referral as many nonradiologist physicians have a financial conflict of interest in using their own office-based diagnostic imaging equipment. Radiologists have several roles to play in dealing with overutilization; they should recommend additional imaging tests in their reports only when they conform to published guidelines and avoid generic recommendations about additional testing that tie the hands of the ordering physicians compelling them to order further tests largely for defensive purposes.

THE RISE OF THE INCIDENTALOMA

The growing use of cross-sectional imaging, particularly CT, has resulted in an increase in the detection of incidental findings that are unrelated to the clinical indication for which the exam is performed—**incidentaloma**. The prevalence of an adrenal incidentaloma on CT in older patients is 10%. Renal cysts are found in more than 40% of abdominal CTs. The vast majority of incidentalomas are benign but present a challenge, both to physicians and patients on their clinical significance and subsequent management. If a radiologist believes an incidentaloma is of no clinical significance but includes it in the radiology report, a cascade of tests, biopsies, and other procedures may follow, all of which have a financial cost and a risk of complications. If a radiologist believes an incidentaloma is of no clinical significance but includes it in a radiology report, further testing, with the financial cost and risk of complications may follow. However, if the incidentaloma is not reported by the radiologist but later turns out to be an early carcinoma, a malpractice lawsuit may be filed. The rise of incidentaloma's in the workup has been partially blamed for the increased utilization of cross-sectional imaging and can also result in unnecessary testing and treatment. To address this problem, the American College of Radiology (ACR) Incidental Findings Committee have published a series of guidelines and white papers on managing incidental findings.

APPROPRIATE CRITERIA

The ACR, which has been an advocate for radiation safety since its inception in 1924, first developed **appropriateness criteria (AC)** in 1994 to primarily address the use of imaging technology. Currently, these appropriateness criteria cover 215 diagnostic radiology topics with more than 1080 clinical variants. The goal of this program is to allow a group of experts and stakeholders to objectively determine the benefits and harms of performing imaging based on a systematic review of the evidence. The AC committees (expert panels totaling more than 300 physicians, including some 80 clinical specialists from 20 nonradiologic medical organizations) systematically review evidence to develop guidelines to assist referring clinicians in ordering the most appropriate imaging for specific clinical conditions. The ACR AC methodology is based on the RAND/University of California at Los Angeles (UCLA) Appropriateness Method User's Manual where "the expected health benefit (e.g., increased life expectancy, relief of pain, reduction in anxiety, improved functional capacity) exceeds the expected negative consequences (e.g., mortality, morbidity, anxiety, pain, time lost from work) by a sufficiently wide margin that the procedure is worth doing, exclusive of cost." Each AC review assesses the risks and benefits of the imaging tests for several indications or clinical scenarios and score them based on a scale of 1 to 9, where the upper range (7–9) implies that the test is generally acceptable and is a reasonable approach and the lower range (1–3) implies that the test is generally not acceptable and is not a reasonable approach. The midrange (4–6) indicates an uncertain clinical scenario. By developing these guidelines and encouraging their use, the ACR is promoting the best use of radiological resources and enhancing the quality of patient care. Many of these guidelines are incorporated in this book. They are available free online and well worth reviewing (www.acr.org)

One way to decrease inappropriate imaging and promote judicious use of imaging resources is the implementation of clinical decision support (CDS) when ordering examinations. The use of imaging CDS, which provides evidence-based feedback to ordering physicians at the time of order entry, has resulted in substantial decreases in the utilization rates of lumbar MRI for low-back pain, head MRI for headache, and sinus CT. The odds of an acute pulmonary embolism (PE) finding in patients when providers adhered to evidence presented in the CDS were nearly double those seen when providers overrode the CDS alerts. Starting in January 2020, the adoption of CDS for advanced imaging (CT, MR, nuclear medicine including PET) will be incentivized for Medicare reimbursement, almost certainly to be followed shortly thereafter by other insurance providers in the United States. The ACR AC will form the basis for software that can be used to fulfill the criteria for CDS which will affect how imaging examinations are ordered. In summary, CDS based on the ACR's AC will change the practice of the ordering diagnostic imaging tests.

IMAGE GENTLY

Children have a lifetime to either derive benefit from or be harmed by the imaging choices made on their behalf. Children are more susceptible to the potential increased risk of cancer from ionizing radiation because of the following: (1) They are smaller, so for any given set of CT scanning parameters, the effective radiation dose is higher for smaller cross-sectional areas, an effect most pronounced in the youngest patients with smaller body mass and radius. (2) They are growing, so their tissues are more radiosensitive than adult tissues. (3) They have longer remaining lifespans, allowing a sufficient time for a latency period during which malignancy may develop.

In 2007, a coalition of healthcare organizations led by ACR and Society for Pediatric Radiology was formed to promote safe, high-quality pediatric imaging. The primary objective was to raise awareness in the imaging community of the need to adjust radiation dose when imaging children. The resulting **"Image Gently"** campaign initially focused on dose optimization for CT but now includes other imaging modalities such as interventional radiology, fluoroscopy, and nuclear medicine. Current recommendations include the following: (1) Review of the standard adult CT protocols by a medical physicist and then modifying the exposure parameters to "right-size" the protocols for children. (2) Avoiding pre and postcontrast and delayed CT scans as they rarely add information in children. Single-phase scans are usually adequate in children. (3) Scanning only the indicated area to obtain the necessary information.

These three recommendations follow the **ALARA** principal of radiation safety. ALARA is an acronym for "as low as (is) reasonably achievable," which means making every reasonable effort to maintain exposures to ionizing radiation as far below the dose limits as practical, consistent with the purpose for which the licensed activity is undertaken, This principle means that even if it is a small dose, if receiving that dose has no direct benefit, you should try to avoid it.

IMAGE WISELY

The ACR and Radiological Society of North America formed a task force to address adult radiation protection by building on the success of the Image Gently campaign for children. The aim of the task force was to educate providers of the need and the opportunities to eliminate unnecessary imaging examinations and to lower the amount of radiation used during imaging to only that needed to capture optimal medical images. In 2010, the task force expanded with involvement of the American Society of Radiological Technologists and American Association of Physicists in Medicine and developed a campaign called **"Image Wisely"** which provides educational resources on the subject. Since its inception, Image Wisely has stressed the ALARA principle by focusing on appropriate examination indications and optimization of imaging techniques to achieve diagnostic quality examinations. Over 50,000 pledges have been made, mostly by radiology technologists to achieve these goals.

In 2012, the American Board of Internal Medicine Foundation collaborated with *Consumer Reports*, a nonprofit advocacy organization, to develop the **Choosing Wisely** initiative. The Foundation invited nine medical organizations including the ACR, the American College of Cardiology, and the American Society of Nuclear Cardiology to each pick five tests or treatments within their purview that they believed were overused. The Choosing Wisely website lists these 45 tests and treatments, 24 of which are directly related to diagnostic imaging. The medical organizations involved in this initiative deserve credit for their participation in the campaign as their members perform the very tests that they included on their lists and this could adversely affect their practices. The ACR's first set of Choosing Wisely recommendations were based on five of the overused imaging tests that could be safely targeted for refinement, as supported by published evidence (Table 1.1).

TABLE 1.1	American College of Radiology's *Choosing Wisely*: First Slate of 5 Recommendations

1. Do not image for complicated headache.
2. Do not image for suspected PE without moderate or high pretest probability.
3. Avoid admission or preoperative chest radiography for ambulatory patients with unremarkable findings on history and physical examination.
4. Do not do CT to evaluate suspected appendicitis in children until ultrasound is being considered as an option.
5. Do not recommend follow-up imaging for clinically inconsequential adnexal cysts.

Used with permission from Johnson PT, Bello JA, Chatfield MB, et al. New ACR choosing wisely recommendations: judicious use of multiphase abdominal CT protocols. *J Am Coll Radiol.* 2019;16:56-60. doi:10.1016/j.jacr.2018.07.026.

In its second slate of ACR Choosing Wisely recommendations (2017), three recommendations guide the management of incidental findings (thyroid nodules, pelvic congestion syndrome, and small bowel intussusception in adults) and two recommendations focus on IV contrast-enhanced abdominal CT protocols that include a precontrast acquisition or delayed acquisition (after the portal venous or nephrographic phases) (see Tables 3.8 and 3.9).

While the benefits of diagnostic imaging are immense and certainly exceed the risks, this is only true when the tests are ordered appropriately and studies are optimized to obtain the best image quality with the lowest radiation dose. In addition to the financial cost incurred, unnecessary and inappropriately performed imaging tests harm patients by exposing them to ionizing radiation and by discovering incidentalomas, the workup of which may cause discomfort and complications. The radiologist has a central role in selecting the most appropriate imaging examination and indication-based protocol for each patient, timely reporting of results, and indicating follow-up testing. As radiologists, we can either be part of the problem or part of the solution—the choice is ours. Here's to the next century of diagnostic imaging.

References

1. www.acr.org/Clinical-Resources/ACR-Appropriateness-Criteria.
2. www.imagegently.org.
3. www.choosingwisely.org.
4. www.Imagewisely.org.

Further Reading

1. Berlin L. The incidentaloma: a medicolegal dilemma. *Radiol Clin North Am.* 2011;49:245-255.
2. www.acr.org/Clinical-Resources/Incidental-Findings.

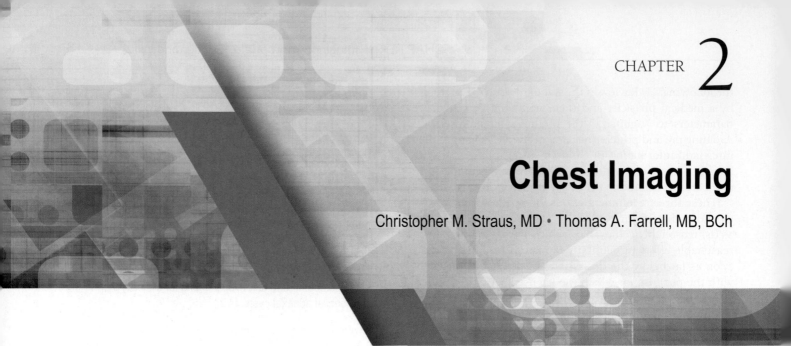

CHAPTER 2

Chest Imaging

Christopher M. Straus, MD • Thomas A. Farrell, MB, BCh

The chest radiograph accounts for approximately 45% of all radiographic examinations in the United States and is an essential tool in the management of patients with cardiorespiratory disorders. This chapter will serve two purposes: Firstly, to provide a logical approach to the interpretation of chest imaging studies with emphasis on chest radiographs and CT and secondly to review the imaging findings of common diseases of the chest.

RADIOGRAPHIC TECHNIQUE

The standard chest radiograph exam consists of two projections, namely **posteroanterior** (PA) and **lateral** views. (We use the terms radiograph and film interchangeably,

but we avoid the term "X-ray"). When the patient's clinical condition prevents obtaining a PA view, a single portable **anteroposterior (AP)** view can be done with the understanding that portable films of the chest are less sensitive for detecting disease because of technical limitations such as magnification, suboptimal patient positioning, and variation in exam technique. In certain settings, for example, when the patient is unstable, portable exams are acceptable, but, if possible, a standard PA view in the radiology department is preferable because consistency of technique over serial exams is important in the detection of subtle change.

Correct patient identification may seem elementary, but errors do occur. Fortunately, with the advent of the electronic medical record and picture archive and

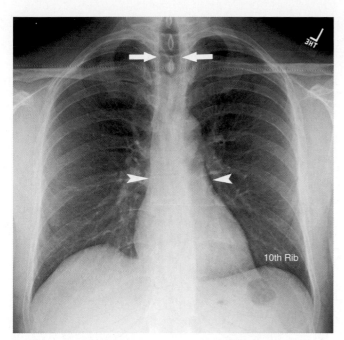

FIGURE 2.1. **Normal chest, PA radiograph.** The vertical trachea (*straight arrows*) should always be midline. The normal mediastinum is of water density (*arrowheads*).

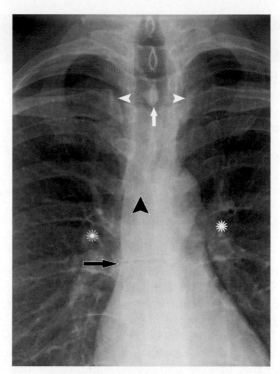

FIGURE 2.2. **Normal chest, PA radiograph. Magnified view showing central structures.** The medial ends of the clavicles (*white arrowheads*) are equidistant from the spinous process, (*white arrow*). The hilar points (*asterisks*) are not at the same level, the right hilar point being higher. The carina (*black arrowhead*) marks the bifurcation of the trachea and is an important landmark for endotracheal tube tip placement. Visualization of the intervertebral disk spaces of the thoracic spine (*black arrow*) is a sign of adequate radiographic exposure.

TABLE 2.1	Technical Adequacy of a PA Chest Film
Rotation	The medial ends of both clavicles should be centered on the thoracic spine
Penetration	The thoracic disk spaces should be visible
Inspiration	8–10 ribs should be visible posteriorly or 6 ribs anteriorly

communication systems, these errors are rare. Identification requires correct left–right annotation, as all images are annotated routinely with either a left or right marker by the technologist. For all frontal chest radiographs (either AP or PA), the right (R) or left (L) markers indicate the patient's right and left side, respectively (Fig. 2.1).

What constitutes a **technically adequate** chest radiograph and why is this important? A technically adequate image is necessary to avoid misidentifying or missing findings that would otherwise be observed. Interpretation is a process that is subject to exam limitations, and the interpreter must have confidence in the image and be able to reason why the image appears as it does or otherwise have to justify a repeat or request more advanced imaging. First, evaluate patient **positioning** to exclude rotation, as the medial ends of the clavicles should be equidistant from the spinous processes (Fig. 2.2). Next check the **exposure**, which is optimal when the thoracic disk spaces are just distinguishable and superimposed on the heart (Fig. 2.2). In addition, the lungs should not be overexposed (black), and the blood vessels in the lung should be defined peripherally but not quite reaching the edge. Finally, the diaphragm should be roughly at the level of the eighth to tenth posterior ribs with a standard **inspiratory effort** (Table 2.1).

The default radiographic chest technique and positioning are designed to optimize evaluation of the lungs and do not generally provide enough diagnostic information of extrapulmonary structures, such as bones or soft tissues. Dedicated rib or spine exams provide better evaluation of these structures.

INTERPRETATION

Frontal

When learning to interpret chest radiographs, it is important to realize that "you will only see what you know." Lack of anatomical knowledge and spatial relationships will hinder your interpretation. Also, the greater number of images you study, the greater your memory bank and expertise becomes. Anatomically there is a right upper, lower, and middle lobe separated by the major and minor fissures and just an upper and lower left lobe separated by a left major

TABLE 2.2	Checklist for Review of Chest Radiographs
PA (or AP) view	**Lateral view**
Patient demographics	
Previous imaging	
Trachea, carina	Trachea
Heart: size, shape, borders	Cardiac outline
Aortic arch, AP window, hila	Hila
Lungs: vasculature and lucency	Retrosternal and retrocardiac lucencies
Diaphragm, gastric bubble	Hemidiaphragms
Bones, soft tissues, 4 corners.	

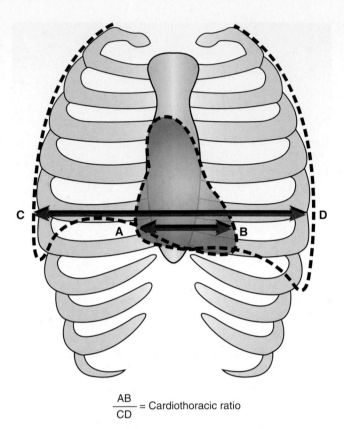

$$\frac{AB}{CD} = \text{Cardiothoracic ratio}$$

FIGURE 2.3. The cardiothoracic ratio (CTR). The CTR is calculated by measuring the transverse diameter of the heart (A–B) and dividing it by the transverse thoracic measurement (C–D).

fissure. Each lobe routinely in turn is divided into as many as five segments, each with its own bronchus and blood supply. The apical segment of both lower lobes can be found as high as the level of the T4 posteriorly.

A logical and methodical approach for review is recommended. Checklists reduce human error and are essential in radiology to avoid overlooking abnormalities. One such checklist is provided in Table 2.2, yet the most important factor in missing abnormalities is lack of consistency. Develop your own checklist and be consistent. Top of any checklist is to **always review previous imaging**. It is useful to start at the top and middle of the radiograph and identify the **trachea**, which on a correctly centered PA film should be near midline, superimposed over the spinous processes of the upper thoracic spine, and minimally deviated away from the aorta arch (usually just to the patient's right of midline). Any deviation or narrowing of the trachea on a properly centered film may indicate a mediastinal or thyroid mass (Fig. 2.1).

Next, follow the trachea inferiorly and identify the **carina,** which serves as a landmark for placement of endotracheal tubes. Evaluate both **contour and width of the mediastinum**. Mediastinal widening (>8 cm) may occur in patients with an aortic aneurysm or dissection, but in the elderly the thoracic aorta may appear tortuous or ectatic, a finding that should not be interpreted as abnormal.

Next evaluate the **cardiac outline, for size and shape**. The transverse diameter of the heart should not exceed 50% of the transverse diameter of the thoracic cage measured at the same level. This is called the **cardiothoracic ratio** (Fig. 2.3). This measurement, however, is only reliable on PA projections as there is approximately a 20% magnification of the cardiac silhouette on AP projections. For this reason, PA (with the anterior chest wall closest to the image cassette) views are preferable. A poor inspiratory effort or recumbent posture can further falsely increase the cardiac size.

Next, evaluate the shape of the **cardiac silhouette**, which has multiple components. The more convex **right cardiac border** represents the right atrial margin, which is just below the vertically straight margin of the superior vena cava (SVC)

(Fig. 2.4). The **left cardiac border** towards the apex represents the left atrial appendage and left ventricle. The superior left cardiac border should be concave and less steeply angled. Given the natural rotation and superimposition of the cardiac chambers, the right ventricle is not a component of the cardiac silhouette on frontal radiographs (Fig. 2.4). Similarly, a normally sized left atrium is also not visible on frontal radiographs. However, in marked left atrial enlargement, the superior left heart border becomes convex and splays the carina with elevation or "horizontal leveling" of the left mainstem bronchus. In severe left atrial enlargement, the right lateral border of the left atrium is superimposed over the right atrial shadow, producing a **double-density sign** (Fig. 2.5). As the left ventricle enlarges, the cardiac apex moves down and out. As the right atrium enlarges, the right heart border becomes convex (Figs. 2.6 and 2.7).

Next, review **the aortic arch, pulmonary arteries, and the mainstem bronchi**. The lung hilum is where the structures such as blood vessels and bronchi enter the lung. These hilar structures are arranged in a similar manner from the front to the back on each side with the upper of the two pulmonary veins in front, the pulmonary artery in the middle, and the bronchus and bronchial vessels posteriorly. Because the left pulmonary artery arches over the left mainstem bronchus, the anatomical arrangements are not symmetrical bilaterally.

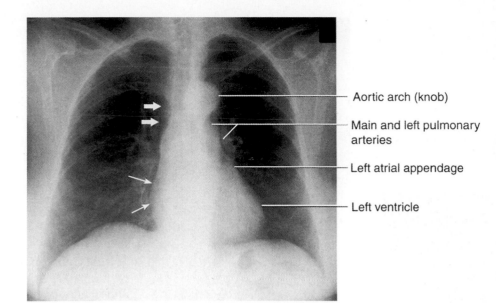

Aortic arch (knob)

Main and left pulmonary arteries

Left atrial appendage

Left ventricle

FIGURE 2.4. **Normal chest, PA radiograph.** The convex right cardiac border is formed by the right atrium (*thin arrows*) and the superior vena cava is indicated by the *heavy arrows*. The left border is composed of four "bumps," from cephalad to caudad; these are the aortic arch, the main and left pulmonary arteries, the left atrial appendage, and the left ventricle.

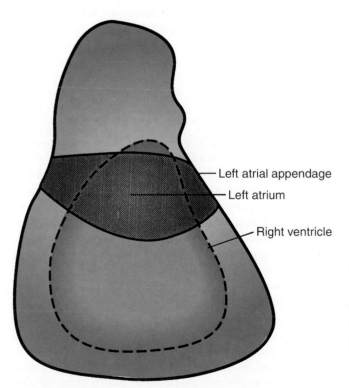

Left atrial appendage

Left atrium

Right ventricle

FIGURE 2.5. **Locations of the left atrium and right ventricle** on a normal PA or AP chest radiograph. This diagram shows the locations of the left atrium and right ventricle superimposed on the cardiac shadow emphasizing that neither of these chambers can be seen on a normal frontal view.

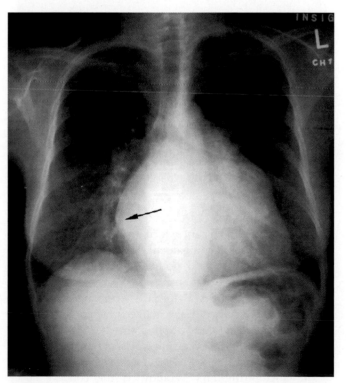

FIGURE 2.6. **Left atrial enlargement.** PA radiograph. This film shows the double density sign (*arrow*) produced by the overlapping of the left atrium with the right heart border (right atrium). Also, note the outward convexity of the upper left heart border typically seen with left atrial enlargement.

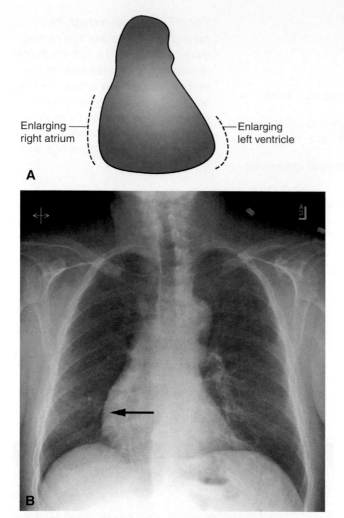

FIGURE 2.7. Right atrial and left ventricular enlargement.
Cardiac silhouette changes during right atrium and left ventricle
enlargement. **A:** As the right atrium enlarges, the convex right heart
border enlarges to the patient's right. As the left ventricle enlarges,
the cardiac apex moves to the patient's left and downward. **B:** PA
chest radiograph showing right atrial enlargement (*arrow*).

Additional components of the hilum include lymph nodes
and a layer of parietal pleura, which folds inferiorly to become
the **inferior pulmonary ligament**, which secures the lower
lobe in position. The **hilar point** (best seen on a PA view)
is where the superior pulmonary vein crosses the descending
pulmonary artery and is useful in determining the position
of the hilum. On normal chest radiographs, the left hilum is
higher than the right hilum in approximately 70% of films and
is at the same level in the remaining 30% of cases (Fig. 2.2). A
lower left than right hilum indicates left lower lobe collapse.

The **aortopulmonary window** is the concave space
immediately below the aortic arch and above the left pulmonary artery (Fig. 2.2). Loss of this concavity may be due
to a mass or lymphadenopathy.

The **pulmonary arteries** and their adjacent **bronchi**
radiate outward from the hila, with the **pulmonary veins**
returning blood back to the left atrium. The angle of the

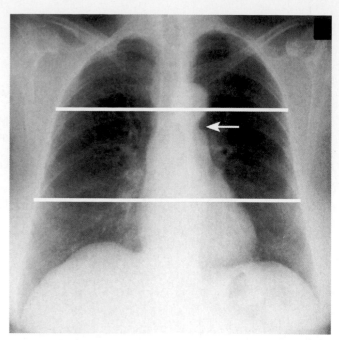

FIGURE 2.8. Normal lung lucency. Chest PA radiograph.
Divide the PA or AP chest radiograph into horizontal thirds and
compare the right and left lung fields moving in a head to foot
direction. Note the aortopulmonary window (*arrow*).

vessel can at times indicate which vessels are arteries and
which are veins, trace a vessel in question to a point of
intersection with other tissues to help assist you in identifying which one it is. That is often the more horizontal
vessels are usually projected in towards the left atrium and
represent returning pulmonary veins In an upright person, the pressure differential and difference in lung volume (lungs are deeper at the bases) are both enough that
the lower lobe pulmonary vessels should be both larger
in size and number as compared to those extending into
the upper lobes. Vessels serving the upper and lower lobes
respectfully are approximately observed in a 1:3 ratio, both
for diameter and number. Alteration in this appearance can
be helpful in determining *vascular redistribution or shunting* and evaluation can be achieved by dividing the lungs
into horizontal thirds, comparing the both the right and
left lungs for symmetry and vascularity (Fig. 2.8). The pulmonary vessels and bronchi are normally almost invisible
in the peripheral 2cm of the lung on a chest radiograph.

Next, evaluate both **diaphragms**; the right hemidiaphragm is often about 1 to 2 cm higher than the left because
of the presence of the liver, yet there is considerable variability. The lateral recesses of the diaphragms form the lateral
costophrenic angles, which should be sharp, where the diaphragms insert laterally to the chest wall. Finally, determine
the location of the **gastric air bubble** (if present), which
should be underneath the left hemidiaphragm (Fig. 2.9).

Evaluation of the **bones** includes the lower cervical spine,
thoracic spine, shoulders, and ribs. On a PA radiograph, the
scapulae should be rotated off the lungs. The posterior portions

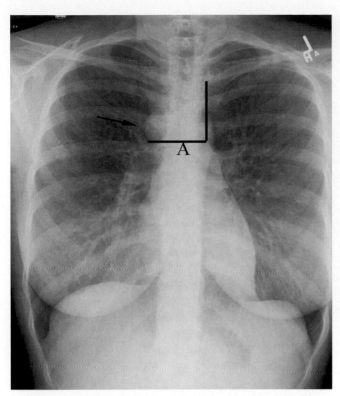

FIGURE 2.9. Normal vascular pedicle. The vascular pedicle is determined by drawing a horizontal line (*A*) from the junction of the azygos vein (*arrow*) and SVC over to a perpendicular line drawn from the left subclavian artery inferiorly along the transverse portion of the thoracic aorta (aortic arch).

of each rib are horizontally oriented and the anterior ribs are usually angled inferiorly (Fig. 2.10). Rib abnormalities may be easier to detect by rotating the image 90 degrees (clock- or counterclockwise). Although bony structures are not as well delineated on chest radiographs, significant abnormalities

can be seen, emphasizing the need for review of all aspects of the image including all four corners (Fig. 2.11).

In addition to the "four corners" of the chest film, four other areas where abnormalities are commonly missed are in the hila, apices, behind the heart, and adjacent to the diaphragm.

Lateral View

The frontal view represents only 70% of the total lung volume, reinforcing the radiological truism that "one view is no view" when interpreting chest films. The lateral view allows confirmation of the location and nature of abnormalities seen on the frontal view. Even if you can make a confident diagnosis on the frontal view, it is an excellent habit to correlate and confirm the findings on the lateral view. For lateral chest radiographs, it is customary to have the film oriented such that the patient is facing toward your left because magnification of the heart is minimized when the heart is closest to the film or detector (Fig. 2.12). Consistent and methodical search patterns are again paramount in developing your detection skills. As with the frontal view, evaluate the size and shape of the cardiac silhouette, the anterior border of which is formed by the right ventricle. The left ventricle forms most of the inferior–posterior cardiac border, and the left atrium forms the superior–posterior cardiac border. Normally there is a single vertebral body width of clear lung between the posterior cardiac margin and the anterior osseous spine.

Often the posterior wall of the inferior vena cava (IVC) can be seen inferiorly as it enters the right atrium (Fig. 2.12, *arrows*). The IVC outline can be useful in the determination of left ventricular size, given that the posterior border of the left ventricle should be 2 cm or less from the inferior vena cava. The right atrium is a superimposed cardiac chamber and is not seen on the lateral view

The lateral chest radiograph provides an excellent view of both **hila**, which can be located by drawing a vertical line

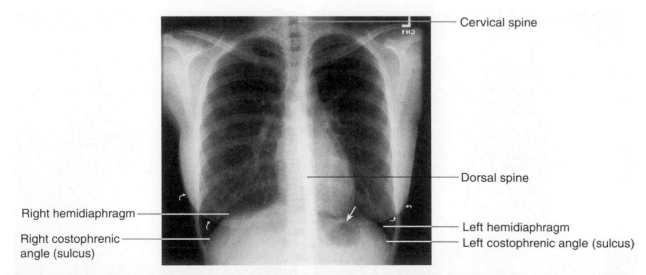

— Cervical spine

— Dorsal spine

Right hemidiaphragm —

Right costophrenic — angle (sulcus)

— Left hemidiaphragm
— Left costophrenic angle (sulcus)

FIGURE 2.10. Normal PA chest radiograph. After comparing the lung fields, you next view the diaphragms, costophrenic angles, and lower dorsal spine. Note the close proximity of the gastric fundus air to the left hemidiaphragm (*straight arrow*). Always remember to identify both breast shadows in female patients (*curved arrows*).

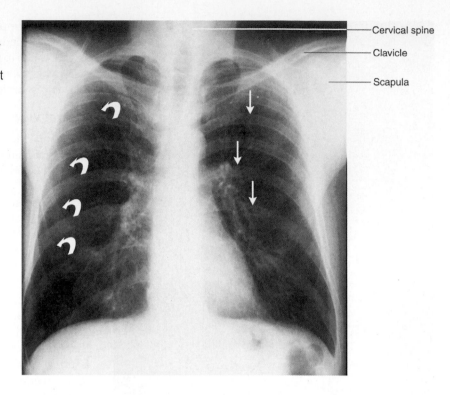

FIGURE 2.11. **Normal PA chest radiograph.** The posterior ribs (*straight arrows*) are horizontal and anterior ribs (*curved arrows*) are angled caudad or inferiorly. All of these structures must be included in your checklist as well as the shoulder girdles and cervical and dorsal spine areas.

Cervical spine

Clavicle

Scapula

down the trachea (Fig. 2.13). There is considerable variability in the **pulmonary venous drainage** patterns, but usually they drain into the left atrium bilaterally through two main trunks. Both upper lobe bronchi are seen on end in the lateral view. The **left pulmonary artery** is a direct continuation of the main pulmonary artery, continuing posteriorly and somewhat laterally as it passes first above and then behind the left upper lobe bronchus and extends well into the left lung where it is surrounded by air, enhancing its conspicuity. The dominant density anteriorly is largely **the right**

pulmonary artery. Even minimal rotation from a true lateral view changes the appearance of the hila, causing vascular structures to be mistaken for tumors and underlines the need for high technical standard when obtaining this view.

Next on the lateral view, locate the sternum, retrosternal aerated lung, and precardiac spaces (Fig. 2.14). The **retrosternal lucency** is due to the superimposition of the aerated upper lobes, whereas the right middle lobe and the lingular segment of the left lobe are obscured by the cardiac silhouette. The lower lobes are superimposed and located in

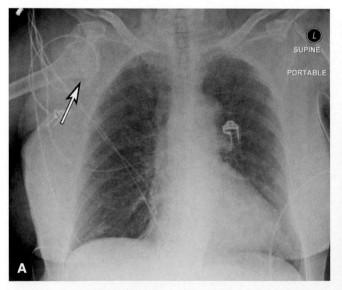

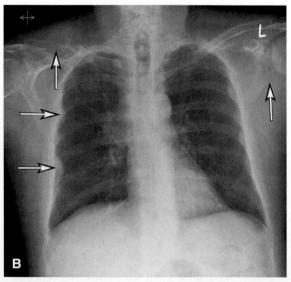

FIGURE 2.12. **Do not forget the four corners! A:** Anterior dislocation of the right humeral head (*arrow*). **B:** Several lytic bony lesions reflecting metastatic disease including the left scapula, right clavicle, and several ribs on the right side (*arrows*).

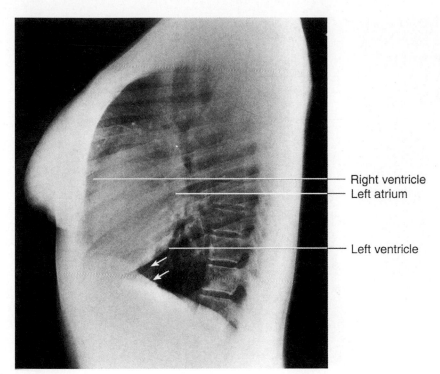

FIGURE 2.13. **Normal lateral chest radiograph.** The cardiac silhouette makes an excellent starting point for your evaluation. The faint vertical water density line (*arrows*) represents the inferior vena cava.

— Right ventricle
— Left atrium

— Left ventricle

the retrocardiac space, overlying the spine extending to the diaphragms (Fig. 2.14). Identification of the major fissures confirms the pulmonary lobar spatial relationships and is necessary to locate pathologic processes. The right major fissure usually can be differentiated from the left by either the intersection of the minor fissure or tracing the fissure to the diaphragm that can be traced anteriorly to the chest wall. The minor fissure (between the right upper and middle lobes) runs anteriorly to the fourth rib on the lateral view. The thoracic spine becomes more radiolucent (darker) as one moves inferiorly because of soft tissues superiorly in the chest.

Finally, on the lateral view, check the contours of both **hemidiaphragms** and the **posterior costophrenic angles**. There is considerable variability, but air in the right lower lobe is expected to abut the soft tissue density hemidiaphragm, forming a sharp interface. On the left side, only the cardiac apex and posterior hemidiaphragm are generally demonstrated, so the anterior aspect of the left diaphragm is usually obscured by its contiguity with the heart and pericardial fat (Fig. 2.15). The presence of acute angles posteriorly in both costophrenic recesses excludes small pleural effusions (<50 mL), which can be missed on the frontal view.

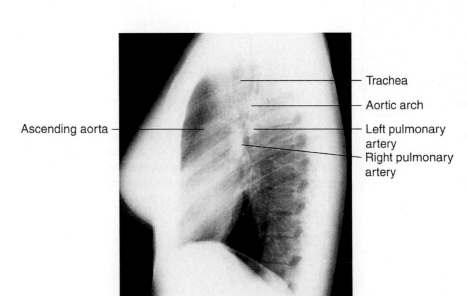

Ascending aorta —

— Trachea

— Aortic arch

— Left pulmonary artery
— Right pulmonary artery

FIGURE 2.14. **Normal lateral chest radiograph.** The oval-shaped right pulmonary artery lies anterior and inferior relative to the left pulmonary artery. The left pulmonary artery crosses cephalad over the left main stem bronchus and it lies inferior to the aortic arch.

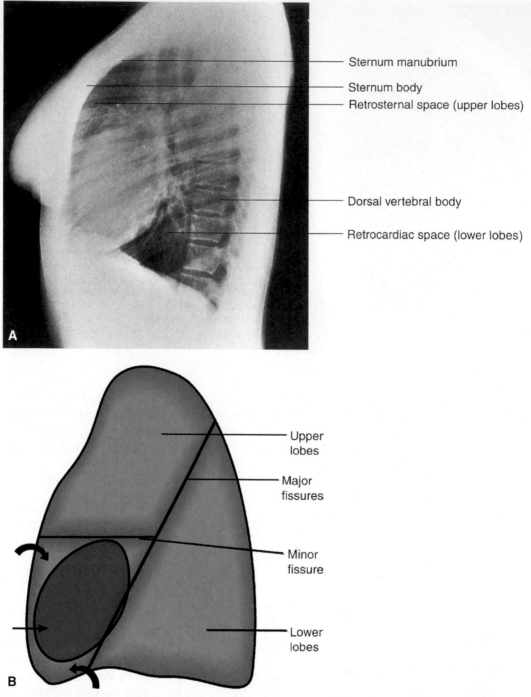

Sternum manubrium

Sternum body

Retrosternal space (upper lobes)

Dorsal vertebral body

Retrocardiac space (lower lobes)

Upper lobes

Major fissures

Minor fissure

Lower lobes

FIGURE 2.15. **A: Normal lateral chest radiograph.** The anterior and posterior bony structures should always be routinely viewed. The spine appears *less* dense as you proceed caudally because of attenuation by the shoulders. **B:** Illustration of the spatial relationships of the pulmonary lobes on the lateral view. Note that the right middle lobe and the lingular segments of the left upper lobe (*curved arrows*) project over the heart (*straight arrow*). The lower lobes are primarily posterior structures. The major fissures extend obliquely up to approximately the T4 level.

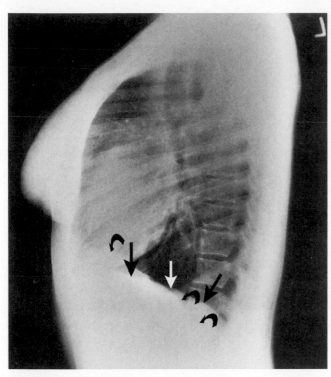

FIGURE 2.16. Normal lateral radiograph. Note that the left hemidiaphragm (*straight arrows*) is not visible anteriorly where it abuts the heart (water density). This is an excellent example of the silhouette sign. On the other hand, the entire right hemidiaphragm (*curved arrows*) is visible.

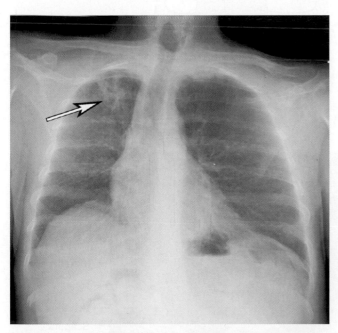

FIGURE 2.17. Apicolordotic view. This view is obtained with the patient leaning backward. Note how the clavicles project above the lung apices allowing better visualization of the upper lobes. This film shows a cavitary lesion in the right upper lobe (*arrow*) due to an atypical mycobacterial infection.

Additional Views of the Chest

The **AP lordotic view** is an AP view taken with the patient leaning back (or the X-ray source angled cranially) and is useful for visualization of upper lobes (Fig. 2.16). This view displaces the clavicles superiorly for better visualization of the lung apices.

Placing a patient on their side (decubitus position) and obtaining a film across the chest in the AP direction is described as a **decubitus view**, either right or left depending on which side is down. This view is helpful for detecting small amounts of free-flowing pleural air or fluid, which may not be seen on the standard views described above (Fig. 2.17).

NORMAL THORACIC CROSS-SECTIONAL ANATOMY

Anatomic Planes

The **axial** plane (or transaxial plane) is a plane that divides the body into superior and inferior parts. It is perpendicular to the coronal plane and sagittal plane. CT is performed in the axial plane.

A **sagittal** plane is the anatomical plane, which divides the body into right and left parts. The plane may be in the center of the body and split it into two halves (midsagittal) or away from the midline and split it into unequal parts (**parasagittal**). The term parasagittal is used to describe any plane parallel to the sagittal plane. In practice, such a section is often referred to simply as a "sagittal" view because viewing is achieved along the sagittal axis.

A **coronal** plane divides the body into ventral and dorsal (front and back) parts.

Multidetector CT (MDCT) allows imaging of the chest within one breath hold (5–10 seconds). CT anatomy is demonstrated in axial, coronal, sagittal, and sagittal oblique planes (Figs. 2.18-2.25). As CT is performed in the axial plane, the coronal, sagittal, and sagittal oblique views are reformatted from the data set acquired in the axial plane. Note how the sagittal oblique view allows visualization of the entire thoracic aorta. Some MDCT scanners are capable of imaging the heart in less than a second with excellent spatial and temporal resolution allowing three-dimensional (3D) visualization of the coronary arteries (Fig. 2.26).

To compensate for motion during the cardiac cycle, cardiac imaging (CT or MR) is best performed using **ECG gating**, which allows data acquisition typically during diastole when the heart is not moving. The R wave of the ECG is used as a reference point with data acquisition being triggered following a given delay after the R wave. Images are subsequently created from data collected over a series of cardiac cycles (R to R intervals). In general, CT is preferable to MR for chest and pulmonary imaging because of faster examination times and less susceptibility to motion and respiratory artifacts (Fig. 2.27). **Cardiac MRI** is used to evaluate the aorta and myocardium where it is helpful in the diagnosis of cardiac masses and cardiomyopathy.

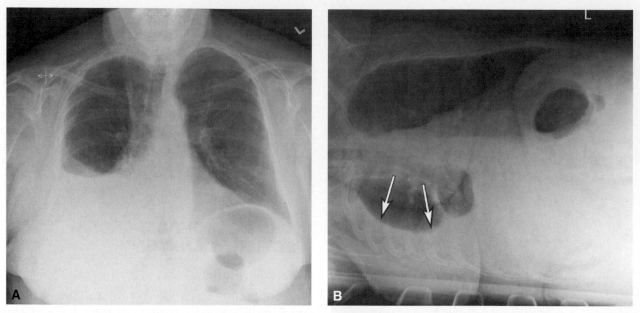

FIGURE 2.18. Right pleural effusion. A: PA chest film shows a moderate right pleural effusion. **B:** Right lateral decubitus film confirms that the right pleural effusion (*arrows*) is free flowing and not loculated.

FIGURE 2.19. Normal axial cross-sectional anatomy. A: Approximate axial anatomic level through the aortic arch for (**B**). **B:** Normal chest CT image at the aortic arch level with mediastinal windows.

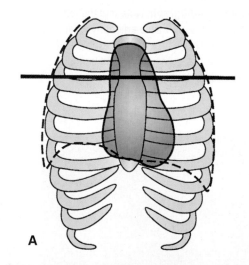

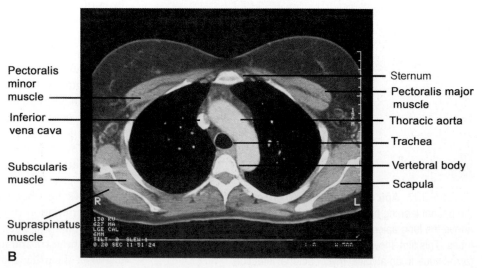

Pectoralis minor muscle

Inferior vena cava

Subscularis muscle

Supraspinatus muscle

Sternum

Pectoralis major muscle

Thoracic aorta

Trachea

Vertebral body

Scapula

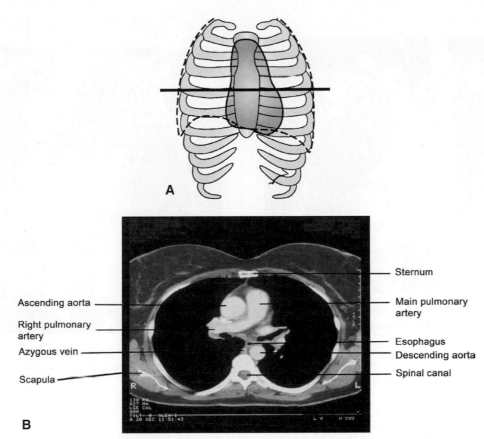

FIGURE 2.20. Normal cross-sectional anatomy. A: Approximate axial anatomic level through the pulmonary arteries for (**B**). **B:** Chest axial CT images at the level of the pulmonary arteries in mediastinal windows.

FIGURE 2.21. Normal cross-sectional anatomy. A: Approximate axial anatomic level through the right and left atria for (**B**). **B:** Chest axial CT images at the level of the atria in mediastinal windows.

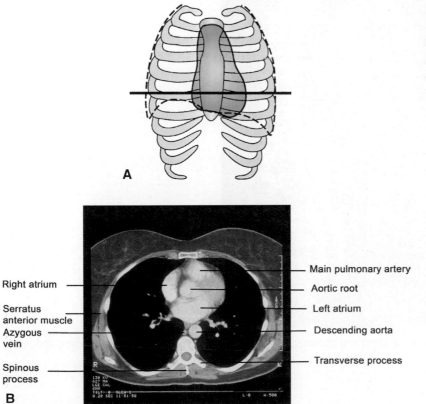

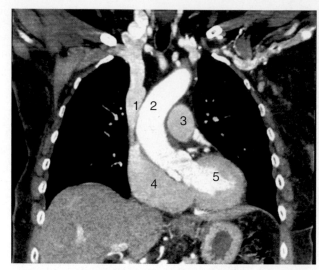

FIGURE 2.22. Normal anatomy. CT coronal view of the chest showing the (1) inferior vena cava, (2) ascending aorta and (3) pulmonary trunk.

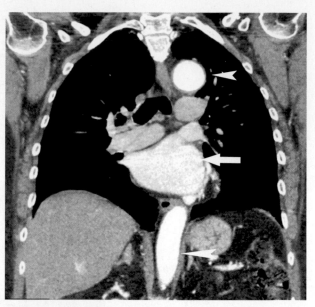

FIGURE 2.23. Normal anatomy. CT coronal view of the chest showing the left atrium and descending thoracic aorta.

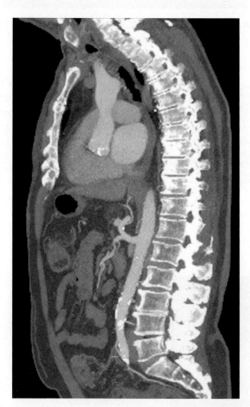

FIGURE 2.24. Normal anatomy. CT sagittal view of the chest and abdomen. Note, only partially visualization of the thoracic and abdominal aorta.

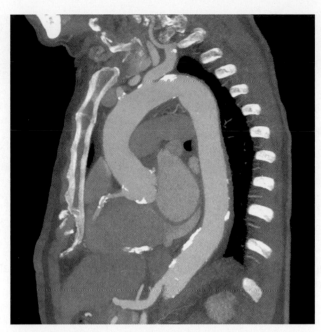

FIGURE 2.25. **Normal anatomy**. CT sagittal oblique view of the thoracic aorta. Note this view visualizes the entire thoracic aorta

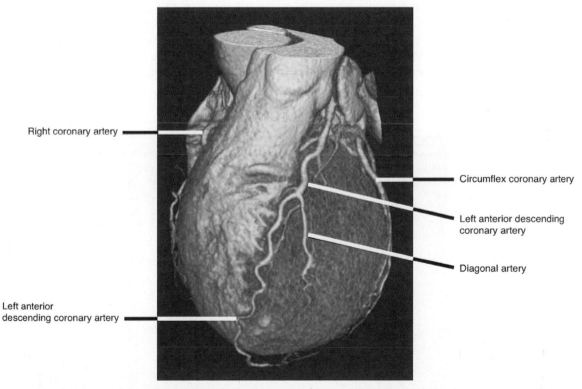

FIGURE 2.26. **CTA surface rendered volumetric image of the left coronary circulation** provides a 3D perspective and demonstrate the left coronary arteries relative to underlying cardiac structures. The left anterior descending coronary artery supplies most of the left ventricle while the circumflex artery runs in the left atrio-ventricular groove. A portion of the right coronary artery is visible along the left side of the image.

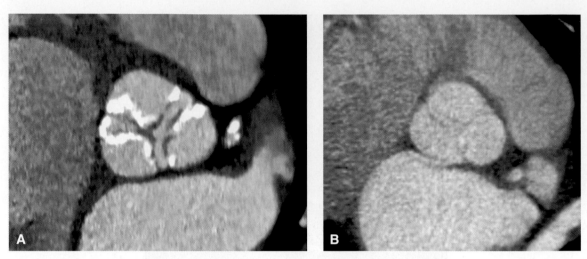

FIGURE 2.27. ECG gated and nongated CT images of the aortic valve. Note the improved spatial resolution of the aortic valve on the gated image compared with the nongated image.

CONGENITAL VASCULAR ANOMALIES

Embryonic lateral migration of the azygos vein from the midline such that it splits the right upper lobe generating a vertical linear opacity and a distinct separate lobe (Fig. 2.28) is known as an **azygos lobe**. Unlike the other lung fissures this fissure is lined with both visceral and parietal pleura, each displaced by the azygos vein running inferiorly to the posterior aspect of the SVC. The azygos fissure, which is only seen on the PA view as a thin curvilinear line, is one of the more common normal variants and is of no clinical significance.

The most common thoracic aortic anomaly is a **right-sided aortic arch** (Fig. 2.29). On the PA view, the right-sided arch appears more cephalad (higher) than a normal left-sided arch. The most common types are right-sided aortic arch with aberrant left subclavian artery and the mirror-image type. The variant with aberrant left subclavian artery is rarely

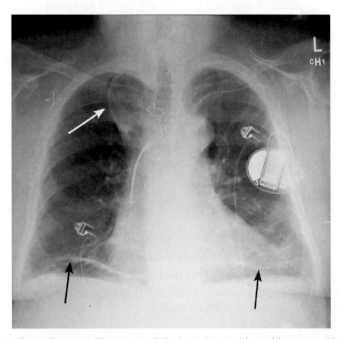

FIGURE 2.28. Azygos lobe. Chest PA radiograph. The azygos lobe is outlined with a *white arrow*. Also note the areas of discoid atelectasis in the lower lobes (*black arrows*) in the basilar regions of both lungs.

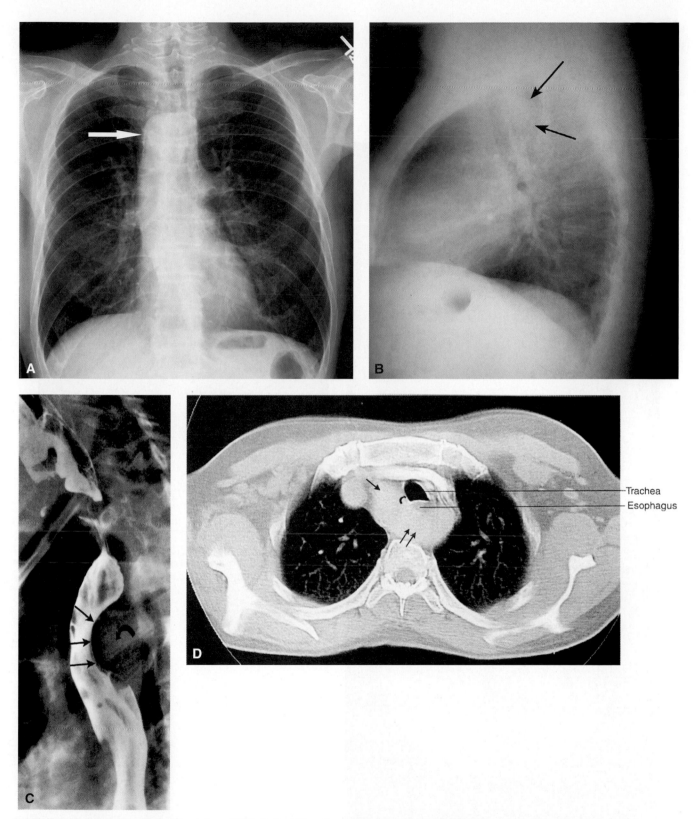

FIGURE 2.29. Right-sided aortic arch and left descending thoracic aorta. Chest PA (**A**) and lateral (**B**) radiographs, barium swallow (**C**), and chest CT (**D**). This 42-year-old male smoker was suspected of having cancer of the lung. **A:** A neoplastic mass was suspected on the PA radiograph, but this proved to be an ill-defined aortic knob to the right of the midline (*arrow*). The right aortic arch is indenting the right side of the trachea. **B:** The right-sided aortic arch indents the posterior aspect of the trachea (*arrows*) on the lateral radiograph. **C:** Barium swallow confirms a significant indentation on the posterior aspect of the barium-filled esophagus (*straight arrows*) secondary to the crossing aortic arch (*curved arrow*). **D:** The diagnosis is confirmed by chest CT that shows the right-sided aorta (*single straight arrow*) passing posterior to the esophagus and trachea (*double straight arrows*) to reach the left side of the thorax. Again, note the indentation on the right side of the trachea (*curved arrow*) secondary to the right-sided aortic arch.

associated with congenital heart disease, whereas the mirror-image type of right aortic arch is strongly associated with congenital heart disease, most commonly tetraology of Fallot.

Coarctation of the aorta is a stenosis at the junction of the aortic arch and the descending thoracic aorta (Fig. 2.30A, B).

The severity of stenosis is variable and the location of the coarctation is described in relation to the ductus arteriosus (preductal, ductal, or postductal). Associated rib notching along the inferior aspect of the ribs reflects collateral flow through dilated intercostal arteries (Fig. 2.30C).

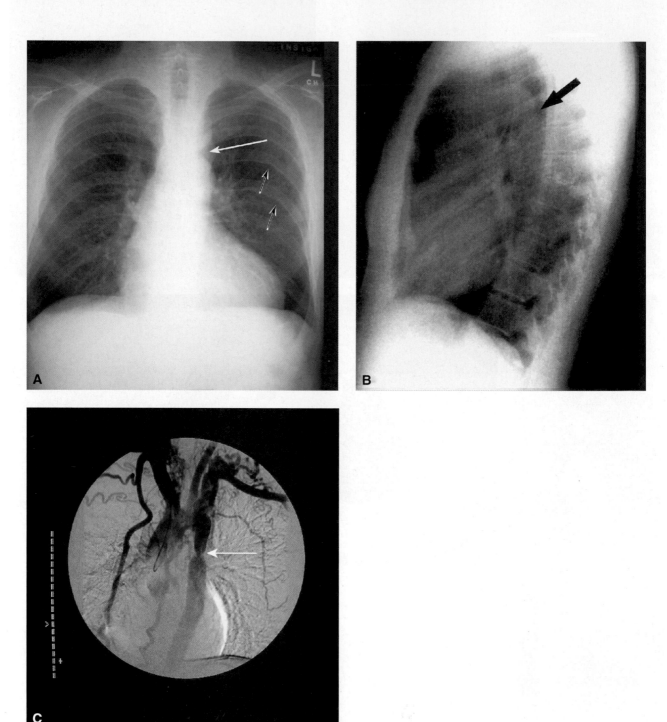

FIGURE 2.30. Coarctation of the aorta. The classical radiographic appearance is an indentation (*arrow*, **A**) involving the lateral aspect of the proximal descending aorta on PA radiograph, and a posterior indentation (*arrow*, **B**) involving the posterior aspect of the proximal descending aorta on the lateral radiograph. These indentations represent the site of coarctation in the proximal descending aorta. Rib notching (*small arrows*, **A**) is also evident along the inferior margins of several ribs. This notching represents collateral blood flow through dilated intercostal arteries. **C:** Aortic angiogram shows the classic appearance of coarctation (*arrow*).

FOREIGN BODIES, LINES, AND TUBES

Objects on the skin surface such as nodules and hair braids may be mistaken for chest pathology (Figs. 2.31-2.34). Characteristically these are **very well defined** on the image. An innocuous skin fold that appears as a well-defined line traversing the lung may be mistaken for a pneumothorax. It is important to recognize and document the course and location a variety of lines (catheters and tubes) when caring for acutely ill patients. For IV access, the optimal location of **central venous lines** is between the mid-SVC and the mid–right atrium. The correct position of the **endotracheal tube (ETT)** is determined by the distance between its tip and the carina. The optimal location of the tip is in the mid trachea, approximately 5 cm above the carina if the patient's neck is in the neutral position (Fig. 2.35). Flexion of the neck causes a 2-cm descent of the tip of the tube, whereas extension of the neck causes a 2-cm ascent of the tip.

When long-term intubation is required, a tracheostomy tube is used, the tip of which should be one-half to two-thirds of the distance from the stoma to the carina. Unlike the ETT's position, the tracheostomy tubes position is not changed by extension or flexion of the patient neck. Long-term complications of tracheostomy tubes include ulceration, stenosis, and perforation.

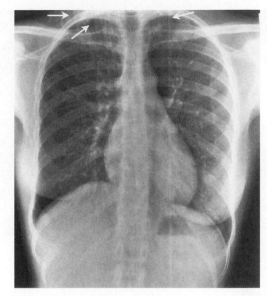

FIGURE 2.31. Hair braid. A soft tissue shadow (*arrows*) projects over the right supraclavicular region.

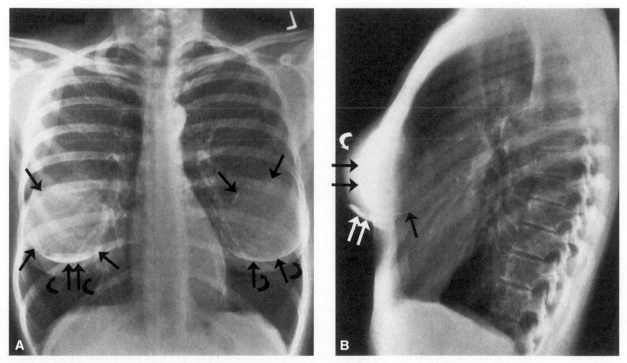

FIGURE 2.32. Bilateral breast implants. PA (**A**) and lateral (**B**) chest radiographs. The breast implants (*arrows*) exhibit peripheral calcifications along the capsules of each prosthesis.

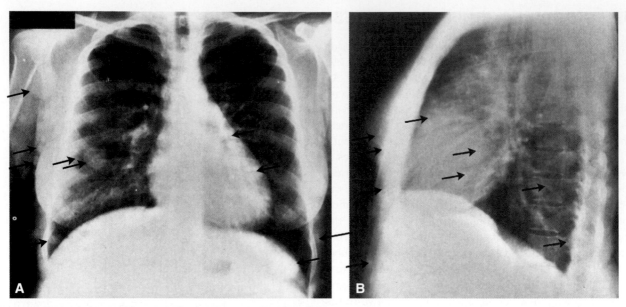

FIGURE 2.33. Neurofibromatosis. Chest PA (**A**) and lateral (**B**) radiographs. Multiple well-defined subcutaneous soft tissue nodules (*arrows*) project over the thorax which should not be mistaken for pulmonary nodules.

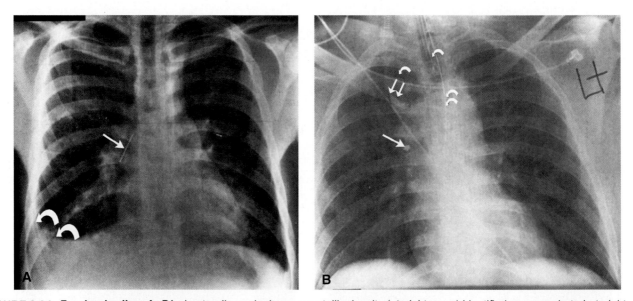

FIGURE 2.34. Foreign bodies. A: PA chest radiograph shows a metallic density (*straight arrow*) identified as an aspirated *straight pin* in the right bronchus intermedius. Note the right pleural effusion (*curved arrows*). It has been estimated that there must be at least 125 mL of pleural fluid before it is recognized on PA and AP views. **B:** Chest portable AP radiograph reveals a *tooth fragment* (*straight arrow*) in the right bronchial tree. The patient was involved in a motor vehicle accident, and a portion of a tooth was missing. The chest radiograph shows the tooth fragment projecting over the right upper bronchial tree. Note that the endotracheal tube (*single curved arrow at top*) lies to the patient's right of the nasogastric tube (*double curved arrows*). An azygos lobe is present, and the position of the azygos vein is more lateral and cephalad than normal (*double straight arrows*). The azygos lobe (*single curved arrow at left*) is visible.

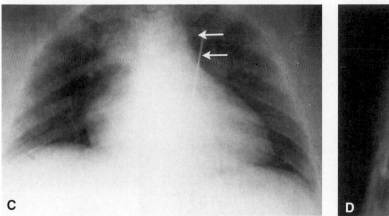

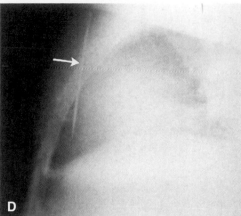

FIGURE 2.34. *(Continued)* **C and D:** Chest AP (**C**) and lateral (**D**) radiographs reveal a *darning needle lodged in the right ventricle.* The child of this young mother accidentally stabbed her with a darning needle. The needle (*arrows*) projects over the right ventricle region in both views. It was successfully removed at thoracotomy.

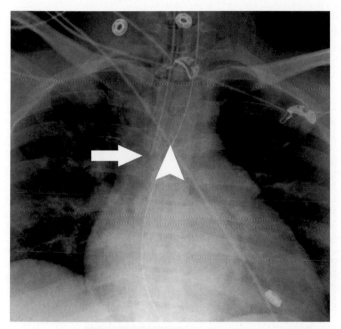

FIGURE 2.35. Endotracheal tube inadvertently placed in the right bronchus intermedius (*arrow*), below the carina (*arrowhead*).

AIR IN THE WRONG PLACES

A pneumothorax is an accumulation of air within the pleural space, and it is most often spontaneous or due to trauma or iatrogenic causes such as lung biopsy or catheter placement. The diagnosis is made by identifying the visceral pleura of the collapsed lung (Fig. 2.36) in combination with a lack of peripheral lung markings. Hyperlucency due to lack of lung vasculature may also occur. Semirecumbent and supine films are unreliable for diagnosing pneumothoraces because pleural air may accumulate in front of and behind the lung, and not be seen on a frontal view. Expiratory films accentuate air trapped in the pleural space and may make small and subtle pneumothoraces more conspicuous.

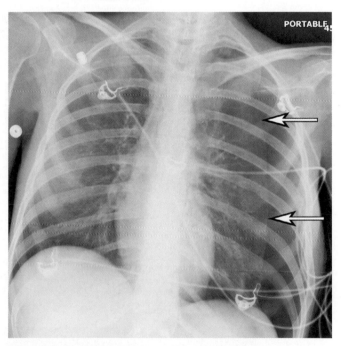

FIGURE 2.36. Left pneumothorax. AP chest radiograph shows a moderate left pneumothorax (*arrows*). Note the clear demarcation of the visceral pleural surface of the left lung.

A **tension pneumothorax** occurs when the pneumothorax is sufficiently large and under pressure, causing mass effect upon the mediastinal structures and ipsilateral diaphragm, resulting in a reduced cardiac output and ultimately acute cardiovascular collapse (Fig. 2.37). A tension pneumothorax represents an emergency requiring immediate placement of chest tube to decompress the pleural space. For most pneumothoraces, the optimal location for chest tube placement is the second intercostal space in the mid-clavicular line anteriorly, in contrast to most pleural effusions, which are percutaneously drained (thoracentesis) posteriorly at or below the seventh intercostal space (Fig. 2.38).

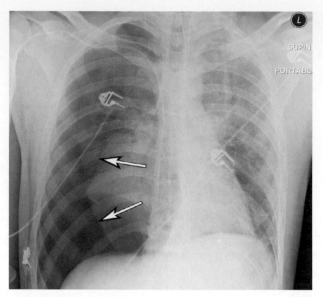

FIGURE 2.37. Right tension pneumothorax. Portable AP radiograph shows a large right pneumothorax with near complete collapse of the right lung (*arrows*). Note the depression of the right diaphragm and the deep right lateral costophrenic sulcus or angle (deep sulcus sign). Also, note the slight deviation of the cardiac silhouette to the left side.

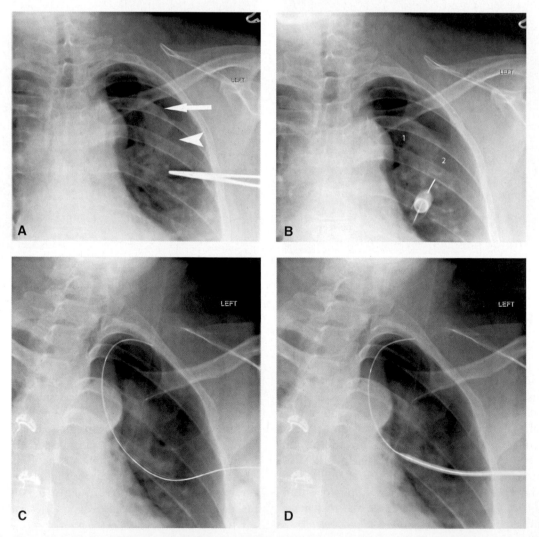

FIGURE 2.38. Placement of chest tube for left-sided pneumothorax. **A:** Localization of second left interspace in the mid clavicular line with forceps (first rib = *arrow*, second rib = *arrowhead*). **B**: Injection of local anesthetic and accessing the pleural space in the 2nd left interspace using the Seldinger technique.

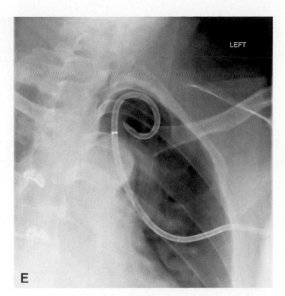

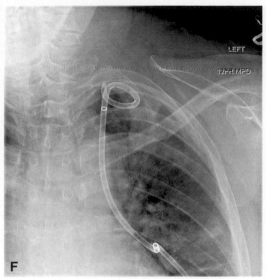

FIGURE 2.38. *(Continued)* **C-E:** Dilation of the percutaneous tract over a guidewire, and placement of a locking 10 French pigtail catheter in the pneumothorax. **F:** Note reduction in size of pneumothorax.

Pneumomediastinum is a collection of air within the mediastinum, the significance of which is variable but can be ominous in patients with a history of trauma or vomiting, suggesting rupture of either the esophagus or trachea (Figs. 2.39–2.41). Spontaneous self-limiting pneumomediastinum may occur in young adults with asthma. Complications of positive pressure ventilation are listed in Table 2.3.

Hiatal hernias may be seen as an incidental retrocardiac lucency or density depending on the amount of air within (Fig. 2.42). Other less common diaphragmatic hernias are Bochdalek and Morgagni occurring in the posterior and anterior diaphragm, respectively.

Gas within the chest wall may be due to infection or subcutaneous emphysema after pneumothorax or barotrauma (Fig. 2.43). Finally, as little as a few milliliters of free intraperitoneal air (**pneumoperitoneum**) may be

FIGURE 2.39. Pneumomediastinum due to esophageal perforation. PA chest radiograph shows extensive air within the mediastinum, as well as lucencies around the aortic arch and along the tracheal air column and associated subcutaneous air.

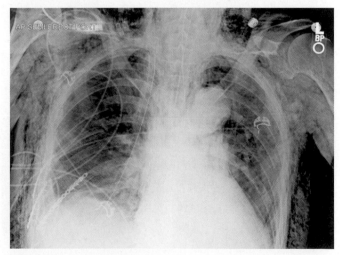

FIGURE 2.40. Pneumomediastinum and subcutaneous emphysema developed postthoracotomy for trauma.

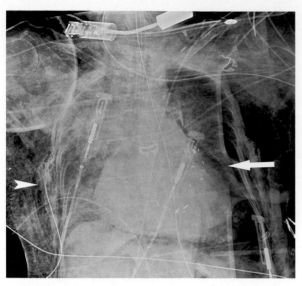

FIGURE 2.41. **Pneumopericardium** *(arrow)* **and subcutane-ous emphysema** *(arrowhead)* following vigorous cardiopulmonary resuscitation. The pericardial cavity is outlined by air.

TABLE 2.3	Complications of Positive Pressure Ventilation
Pneumothorax	
Pneumomediastinum	
Interstitial emphysema	
Subcutaneous emphysema	

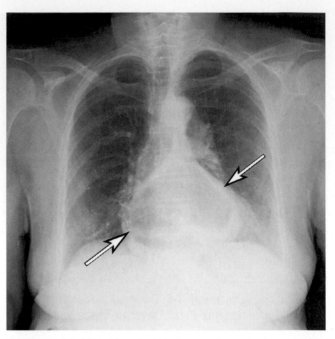

FIGURE 2.42. **Hiatal hernia.** PA chest radiograph shows a large air-filled bubble *(arrows)* overlying the cardiac silhouette reflecting a herniation of the stomach up into the chest.

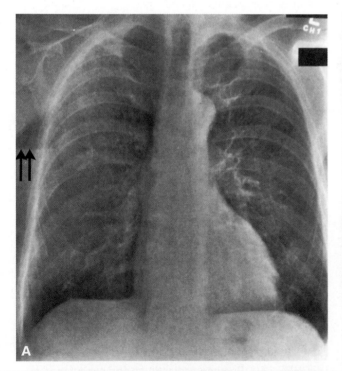

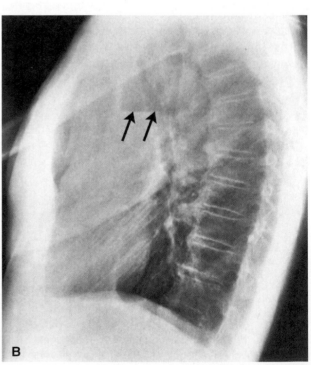

FIGURE 2.43. **Right axillary abscess.** PA (**A**) and lateral (**B**) chest radiographs. This patient developed an abscess after a right axillary node dissection. An air–fluid level *(arrows)* is seen on both views.

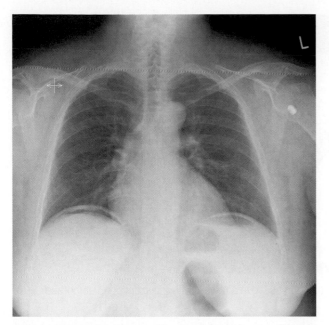

FIGURE 2.44. Free intraperitoneal air. PA chest radiograph showing crescentic air under both diaphragms due to a perforated gastric ulcer.

detected under the diaphragm on upright radiographs (Fig. 2.44). This is a significant finding if spontaneous and often indicating visceral perforation if not immediately post abdominal surgery.

HYPERLUCENT LUNG

Emphysema is characterized by the destruction of the alveoli distal to the terminal bronchioles with loss of surface area. Radiographically, air trapping and parenchymal loss appear as hyperinflation (flattening of the diaphragm) or hyperlucency (darker) on a chest radiograph (2.45A and B). High-resolution CT (HRCT) is the best technique for detecting and quantifying emphysema and/or bullous lung disease as chest radiography is relatively insensitive for screening mild and moderate emphysema (Fig. 2.45C). Blebs (<2 cm) or bullae (>2 cm) are thin-walled pleural "cysts" that may also contribute to the findings of hyperinflation and hyperlucency (Fig. 2.46). Other causes of lung hyperinflation are asthma (bilateral) and inhaled foreign body (unilateral).

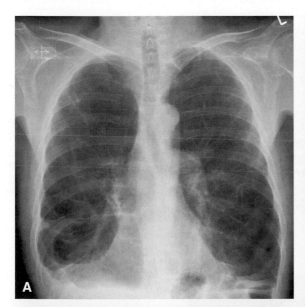

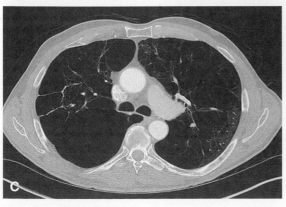

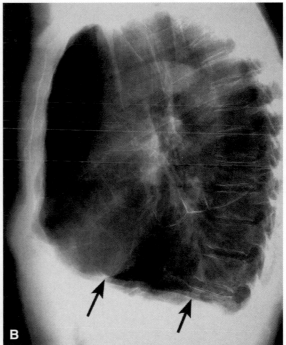

FIGURE 2.45. Chronic obstructive pulmonary disease (COPD). PA (**A**) and lateral (**B**) chest radiographs. The lungs are hyperlucent and hyperinflated. The diaphragms are flattened on both projections reflecting the increase in lung volumes (*arrows*). The retrosternal airspace is expanded and the AP dimension of the chest is greater than normal. **C:** The emphysematous and bullous changes, are demonstrated on the corresponding chest CT.

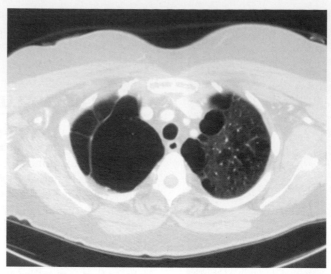

FIGURE 2.46. **Biapical blebs and bullae**. Axial CT showing blebs and bullae in a patient with recurrent pneumothoraces.

AIR SPACE AND INTERSTITIAL LUNG DISEASE

On a chest radiograph, distal bronchi are not usually visible because they are thin walled, contain air and are surrounded by air. However, when the adjacent alveoli fill with fluid as occurs in pneumonia, edema, or hemorrhage, the bronchi become more conspicuous producing an **air bronchogram** seen as a linear lucency (tube of air) within the adjacent denser fluid-filled space and is a **hallmark of airspace disease** (Fig. 2.47). The pattern of airspace (alveolar) disease is typically one of fluffy, ill-defined, and confluent opacification (density) on a chest film. In contrast, thickening of the lung interstitium or interlobular supporting structures is seen as an **interstitial** pattern, which can

be subclassified into nodular (metastases, sarcoidosis, silicosis) or reticular (linear) (pulmonary interstitial edema, idiopathic pulmonary fibrosis) or a combination of both (reticulonodular) (Fig. 2.48). Most interstitial patterns are inhomogeneous and in contrast to airspace disease often do not respect lobar boundaries.

A third pattern of note is **groundglass opacity (GGO)** which is a CT pattern of a hazy opacity that does not obscure the underlying bronchial structures or pulmonary vessels (Fig. 2.49A and B). The differential diagnosis for GGO is extensive and includes malignancies and benign conditions, such as interstitial fibrosis, inflammation and hemorrhage.

A structure's outline is only seen when an adjacent structure in the same anatomic plane is of a different radiographic tissue density giving rise to **the silhouette**

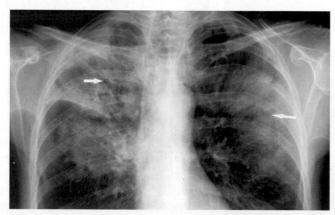

FIGURE 2.47. **Airspace disease**. PA chest radiograph showing bilateral air bronchograms (*arrows*) and confluent opacification consistent with airspace disease due to pneumonia.

sign. Conversely, when two structures of the same or similar radiographic tissue density are adjacent to each other, the margin between them is indistinct. For example, left lower lobe collapse or consolidation obscures the adjacent medial margin of the left hemidiaphragm. Similarly, since the right middle lobe is adjacent to the right cardiac border, right middle lobe collapse or consolidation obscures the right cardiac border on the frontal radiograph (Fig. 2.50C and D). The same observation also holds true for disease processes within the lingular segment of the left upper lobe, which will obscure the adjacent left heart border.

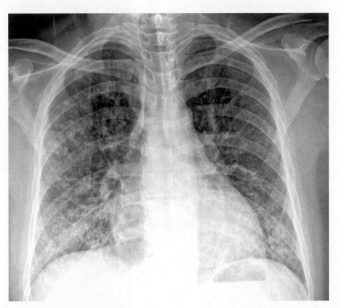

FIGURE 2.48. **Interstitial (nodular) lung disease**. PA chest radiograph showing extensive increased nodular markings consistent with interstitial lung disease.

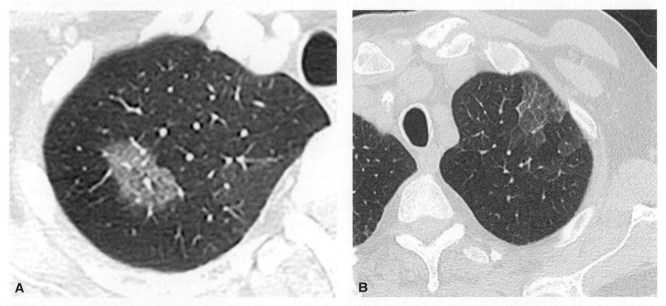

FIGURE 2.49. **Groundglass opacity.** Axial CT in two different patients showing confluent attenuation with visualization of the underlying normal vascular shadows.

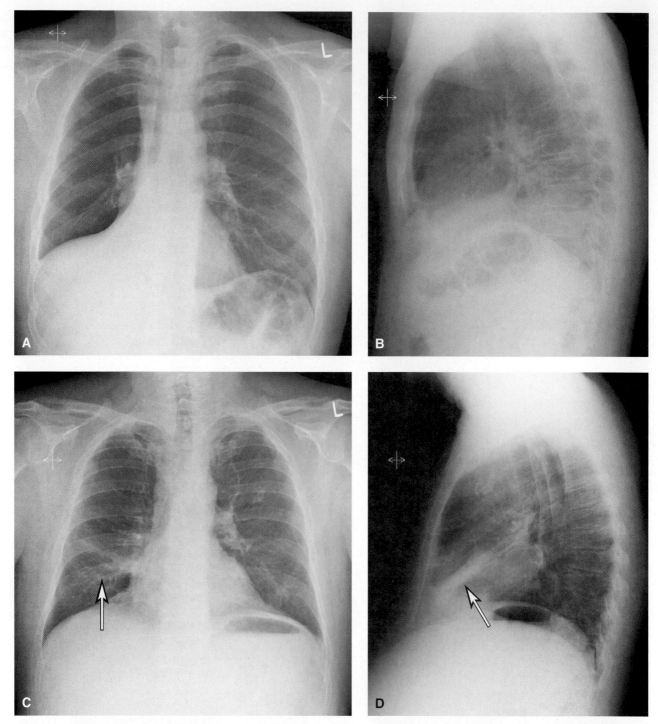

FIGURE 2.50. Lobar (collapse). A and B: PA and lateral views of the chest showing combined *right lower and middle* lobe collapse. The frontal projection shows obscuration of both the right diaphragm and right heart border (silhouette sign) and the lateral projection shows opacity overlying the lower thoracic spine due to the collapsed lower lobe (spine sign). **C and D:** *Right middle lobe* collapse. Note the partial obscuration of the right heart border on the frontal film due to atelectasis (*arrow*, **C**) and the band of atelectasis overlying the heart shadow on the lateral film (*arrow*, **D**).

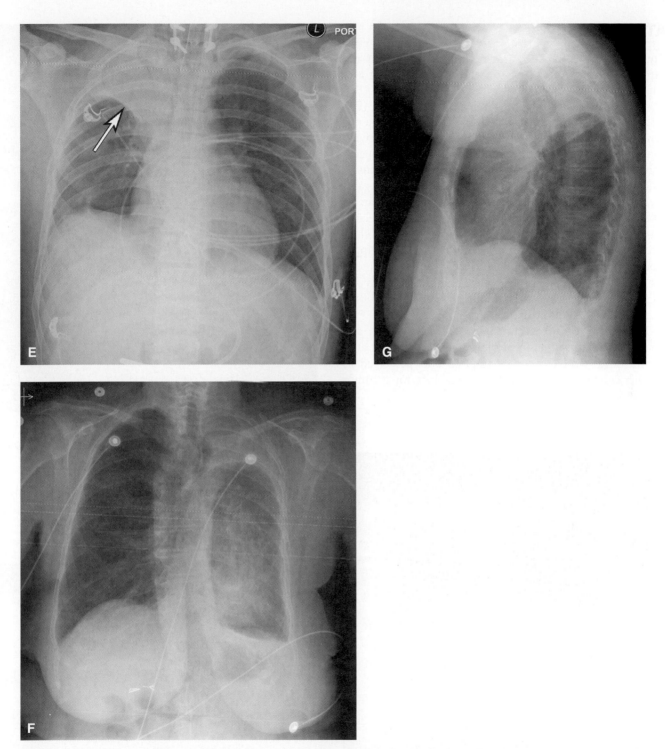

FIGURE 2.50. *(Continued)* **E:** *Right upper lobe* collapse. AP chest radiograph showing the typical-wedge shaped appearance of right upper lobe collapse (*arrow*). Note the elevation of the right diaphragm reflecting the associated volume loss. **F and G:** *Left upper lobe* collapse. PA and lateral chest films show veil-like volume loss of the left lung due to complete left upper lobe collapse with associated deviation of the trachea and the heart to the left side. On the lateral film, the collapsed left upper lobe which resides anteriorly, produces the generalized groundglass changes of the left lung, which are apparent on the frontal projection.

ATELECTASIS

Atelectasis or collapse represents a loss of aeration and varies in extent from being subsegmental appearing as a linear density (subsegmental or discoid atelectasis) (Fig. 2.51) to a complete collapse of a lobe or entire lung (Fig. 2.52). Atelectasis is not permanent and by itself is not a primary disease process but rather an indicator of underlying abnormality. Contributory factors to postoperative atelectasis include accumulation of secretions, reduced inspirational effort and the type of anesthetic drugs and gases used. The classical appearance of each of the collapsed lobes is shown in Figure 2.52 and should be correlated with relative volume loss within the lung. Note the characteristic veil-like appearance associated with left upper lobe collapse. While volume loss, opacity, and fissural shift should be relatively easy to detect, compensatory hyperinflation of an adjacent normal lobe or lung can be subtle. The signs of atelectasis are listed in Table 2.4.

The term **"round atelectasis"** is a misnomer and describes the invagination of pleural surface around atelectatic lung, which becomes trapped and perceived as a spherical mass, which may be mistaken for a tumor (Fig. 2.53).

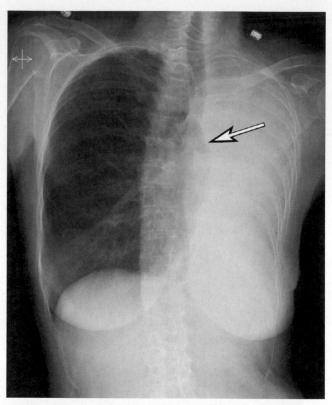

FIGURE 2.52. Complete left lung collapse. AP chest film shows complete collapse of the left lung, which is due to mucous plugging in the left mainstem bronchus. Note how there is an abrupt loss of the normal pneumatization of the left mainstem bronchus (*arrow*) at the site of the mucous plug. This is known as the bronchial cutoff sign.

TABLE 2.4	Signs of Atelectasis
Opacity	
Volume loss	
Shift of fissures and/or trachea, heart to hemidiaphragm toward volume loss	
Compensatory hyperinflation of normal lung	

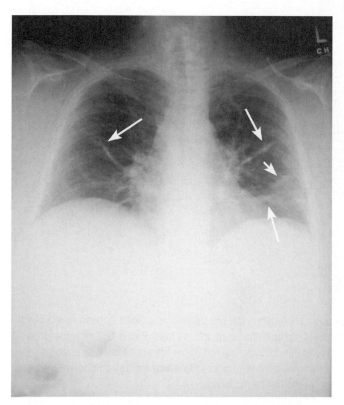

FIGURE 2.51. Bilateral discoid (plate-like) atelectasis. PA chest radiograph. The *arrows* indicate the typical appearance of regions of discoid atelectasis, which are commonly found in postoperative, posttrauma, severely ill, or debilitated patients.

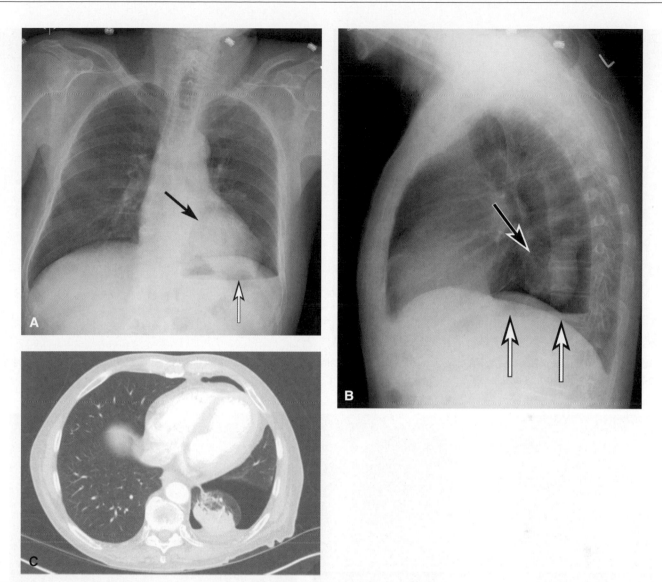

FIGURE 2.53. Round(ed) atelectasis. PA (**A**) and lateral films (**B**) of the chest show a spherical opacity in the left lower lobe postero-medially (*black arrows*), which, on the corresponding chest CT (**C**), reflects an area of round atelectasis. Note the conspicuous volume loss of the left lower lobe. Also, note on the CT the presence of both air and fluid in the left pleural space (*white arrows*). This hydropneu-mothorax occurred after transbronchial biopsies of the left lower lobe.

PLEURAL DISEASE

A **pleural effusion** is an abnormal collection of fluid in the pleural space due either to increased production or reduced absorption. Normally a small amount of fluid (5 mL) is present to lubricate movement of the pleural surfaces during respiration. On a PA film, up to 200 mL of pleural fluid can be missed if it occur in the subpulmonic and costophrenic spaces. Lateral tenting of the "hemidiaphragm" may be seen in a subpulmonic effusion. As the volume of pleural fluid increases, the hemidiaphragm and costophrenic angle are obscured, leading to the characteristic **meniscus sign** in the lateral margin (Fig. 2.54A and B). Pleural effusions can

opacify the entire hemithorax and can cause displacement of the mediastinum and hemidiaphragm away from the effusion. The meniscus sign is lost with a distinct flat line intersecting the lateral margin in a **hydropneumothorax**, which is a combination of fluid and air in the pleural space (Fig. 2.55A and B).

Pleural effusions occurring within **interlobar fissures** have a characteristic appearance of a spindle-shaped opacity within the plane of the fissure, which is continuous with a line of thickened pleura at one or both ends. Treatment of the underlying condition, usually congestive heart failure, causes the interlobar effusion, sometimes known as pseudotumor, to resolve promptly (Fig. 2.56A and B).

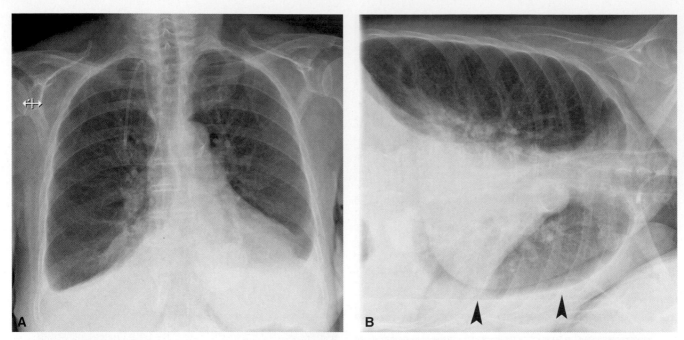

FIGURE 2.54. Pleural effusion. A: PA view showing moderate bilateral effusions, greater on the left. **B:** A left decubitus view shows a free-flowing, effusion (*arrowheads*).

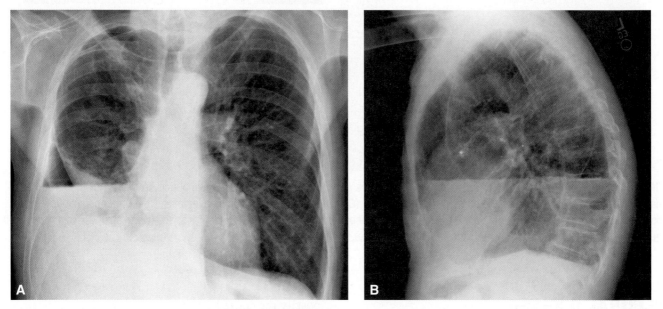

FIGURE 2.55. Hydropneumothorax. A and B: PA and lateral views showing lack of the meniscus sign with a straight horizontal air-fluid level.

Pleural effusions are generally classified as transudates or exudates, depending on the mechanism of fluid formation and their albumin and LDH (lactate dehydrogenase) contents. **Transudates** result from an imbalance in oncotic and hydrostatic pressures and have a serum albumin and LDH level less than that of **exudates**, which are usually the result of inflammation or reduced lymphatic drainage. A pleural effusion associated with pneumonia is called **a parapneumonic effusion**, which if secondarily infected will result in the accumulation of pus within the pleural space and it is then termed **empyema**, which require percutaneous drainage. Biochemically empyemas have a pH <7.2 and a glucose level <60 mg/dL. Table 2.5 lists the CT features.

On a decubitus chest film, the inability of an effusion to flow freely and layer inferiorly may be diagnostic of a **loculated effusion**, which occurs most commonly as result of adhesions in the pleural space. The presence of loculations can be confirmed on ultrasound (Fig. 2.57). Empyema

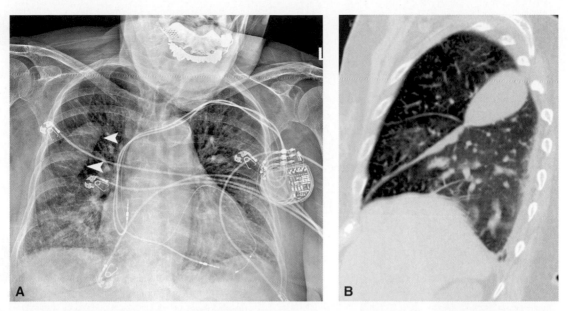

FIGURE 2.56. **Encysted pleural effusion. A:** AP view showing well defined, opacity over the right lung (*arrowheads*), which represents encysted fluid in the right major fissure. **B**: Sagittal reformatted of CT chest showing well defined, encysted pleural effusion in the major fissure.

TABLE 2.5	CT Features of Parapneumonic Pleural Effusion, Empyema, and Lung Abscess		
Features on CT	**Parapneumonic Effusion**	**Empyema**	**Lung abscess**
Wall thickness	Minimal	Thicker, split pleural sign	Thickest irregular
Wall contrast enhancement	None	Present	Present
Shape	Lentiform	Lentiform	"Round"
Angle with pleura	Obtuse	Obtuse	Acute
Volume of fluid as measured by thickness on CT	Less than 30 mm	Greater than 30 mm	
Treatment	Thoracentesis	Percutaneous drainage and intrapleural lytics.	Antibiotics

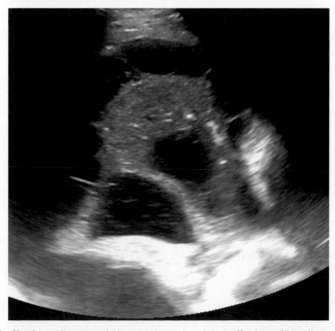

FIGURE 2.57. **Loculated pleural effusion.** Ultrasound shows a large loculated effusion with collapsed lung centrally.

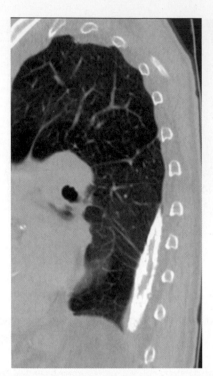

FIGURE 2.58. Calcified pleural plaques. Pleural calcification due to previous hematoma.

TABLE 2.6	Causes of Pulmonary Edema

1. Cardiogenic (heart failure)
2. Neurogenic (head injury)
3. Noncardiogenic (increased permeability > injury > edema)
   a. Toxic gas or smoke inhalation
   b. High-altitude sickness
   c. Aspiration
   d. Contusion
   e. Fat embolism
   f. Sepsis

TABLE 2.7	Radiographic Appearance of Pulmonary Edema

1. Vascular redistribution (increase size of vessels in the upper lobes)
2. Kerley B lines (interstitial edema)
3. Vascular congestion
4. Central peribronchial cuffing
5. Airspace disease/edema (batwing or diffuse and gravitational)
6. Pleural effusions (usually bilateral and symmetric in size)

and loculated effusions may be treated with percutaneous catheter drainage combined with intrapleural injection of thrombolytics such tissue plasminogen activator.

Pleural calcifications or calcified pleural plaques are often benign, especially when bilateral, indicating asbestos exposure (Fig. 2.58). More extensive and unilateral pleural calcification may be due to healed empyema or tuberculosis. Causes of solid and irregular pleural masses include lung carcinoma and mesothelioma for which biopsy is needed for confirmation.

PULMONARY EDEMA

Although there are many causes of pulmonary edema (Table 2.6), the most common, is **left ventricular failure (cardiogenic pulmonary edema).** The various radiographic appearances of pulmonary edema depend on the hydrostatic effects of left ventricular failure and pulmonary venous hypertension (Table 2.7). Normally on upright films, flow (and vessel prominence) is greater in the lower lobes than in the upper lobes (Table 2.12). The first radiographic sign of left ventricular failure is **cephalad redistribution** of blood flow to the upper lobes, recruiting underused capacity in response to impaired oxygen diffusion across the capillary–alveolar interface. At this stage, the pulmonary vessels should still remain sharp in outline (Fig. 2.59A).

With further deterioration in left ventricular function and increase in pulmonary venous pressure, there is transudation of intravascular fluid into the adjacent perivascular connective tissues producing **interstitial edema** (formally known as "Kerley lines"), which are identified on chest films as small perpendicular lines at the lung periphery, most commonly in the lower zones (Fig. 2.59B). In addition, because interstitial fluid extends into interlobular spaces, which include the pulmonary vessels and smaller bronchi, these structures become less sharp, causing **peribronchial cuffing**. As left ventricular failure worsens, extravascular fluid accumulates in alveoli as **bilateral symmetric airspace pattern disease** but one which may initially be in a perihilar or batwing distribution (Fig. 2.59C).

Additional findings in left ventricular failure with fluid overload reflect increased circulating intravascular volume such as **widening of the vascular pedicle and enlargement of the SVC and azygos veins**. The vascular pedicle width is measured from the lateral aspect of the SVC at the insertion of the azygos vein horizontally to a line drawn vertically from the origin of the left subclavian artery. The azygos vein diameter is particularly sensitive to changes in intravascular volume. On upright films, the azygos vein is usually collapsed measuring no wider than 1 cm.

In contrast, **noncardiogenic pulmonary edema**, such as adult respiratory distress syndrome (ARDS), lacks most of the features of hydrostatic edema (Table 2.8). In ARDS, airspace opacification results directly from lung injury and loss of integrity of the alveolar epithelium. Fluid and cellular

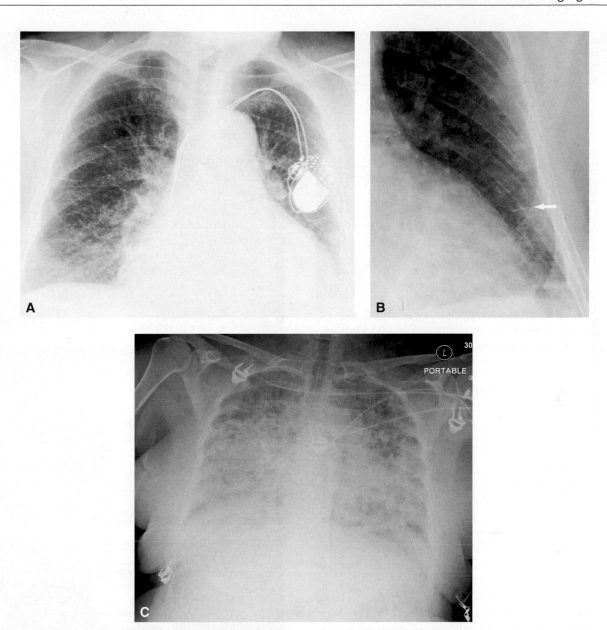

FIGURE 2.59. **Cardiogenic pulmonary edema. A:** Upper lobe venous diversion. **B:** A magnified view of the left lung shows interstitial edema (*arrow*) due to transudation of fluid into the avascular connective tissues. **C:** Bilateral extensive airspace disease due to pulmonary edema.

TABLE 2.8	Comparison of Findings of Cardiogenic Pulmonary Edema and Adult Respiratory Distress Syndrome (ARDS) (noncardiogenic)	
Feature	**Cardiogenic pulmonary edema**	**ARDS**
Heart size	Enlarged	Often normal
Location of pulmonary opacification	Perihilar (batwing)	Extends to subpleural
Pleural effusions	Common	Unusual, delayed

components accumulate within the alveoli, but without the vascular redistribution or interstitial edema seen in cardiogenic pulmonary edema (Fig. 2.60). Furthermore, the distribution is often patchy and asymmetric at onset, eventually becoming more uniform in distribution and increasingly dense b cellular content. ARDS results in considerable respiratory dysfunction, stiff lung compliance, and greater morbidity. Because of the highly cellular composition of alveolar fluid, the overall course of noncardiogenic pulmonary edema is protracted taking up to several weeks to months to resolve in contrast to cardiogenic pulmonary edema, which typically responds promptly to appropriate treatment.

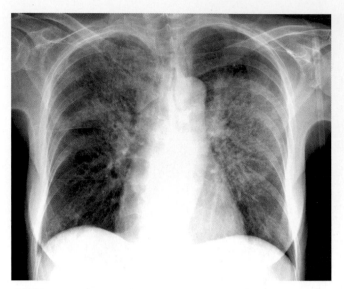

FIGURE 2.60. Noncardiogenic pulmonary edema. Similar appearance with increase in perihilar airspace disease to cardiogenic pulmonary edema, but with a normal heart size.

Transfusion-related acute lung injury (TRALI) is a rare but serious syndrome characterized by sudden acute respiratory distress following transfusion and is the leading cause of blood product transfusion–related mortality in the United States. Chest film shows noncardiogenic pulmonary edema with bilateral patchy infiltrates, which may rapidly progress to complete "white out" indistinguishable from ARDS.

PULMONARY EMBOLISM

Pulmonary embolism is the third most common cause of death in hospitalized patients, with over 650,000 cases occurring annually in the United States. Typically, a **deep venous thrombus (DVT)** originating in lower extremity or pelvis migrates to the pulmonary arteries, causing acute chest pain, dyspnea, and right-sided heart failure. Pulmonary embolism is present in 60% to 80% of patients with DVT, even though more than half of these patients are asymptomatic.

Less than 10% of chest radiographs are abnormal in patients with acute PE with findings that include atelectasis, effusion, and pulmonary infarction (Fig. 2.61A). A CT angiogram (CTA) of the chest is the most commonly used imaging test for diagnosing PE (Fig. 2.61C), and this test has largely replaced ventilation/perfusion (V/Q) scanning and pulmonary angiography (Fig. 2.62). CT PE protocol requires timing to ensure maximum opacification of the pulmonary arteries by the contrast bolus in addition to image reconstructions/reformats. Pulmonary emboli appear as filling defects within the opacified pulmonary arteries. A **saddle embolism** describes the continuous extension of thrombus into both pulmonary

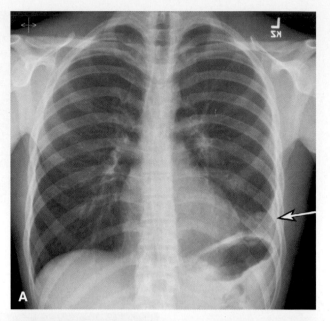

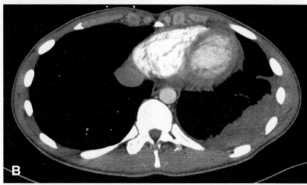

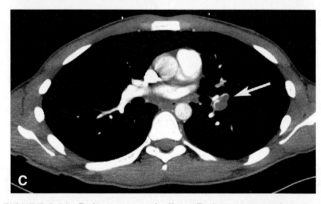

FIGURE 2.61. Pulmonary embolism. Patient presented with acute shortness of breath and chest pain. The PA film (**A**) shows a subtle peripheral pleural-based opacity in the left lower lobe (*arrow*), which on corresponding chest CT (**B**) relates to a large area of peripheral left lower lobe consolidation/infarction (Hampton hump). **C:** CT angiography revealed a large occlusive left lower lobe acute pulmonary embolus (*arrow*).

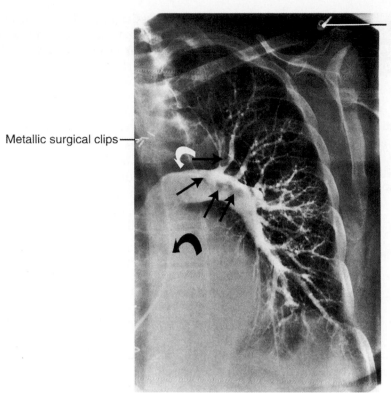

External monitoring electrode

Metallic surgical clips—

FIGURE 2.62. Acute pulmonary embolism: Pulmonary angiogram. This 72-year-old woman had 72-hour status post coronary artery bypass grafting and developed acute shortness of breath and hypoxia. There are multiple pulmonary emboli (*straight arrows*) within the left main pulmonary artery and its branches secondary to lower extremity deep vein thrombosis. The angiographic catheter (*curved arrows*) is visible in the left pulmonary artery.

arteries (Fig. 2.63). CTA is also useful for evaluating the degree of **right ventricular strain** or overload, which is one of the factors determining the severity and prognosis of PE. The ratio of right ventricular diameter to left ventricular diameter as measured on a four-chamber view of the heart on a CTA is normally 0.8, but an RV/LV ratio of greater than 0.9 is associated with a 2.8- to 7.4-fold increase in short-term mortality (Fig. 2.64).

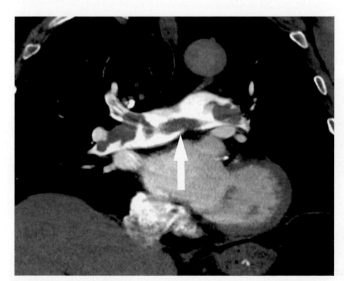

FIGURE 2.63. Saddle embolism. Coronal reformat of CT PE protocol showing embolism extending into both right and left main pulmonary arteries.

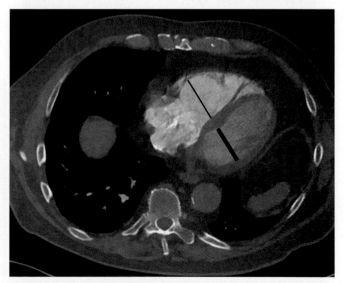

FIGURE 2.64. Right ventricular overload. Axial CT of the heart (Four chamber view), showing a right ventricular to left ventricular ratio of 1.2. Normal RV to LV ratio is 0.9 or less.

TABLE 2.9	Definitions of Massive, Submassive, and Low-Risk Pulmonary Embolism (PE) and Associated Mortality	
PE Classification	Definition	30-Day Mortality
Massive	Acute PE with sustained hypotension (<90 mm Hg)	25%-65%
Submassive	Systolic pressure > 90 mm Hg **and** either RV dysfunction (CT, BNP, ECG) or myocardial necrosis (elevated troponins)	3%
Low risk	Absence of hypotension, RV dysfunction and myocardial necrosis	<1%

(1) After Jaff, Circulation 2011

Patient stratification based on mortality risk allows early treatment, which ranges from heparinization in low-risk patients to thrombolysis (IV or catheter directed) and thrombectomy in high-risk patients (Table 2.9). Catheter-directed thrombolysis involves placement of an infusion catheter in the pulmonary arterial clot and infusing a thrombolytic drug such as tissue plasminogen activator.

False-positive readings for PE should be considered when only a single embolism or only subsegmental emboli are reported on CTA as diagnostic difficulty may occur with artifacts due to breathing motion and CT beam-hardening.

Ventilation/perfusion (V/Q) scans are still useful in patients who cannot receive IV contrast because of impaired renal function or those with a history of contrast allergy. See Chapter 10 for more on V/Q scanning. Rarely, thrombus may originate from central venous lines, which when infected can cause septic pulmonary emboli, which result in cavitary lung abscesses (Fig. 2.65).

In patients with low or intermediate clinical probability of PE, a negative D-dimer test effectively excludes PE or DVT. D-dimer levels will be elevated in any significant thrombotic process, so this test is of limited value in pregnant and postoperative patients. PE is a leading cause of pregnancy-related mortality in the developed world, accounting for 20% of maternal deaths in the United States. Lower-extremity duplex ultrasonography for assessment of DVT is recommended in pregnant patients with suspected PE and signs and symptoms of lower-extremity DVT. There is still debate over the optimal imaging of PE during pregnancy (see Chapter 10).

Triple-rule-out (TRO). The ability of chest CTA to simultaneously examine the coronary arteries, the thoracic aorta, and the pulmonary arteries may be beneficial in the evaluation of patients with chest pain for whom additional diagnoses other than acute coronary syndrome are considered, such as pulmonary embolism or aortic dissection. Typically, intravenous β-blocker and sublingual nitroglycerin are given. For the diagnosis of coronary artery disease, TRO CT has a sensitivity of 94.3%, a specificity of 97.4%, and a negative predictive value of 99%.

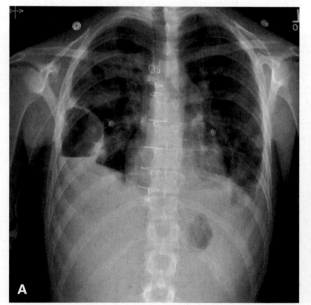
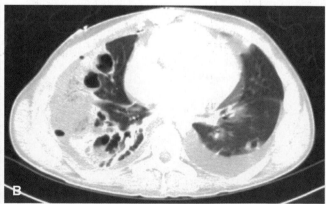

FIGURE 2.65. Septic pulmonary emboli. A: PA chest film shows numerous cystic lung lesions (abscesses) on the right side along with a right pleural effusion. **B:** Corresponding chest CT image shows to better advantage these scattered pulmonary abscesses, which are bilateral and which have the peripheral distribution typical of septic embolic disease.

TABLE 2.10	Nice Classification of Pulmonary Hypertension (2013)
Category	**Causes**
1. PAH	Idiopathic, heritable, drugs, connective tissue disease, HIV
2. PH due to left heart disease	Left ventricular dysfunction, valvular, congenital heart.
3. PH due to lung disease	COPD, interstitial lung disease
4. Chronic thromboembolic	
5. Multifactorial	Myeloproliferative, sarcoidosis

PAH, pulmonary arterial hypertension; PH, pulmonary hypertension.

Pulmonary hypertension (PH) is defined as mean pulmonary arterial pressure of 25 mm Hg or more at rest. Without treatment, PH has a poor prognosis and may progress to right ventricular failure and death. The terms "primary PH" and "secondary PH" have been replaced by the Nice Classification (Table 2.10). Idiopathic PAH is diagnosed only in the absence of any other cause of PH and in the absence of any pulmonary or mediastinal finding that may be a cause of PH. The term pulmonary arterial hypertension (PAH) should be reserved for those cases that fall into Category 1. Chest radiographs are abnormal in most patients with idiopathic PAH at the time of diagnosis. Echocardiography is useful for measuring arterial and cardiac chamber pressures, ejection fractions, and shunts but has limited diagnostic capability beyond the main pulmonary artery. In the initial diagnosis, an enlarged pulmonary artery diameter greater than 29 mm is seen on CT

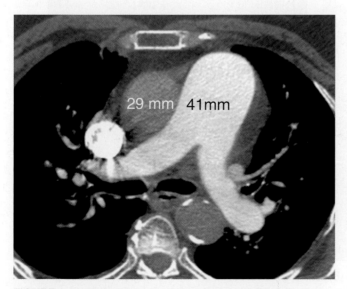

FIGURE 2.66. Pulmonary hypertension. Axial CT shows a large pulmonary trunk measuring 41 mm compared with an ascending, aortic diameter of 29 mm.

(Fig. 2.66). Findings such as increased segmental artery-to-bronchus ratio of greater than 1:1 in three or more lobes increase the specificity for diagnosis of PH.

INFECTIONS

Pneumonias may occur as an airspace or interstitial disease with findings ranging from focal to complete opacification of both lungs (Figs. 2.67–2.70). Given the extensive overlapping appearance of numerous pathogens, it is difficult to determine the microbiologic cause of pneumonia based on the radiographic appearances alone. The main goal of imaging is to distinguish bacterial pneumonias, which respond to antibiotics, from viral infections, which are usually self-limiting. Imaging is not recommended in patients with normal vital signs and physical findings. Exceptions to this rule are the elderly, patients with comorbidities, and those who may not follow up reliably. The standard PA and lateral views should be the initial test. Although CT is more accurate than chest radiographs for the diagnosis of pneumonia, its use should be reserved for patients in whom the initial chest radiograph is negative or equivocal, and in patients with atypical presentations, advanced age, or significant comorbidities. Ultrasound is useful in the evaluation parapneumonic effusions and empyema for its superior visualization of loculations. Lung abscess, a possible complication of pneumonias due to *Staphylococcus aureus*, *Streptococcus pyogenes*, and gram- negative organisms, can appear as a cavitation within the lung consolidation (Figs. 2.71–2.72).

Atypical pneumonias are characterized by a lack of inflammatory exudate into the alveoli, diminishing the "typical" airspace component. Instead, the lung interstitium and interlobar elements become engorged and these imaging findings are disproportionate to the severity of clinical presentation. Table 2.11 lists common causes of atypical pneumonia and an example is shown in Figure 2.73.

Imaging and clinical manifestations of **viral pneumonia** are not reliably predictive of its origin. The spectrum of CT findings encountered in various pulmonary viral diseases encompasses five main categories: (1) parenchymal attenuation abnormality; (2) groundglass opacity and consolidation; (3) nodules, micronodules, and tree-in-bud opacities (Fig. 2.74); (4) interlobular septal thickening (measles); and (5) bronchial and/or bronchiolar wall thickening (RSV, measles, adenovirus). There are many noninfectious or different infectious disorders that should be differentiated from viral pneumonia.

Immunosuppressed patients are particularly susceptible to infections, and pneumonia occurs in up to one-quarter of patients with neutropenia following chemotherapy. These pneumonias may have multiple causes including resistant bacteria, filamentous fungi, mycobacteria, *Pneumocystis jiroveci*, and viruses although in one-third of patients no infectious cause can be identified. The differential diagnosis includes bleeding, progression of malignancy, and injury

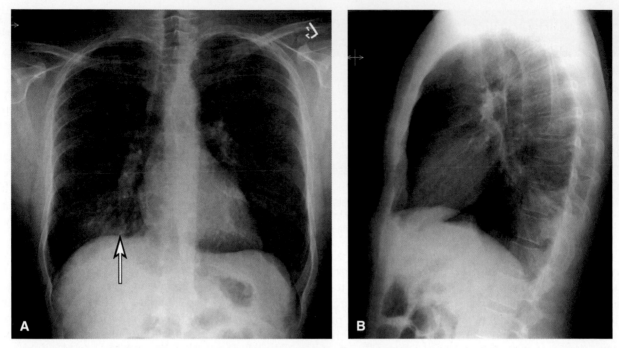

FIGURE 2.67. Right lower lobe pneumonia. PA (**A**) and lateral (**B**) views of the chest show airspace disease in the right lower lobe (*arrow*, **A**). Note on the lateral projection the corresponding "spine sign" produced by the infiltrate which overlies the lower thoracic spine. The spine sign refers to additional density overlying the spine by a superimposed opacity which in this case was due to the right lower lobe infiltrate.

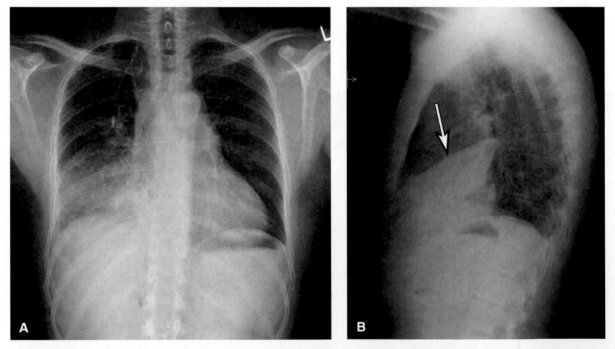

FIGURE 2.68. Right middle lobe pneumonia. PA (**A**) and lateral (**B**) films show a confluent opacity in the right middle lobe (*arrows*).

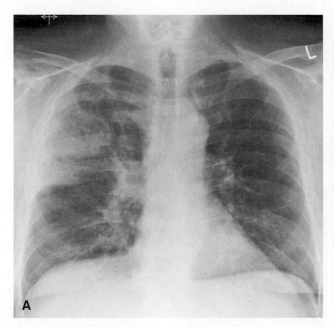 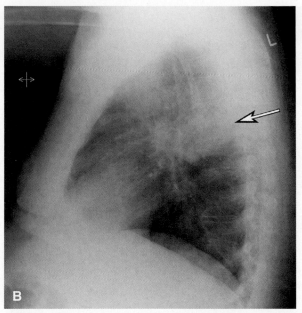

FIGURE 2.69. **Right upper lobe pneumonia.** PA (**A**) and lateral (**B**) films show pneumonia in the posterior segment of the right upper lobe (*arrow*, **B**).

caused by chemotherapy or radiation. Prompt CT and bronchoscopy with bronchoalveolar lavage (BAL) are necessary for diagnosis (Fig. 2.75).

Cytomegalovirus (CMV) pneumonia is a major cause of morbidity and mortality following hematopoietic stem cell and solid organ transplantation and in patients with HIV in whom CD4 cell count is less than 100/ mm³. CMV infection occurs in up to 70% of bone marrow transplant recipients, and approximately one-third of patients develop CMV pneumonia, which characteristically occurs 50 to 60 days after transplantation.

Pneumocystis jirovecii is a yeast-like fungus, which is specific to humans and most often occurs in immunocompromised patients. Pneumocystosis or now PJP (previously known as pneumocystis pneumonia or PCP) causes thickening of alveolar septa in combination with the development of an eosinophilic alveolar exudate. Both the thickened septa and the exudate contribute to the reduced oxygen diffusion, which is characteristic of this pneumonia. Chest imaging initially shows bilateral, diffuse, and often perihilar, fine, reticular, or reticulonodular interstitial changes. This interstitial pattern progresses to airspace pattern disease over

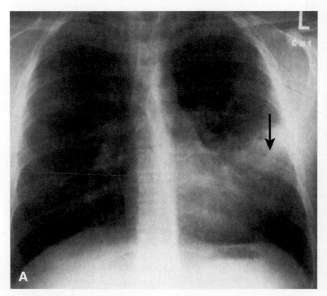 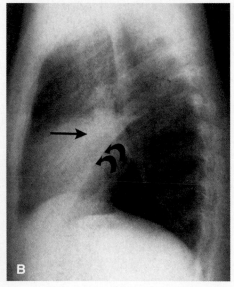

FIGURE 2.70. **Lingular pneumonia.** PA (**A**) and lateral (**B**) films show an infiltrate in the lingula (*arrows*). Note the obscuration of the left heart border on the PA projection (silhouette sign).

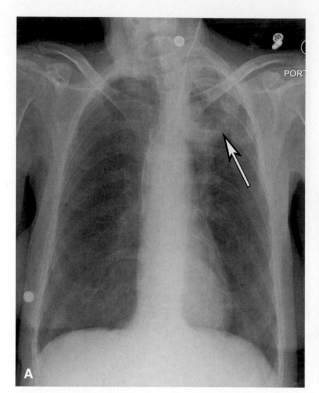

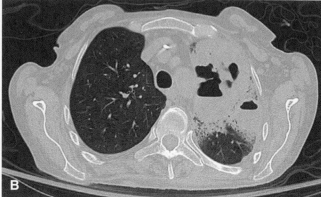

FIGURE 2.71. **Pulmonary abscess.** PA chest radiograph (**A**) and chest CT image (**B**) show a large left upper lobe consolidation with cavitation (*arrow*, **A**) typical of a pulmonary abscess, which in this case was due to *Staphylococcus aureus*.

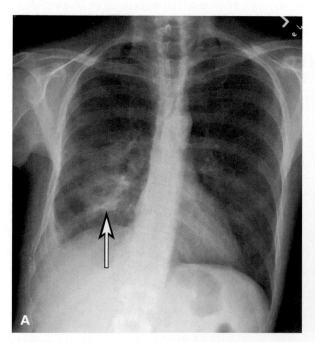

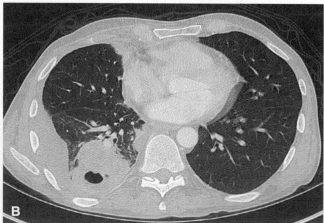

FIGURE 2.72. **Pulmonary abscess. A:** PA chest radiograph shows a cavitary right lower lobe abscess (*arrow*). **B:** CT confirms the cavitation.

TABLE 2.11 Causes of Atypical Pneumonia

Cytomegalovirus
Legionnaires disease
Measles
Mycoplasma
Pneumocystis
Tuberculosis
Varicella

several days, which may then be followed by coarse reticulation as the infection resolves (Fig. 2.76). Chest films are normal in up to 20% of PJP patients, with CT imaging showing GGO, which describes an airspace density, which does not obscure the underlying pulmonary architecture.

Despite new therapies and improved public health measures, **pulmonary tuberculosis** remains problematic with as much as one-third of the world's population having been infected with *Mycobacterium tuberculosis,* which typically involves the lungs but can also affect other organs. **Primary TB** presents as a lobar pneumonia or mediastinal/hilar adenopathy usually in children and immunocompromised adults within 1 year of exposure. Most tuberculous infections in adults are asymptomatic and **latent (primary)**, but about 1 in 10 latent infections reactivates and progresses to **reactivation TB** which, if untreated has a 50% mortality rate. Reactivation TB typically occurs after 1 year of exposure with characteristic

apical posterior upper-lobe or apical segment lower-lobe fibrocavitary disease and bronchiectasis Table 2.12 shows a comparison of primary and reactivation tuberculosis. The chest radiograph is the most appropriate initial imaging test for pulmonary tuberculosis. CT may be able to better show distinct findings such as cavitation or endobronchial spread with tree-in-bud nodules (Fig. 2.77).

Miliary TB is characterized by a multisystem hematogenous dissemination any time after the primary infection and is often associated with immunosuppression. It is characterized by numerous small (1 to 3 mm) punctate lesions of soft tissue density that are often detectable on CT before a chest film (Fig. 2.78). In disease-endemic areas, river valleys such as Ohio River, Lower Mississippi River, histoplasmosis is the main differential diagnosis for tuberculosis among human immunodeficiency virus (HIV)–infected patients.

Bronchiectasis is an irreversible dilatation of the bronchi and is usually a complication of necrotizing pneumonia. The process may be focal following staphylococcal and *Klebsiella pneumonia* or generalized as in cystic fibrosis. On a normal chest film, most of the lung markings are blood vessels because bronchi are air-containing thin-walled structures surrounded by air, rendering them almost invisible. In contrast, features of bronchiectasis include bronchial wall thickening (tram tracks), fluid-filled bronchi, and cysts (Fig. 2.79A). In addition, a classic CT feature of bronchiectasis is a relative increase in the bronchial diameter compared with the adjacent pulmonary artery branch, **the signet ring sign** (Fig. 2.79B).

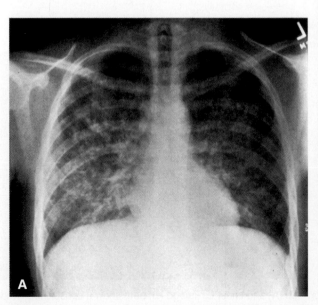
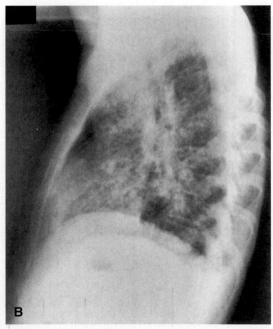

FIGURE 2.73. Atypical pneumonia due to varicella (chicken pox). Chest PA (**A**) and lateral (**B**) radiographs showing diffuse reticulonodular infiltrates throughout both lung fields. These patients are acutely ill, and the presence of skin lesions is diagnostically helpful.

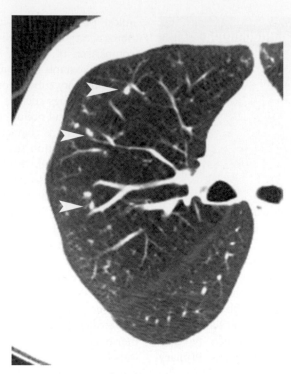

FIGURE 2.74. **Tree-in-bud pattern**. There are multiple centrilobular nodules with a linear branching pattern (*arrowheads*). Causes include mycobacteria, bacteria, and viruses.

Sarcoidosis is a multisystem disorder of unknown etiology characterized by noncaseating granulomas. Chest involvement occurs in over 90% of patients, which also accounts for most of its long-term morbidity and mortality (5%). Granulomas occur in a characteristic lymphatic and perilymphatic distribution, and biopsy (mediastinal or transbronchial) is usually diagnostic. Most patients present with bilateral hilar and right paratracheal adenopathy (stage I) (Fig. 2.80). Reticular or reticulonodular interstitial changes in a middle and upper zone distribution occur

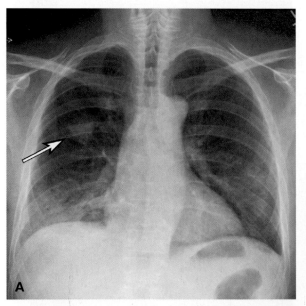

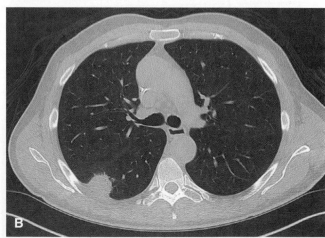

FIGURE 2.75. **Acute pulmonary aspergillosis.** PA chest radiograph (**A**) and chest CT image (**B**) both show a conspicuous nodule (*arrow*, **A**) in a patient with profound neutropenia after bone marrow transplant for leukemia. The nodules in aspergillosis have a solid and slight spiculated morphology mimicking a bronchogenic carcinoma.

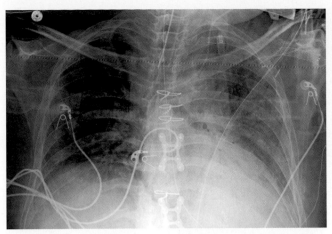

FIGURE 2.76. **Pneumocystis pneumonia.** Portable chest film in an intubated patient shows extensive airspace disease with air bronchograms the left lower lobe.

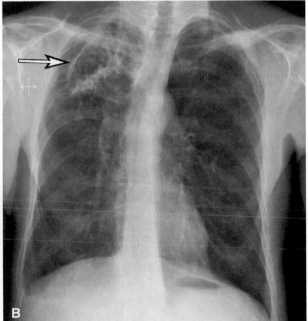

TABLE 2.12	Comparison of Primary and Reactivation TB findings	
	Primary TB	**Reactivation TB**
Hilar adenopathy	Very common	Rare
Cavitation	Rare	Common
Pleural effusion	Rare	Common

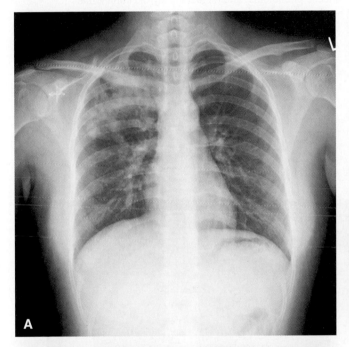

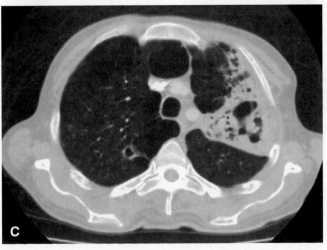

FIGURE 2.77. **Mycobacterial infections. A:** PA chest radiograph shows a large area cavitating acute tuberculosis pneumonia in the right upper lobe. Although this could represent a bacterial pneumonia with abscess, cultures were positive for *Mycobacterium tuberculosis.* **B:** Tuberculous pneumonia in a different patient which evolved into irregular thick-walled cavity (*arrow*). **C:** Chest CT in a different patient shows a left upper lobe cavitary pneumonia due to *M. tuberculosis.*

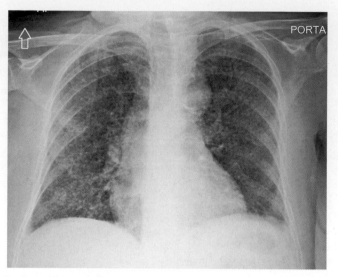

FIGURE 2.78. **Miliary tuberculosis:** Portable chest film showing diffuse fine nodular opacities measuring 1 to 3 mm. The differential diagnosis includes fungal infection (histoplasma, blastomycosis), varicella pneumonia, and metastatic thyroid carcinoma.

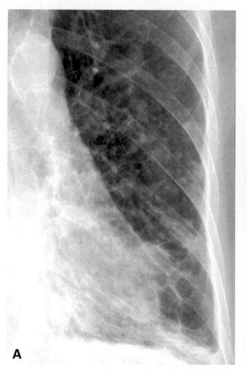

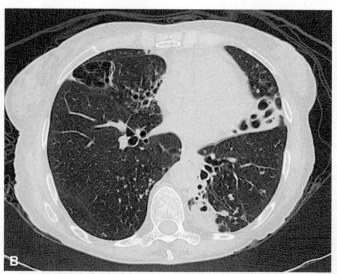

FIGURE 2.79. **Bronchiectasis. A:** Frontal chest film, magnified view of the left lung showing bronchial wall thickening and fluid-filled cysts. **B:** Axial CT showing bilateral bronchial wall thickening and fluid-filled cysts.

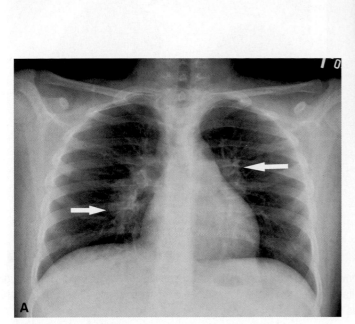

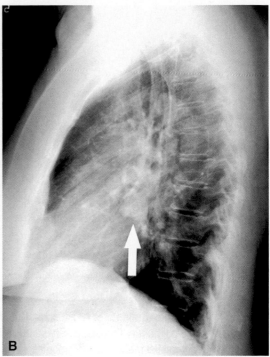

FIGURE 2.80. **Sarcoidosis. A and B:** PA and lateral chest views showing bilateral hilar adenopathy (*arrows*) (stage I disease).

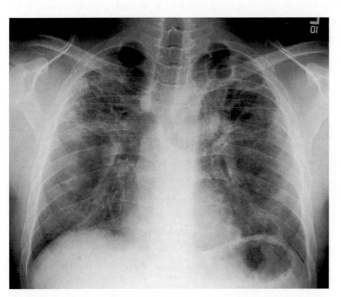

FIGURE 2.81. **Sarcoidosis A**. PA chest showing bilateral upper lobe, fibrosis, indicating end-stage, sarcoidosis (stage IV).

TABLE 2.13	**Interstitial Lung Disease by Location**
Predominantly Upper Lobe Zones	**Predominantly Lower Lobe**
Sarcoidosis	Collagen vascular disease
Silicosis	Idiopathic pulmonary fibrosis /UIP
Tuberculosis	Drugs
Extrinsic allergic alveolitis (chronic)	
Ankylosing spondylitis	

UIP, usual interstitial pneumonitis.

in half of patients in combination with adenopathy (stage II). Spontaneous remission occurs in most stage I and stage II patients. Stage III patients have interstitial change alone although progression to fibrosis (stage IV) occurs in up to 25% of all patients (Fig. 2.81).

Interstitial lung disease (ILD) is a spectrum of disorders of various etiologies (many unknown) that are usually progressive and characterized by the presence of superimposed lung fibrosis or distinctive scarring (Table 2.13). The most common cause of pulmonary fibrosis is **idiopathic pulmonary fibrosis**, the imaging and histological correlate of which is **usual interstitial pneumonitis** (UIP). Two CT findings most predictive of UIP are basal-predominant honeycombing with lung volume loss and the presence of some reticulation in the upper lobes (present in the vast majority of the patients with UIP and in only a third of those with other interstitial lung diseases) (Fig. 2.82). Additional diagnostic criteria are distortion of the secondary lobules, and a nonsegmental distribution (crosses fissures) MDCT, which has replaced open lung biopsy for diagnosis of ILD, involves scanning the patient while prone both in maximal inspiration and expiration with the use of dedicated reconstruction algorithms.

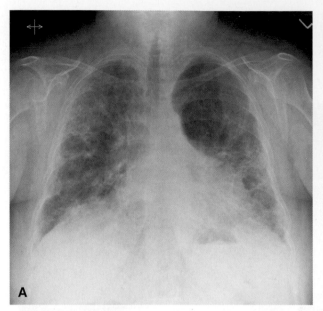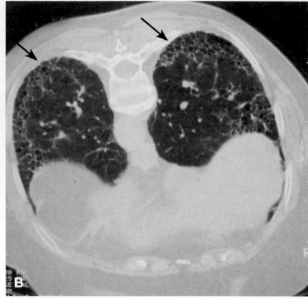

FIGURE 2.82. Interstitial lung disease. A: PA chest film shows extensive bilateral symmetric interstitial or reticular changes throughout both lungs reflecting pulmonary fibrosis. **B:** These interstitial changes are better demonstrated on the corresponding prone chest CT, which shows the fine interstitial markings of pulmonary fibrosis (*arrows*).

PULMONARY NODULES, MASSES, AND CARCINOMA

A solitary pulmonary **nodule** (SPN) is a discrete, focal lung opacity less than or equal to 3 cm in diameter (Fig. 2.83). Soft-tissue lesions larger than 3 cm are referred to as **masses**. The most common causes of lung nodules and masses are listed in Table 2.14. The workup of an SPN includes review of previous imaging and depends on many factors including the pretest probability of malignancy, size, multiplicity, density, and morphology of the nodule as well as identification of related findings such as adenopathy, air-space involvement, or pleural effusion.

Clearly, there is considerable difference in the likelihood of malignancy when dealing with a smooth 1-cm nodule in a 30-year-old nonsmoker compared with a 2-cm spiculated nodule in a 60-year-old lifetime smoker. First, the larger the nodule the greater the chance that it will be malignant (Fig. 2.84). Second, interval growth of a pre-existing nodule also supports malignancy, so review of previous imaging is essential (Fig. 2.85). A 9-mm SPN with a (volume) doubling time of 100 days will measure 1.1 cm at 3 months and 1.4 cm at 6 months. The presence of spiculation and interstitial changes is concerning for primary malignancy in contrast to secondary malignant lung nodules or metastases from either a primary lung or extrathoracic source that are often smoothly marginated and well circumscribed (Fig. 2.86). Other features associated with increased likelihood of malignancy include pleural effusions, hilar or mediastinal adenopathy, or presence of bone, adrenal gland, or liver lesions, all common sites of metastatic disease. Primary lung

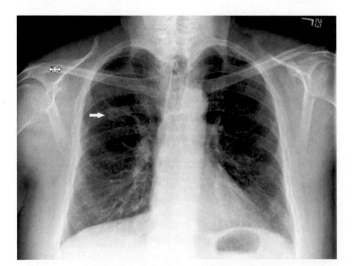

FIGURE 2.83. Solitary pulmonary nodule. There is a solitary 2 cm nodule in the right upper lobe. The differential diagnosis includes hematoma, granuloma, and carcinoma.

TABLE 2.14	Causes of Solitary and Multiple Pulmonary Nodules/ Masses	
Single		Multiple
Granuloma		Metastases
Carcinoma		Histoplasmosis
Hamartoma		Sarcoidosis

MacMahon H, Naidich DP, Goo JM, et al. Guidelines for management of incidental pulmonary nodules detected on ct images: From the fleischner society 2017. *Radiology* 2017; 284: 228–243.10.1148/radiol.2017161659

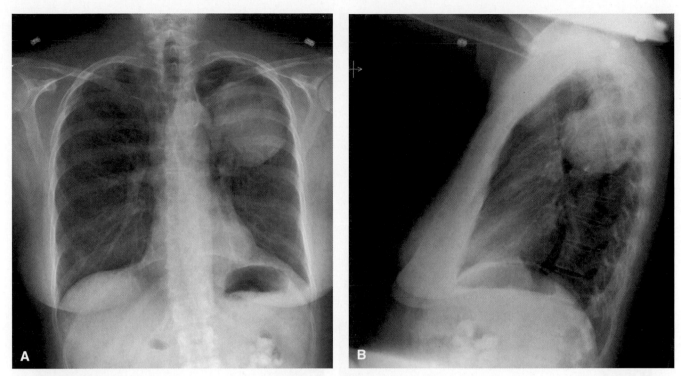

FIGURE 2.84. **Squamous cell lung carcinoma.** PA (**A**) and lateral (**B**) radiographs show a large mass in the left upper lobe. The risk of malignancy increases with lesion size.

malignancies, especially squamous cell, may present as a cavity which may be mistaken as a lung abscess (Fig. 2.87).

Calcifications in a hamartoma are scattered resembling calcified cartilaginous matrix. The presence of fat within the mass confirms the diagnosis of hamartoma. Dystrophic and bulky **calcifications** also favor a benign diagnosis, specifically granulomatous disease. Calcifications within granulomas are highly variable including solid, centrally located

nidus, or laminar patterns. If there is doubt as to whether a nodule contains calcification, CT should be used to measure its density. When the CT density of a pulmonary nodule measures greater than 200 Hounsfield units, and the calcification composes most of the nodule, a benign entity is confirmed and no further evaluation or surveillance is required. Biopsy is usually necessary when imaging alone cannot distinguish benign from malignant lung lesions.

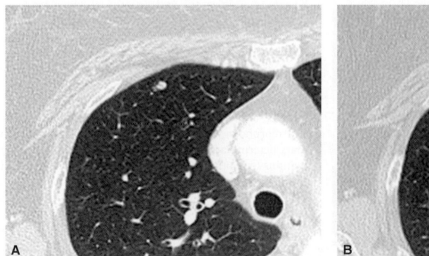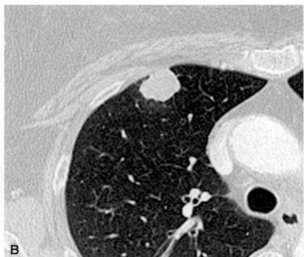

FIGURE 2.85. **Lung carcinoma, lesion growth. A:** Low-dose CT shows a 5 mm subpleural nodule in a cigarette smoker. **B:** Two years later low-dose CT shows, interval growth to a 27 millimeter nodule. Biopsy confirmed carcinoma.

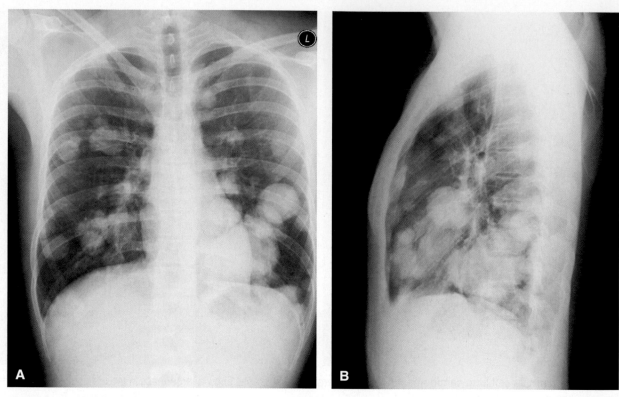

FIGURE 2.86. Metastatic disease. Chest PA (**A**) and lateral (**B**) radiographs show numerous bilateral soft tissue nodules consistent with metastases in a patient with testicular cancer.

Screening chest radiography programs have not been effective in reducing mortality from lung cancer. Based on recent large studies, the USPSTF recommends annual screening for lung cancer with low-dose computed tomography (LDCT) in adults aged 55 to 80 years who have a 30 pack-year smoking history and currently smoke or have quit within the past 15 years. CT screening should be discontinued once a person has not smoked for 15 years

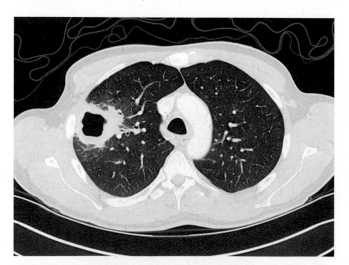

FIGURE 2.87. Cavitating lung carcinoma. Axial CT of the chest showing a thick-walled cavity in the right upper lobe. The differential diagnosis includes lung abscess.

or develops a health problem that substantially limits life expectancy or the ability or willingness to have curative lung surgery. The use of thin (1.0–1.5 mm) sections is essential for the characterization of solid and subsolid pulmonary nodules and the detection of calcium or fat components; these features can lead to different management options. A screening low-dose CT scan involves one-fifth of the dose of a standard CT chest.

On CT screening for lung cancer, 70% of smokers will have lung nodules, the vast majority of which are benign. Percutaneous biopsy has a small but definite morbidity risk (pneumothorax, hemothorax, conscious sedation), as does surgical resection so either option is not suitable for all lung nodules. The **Fleischner Society's guidelines for management of nodules** detected on CT are based on their appearance (solid versus subsolid, groundglass), size, number, and risk category of patient (Table 2.15). The size and morphology of a pulmonary nodule are the two primary determinants of cancer risk. Morphology refers to the margins (smooth, lobulated, or spiculated) and attenuation (solid, partly solid, or purely groundglass) of the nodule (Fig 2.88). Single solid noncalcified nodules smaller than 6 mm do not require routine follow-up in patients at low risk. Of interest are the various patient categories excluded from the Fleischner Criteria (Table 2.16).

Generally, biopsy of an SPN is not indicated in the initial course of management. In the absence of prior imaging, and depending on the lesions size, PET scanning should be

TABLE 2.15   Fleischner Society 2017 Guidelines for Management of Incidentally Detected Pulmonary Nodules in Adults

A: Solid Nodules[a]

Nodule Type	<6 mm (<100 mm³)	6–8 mm (100–250 mm³)	>8 mm (>250 mm³)	Comments
Single				
Low risk[b]	No routine follow-up	CT at 6–12 months, then consider CT at 18–24 months	Consider CT at 3 months, PET/CT, or tissue sampling	Nodules <6 mm do not require routine follow-up in low-risk patients (recommendation 1A).
High risk[b]	Optional CT at 12 months	CT at 6–12 months then CT at 18–24 months	Consider CT at 3 months, PET/CT, or tissue sampling	Certain patients at high risk with suspicious nodule morphology, upper lobe location, or both may warrant 12-month follow-up (recommendation 1A).
Multiple				
Low risk[b]	No routine follow-up	CT at 3–6 months, then consider CT at 18–24 months	CT at 3–6 months, then consider CT at 18–24 months	Use most suspicious nodule as guide to management. Follow-up intervals may vary according to size and risk (recommendation 2A).
High risk[b]	Optional CT at 12 months	CT at 3–12 months, then CT at 18–24 months	CT at 3–6 months, then at 18–24 months	Use most suspicious nodule as guide to management. Follow-up intervals may vary according to size and risk (recommendation 2A).

B: Subsolid Nodules[a]

Nodule Type	<6 mm (<100 mm³)	≥6 mm (>100 mm³)	Comments
Single			
Ground glass	No routine follow-up	CT at 6–12 months to confirm persistence, then CT every 2 tears until 5 years	In certain suspicious nodules <6 mm, consider follow-up at 2 and 4 year. If solid component(s) or growth develops, consider resection (recommendation 3A and 4A).
Part solid	No routine follow-up	CT at 3–6 months to confirm persistence. If unchanged and solid component remains <6 mm, annual CT should be performed for 5 years	In practice, part-solid nodules cannot be defined as such until ≥6 mm, and nodules <6 mm do not usually require follow-up. Persistent part-solid nodules with solid components ≥6 mm should be considered highly suspicious (recommendation 4A-4C).
Multiple	CT at 3–6 months. If stable, consider CT at 2 and 4 years.	CT at 3–6 months. Subsequent management based on the most suspicious nodule(s)	Multiple <6 mm pure ground glass nodules are usually benign, but consider follow-up in selected patients at high risk at 2 and 4 years (recommendation 5A).

Note—These recommendations do not apply to lung cancer screening, patients with immunosuppression, or patients with known primary cancer.
[a]Dimensions are average of long and short axes, rounded to the nearest millimeter.
[b]Consider all relevant risk factors (see Risk Factors).
Reproduced from MacMahon H, Naidich DP, Goo JM, et al. Guidelines for management of incidental pulmonary nodules detected on CT Images: From the Fleischner Society 2017. Radiology. 2017;284:228-243.

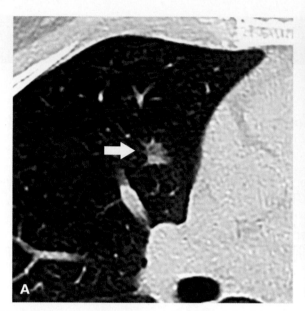
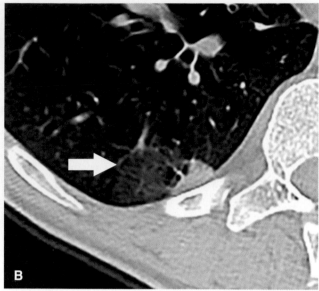

FIGURE 2.88. Subsolid pulmonary nodules. Axial CT showing subsolid (groundglass and solid components) pulmonary nodules (*arrows*) in the **(A)** right middle and **(B)** right lower lobes.

TABLE 2.16	Patient Categories Excluded from Fleischner Criteria
Patient Category	**Reason for Exclusion**
Under 35 years of age	Low risk
Known malignancy	High risk
Immunocompromised	Most lung nodules (70%) are infectious
Lung cancer screening population	Annual screening protocol applies even if negative

After Bueno J. (2018). Updated Fleischner Society Guidelines for Managing Incidental Pulmonary Nodules: Common Questions and Challenging Scenarios. Radiographics, 38. 1337-1350.

TABLE 2.17	Radiological Appearances of Lung Carcinoma
Solitary pulmonary nodule	
Central/mediastinal/hilar mass	
Persistent infiltrate	
Cavity	
Atelectasis	
Pleural effusion	
Calcification	
Bone erosion (rib/vertebral body)	

considered for lesions over 1 cm. Nodules under 1 cm often are followed with repeat CT. If the level of suspicion or pretest probability is relatively high, surgical resection rather than biopsy is the best course of action. Biopsy of a solitary nodule should be considered under the following two exceptions: (1) Patients who are nonsurgical candidates (owing to coexisting morbidities) and a tissue diagnosis is needed prior to instituting therapy, or (2) a new pulmonary nodule is discovered in the setting of a known primary cancer. In the latter case, biopsy determines whether the nodule is a second primary lung carcinoma or a metastasis, given that in many circumstances second de novo cancers in patients with known malignancies are more common than not.

Staging: A solitary lung nodule or mass is the most common radiologic presentation of lung carcinoma; however, other potential radiologic appearances must also be considered (Table 2.17). All lung tumors are initially staged with F-18 FDG PET/CT, which detect the distribution and all primary lung carcinomas can be additionally staged with F-18 FDG PET/CT, which detect the distribution and extent of disease, referred to as TNM staging, tumor size (T), nodal involvement (N), and metastatic spread of tumor (M) (Fig. 2.89). Small-cell lung carcinoma (SCLC) should be regarded as a systemic disease and is rarely operable at diagnosis.

SVC syndrome is an oncologic emergency, due to extrinsic compression of the SVC by tumor or mediastinal nodes. Eighty percent of SVC syndrome cases are due to lung cancer. Typically, the patient presents with dyspnea, facial fullness, which eventually progresses to hoarseness, and chest pain. CT reveals narrowing or occlusion of the SVC with multiple chest wall and mediastinal collaterals. Treatment options include emergent radiotherapy to reduce the mediastinal mass or placement of an SVC stent from a common femoral approach to relieve the obstruction (Fig 2.90).

The lungs are the most frequently targeted organs for **metastatic disease,** CT scanning of which is superior to chest radiography. In addition to nodules and masses, pulmonary metastatic disease may also appear as lymphangitic carcinomatosis (most commonly tumors of the lung, stomach, breast, pancreas, uterus, rectum, and prostate).

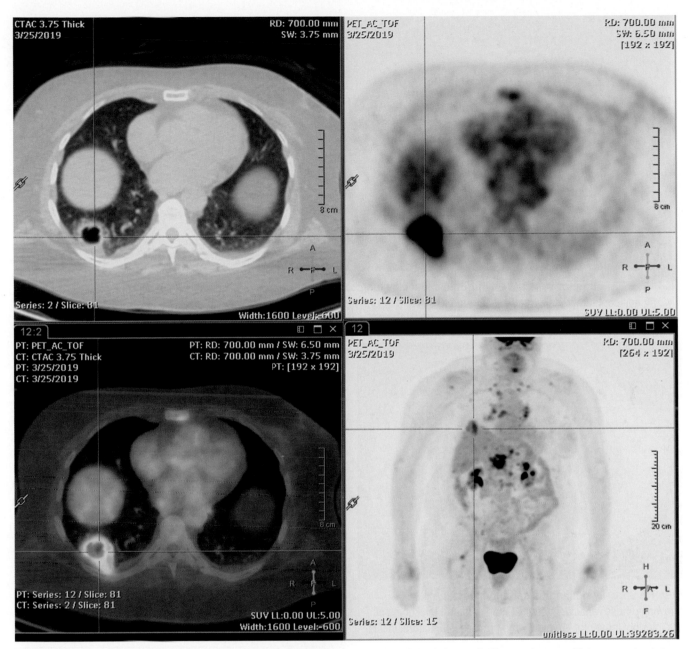

FIGURE 2.89. **Lung carcinoma staging with F-18 FDG PET/CT** showing right lower lobe cavitating carcinoma with increased uptake in multiple lymph nodes including bilateral supraclavicular; right peritracheal; precarinal; subcarinal; bilateral pulmonary hilar; gastrohepatic; periportal nodes. Note normal uptake in both kidneys, bladder, and brain.

Plain film findings of lymphangitic carcinomatosis include diffuse reticular or in later stages reticulonodular interstitial markings, usually with irregular contours, and thickening of the interlobular septa which contain lymphatics (formerly Kerley B lines). CT is sensitive in the detection of lymphangitic patterns, including thickened core structures in the central portions of the secondary pulmonary lobules. This is usually bibasal process (Fig 2.91). Table 2.18 lists the patterns of metastatic disease to the lung.

Metastases to the pleura from cancers of the lung, breast, pancreas, and stomach occur because of hematogenous dissemination with extension to the pleura, with lymphangitic spread, or originating from established hepatic metastases. Metastases may appear as nodules or plaques on plain films and CT scans. Malignant pleural effusions most commonly arise from primary tumors of the lungs, the breast, and the ovaries, and from lymphoma.

Lung cancer is the third most common malignancy among HIV-infected patients, following Kaposi sarcoma and non-Hodgkin lymphoma. With prolonged survival due to the use of HAART, the morbidity and mortality attributable to lung cancer in HIV-infected patients may increase.

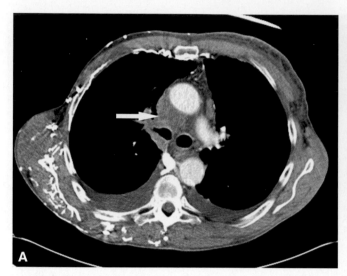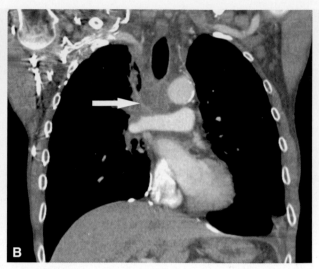

FIGURE 2.90. Superior vena cava syndrome caused by lung carcinoma. Axial (**A**) and coronal CT (**B**) showing occlusion of the SVC by adjacent tumor in the mediastinum (*arrows*). Note extensive, right posterior chest wall collaterals.

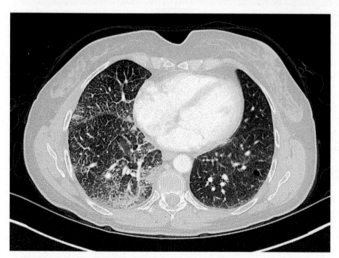

FIGURE 2.91. Lymphangitis carcinomatosis. Axial CT showing diffuse reticular interstitial markings and thickening of the interlobular septal. Atypically the process is unilateral in this patient.

TABLE 2.18	Patterns of Metastatic Spread to the Lungs	
Fine nodular	**Fine reticular**	**Multiple Nodules and Masses**
Thyroid	Lymphangitic spread from adenocarcinoma	Kidney, GI, melanoma,
Melanoma	(Breast, colon, stomach, pancreas)	Uterus, ovary, testis
Breast		Sarcoma

Chest Radiograph Appearances Post Lung Resection

In a traditional non–video-assisted thoracoscopic surgical (VATS) resection, the fourth or fifth rib is resected posteriorly and the pneumonectomy space fills in with mediastinal shift to the *same* side within 4 to 8 weeks. Following lobar resection, the remaining lobe(s) expand to fill the space formerly occupied by the resected lobe. With segmental or subsegmental resection, the cut surface of the lung is oversewn or stapled through which air leaks may occur causing a pneumothorax or bronchopleural fistula. An empyema may present as a rapid accumulation of fluid in the postpneumonectomy space with mediastinal shift to the *opposite* side. If a fistula develops between the bronchus and pneumonectomy space, the air–fluid level will suddenly drop.

MEDIASTINAL COMPARTMENTS AND PATHOLOGY

The mediastinum is the space between the pleura of the lungs that contains all the viscera of the chest except the lungs and pleura. On a chest film, mediastinal masses characteristically form an **obtuse angle** rather than an acute angle with lung tissue. The concept of an obtuse angle is best described using the analogy of a "ball under a rug," where the rug which is draped over the ball forming sloping sides to the floor upon which it rests represents the lung pleura and the ball is the tumor. If an **acute angle** is observed, this would be as if the ball was placed on the surface of the rug, where there is air undercutting the ball and represents an **intrapulmonary process** abutting the pleura, and not pushing from the mediastinal space in toward the aerated lung. The same principle applies for pleural and chest wall versus intrapulmonary masses.

TABLE 2.19 Mediastinal Masses by Location

Anterior
1. Thyroid and parathyroid masses
2. Thymic gland tumors (thymomas, cysts, thymic carcinoma/ sarcoma)
3. Teratoma
4. Lymphadenopathy/lymphoma and leukemia
5. Aneurysms, especially of ascending thoracic aorta
6. Chest wall/bone tumor (i.e., sarcomas, metastatic disease)

Middle Mediastinum (90% of masses are malignant)
1. Bronchogenic carcinomas and bronchogenic cyst
2. Lymphadenopathy/lymphoma/leukemia
3. Pericardial fat pad and pericardial cyst
4. Diaphragm (Morgagni) hernia
5. Aneurysms
6. Esophageal neoplasms and masses

Posterior Mediastinum
1. Neurogenic tumors (30% are malignant)
2. Duplication cysts
3. Lymph node enlargement
4. Esophageal lesions
5. Diaphragmatic (Bochdalek) hernias
6. Extramedullary hematopoiesis

The differential diagnosis of a mediastinal mass depends on its location. Table 2.19 lists the contents of the mediastinal compartments which can be thought of as three potential spaces: **anterior, middle, and posterior**. The anterior mediastinum extends from the posterior margin of the sternum back to the anterior surface of the pericardium and it contains mediastinal fat, thymus gland, lymphoid tissue, and the ascending thoracic aorta, all covered anteriorly by the anterior chest wall. Retrosternal extension of the thyroid gland must also be considered within the anterior compartment given its embryonic development. A useful mnemonic for anterior mediastinal masses is the "4 T's" which include **thymoma, thyroid tumors, (terrible) lymphoma, and** occasionally germ cell tumors such as **teratomas** (Fig. 2.92).

The **middle mediastinum** extends from the ventral pericardial surface posteriorly to the ventral surface of the thoracic spine and includes the heart, pericardium, aortic arch, hila, esophagus, lymph nodes, and nerves (Fig. 2.93). Pulmonary arterial aneurysms may present as hilar enlargement, which is a common finding in patients with pulmonary hypertension. Table 2.20 lists the causes of hilar enlargement.

The **posterior mediastinum** extends from the ventral border of the thoracic spine posteriorly to the posterior

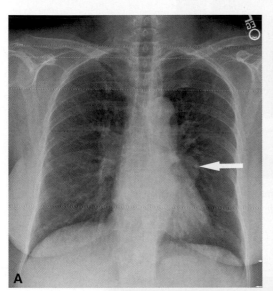

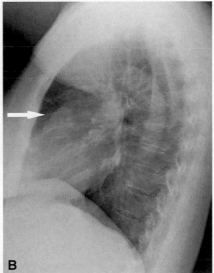

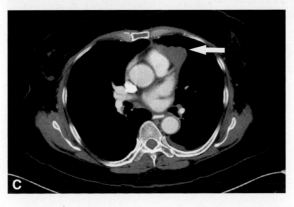

FIGURE 2.92. Anterior mediastinal mass. A and B: PA and lateral chest films demonstrating an anterior mediastinal mass (*arrows*). **C:** Axial CT showing soft tissue mass (*arrow*) anteriorly. Biopsy confirmed lymphoma.

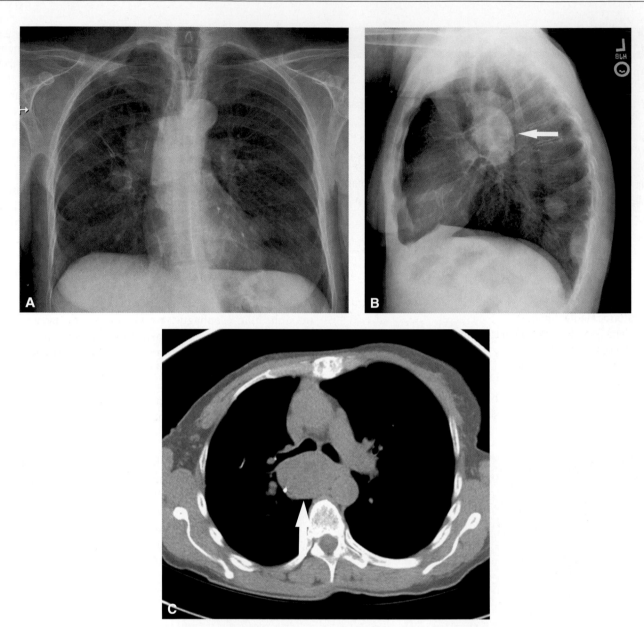

FIGURE 2.93. **Middle mediastinal mass. A and B:** PA and lateral chest films demonstrating a middle mediastinal mass (*arrow*). **C:** Axial CT shows a predominantly cystic mass (*arrow*) consistent with a bronchogenic cyst. Note how the right hilum is not clearly seen on the plain film.

TABLE 2.20	Causes of Hilar Enlargement
Unilateral Hilar Enlargement	**Bilateral Hilar Enlargement**
Lung carcinoma	Sarcoidosis
Infection (primary TB, histoplasmosis)	Lymphoma (asymmetrical)
Pulmonary artery aneurysm	Infection (viral, fungal)
Superimposed mediastinal mass	Pulmonary Arterial hypertension

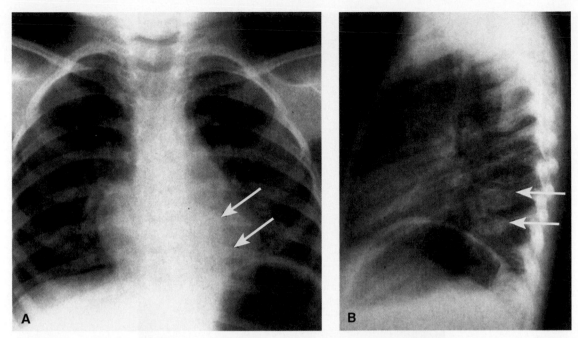

FIGURE 2.94. Posterior mediastinal mass: neuroblastoma. A: On the PA view, a paraspinal mass can be seen projecting through the cardiac shadow (*arrows*). **B:** On the lateral film, the mass is posterior in location along the spine, producing a small "spine sign" (*arrows*).

chest wall and includes the spine and the descending thoracic aorta (Fig. 2.94). Although CT is useful for workup of anterior and middle mediastinal masses, MRI is more helpful for posterior masses given that the majority of these turn out to be neurogenic in nature.

If the hilar vessels can be seen separately from a mediastinal mass, it is very unlikely that the mass arises from the hilum, which is in the middle mediastinum given the anticipated distortion and silhouette sign. This is known as the **hilum overlay sign.** The majority are mediastinal masses that on a lateral view will displace the middle mediastinal structures posteriorly. Because the anterior mediastinum ends at the upper margin of the clavicle, any mass that extends above the clavicle must be in the posterior mediastinum. When lung tissue is seen between the mass and the neck, the mass is probably in the posterior mediastinum. This is known as the **cervicothoracic sign.**

CARDIAC CHAMBER ENLARGEMENT

Although the radiographic appearance of the heart correlates poorly with overall cardiac function, enlargement of individual cardiac chambers on the PA and lateral views

can be useful in diagnosing certain cardiopulmonary diseases. Echocardiography is recommended in patients with suspected pericardial effusion, valve malfunction, and infective endocarditis.

Left ventricular enlargement appears with the cardiac apex displaced down and lateral (Fig. 2.95 A), and on the lateral projection one there is posterior displacement of the left ventricular border (Fig. 2.95 B). When the **right ventricle** enlarges, the cardiac apex is displaced superiorly, and the heart appears somewhat boot-like in configuration on the PA view (Fig. 2.96A) and there is increased retrosternal opacity on the lateral view (Fig.2.96B).

Left atrial enlargement occurs in mitral valve disease and produces the classic findings on a PA film of bulging of the upper left heart border below the main pulmonary artery (Figs. 2.97 and 2.6), and if severe enough, can displace or elevate the left mainstem bronchus into a more horizontal configuration and provide a double density sign to the right heart border. Examples of mitral and aortic valvular disease are illustrated on Figures 2.98 and 2.99, respectively.

Right atrial enlargement will produce a conspicuous right heart shadow (Fig. 2.7) and occurs in patients with tricuspid valve disease or right heart failure.

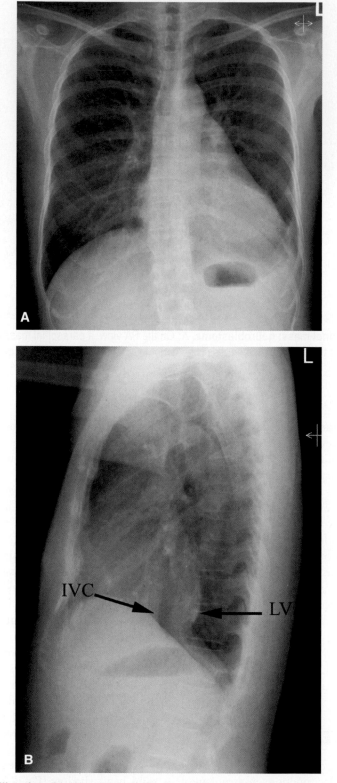

FIGURE 2.95. Left ventricular dilatation. PA (**A**) and lateral (**B**) views of the chest show the characteristic morphologic changes in the cardiac silhouette in a patient with left ventricular dilatation. **A:** Note on the PA film that the apex of the heart is displaced down and out. **B:** On the lateral film, note how the posterior margin of the left ventricle (LV) projects unusually posterior to the IVC. Normally, the posterior border of the left ventricle should be within 2 cm of the posterior border of the IVC.

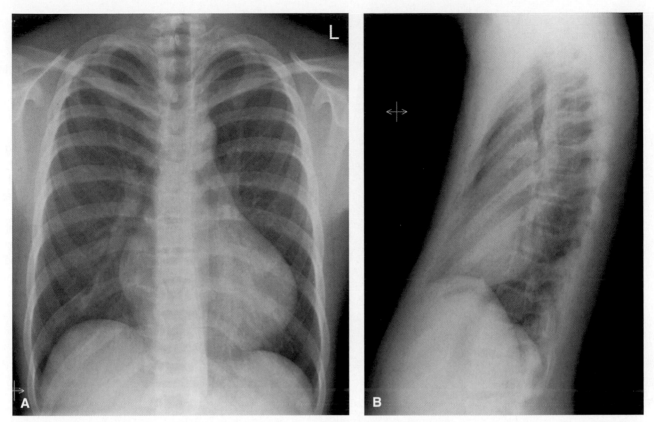

FIGURE 2.96. **Right ventricular enlargement. A:** PA film of the chest shows the characteristic upward pointing of the cardiac apex characteristic of right ventricular dilatation. **B:** On the lateral film, note how the retrosternal region is more opacified than usual reflecting the corresponding dilatation of the right ventricle.

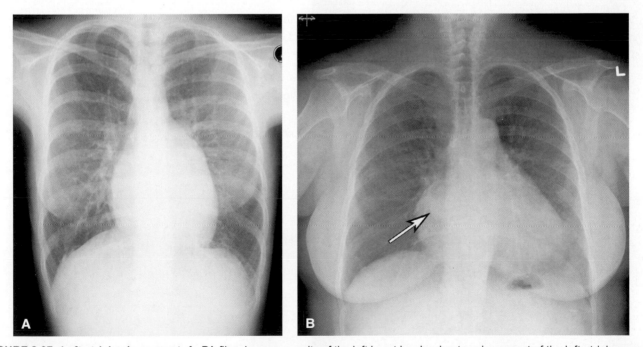

FIGURE 2.97. **Left atrial enlargement. A:** PA film shows convexity of the left heart border due to enlargement of the left atrial appendage. **B:** The double density sign of left atrial enlargement can be seen, which corresponds to the overlap of the right atrial shadow and the right lateral wall of the left atrium (*arrow*).

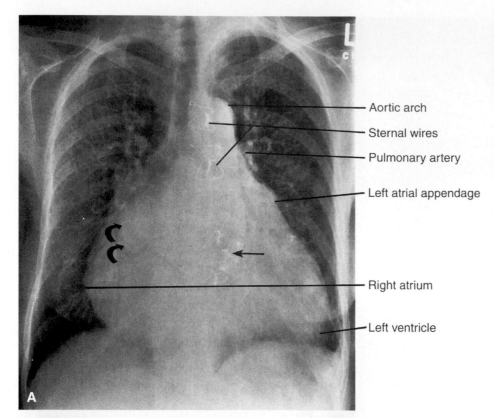

Aortic arch

Sternal wires

Pulmonary artery

Left atrial appendage

Right atrium

Left ventricle

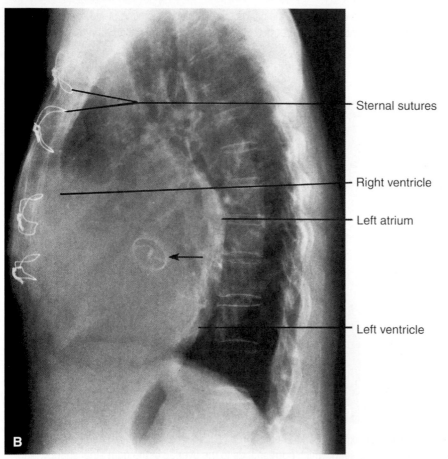

Sternal sutures

Right ventricle

Left atrium

Left ventricle

FIGURE 2.98. Multichamber enlargement: Mitral stenosis. PA (**A**) and lateral (**B**) chest films show severe cardiomegaly and a prosthetic mitral valve (*straight arrows*). On the PA view, the enlarged left atrium creates the double density indicated by the *curved arrows*, and the left atrial appendage is prominent along the left cardiac border. Also, on the PA view, there is right atrial and left ventricular enlargement. On the lateral view, right ventricular enlargement results in fullness of the retrosternal space. Also, on the lateral view, there is enlargement of the left atrium and ventricle.

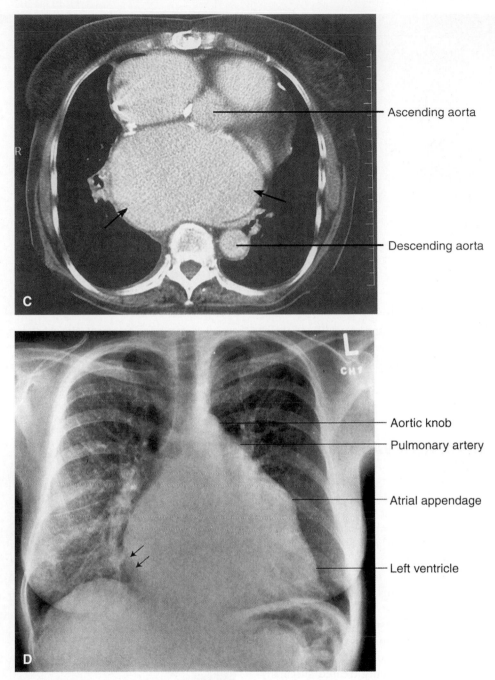

FIGURE 2.98. *(Continued)* **C:** Chest axial CT image through the atrial level. Left atrial enlargement (*straight arrows*). **D:** Shows typical changes in the morphology of the heart of left atrial enlargement in a patient with mitral stenosis. Again note the bulging left heart border and the double density sign (*arrows*).

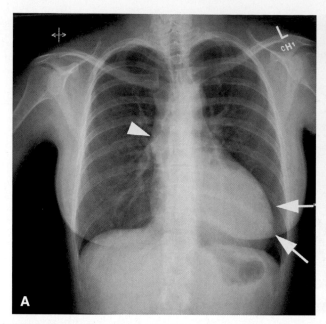

FIGURE 2.99. Aortic stenosis. PA (**A**) and lateral (**B**) radiographs show left ventricular enlargement (*straight arrows*) manifested by rounding of the cardiac apex on the PA view, and on the lateral view the enlarged left ventricle projects more than 2 cm posterior to the inferior vena cava). The ascending aorta is dilated (*arrowheads*), and this is often encountered in patients with severe aortic stenosis reflecting poststenotic dilatation.

AORTIC DISEASE AND VASCULAR CALCIFICATIONS

The thoracic aorta is divided into three parts, ascending aorta, aortic arch, and descending aorta. Aneurysm of the thoracic aorta is defined as a diameter of greater than 4.5 cm and yet its appearance on a chest film depends on its location. Aneurysms of the aortic arch distort the middle mediastinum (Fig. 2.100). An intramural hematoma is thought to predispose to **aortic dissection**, which occurs when there is a tear in the medial layer of the vessel wall (Fig 2.101). Aortic dissections are classified if the tear involves the ascending aorta (Stanford type A) or is confined to the descending thoracic aorta (Stanford type B). Type A dissections are usually treated surgically and often. Emergently, while most type B dissections are managed medically. Indications for surgical or endovascular treatment of type B dissections include organ or limb ischemia and impending rupture (Fig. 2.102).

In patients with acute chest pain and suspected aortic dissection, CTA chest and abdomen is recommended. MRA may be used as an alternative in patients who were hemodynamically stable, but takes longer and depends on scanner availability.

Atherosclerotic calcification of thoracic vessels occurs commonly with advancing age, usually without associated vascular

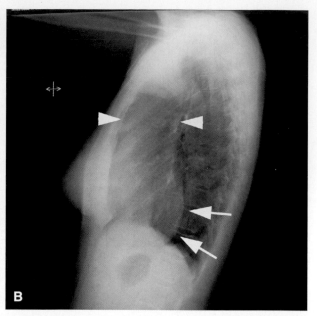

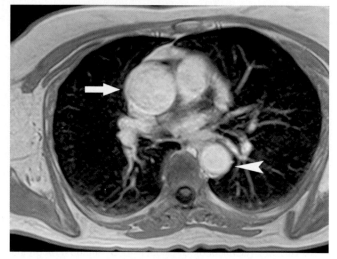

FIGURE 2.100. Aneurysm of ascending thoracic aorta. Axial MRI showing an aneurysm of the ascending thoracic aorta without dissection rupture (*arrow*). The descending thoracic aorta is unremarkable (*arrowhead*)

aneurysm. Premature vascular calcifications, especially when discovered in younger patients can be indicators of hyperlipidemia or diabetes mellitus. Coronary artery calcium scoring on either an electron beam CT or MDCT is a proven predictor

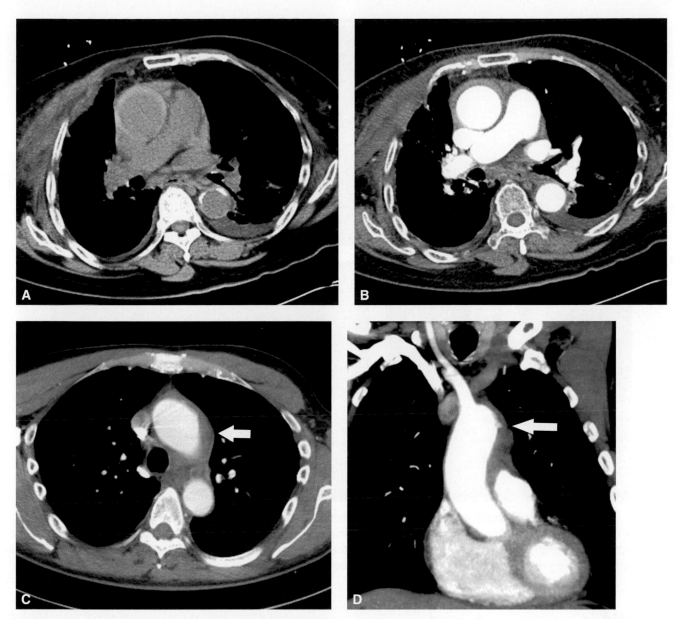

FIGURE 2.101. Intramural hematoma of the ascending thoracic aorta. A and B: Axial CT shows a hyperdense band within the aortic wall, better seen on the noncontrast images. **C and D:** Different patient, axial and coronal CT reformats show a focal dissection in the aortic arch causing intramural hematoma (*arrows*).

of future cardiovascular events and its use is appropriate in asymptomatic, intermediate-risk patients and in low-risk patients who had a family history of premature CAD.

Coronary CT angiography (CCTA) noninvasively assesses the coronary arteries, the presence of plaques (calcified and noncalcified), and ventricular function. The technique is highly sensitive for detecting a 50% stenosis and has a negative predictive value of up to 99%.

Cardiac MR is the current standard for imaging myocardial anatomy, regional and global function, and viability. It has a central role in the work up of heart failure due to ischemic and nonischemic cardiomyopathies. In nonischemic cardiomyopathy, delayed myocardial enhancement with gadolinium usually does not occur in a coronary artery distribution and is often mid-wall or subepicardial rather than subendocardial or transmural.

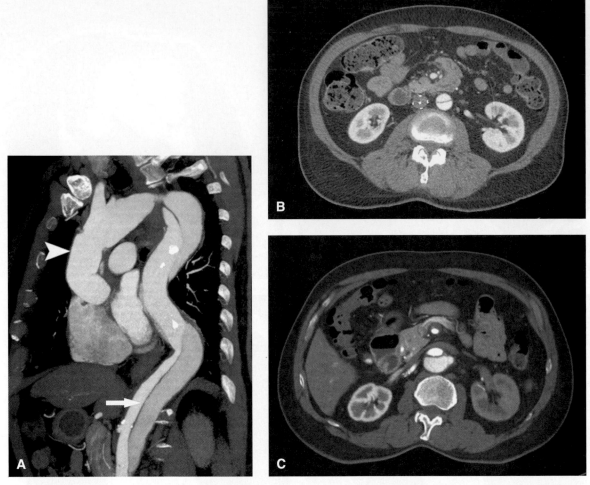

FIGURE 2.102. Type A aortic dissection. A: Sagittal oblique CT reformat of the thoracic aorta shows a type. A dissection after placement of an interposition graft (*arrowhead*) in the ascending aorta. The dissection flap (*arrow*) extends inferiorly to the common iliac arteries (not seen). **B.** Axial CT showing aortic dissection involving the abdominal aorta with equal perfusion to both kidneys. **C:** Different patient, axial CT showing aortic dissection involving the abdominal aorta with the left renal ischemia.

TRAUMA

Penetrating chest trauma (gun shot, stabbing) is generally less common but potentially more fatal than **blunt** chest trauma, and proportionally more patients require surgery. The imaging algorithm for both types of chest trauma is similar and involves the use of chest radiography and CT and to a lesser degree US or echocardiography.

Chest radiography allows a rapid evaluation for the presence of pneumothorax, pleural fluid, mediastinal widening, and lung contusion (Figs. 2.103, 2.104). However, for technical reasons, as many as half of all pneumothoraces, rib fractures, and pulmonary contusions may not be apparent on a portable AP chest radiograph performed emergently for chest trauma, so reliance on this modality to exclude significant traumatic thoracic injuries is not recommended. Many view chest radiography and CTA as complementary tests with the major advantage of obtaining a portable AP chest

radiograph depending on the ease and speed with which it can be done in the initial assessment of a patient with chest trauma.

Where there is concern for vascular injury due to high impact mechanism (motor vehicle, motor cycle, fall from a height), emergent CTA of chest and abdomen is recommended. The most serious injury following blunt chest trauma is acute **aortic transection** (traumatic dissection), which most commonly occurs adjacent to the origin of the left subclavian artery (Fig. 2.105). Echocardiography is recommended if cardiac injury is suspected.

Rib fracture is one of the more common blunt thoracic injuries and can predict the severity of trauma (Fig. 2.106). Studies have correlated the number of ribs fractured with a higher morbidity and mortality. Additionally, a first rib fracture is especially significant because of the force necessary for it to occur and the increased likelihood of additional visceral and vascular injury. A **flail chest** is described as a

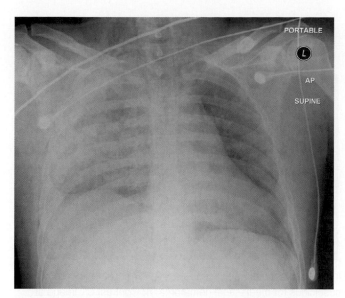

FIGURE 2.103. Pulmonary contusion. AP chest film on a patient following blunt trauma shows extensive unilateral airspace disease in the right lung reflecting pulmonary contusion or hematoma. Also, note the associated pleural effusion on the right reflecting a right hemothorax.

free-floating segment of ribs where three or more fractured ribs broken in two places, allowing paradoxical movement of the chest wall opposite to the adjacent chest wall during respiration. This reverse direction negates the volume change, thus preventing adequate gas exchange.

Pneumothorax is the most common serious injury associated with penetrating chest trauma, and a chest tube should be considered for symptomatic cases, often observed when the pneumothorax is approximately 15% or more in volume, as these are not likely to resolve spontaneously. Placement of a chest tube alone is usually sufficient to manage 85% of these cases (Fig. 2.106). Hemothoraces of volumes greater than 300 to 500 mL also require a chest tube.

Emergent tracheal intubation of patients with pericardial tamponade or a tension pneumothorax can worsen hypotension and cause cardiovascular collapse. Therefore, percutaneous drainage of the pericardial effusion or decompression of the pneumothorax (both of which are feasible at the bedside in the ER) should be done *before* the patient is intubated.

Focused assessment with sonography for trauma (**FAST**), in which US is used to detect free fluid in the abdomen and pericardium, is used in some centers, but its accuracy is subject to the training and expertise of those performing the test, which may be associated with a high false negative rate.

Finally, **hemodynamically unstable patients** do not belong in radiology departments and hemodynamically unstable patients should not be long in radiology departments. The trade-off of time versus accuracy is important because unstable patients may have their survival compromised in the time it takes to get a CT. Chest radiography to localize bullet fragments, diagnose pneumothorax, and determine trajectory and a bedside US to evaluate for hemothorax, hemopericardium, and cardiac tamponade may be sufficient in unstable patients. One should resist the temptation to get one more scan or view as unstable patients have died in radiology departments when they should have been in the OR.

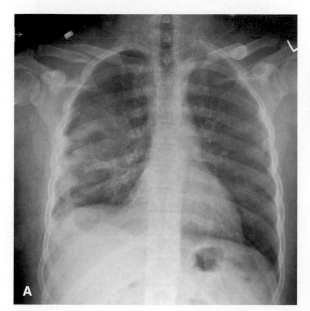

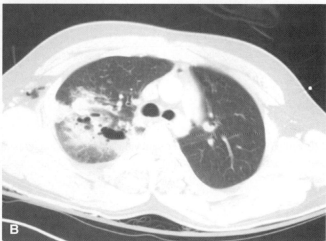

FIGURE 2.104. Pulmonary lacerations. Motor vehicle accident victim. **A:** AP chest film shows extensive airspace disease/hemorrhage in the right lung consistent with pulmonary contusion. Careful examination of the right lung also shows multiple lucencies. **B:** CT shows both the contusion (airspace opacities) with associated lacerations, which appear as lucencies or tears within the lung tissues.

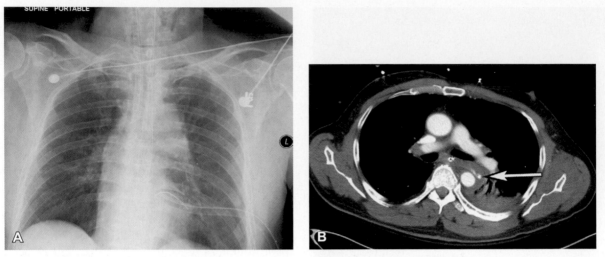

FIGURE 2.105. Aortic transection (traumatic dissection). Patient involved in a motor vehicle collision. **A:** AP chest radiograph obtained in the emergency room shows widening of the mediastinum suspicious for mediastinal hematoma. **B:** Contrast CT image at the level of the aortic arch showed a transection or traumatic dissection of the level of the ligamentum arteriosum with extravasation of contrast (*arrow*) from the aorta.

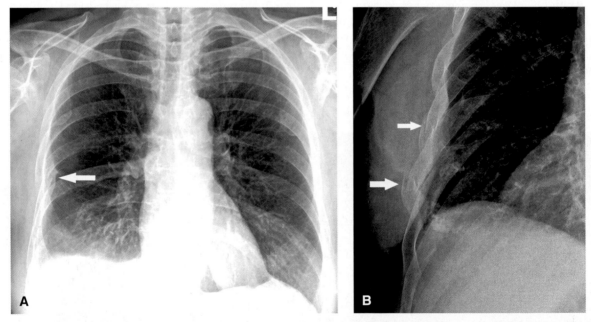

FIGURE 2.106. Rib fractures. A: Frontal views of right rib fractures (*arrow*), and associated hematoma. **B:** Oblique views of right rib fractures (*arrows*), in a different patient.

KEY POINTS

A technically adequate PA and lateral chest film is an essential component in the diagnosis of many diseases of the chest.

Review of previous imaging is mandatory.

Check the four corners of a chest radiograph, in addition to the hila, apices, behind the heart, and adjacent to the diaphragm.

On radiography, a structure's outline is only seen when an adjacent structure in the same anatomic plane is of a different tissue density giving rise to **the silhouette sign**. Conversely, when two structures of the same or similar radiographic tissue density are adjacent to each other, the margin between them is indistinct.

Multidetector CT (MDCT) allows scanning of a greater volume of tissue, which when combined with intravenous contrast allows visualization of the arterial system to produce a CT angiogram (CTA).

CTA of the chest to diagnose pulmonary embolism may also be used to evaluate right ventricular overload.

A limited V/Q scan may be a more appropriate exam to diagnose pulmonary embolism during pregnancy.

Screening low-dose chest CT is recommended in adults aged 55 to 80 years who have a 30 pack-year smoking history and currently smoke or have quit within the past 15 years.

All primary lung carcinomas are increasingly staged with F-18 FDG PET/CT, which detect the distribution and extent of disease

The differential diagnosis of mediastinal masses varies according to location.

Although CT is useful for workup of anterior and middle mediastinal masses, MRI is more helpful for posterior masses given that the majority of these turn out to be neurogenic in nature.

The most serious injury following blunt chest trauma is acute aortic transection (traumatic dissection), which most commonly occurs adjacent to the origin of the left subclavian artery.

The choice of imaging in hemodynamically unstable patients is a trade-off of time versus accuracy because unstable patients may have their survival compromised in the time it takes to get a CT. Chest radiography and bedside ultrasound may be sufficient.

Questions

1. The silhouette sign refers to
   a. The presence of air within the mediastinum.
   b. Loss of the normal radiographic border due to adjacent abnormal lung or pleura.
   c. Enlargement of the cardiac silhouette.
   d. Tension pneumothorax.

2. Which of the following radiographic findings is not associated with a tension pneumothorax?
   a. Pulmonary laceration.
   b. Depression of ipsilateral diaphragm.
   c. Displacement of the mediastinum away from the pneumothorax.
   d. Hyperlucency.

3. A hydropneumothorax
   a. May occur after thoracentesis.
   b. Is associated with the meniscus sign.
   c. Always requires percutaneous treatment.

4. The differential diagnosis of fine, reticular opacities includes
   A. Lymphangitis carcinomatosa
   B. Pulmonary edema
   C. Interstitial pneumonia
   D. Collagen vascular disease

   Options
   a. A and C
   b. A, B, and C
   c. B and D
   d. All

5. True or False: CT chest is mandatory in all hemodynamically unstable patients with suspected chest trauma.

6. True or False: CT angiography is clearly superior to V/Q scanning in pregnant patients.

7. True or False: MRI is the preferred modality for imaging posterior mediastinal masses.

8. True or False: Typically, type A aortic dissections are treated surgically and type B dissections are treated medically.

9. True or False: Treatment options for SVC syndrome due to lung carcinoma include radiation treatment and stent placement.

10. True or False: The hilum overlay sign indicates a high likelihood of a mass being in the middle mediastinum.

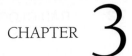

Abdominal Imaging

Thomas A. Farrell, MB, BCh

Obtaining a history, physical examination, and basic laboratory tests allows diagnosis of most abdominal conditions. When the diagnosis remains uncertain, imaging may be helpful, bearing in mind the consideration of possible pregnancy should precede the use of ionizing radiation in women of childbearing age.

PLAIN FILMS

Despite the exponential growth in the use of cross-sectional imaging (ultrasound [US], CT, and MRI), plain radiographs in the form of an AP view of the abdomen (plain film of abdomen [PFA] or kidney, ureter, bladder [KUB]) are still useful. The examination is performed with the patient supine (Fig. 3.1). An additional upright radiograph is useful in searching for free intraperitoneal air and/or intestinal air–fluid levels. If the patient cannot stand, a decubitus view obtained with the patient lying on either the right or, preferably, the left side can be substituted. All patients having a CT of the abdomen routinely get scout scans which can provide the same information as plain films. Examples of these are included in the section and should also be reviewed.

FIGURE 3.1. Normal supine abdominal radiographs. A: Abdomen AP supine radiograph. Normal. The psoas muscles (*straight arrows*) and the right kidney (*curved arrows*) are visible. The left renal silhouette is obliterated by intestinal gas. It is common to have intestinal gas and contents obliterating the renal shadows (L, liver; S, spleen). **B:** Abdomen AP supine radiograph. Normal. Representative vertebral pedicles are shown by *straight arrows*. The water density urinary bladder is shown by *curved arrows*.

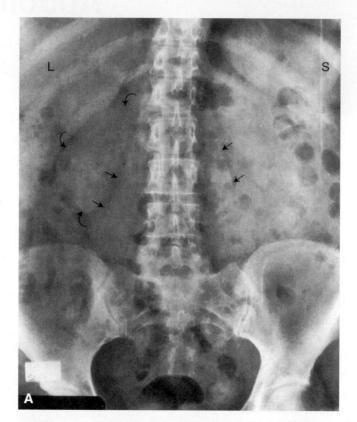

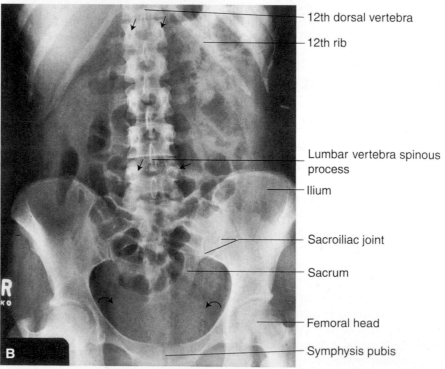

12th dorsal vertebra

12th rib

Lumbar vertebra spinous process

Ilium

Sacroiliac joint

Sacrum

Femoral head

Symphysis pubis

TABLE 3.1	Checklist for Review of Abdominal Plain Films

Patient Demographics

Old films

Liver, spleen, and psoas outlines

Opacities (stones, surgical clips and sponges, drains and stents)

Bowel gas (too much, too little, distribution, intraluminal, extraluminal, retroperitoneal)

Bone and soft tissues

Technique for Viewing Plain Films

Table 3.1 will work, until you develop your own.

Step 1: Check the patient demographics, location of side marker, and confirmation of correct technique (supine, erect, decubitus). Comparison with old films is mandatory.

Step 2: Locate the liver and spleen (**water density**) silhouettes. One clue to locating hepatic and splenic edges in the location of bowel gas in the right and left upper abdominal quadrants respectively. Such bowel gas permits an indirect estimate of the location of the hepatic and splenic borders because the gas is located at the lower edges of the liver and spleen. When either the liver or splenic shadow extends to the iliac crest, the organ is usually enlarged (Figs. 3.2 and 3.3).

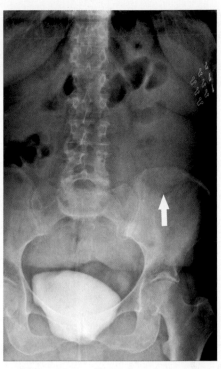

FIGURE 3.3. **Splenomegaly.** The spleen is markedly enlarged extending into the left flank (*arrow*). Unremarkable bowel gas pattern.

Both psoas major muscle margins are usually visible, extending inferolaterally from T12. A nonvisible psoas margin may indicate retroperitoneal pathology such as a ruptured abdominal aortic aneurysm, but may also occur in up to 30% of the normal population. Next evaluate the size, shape, and position of the renal outlines which are visible because they are of water density (gray) surrounded by variable amounts of retroperitoneal fat (black). Identification of the upper renal poles may be difficult because of the adjacent liver and stomach.

Step 3: Search for **calcifications** in the region of the kidneys, ureters, bladder, and gallbladder, as they may represent stones. The presence of an appendicolith in patients with acute appendicitis indicates a greater likelihood of perforation and abscess formation. Additional **opacities** of plastic (stents and drains) or metallic density (IVC filter, surgical clips, or retained surgical sponge) should be noted (Figs. 3.4-3.8).

Step 4: Evaluate the bowel **gas pattern** which will be discussed in more detail in the next section.

Step 5: Finally, examine the **bones and associated soft tissues**, beginning with ribs, spine, and vertebral bodies. Check vertebral body alignment and presence of spinous processes and pedicles throughout. Scoliosis of the lumbar spine on the AP view may indicate adjacent abdominal pathology while loss of the normal lumbar scoliosis on the lateral view may indicate acute pathology in the lumbar

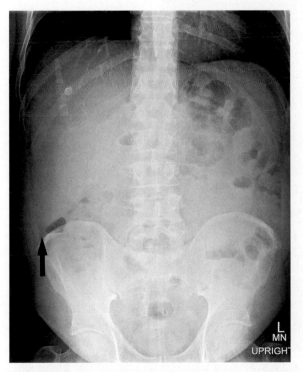

FIGURE 3.2. **Hepatomegaly.** The liver is markedly enlarged, extending to the right lower quadrant (*black arrow*). Unremarkable bowel gas pattern.

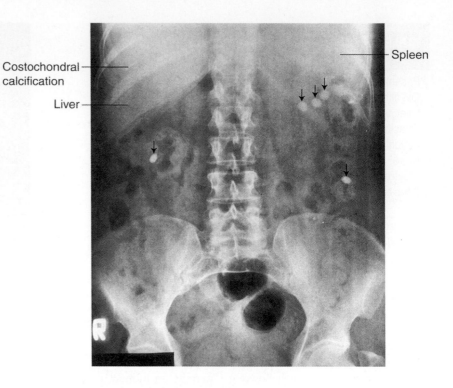

FIGURE 3.4. Abdomen AP supine radiograph. Classic appearance of tablets or pills (*arrows*) in the GI tract. All the tablets are the same size and shape with homogeneous density. (Not all tablets or pills can be visualized on a radiograph.)

Costochondral calcification

Liver

Spleen

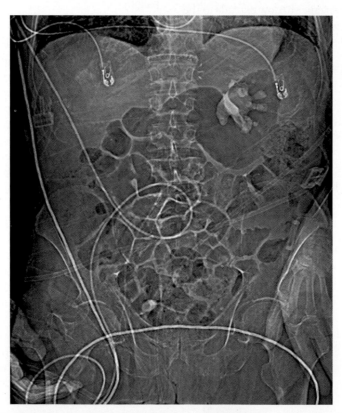

FIGURE 3.5. Left renal staghorn calculus and right lower ureteral calculus. AP scout films from CT scan showing a large left staghorn calculus. A smaller opacity in the right lower quadrant is a ureteral calculus.

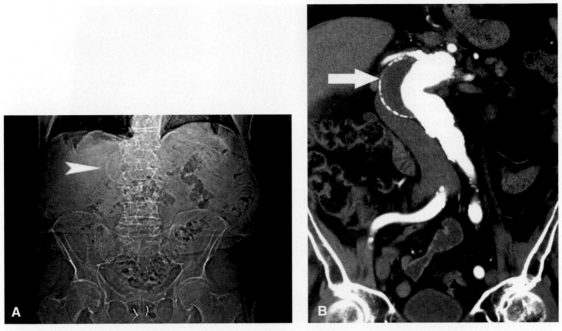

FIGURE 3.6. **Calcification of aortic aneurysm wall. A:** Supine abdominal film shows curvilinear calcification (*arrowhead*) of aortic aneurysm wall. **B:** Coronal reformat of abdominal CT showing suprarenal abdominal aortic aneurysm (*arrow*).

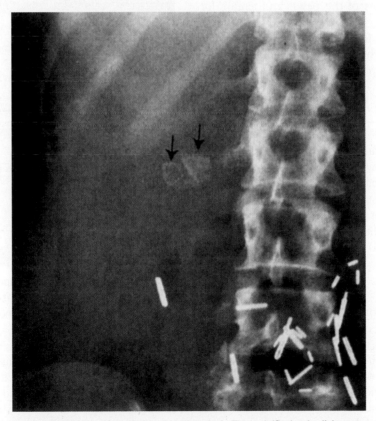

FIGURE 3.7. **Abdomen AP supine radiograph.** Cholelithiasis (gallstones). The calcified calculi (*arrows at center*) are faceted. Surgical metallic clips (*arrow at right*) are secondary to previous abdominal surgery.

FIGURE 3.8. **Abdomen AP upright radiograph.** Surgical laparotomy pad in a postoperative abdomen. The radiograph was obtained when the patient experienced severe postoperative abdominal pain and distention. The *straight arrow* indicates the opaque strip in the laparotomy pad, and the *curved arrow* indicates the metallic ring attached to the laparotomy pad. Note the mottled black appearance of the air trapped in the laparotomy pad. The air–fluid level in the gastric fundus gives a clue to the upright position of the patient.

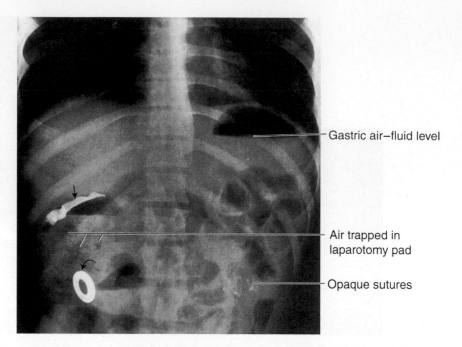

Gastric air–fluid level

Air trapped in laparotomy pad

Opaque sutures

spine. A missing vertebral pedicle may be an evidence of a metastasis. Evaluate bones of the pelvis and femurs for density.

A similar review system for evaluating **upright** abdominal radiographs is useful while specifically looking for free air under the diaphragms (pneumoperitoneum).

EVALUATING THE BOWEL GAS PATTERN

Bowel gas provides a natural contrast medium that can be useful for detecting abdominal disease (Fig. 3.9). When evaluating the bowel gas pattern, remember that there is normally some gas in the stomach, small intestine, colon, and rectum (Fig. 3.10). If the gas pattern is abnormal, decide if there is too much or too little bowel gas and if it is in the right location (intraluminal) or wrong location (extraluminal or intramural).

Too Much Bowel Gas

The differential diagnosis for too much bowel gas includes **adynamic ileus** and **bowel obstruction**. In adynamic ileus (also referred to as paralytic ileus or ileus), there is too much bowel gas overall with comparable amounts of gas in the small and large intestines and in the rectum due to reduced motility. The common causes of adynamic ileus are in Table 3.2. A localized ileus of persistently dilated small bowel known as a **sentinel loop** may occur adjacent to focal inflammation such as acute pancreatitis, cholecystitis, appendicitis, and diverticulitis.

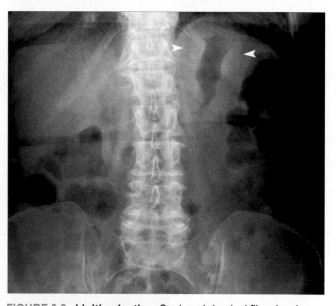

FIGURE 3.9. **Linitis plastica.** Supine abdominal film showing circumferential thickening of the gastric wall (*arrowheads*) consistent with gastric carcinoma, also known as linitis plastica.

In bowel obstruction, by contrast there are usually loops of dilated gas-filled bowel proximal to the site of obstruction and little or no gas distal to the obstruction (Figs. 3.11 and 3.12). In both ileus and obstruction, air–fluid levels are seen on upright and decubitus radiographs. If a diagnosis of obstruction versus adynamic ileus is not readily apparent on plain film, CT may be necessary.

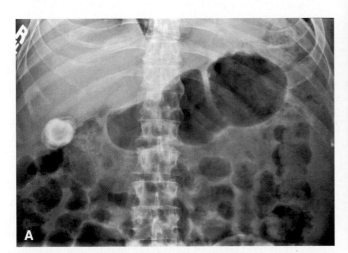

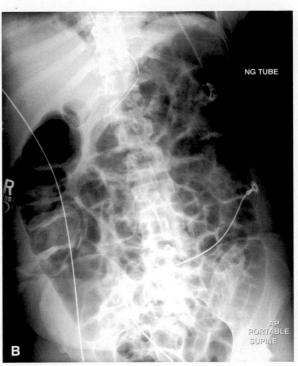

FIGURE 3.10. **Normal air swallowing. A and B:** Two supine films showing gas-filled stomach, small and large bowel, all of normal diameter.

TABLE 3.2	Causes of Adynamic Ileus
Postoperative	
Postinflammatory	
Narcotics	
Metabolic: hyperkalemia, uremia	

Determination of the location of the obstruction is important as there are different causes, depending on whether it is small or large bowel (Table 3.3). In small bowel obstruction (SBO), there are loops of dilated small bowel proximal to the obstruction site and little or no gas in the colon or the rectum. In large bowel obstruction (LBO), there is dilated colon proximal to the obstruction site but little or no air distally and minimal air in the rectum. If the ileocecal valve is competent, cecal dilatation may occur. An incompetent ileocecal valve allows retrograde decompression into the small bowel.

Differentiation between dilated small bowel and large bowel may be difficult. Dilated small bowel tends to be central, and dilated large bowel lies more peripherally in the abdomen. Another useful sign is to distinguish between valvulae conniventes and colon haustra. Valvulae conniventes are regularly spaced, thin mucosal folds that extend across the entire small bowel lumen (Fig. 3.11A). On the other

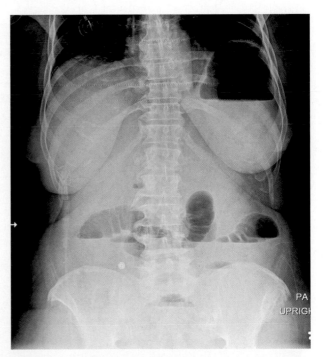

FIGURE 3.11. **Small bowel obstruction. A:** Upright abdominal film showing multiple small bowel fluid levels and a fluid level in the stomach consistent with small bowel obstruction. Note the absence of gas in large bowel. See Figure 3.77 for CT correlation.

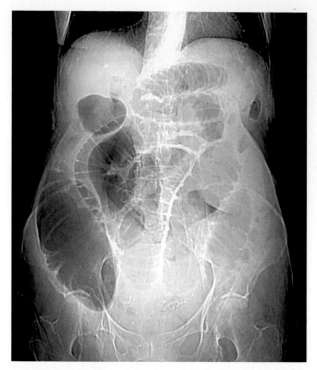

FIGURE 3.12. Large bowel obstruction. CT scout film (supine) showing multiple loops of dilated small bowel and ascending colon in a patient who had an obstructing carcinoma in the transverse colon. Note the paucity of gas in the descending colon.

TABLE 3.3	Causes of Bowel Obstruction
Small Bowel Obstruction	**Large Bowel Obstruction**
Adhesions	Tumor
Hernia	Volvulus
Tumor	Diverticular stricture

hand, the colon can usually be identified by the somewhat irregularly spaced transverse bands, called colon haustra or haustral folds, that do not extend completely across the colon lumen (Fig. 3.12)

Sigmoid volvulus occurs predominantly in elderly patients with a history of chronic constipation in which redundant sigmoid mesentery twists on itself like a garden hose. Twisting or volvulus of the bowel causes partial or complete obstruction, with a dramatically dilated sigmoid colon (Fig. 3.13A). Barium enema is confirmatory with complete obstruction to retrograde flow of barium at the site of volvulus (Fig. 3.13B). Colonic volvulus may also occur in the cecum or transverse colon.

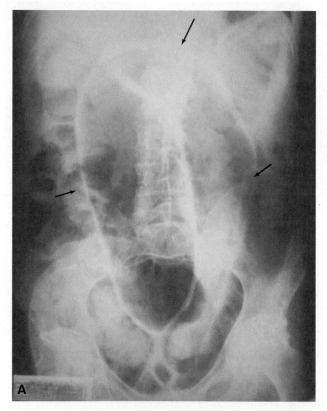

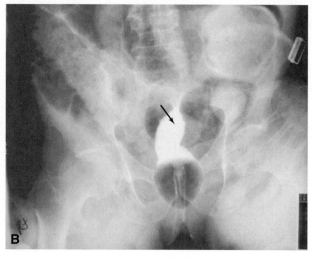

FIGURE 3.13. Sigmoid volvulus. A: Abdominal radiograph. The air-filled, obstructed sigmoid colon (*arrows*) arises from the pelvis. **B:** Barium enema. Contrast introduced per rectum shows obstruction and a twist (*arrow*) at the sigmoid colon. (Courtesy of Bruce Brown, M.D.)

TABLE 3.4	Causes of a Paucity or Absence of Bowel Gas

Proximal small bowel obstruction
Gastroenteritis
Enlarged abdominal organs
Abdominal tumor

TABLE 3.5	Causes of Pneumoperitoneum

Perforation of a hollow viscus: Peptic Ulcer disease, ischemic Bowel, Diverticulitis
Postoperative
Peritoneal dialysis

Too Little Bowel Gas

The differential diagnosis for a paucity or absence of bowel gas is listed in Table 3.4.

GAS IN THE WRONG PLACES

There are several conditions in which air is found outside of the intestinal lumen. Free air in the peritoneal cavity (**pneumoperitoneum**) results from any process that perforates the intestinal tract (Table 3.5). Supine and upright abdominal radiographs should be performed if there is clinical suspicion of bowel perforation. The upright position allows the free intraperitoneal air to rise outlining the undersurface of the diaphragm (Fig. 3.14). If an upright view is not possible, a decubitus view will suffice in which the free intraperitoneal air rises to the nondependent portion of the peritoneal cavity (Fig. 3.15). Either technique may be used to identify

as little as 2 mL of free air, provided the patient is in the upright or decubitus position for at least 5 minutes before the radiograph. Larger amount of free air may outline the falciform ligament. Another example of air in the wrong place is **pneumatosis intestinalis** in which gas occurs in the wall of small bowel (Fig. 3.16), the causes of which are listed in Table 3.6. Pneumatosis indicates breach of bowel mucosal integrity and not necessarily bowel necrosis. Gas-filled abscesses can be found in any location, including the abdomen (Fig. 3.17).

Retroperitoneal air, common cause of which is perforation of the duodenum (parts 2–4) or colon, is poorly defined and fixed as it tends to collect a linear fashion along the margins of the kidneys and psoas muscles (Fig. 3.18). Gas from a duodenal perforation tends to collect in the right anterior prior renal space. Retroperitoneal abscesses may be pancreatic or renal in origin. Psoas abscesses may occur as a complication of vertebral discitis. Retroperitoneal air may extend superiorly causing a pneumomediastinum.

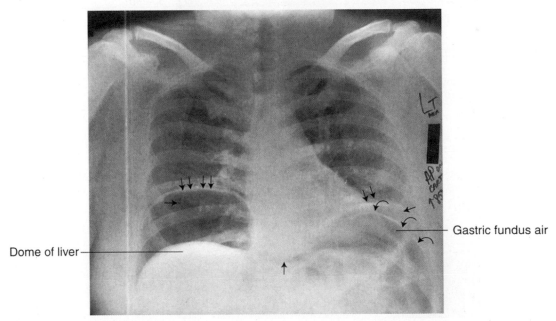

Dome of liver

Gastric fundus air

FIGURE 3.14. Chest AP upright radiograph. Free intraperitoneal air. The right and left hemidiaphragms (*double straight arrows*) are elevated owing to bilateral subdiaphragmatic air (*single straight arrows*). The black zone between the right hemidiaphragm and the dome of the liver represents free intraperitoneal air. On the left, there is air in the gastric fundus as well as free air surrounding the gastric fundus, allowing visualization of both sides of the stomach wall (*curved arrows*). When you see both sides of the gut wall, this represents free intraperitoneal air (Rigler sign).

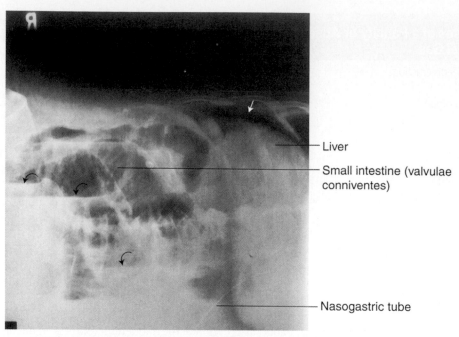

FIGURE 3.15. Abdomen left lateral decubitus radiograph (left side down). Free intraperitoneal air in a patient with small bowel obstruction and perforation. The free intraperitoneal air (*white arrow*) is between the right rib cage and the liver. The dilated small bowel contains multiple air–fluid levels (*black arrows*).

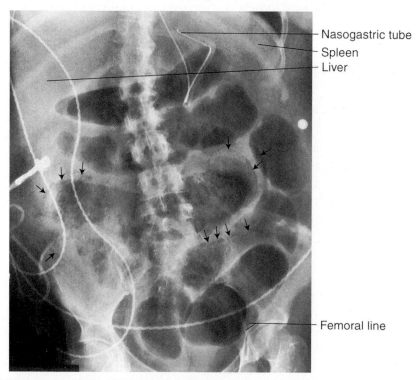

FIGURE 3.16. Abdomen AP supine radiograph. Pneumatosis intestinalis (air in the bowel wall). There is widespread bubbly air within the small intestine walls (*arrows*).

TABLE 3.6   Causes of Pneumatosis Intestinalis/ Coli

Bowel ischemia
Colitis nonischemic causes—infection, inflammatory bowel disease
Collagen vascular disorders
Primary pneumatosis—rare (benign)

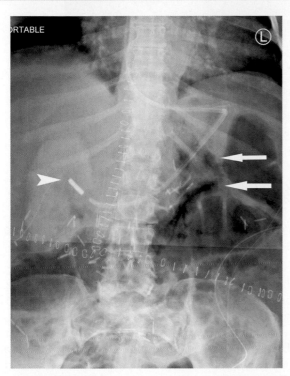

FIGURE 3.17. Retroperitoneal gas collection. Supine abdominal film showing an irregular fixed mottled gas collection in the left retroperitoneum (*arrows*) due to duodenal perforation. Note the radiodense tip of a Dobhoff feeding tube (*arrowhead*) in the proximal duodenum.

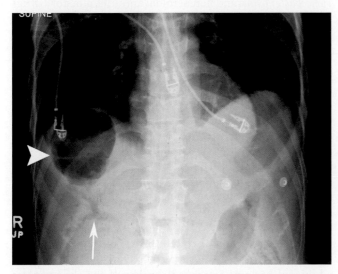

FIGURE 3.18. Gas in hepatic abscess. Supine abdomen film showing well-defined lucency (*arrowhead*) in the liver due to a gas-containing abscess. Air also outlines the intrahepatic bile ducts (*arrow*).

Pneumobilia or gas in the bile ducts is seen as branching tubular lucencies in the central liver. The origin of the gas is usually the intestine, either following an endoscopic retrograde cholangiopancreatography (ERCP) or surgically created hepaticojejunostomy. The important differential diagnosis is portal vein gas, which tends to occur more peripherally.

GASTROINTESTINAL CONTRAST STUDIES

For evaluation of the upper GI tract (the esophagus, stomach, and duodenum), endoscopy is more commonly performed, although upper GI contrast studies are still accurate and safe.

Upper GI Series (Barium Swallow and Meal)

For an upper GI series, the patient swallows liquid barium sulfate, often combined with gas-producing crystals, to visualize the esophagus, stomach, and small intestine under fluoroscopy (Fig. 3.19). When both barium and air are used, the process is referred to as a **double-contrast** study. When barium is used alone, it is a **single-contrast** study. The main indications for this study are to evaluate swallowing in patients with dysphagia, to diagnoses peptic ulcer disease, and to evaluate post-op anatomy. When perforation or anastomotic leak of the upper GI tract is suspected, water-soluble contrast media is used, as the intraperitoneal leakage of barium is usually fatal.

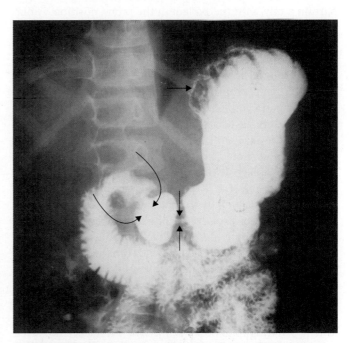

FIGURE 3.19. Normal upper GI series. Barium-filled stomach and duodenum. The patient is in the prone position. Gas (*horizontal arrow*) is seen in the gastric fundus; a peristaltic wave (*vertical arrows*) crosses the gastric antrum; and the pylorus (*curved arrows*) separates the duodenal bulb and stomach.

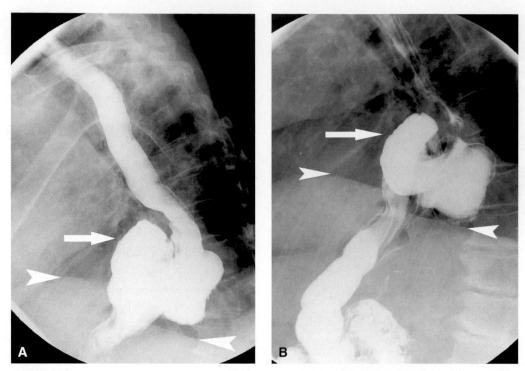

FIGURE 3.20. Hiatal hernia. Two views of a barium swallow showing a large hiatal hernia with the stomach (*arrows*) lying above the diaphragm (*arrowheads*).

An **axial hiatal hernia** occurs when the gastroesophageal junction is above the esophageal hiatus of the diaphragm and is most reliably diagnosed on a single-contrast barium study with the patient in the prone position. A hiatal hernia can often be recognized by the presence of gastric folds within the hernia (Fig. 3.20). In patients with a (less common) **paraesophageal hernia**, the gastric fundus herniates through the diaphragm beside the distal esophagus while the gastroesophageal junction is normally located in the abdomen. Unlike axial hernias, paraesophageal hernias are rarely associated with the reflux and esophagitis. However, they are more likely to twist and obstruct causing infarction and should be repaired prophylactically.

Gastroesophageal reflux occurs when the lower esophageal sphincter pressure is decreased or absent allowing reflux of gastric contents into the esophagus causing esophagitis and eventual stricture. The severity of reflux depends both on its frequency and duration. Although reflux is often accompanied by a hiatal hernia, the relationship between the two is not constant. Double-contrast technique allows detection of esophageal ulceration and Barrett esophagus. **Barrett esophagus** is a premalignant condition that occurs when there is progressive columnar metaplasia of the distal esophagus secondary to long-standing reflux esophagitis. The prevalence of Barrett esophagus in patients with reflux is about 10%, and the prevalence of adenocarcinoma in patients with Barrett esophagus is also 10%. **Adenocarcinoma** with risk factors of reflux esophagitis and Barrett esophagus comprises 50% of all esophageal cancers. Historically, however, **squamous** cell carcinomas

with risk factors of tobacco and alcohol consumption were the most common form of esophageal carcinoma and occur in the upper and middle thirds of the esophagus and rarely in the lower third of the esophagus, in contrast to adenocarcinoma.

Dysphagia is a symptom that should be investigated promptly, as it may be due to esophageal carcinoma. Barium swallow examination shows a typical shouldering appearance in esophageal carcinoma (Fig. 3.21).

Peptic Ulcer Disease

Helicobacter pylori and nonsteroidal anti-inflammatory drugs are responsible for the development of peptic ulcers in most patients. Almost all duodenal ulcers are benign; however, a small percentage of gastric ulcers are malignant and require careful workup including endoscopy and biopsy. Most duodenal ulcers occur in the duodenal bulb, and about half of these are in the anterior wall of the bulb. Ulcer healing may cause a scar manifested by deformity and radiating folds (Fig. 3.22). Complications of peptic ulcers include bleeding, gastric outflow obstruction, and perforation. Perforation of ulcers on the anterior wall of the stomach and duodenum may result in pneumoperitoneum, whereas perforation ulcers on the posterior wall result in a localized collection.

Antegrade Small Bowel Examination

A **small bowel follow-through (SBFT)** examination is performed after an upper GI series by having the patient drink additional barium. Serial radiographs of the abdomen are obtained at 15- to 30-minute intervals to evaluate the small

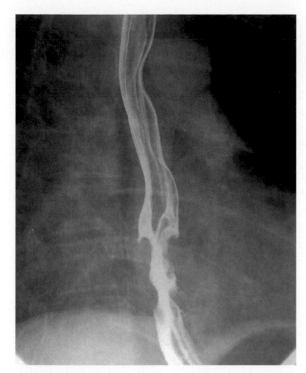

FIGURE 3.21. Esophageal carcinoma. Barium swallow showing a well-defined shouldered narrowing in the distal esophagus consistent with carcinoma.

bowel with attention to mucosal pattern, bowel diameter, and transit time (Fig. 3.23). Fluoroscopy is commonly used as a supplement to study the terminal ileum when barium begins to enter the colon or to further investigate focal abnormalities seen on the serial radiographs. **Enteroclysis** is a focused examination of the small intestine, where air and barium sulfate are introduced directly into the small

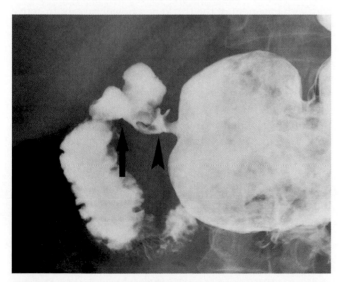

FIGURE 3.22. Duodenal ulcer. Upper GI barium study showing triradiate folds (*arrow*) and deformity of the duodenal bulb (*arrowhead*), consistent with a peptic ulcer.

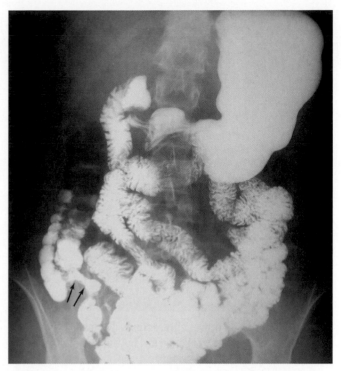

FIGURE 3.23. Normal antegrade small bowel examination. Barium was administered by mouth, and this radiograph was done about 30 min later. Note the barium-filled stomach, duodenal C-loop, feathered jejunum in the upper abdomen, and relatively formless mucosa of the ileum in the lower and right abdomen. The terminal ileum (*arrows*) entering the cecum can be identified. (Courtesy of Bruce Brown, M.D.)

intestine via a nasointestinal tube. Under fluoroscopy, the tip of the tube is placed just beyond the ligament of Treitz (duodenojejunal junction) and contrast is injected (Fig. 3.24). This technique allows better small bowel distention with better visualization of mucosal detail.

Malabsorption may be caused by a variety of diseases in the hepatobiliary system, pancreas, and small intestine. Clinically, malabsorption is characterized by diarrhea, abdominal pain, and weight loss. **Celiac disease** is a chronic inflammatory disease caused by the gliadin fraction of wheat, barley, or rye gluten, which causes damage to the small bowel mucosa resulting in malabsorption. Various degrees of villous atrophy may occur, which is manifested radiologically as a decrease in the number of folds in the proximal jejunum. There is compensatory hypertrophy of the ileal folds termed *jejunization of the ileum*.

Inflammatory Bowel Disease

Crohn's disease (CD) and ulcerative colitis (UC) are the two main forms of inflammatory bowel disease (IBD), accurate diagnosis and disease staging of which rely heavily on imaging.

Crohn's disease is a transmural chronic inflammatory disorder that can affect any part of the gastrointestinal tract

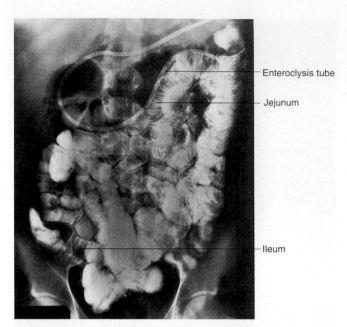

FIGURE 3.24. **Small bowel enteroclysis.** Normal. The naso-intestinal tube has been positioned just beyond the duodenal–jejunal junction. Barium fills the entire small bowel.

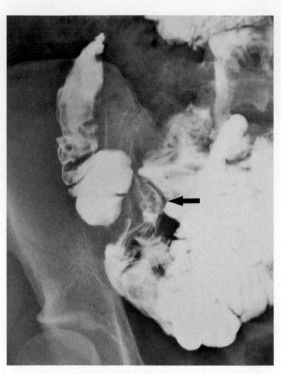

FIGURE 3.25. **Small bowel follow-through examination of the terminal ileum.** Normal terminal ileum (*arrow*).

in a skip-like fashion (Fig. 3.25). Conventional SBFT in which orally ingested dilute barium is imaged as it passes to the small bowel does not reliably exclude early Crohn's disease and has largely been replaced by **CT enterography (CTE)** as the initial test of choice for small bowel CD (Fig. 3.26). Standard CT abdomen with IV contrast may be sufficient in the acute presentation for evaluation of CD complications including bowel obstruction, fistula formation, and abscess formation. Although oral contrast with abdominal CT may decrease evaluation for bowel inflammation, it is helpful for identification of fistulas and abscesses. CT is also effective to assess for possible alternative diagnoses such as appendicitis.

CTE allows visualization of the small bowel lumen, wall, and adjacent tissues by distending the small bowel with large volumes of dilute oral contrast. The technique is useful in patients with known or suspected CD, obscure GI bleeding, malabsorption, or abdominal pain of unknown etiology. Up to 2000 mL of oral contrast is ingested over 1 hour. The patient is scanned approximately 50 seconds after IV contrast injection which corresponds with peak contrast enhancement of the small bowel wall. Normally, the jejunal caliber is slightly greater in the ileum, and the jejunal valvulae conniventes are thicker and more closely spaced than those of the ileum. Bowel wall thickness of 3 mm or greater is abnormal. CT evidence of CD includes mural inflammation which appears as hyperenhancement and thickening, penetrating disease (fistulas, sinus tracks, and abscesses) which occur in approximately 25% of patients and bowel obstruction.

In patients with CD, **MR enterography (MRE)** allows evaluation of the bowel wall thickness, the degree and pattern of gadolinium enhancement, length of the involved diseased segment, and presence of edema in the bowel wall on T2-weighted images in addition to adjacent mesenteric disease. MRE is more sensitive than CTE for diagnosing submucosal pathology. The degree of bowel enhancement with gadolinium correlates with disease activity. By contrast, in chronic inactive Crohn's disease, little or no contrast enhancement of the thickened bowel is seen. In active Crohn's disease, there is enhancement of mucosal and the serosal layers with an intervening nonenhancing layer representing edema in the bowel wall, producing a layered pattern of mural enhancement. Penetrating complications of Crohn's disease, as listed above, can also be seen on MRI.

Three findings occur as a result of **mesenteric inflammation** in patients with Crohn's disease and are seen on both CT and MRI: lymphadenopathy, fat changes, and engorged vasa recta. Reactive lymphadenopathy is characterized by numerous enhancing nodes. Fat changes represent fat stranding, which is a marker of active disease, and fibrofatty proliferation that is usually seen in patients with long-standing disease. Engorged vasa recta, also known as the "comb" sign, can occur in an involved intestinal loop.

While CTE is more widely available, its major limitation is the cumulative ionizing radiation dose. While the availability of MRE expertise and access is limited, this modality is preferred in younger patients with IBD.

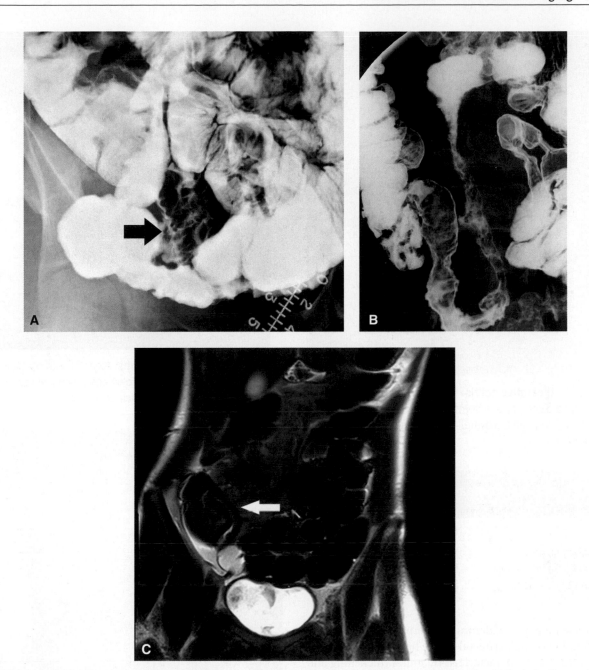

FIGURE 3.26. Crohn's disease. A: Mucosal thickening and transmural ulceration in the terminal ileum due to Crohn's disease (*arrow*). **B:** Extensive mucosal thickening and inflammatory change in the terminal ileum due to Crohn's disease. **C:** MR enterography shows inflammatory change in the terminal ileum due to Crohn's disease (*arrow*).

UC is a diffuse inflammatory disease involving the colorectal mucosa initially but later extending to other layers of the bowel wall. Characteristically the disease begins in the rectum and extends contiguously and proximally to involve part or all of the colon (Fig. 3.27). Table 3.7 lists the barium enema findings in acute and chronic UC. In the acute phase, severe mucosal ulceration can lead to inflammatory pseudopolyps. Other features of acute UC include mural thinning, perforation, pneumatosis, prominence of

vasa recta (Fig. 3.28), and megacolon. Mural thickening and luminal narrowing are common features in chronic UC.

On CT, a target or halo appearance may be seen as the lumen is surrounded by a ring of soft tissue (mucosa, muscularis mucosa) surrounded by a low-density ring (edema of the submucosa) which is in turn surrounded by a ring of soft tissue density (the muscularis propria). This pattern of stratification can also be seen in patients with Crohn's disease and other forms of colitis. Rectal narrowing because of

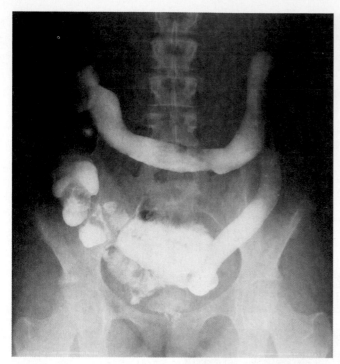

FIGURE 3.27. Ulcerative colitis. Barium enema. The entire colon, except the cecum, is uniformly narrowed; the mucosal surface is irregular; and the overall configuration suggests a lead pipe appearance.

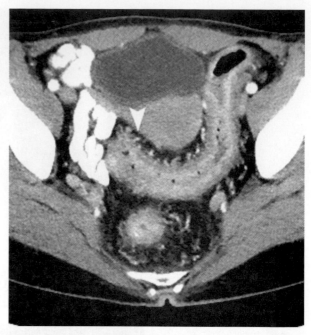

FIGURE 3.28. Ulcerative colitis. Axial CT with contrast shows a diffusely thickened sigmoid colon and prominent vasa recta (*arrowhead*) in a patient with ulcerative colitis.

TABLE 3.7	Barium Enema Findings in Ulcerative Colitis
Acute	**Chronic**
Mucosal granularity	Haustral loss
Haustral thickening or loss	Luminal narrowing
Inflammatory pseudopolyps	Backwash ileitis

mural thickening and widening of the presacral space due to proliferation of the perirectal fat are hallmarks of chronic UC. On MRI, UC is characterized by mural thickening and enhancement.

The risk of developing colorectal cancer is higher in patients with UC than in the general population and is related to the extent, duration, and activity of the disease. Carcinoma associated with UC are multiple in almost 25% of cases.

Lower GI series (barium enema) is a test where barium and/or air are introduced into the colon via a rectal tube. For this study, it is important to have an empty colon, which is best accomplished with oral bowel prep. When both air and barium are used, it is called a double-contrast study (Fig. 3.29), whereas the use of barium alone is a termed single-contrast study. The double-contrast study is preferred to evaluate intraluminal and mucosal diseases, such as small ulcers and polyps (Fig. 3.30). If colonic perforation is suspected, a water-soluble contrast medium is used.

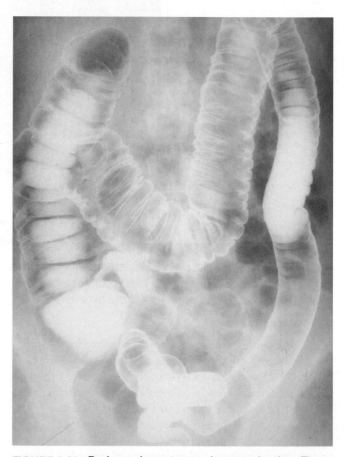

FIGURE 3.29. Barium–air contrast colon examination. The entire colon is filled with barium and air. Films are made in prone, supine, and both decubitus positions so that different parts of the colon can be visualized with the air-contrast techniques. (Courtesy of Bruce Brown, M.D.)

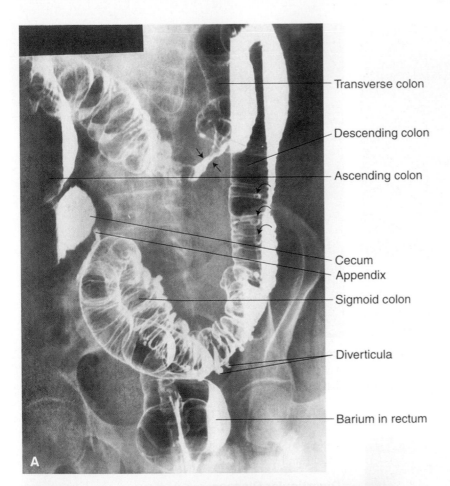

Transverse colon

Descending colon

Ascending colon

Cecum
Appendix

Sigmoid colon

Diverticula

Barium in rectum

A

FIGURE 3.30. A: Adenocarcinoma of the transverse colon. Double-contrast colon examination. Note the classic apple core appearance of the colon cancer. The core represents the patent portion of the bowel lumen (*straight arrows*). Diverticula of the descending colon are seen en face (*curved arrows*). **B:** Close-up view of the tumor in **(A)**. Note the irregular mucosa of the narrowed lumen of the apple core lesion (*white arrows*). The mass creates a shouldering (*black arrows*) deformity in the neighboring transverse colon both proximally and distally.

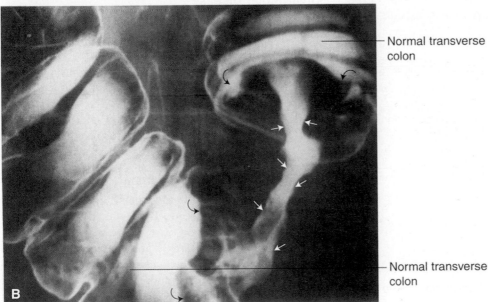

Normal transverse colon

Normal transverse colon

B

CT colonography (CTC) examines the entire colon using multidetector CT (MDCT) and a dedicated software program to detect colorectal polyps and masses. The examination is usually performed after administration of an agent that tags fecal material, which can then be subtracted from the viewed images. Before the examination begins, the colon is insufflated with CO_2 so the images resemble an endoscopic view of the colon. CTC can detect almost all colon cancers (Fig. 3.31) as well as larger polyps (Fig. 3.32), and unlike colonoscopy, conscious sedation

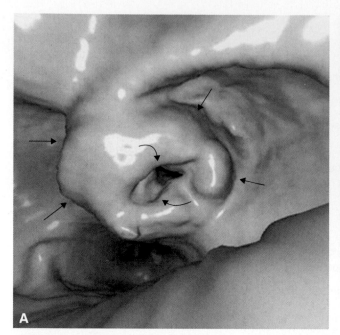
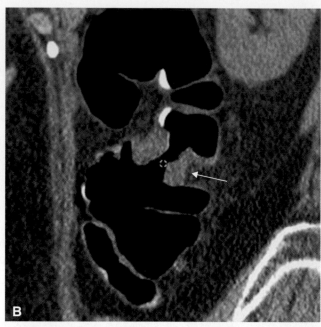

FIGURE 3.31. **"Apple core" invasive cancer discovered on virtual colonoscopy. A:** The virtual colonoscopy image shows a large endoluminal mass (*straight arrows*), associated with narrowing of the colon lumen (*curved arrows*). **B:** Coronal CT reconstruction of the colonoscopic image. The tumor (*arrow*) is noted on both sides of the colon lumen and extrudes into the pericolic space. (Courtesy of J.G. Fletcher, M.D.)

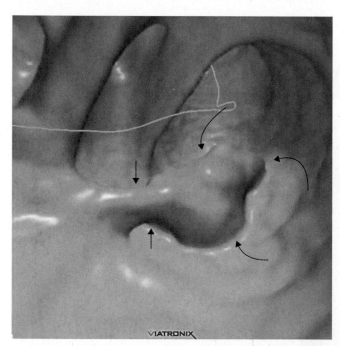

FIGURE 3.32. **Virtual colonoscopy.** Colon polyp detected in virtual colonoscopy. The stalk (*short arrows*) and the polyp (*curved arrows*) are readily apparent. (Courtesy of Wei Chang, M.D.)

is unnecessary. As experience with the technique has increased, CTC approaches the accuracy of colonoscopy for detection and characterization of polyps and masses. The main disadvantage is the use of radiation, although the dose is typically less than 50% of that from a standard abdominal CT.

Diverticular Disease

Colonic diverticula are acquired herniations of the mucosa and submucosa through the muscularis propria which progress to diverticulosis and diverticulitis (perforation and infection). In the Western world, diverticular disease is widely prevalent, occurring in up to one-third of the population older than 50 years. The sigmoid colon is the most common site. On barium enema, diverticulosis is characterized by multiple protrusions ranging in size from several millimeters to 1 cm in size (Fig. 3.33). Diverticulitis and diverticular abscess will be discussed in the Acute Abdomen section of this chapter. Diverticular hemorrhage is one of the most common causes of lower GI bleeding (IR), the treatment of which will be covered in Chapter 12.

CT angiography (CTA) is an accurate test for identifying the source of acute GI bleeding. CTA is more sensitive than catheter angiography for detection of bleeding, but less sensitive than RBC scanning, being able to depict bleeding at a rate of 0.3 to 0.5 mL/min. Three-phase CT is obtained: noncontrast, arterial (+40 seconds), and portal venous (+80 seconds) phases, without oral contrast. Timing is paramount with these examinations as many GI hemorrhages are intermittent. Negative-result CTA yields helpful prognostic information, as patients with negative findings are unlikely to need emergent surgical or angiographic

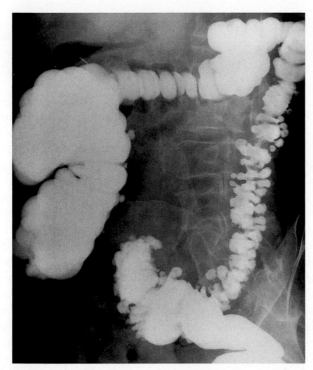

FIGURE 3.33. Diverticulosis. Lower GI contrast study showing extensive diverticular disease.

intervention. **Multiphase CTE** can also be used in stable patients who have negative endoscopic results and are suspected of having small bowel or obscure GI bleeding. Enterographic CT images are acquired during three intravenous contrast enhancement phases—arterial, enteric, and delayed phases, 60 minutes after the administration of 1,500 to 2,000 mL of dilute oral contrast material which distends the bowel.

Rectal Carcinoma

The benefits of using MRI in patients with rectal carcinoma include the ability to identify patients at risk of local recurrence by (1) delineating the tumor location and morphology, (2) accurately staging T and N categories, (3) identifying extramural vascular invasion, and (4) clarifying its relationship with surrounding structures, including the sphincter complex and involvement of the mesorectal fascia (MRF). Poor prognostic factors of rectal carcinoma on MRI include extramural vascular invasion (EMVI), mucin content, and involvement of the MRF. EMVI is suspected if a vascular structure close to the tumor is expanded, irregular or infiltrated by tumor signal intensity. The circumferential resection margin (CRM) is the surface of the non-peritonealized part of the rectum that is resected during surgery. MRI is the most reliable modality to determine potential CRM involvement which can be obtained by measuring the shortest

distance between the outermost part of the rectal tumor and the MRF. The CRM status is potentially positive if this measurement is less than 1 mm and threatened if it is between 1 and 2 mm.

In contrast to patients with stage T1 or T2 rectal carcinoma for whom surgery is the initial treatment, the features outlined above diagnose locally advanced rectal tumors (LARC) (categories T3c-d, T4, N1, and N2), for which neoadjuvant chemoradiotherapy (CRT) is initially given. In restaging after neoadjuvant CRT, in addition to reassessing the features noted above, MRI allows early diagnosis of tumor recurrence and determines surgical planning for resectability (Fig. 3.34). The use of endorectal coils and a bowel prep are not necessary for rectal MRI.

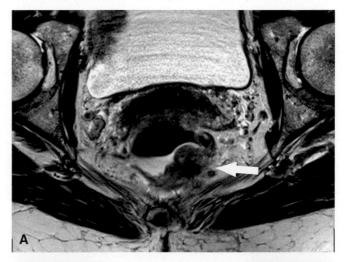

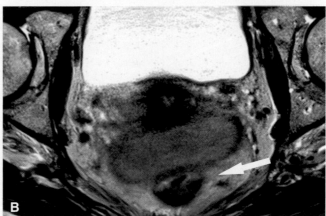

FIGURE 3.34. Rectal carcinoma. MRI before and after neoadjuvant treatment. **A:** Before neoadjuvant treatmentan oblique axial scan showing a left-sided rectal carcinoma and a circumferential resection margin of less than 1 mm, with an adjacent node (4 o'clock position) (*arrow*) in the mesorectal fat. **B:** After neoadjuvant treatment, note reduction in the size of the node and increase in the circumferential margin (arrow)

BASIC CROSS-SECTIONAL (US, CT, AND MRI) IMAGING TECHNOLOGY AND PROTOCOLS

Three anatomic planes are commonly used for cross-sectional imaging and interpretation.

A **sagittal** plane is the anatomical plane which divides the body into right and left parts. The plane may be in the center of the body and split it into two halves (midsagittal) or away from the midline and split it into unequal parts (parasagittal). The term parasagittal is used to describe any plane parallel to the sagittal plane. Technically, the term parasagittal describes any plane parallel to the sagittal plane but in practice, this is often referred to simply as a "sagittal" view because it is along the sagittal axis.

An **axial** plane (or transaxial plane) is one that divides the body into superior and inferior parts. It is perpendicular to the coronal plane and sagittal plane. CT scanning is performed in the axial plane.

A **coronal** plane divides the body into ventral and dorsal (front and back) sections.

Ultrasound

In diagnostic US, a piezoelectric transducer converts electrical energy into high-frequency mechanical vibrations. These US vibrations are focused either by the shape of the transducer or electronically to produce an arc-shaped sound wave which travels into the body. The sound wave is partially reflected or scattered from different tissues depending on their composition. Reflected sound returns to the transducer and is converted back into electrical energy which is processed and converted into an image.

There are three main patterns of reflected US.

1. **No reflection of the sound wave.** Almost all of the sound passes through the object. This is also termed sonolucent and appears black on US images. Fluid, such as in ascites, effusion or cysts is sonolucent.
2. **Partial reflection and transmission of some sound.** US waves are reflected at the boundaries of organs with different acoustic impedance, such as the boundary between the liver and the kidney (Figs. 3.35 and 3.36).
3. **Reflection of all sound.** Bone, air, and calcifications are examples. US is of limited use in this category.

US scan orientation should be provided by the person who performs the scan. By convention, when scanning sagittal, the patient's head is to the left of the image. In general, the area of interest is scanned in two orthogonal planes, typically axial (transverse) and longitudinal (sagittal). Ultrasonography is valuable in the workup of diseases involving the liver, biliary tract, kidneys, abdominal aorta, and abdominal masses. It is particularly useful in defining fluid versus solid (e.g., cyst vs. solid mass) as well as in imaging fluid-filled structures, such as the gallbladder, urinary bladder, and renal pelvis. The abdominal organs and pathologic processes have their own characteristic echo patterns.

Computed Tomography

In a helical or spiral CT scanner, the X-ray tube rotates around the patient while the patient is moving on the scanner table. The combination of continuous patient and X-ray tube movements result in a spiral or helical configuration resulting in a volume of tissue being imaged. By contrast, in a nonhelical scanner, the X-ray tube rotates about the patient

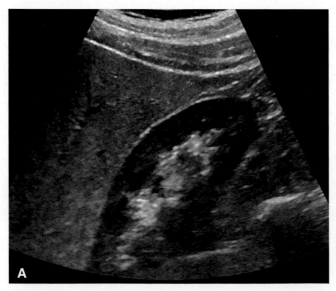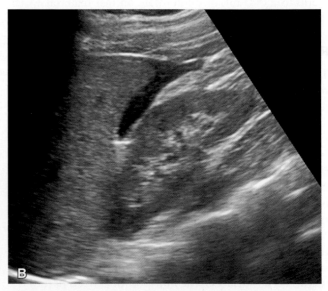

FIGURE 3.35. Ultrasound of the hepatorenal fossa. A: Normal appearance of the liver and kidney and lack of fluid in the hepatorenal fossa. Note the different appearances of the liver and kidney on ultrasound with the renal sinus fat being relatively hyperechoic. **B:** Abnormal: Free fluid in the hepatorenal fossa indicating free intraperitoneal fluid.

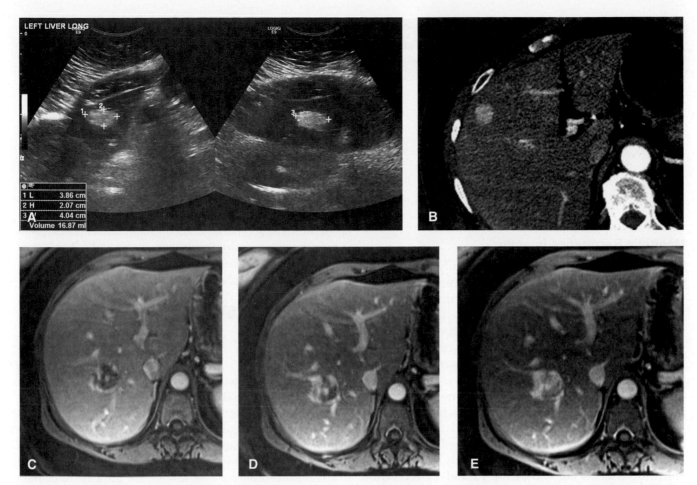

FIGURE 3.36. **Hepatic cavernous hemangioma.** **A:** Ultrasound of liver showing a well-defined hyperechoic lesion. **B:** CT showing a well-defined, enhancing lesion. **C-E:** Sequential MRI showing a peripheral nodule with a centripetal enhancing pattern consistent with cavernous hemangioma.

when the patient is stationary. Once the X-ray tube rotation is complete, the patient moves and the scan process repeats resulting in a slice of tissue being imaged. The current technology standard is MDCT, which has multiple contiguous rows of X-ray detectors that yield multiple tomographic slices with only one rotation of the X-ray tube around the patient. Hence, larger volumes can be scanned in a short period of time. This increased speed of volume coverage by MDCT is utilized when performing a CTA where a bolus of injected IV contrast is followed by the scanner to produce arterial opacification. Scanning can be timed after contrast injection, based on the region of anatomic interest; for example, hepatic arterial opacification is maximal approximately 40 seconds after commencement of injection of IV contrast while portal venous opacification is maximal 80 seconds after commencement of injection. Similarly, the lower extremity arterial system can be imaged by timing the scan to begin once peak opacification of contrast occurs in the lower abdominal aorta, after which the scan table moves to follow the bolus of contrast caudally to the patient's feet. **Delayed images** may be obtained several minutes after contrast injection for optimal opacification of the kidneys, ureters and bladder and for characterization of tumors, which may wash out or retain contrast. Not every patient requires a noncontrast CT scan followed by a contrast CT scan. Similarly, not every patient requires a delayed CT scan after the venous phase. As part of its "Choosing Wisely" initiative, the ACR published recommendations addressing these two issues (Tables 3.8 and 3.9).

TABLE 3.8	Indications for a Noncontrast CT (NCCT) Followed by Contrast-Enhanced CT (CECT)

Renal lesion Characterization
Workup of hematuria
Indeterminate adrenal nodule characterization
Follow-up after endovascular aortic stent graft placement
Gastrointestinal hemorrhage
Focal liver mass characterization

Reproduced from Johnson PT, et al. Recommendations: judicious use of multiphase abdominal CT protocols. *JACR*. 2018.

TABLE 3.9	Indications for Which Delayed CT Scan is Recommended After the Initial Contrast Phase

Renal lesion characterization

Hematuria workup

CT urography

Indeterminate adrenal nodule characterization

Hepatocellular carcinoma and cholangiocarcinoma

Reproduced from Johnson PT, et al. Recommendations: judicious use of multiphase abdominal CT protocols. *JACR.* 2018.

Magnetic Resonance Imaging

Hydrogen is abundant in the human body and is easily manipulated by a magnetic field. Because the hydrogen proton has a positive charge and is constantly spinning at a fixed (spin) frequency, a small magnetic field is created. While in the MRI scanner, short bursts of radiofrequency waves are transmitted at the same frequency as the protons being imaged causing them to become energized or resonate Once the radiofrequency broadcast is discontinued, the protons revert or decay back to their normal or steady state that existed before resonance. During this decay, radio waves can be detected by the receiver coil and are digitized to create images. The received radio wave intensity from the patient is determined not only by the number of hydrogen atoms but also by the **T1 and T2 relaxation times** which are specific to individual tissues and organs. T1-weighted imaging (T1WI) is useful for showing normal anatomy and T2-weighted imaging (T2WI) is useful for showing pathology in which edema causes increased signal due to excess water. For appearances of various tissues on T1- and T2-weighted images, see Table 3.10. Because fat is bright on T1WI, it is sometimes necessary to suppress the signal from it, to improve visualization of adjacent tissue. The ability to suppress fat is also useful when evaluating fat containing tumors such as lipomas

and ovarian dermoids as or appearance will become dark on the fat-suppressed images.

Gadolinium is a rare earth heavy metal, which when chelated forms gadopentetate dimeglumine, the most commonly used MRI contrast agent. Gadolinium reduces T1 relaxation times causing a brighter signal on T1WIs. Inflammation and vascular structures typically enhance after administration of gadolinium. In patients with renal impairment, gadolinium chelates have been associated with **nephrogenic systemic fibrosis (NSF)**, a debilitating and sometimes fatal disease affecting the skin, muscle, and abdominal organs. NSF presumably results from the in vivo release of the gadolinium ion from extra cellular gadolinium chelates. The second-generation gadolinium chelates have a macrocyclic structure that is more stable and at less risk of dissociated toxic free gadolinium than the first-generation linear gadolinium chelates structures.

ORGAN- OR SYSTEM-SPECIFIC IMAGING

Liver

MRI without and with contrast is the technique of choice for the **characterization of focal liver lesions**. In patients who cannot undergo an MRI, CT with contrast is a suitable alternative technique of choice. US has a limited role in the characterization of focal liver lesions apart from differentiating solid from cystic lesions (Tables 3.11 and 3.12). Subcentimeter liver lesions are difficult to characterize on any modality and are often evaluated with follow-up imaging as most are benign. For indeterminate liver lesions >1 cm, a biopsy should be considered when additional imaging tests are inconclusive. Short-term

TABLE 3.10	Comparison of Appearances on T1- and T2-Weighted Imaging	
Object	**T1**	**T2**
Air	Dark	Dark
Fat	Very bright	Less bright
Muscle	Intermediate	Dark
Bone cortex	Bright	Dark
Bone marrow	Intermediate	Bright
CSF	Dark	Bright
Gadolinium	Very bright	Bright

TABLE 3.11	Causes of Liver Hypoechogenicity on US	
Focal		**Diffuse**
Cyst		Acute hepatitis
Metastasis		Metastases
Abscess		
Focal sparing in steatosis		

TABLE 3.12	Causes of Liver Hyperechogenicity on US	
Focal	**Diffuse**	
Hemangioma	Steatosis (alcoholic, nonalcoholic)	
Focal fat	Cirrhosis	
Metastasis	Hepatitis	

TABLE 3.13	Imaging Algorithm for a Jaundiced Patient	
Cause	**Initial Imaging**	**Next Step**
Hepatitis/Sepsis	US ≫ CT, MR	Serology, biopsy
Alcoholic liver disease	US ≫ CT, MR	Biopsy
Obstruction due to stone/tumor	CT, MRCP ≫ US	Drainage by PTC or ERCP
Drugs/toxins	US	Biopsy

ERCP, endoscopic retrograde cholangiopancreatography; PTC, percutaneous transhepatic cholangiography.

imaging surveillance can be useful to monitor lesion stability. Ultimately, US- or CT-guided liver **biopsy** should always be considered to obtain a tissue diagnosis. Table 3.13 shows a simplified algorithm for imaging of a jaundiced patient. Up to 8% of the population have a **hepatic cavernous hemangioma**, which is benign. Typically, these are well defined and uniformly hyperechoic on US. On CT and MRI contrast enhancement of hepatic hemangiomas is usually nodular and centripetal (Fig. 3.35).

Common patterns of **fatty liver disease** include **diffuse fat accumulation, diffuse fat accumulation with focal sparing**, and **focal fat accumulation in an otherwise normal liver**. Unusual patterns that may cause diagnostic confusion by mimicking neoplastic, inflammatory, or vascular conditions include **multinodular and perivascular accumulation**. All these patterns involve the heterogeneous or nonuniform distribution of fat. The two most common conditions associated with diffuse fatty liver are alcoholic liver disease and nonalcoholic fatty liver disease (NAFLD) (Table 3.14). Because of the current epidemic of obesity, NAFLD is the most common chronic liver disease in the United States. In many conditions associated with fatty liver, steatosis may progress to steatohepatitis (with inflammation, cell injury, or fibrosis accompanying steatosis) and then cirrhosis. Up to 7% of patients with NAFLD related cirrhosis will develop hepatocellular carcinoma (HCC) within 10 years.

On US diffuse fatty liver may be diagnosed if the liver's echogenicity exceeds that of the renal cortex and spleen, with attenuation of the US wave, loss of definition of the diaphragm, and poor delineation of the intrahepatic

TABLE 3.14	Causes of Diffuse Fatty Liver

Toxin: Alcohol, chemotherapy, steroids
Infectious: Viral hepatitis
Metabolic: Obesity, total parenteral nutrition

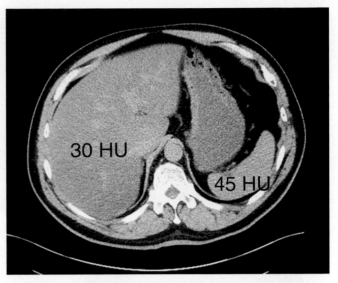

FIGURE 3.37. Diffuse fatty liver. Note the lower attenuation of the liver in Hounsfield Units (HU) compared with the spleen.

architecture. Fatty liver can be diagnosed on CT if the attenuation of the liver is at least 10 HU less than that of the spleen or if the attenuation of the liver is less than 40 HU (Fig. 3.37). Chemical shift gradient-echo (GRE) imaging with in-phase and opposed-phase acquisitions is the most widely used MR imaging technique for the assessment of fatty liver. The signal intensity of the normal liver parenchyma is similar on in-phase and opposed-phase images. Fatty liver may be present if there is a signal intensity **loss on opposed-phase images** in comparison with in-phase images, and the amount of hepatic fat present can be quantified by assessing the degree of signal intensity loss.

Focal fat deposition or **focal fat sparing** characteristically occurs in specific areas, for example, adjacent to the falciform ligament or ligamentum venosum, the porta hepatis, the caudate lobe and the gallbladder fossa (Fig. 3.38). Focal fat has no mass effect and its appearance may be transient. The differential diagnosis of focal fat includes metastases and primary tumors, lesions that exert a mass effect, tend to enhance after contrast and may contain areas of necrosis or hemorrhage.

Ultrasonographic elastography (FibroScan) is an office-based test that measures the velocity of the sound passing through the liver and converts that measurement into a liver stiffness value. Limitations of liver biopsy, the gold standard for staging liver disease include invasiveness with risks of pain and bleeding, sampling error and interpretation error leading to over- or understaging. The FibroScan cannot be done in patients who are obese or in those with ascites. The test is complementary to serum biomarker tests for liver fibrosis, and liver biopsy could be avoided in patients who were shown to not have cirrhosis who are then eligible for treatment for Hepatitis B and C. **MR elastography** measures

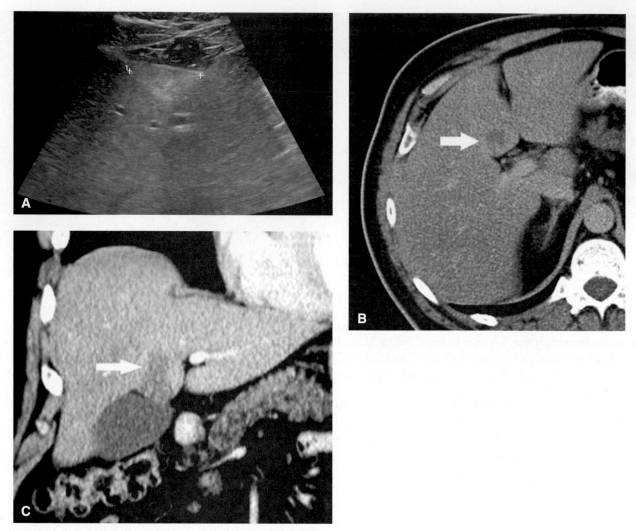

FIGURE 3.38. Focal fat infiltration. A: Ultrasound showing focal fat infiltration adjacent to the falciform ligament of the liver (+-+). Note the well-defined (geographic) border of the focal fat. **B and C:** Axial and coronal CT showing well-defined low attenuation focal fat (*arrows*) adjacent to the gallbladder fossa.

tissue stiffness with similar accuracy to US elastography but is unreliable in patients with hemochromatosis due to low MRI signal.

Cirrhosis is characterized pathologically by necrosis, fibrosis, and regeneration. Common causes include Hepatitis B and C, alcohol, and increasingly nonalcoholic steatohepatitis (NASH). The most accurate ultrasonographic finding is a nodular surface (Fig. 3.39A). CT and MR also show a nodular appearance of the liver surface with a reduction in volume of the right lobe in contrast to the caudate and left lobes which increase in size. Presence of splenomegaly, ascites, and varices indicate the development of portal hypertension (Fig. 3.39B and C).

HCC is the most common primary malignant liver tumor and usually enhances early on CECT because most of its blood supply is from the hepatic artery. HCC has a propensity to invade the portal and hepatic veins. Tumor thrombus in the portal vein is characterized by vein expansion and enhancing thrombus. Surveillance of patients with cirrhosis with MRI may identify hepatic nodules, which are dysplastic, premalignant, or malignant and are classified according to LIRADS criteria (Fig. 3.40A and B). The Liver Imaging Reporting and Data System **(LIRADS)** is a reporting system created for the standardized interpretation of liver imaging findings in adult patients who are at risk for HCC because of cirrhosis, chronic hepatitis B, current or prior HCC with or without cirrhosis, adult liver transplantation candidates, and liver transplant recipients.

Typically, cirrhotic nodules are high signal intensity on T1WI and isodense or hypodense on T2WI in contrast to HCC which is often hyperintense on T2WI (Fig. 3.40C).

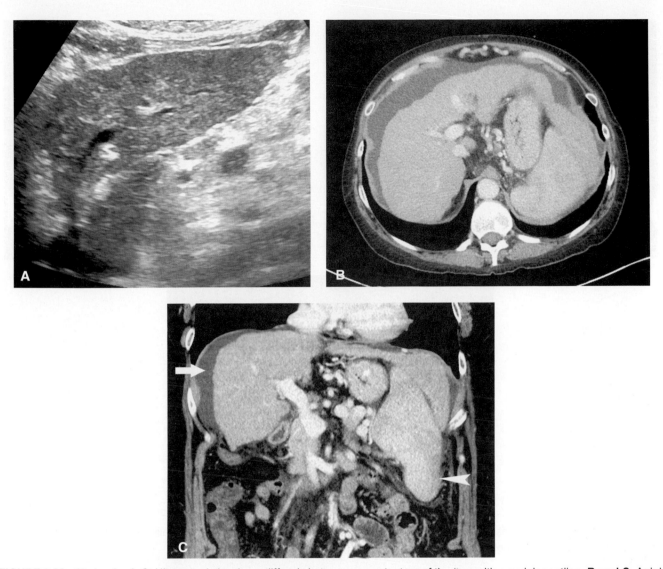

FIGURE 3.39. Cirrhosis. A-C: Ultrasound showing a diffusely heterogeneous texture of the liver with a nodular outline. **B and C.** Axial and coronal CT showing a nodular liver surface and an enlarged left lobe of liver in addition to features of portal hypertension, ascites (*arrow*), and splenomegaly (*arrowhead*).

Metastases are the most common liver malignancy, outnumbering primary tumors by 20 to 1. GI carcinomas, colon, stomach, and pancreas are the most common primary source neoplasms. US is a highly sensitive modality for the detection of liver metastases which may appear hyperechoic, or hypoechoic. Metastases which cause a diffuse permeative infiltrative pattern may be difficult to detect on US and are misdiagnosed as cirrhosis. On CT, most metastases or hypodense and are best visualized in the portal phase (80 seconds after administration of contrast) when the normal liver is maximally enhanced (Fig. 3.41). Image-guided biopsy is usually necessary for confirmation of diagnosis.

Gallbladder and Biliary Tract

Oral cholecystography has been replaced by US which is more accurate for diagnosing gallstones, gallbladder wall thickness as evidence of cholecystitis and pericholecystic fluid collections (Fig. 3.42). While it is accurate for the diagnosis of biliary duct obstruction, the cause of obstruction such as gallstone or tumor is not always visible on US.

While the standard MRI sequences can accurately demonstrate both the site and cause of biliary obstruction, a heavily T2-weighted fluid-sensitive sequence in the coronal plane, **magnetic resonance**

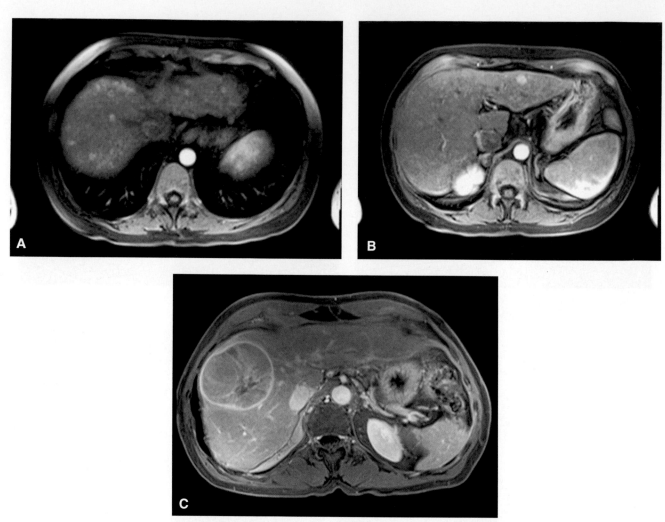

FIGURE 3.40. Cirrhotic nodules and hepatocellular carcinoma. A and B: Axial MRI showing dysplastic liver masses in a patient with cirrhosis. **C:** Large enhancing hepatocellular carcinoma on T2-weighted image.

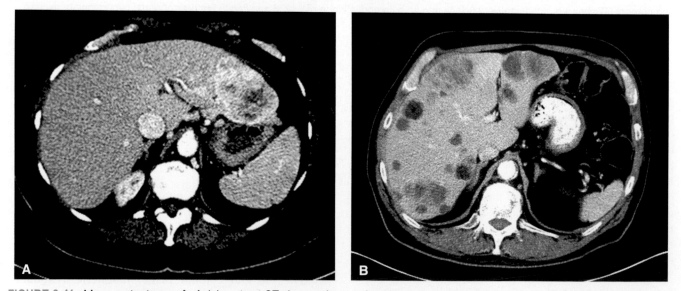

FIGURE 3.41. Liver metastases. A: Axial contrast CT shows a large enhancing mass in the left lobe of liver. **B:** Axial contrast CT shows multiple lesions of various sizes and attenuation.

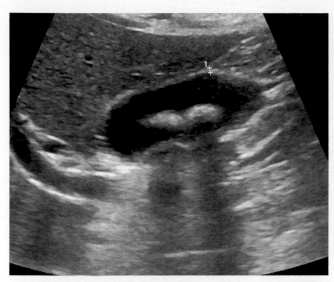

FIGURE 3.42. Gallstones. Ultrasound showing multiple gallstones with echogenic shadowing. No evidence of cholecystitis is seen.

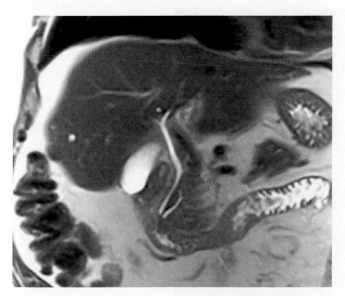

FIGURE 3.43. Magnetic resonance cholangiopancreaticography (MRCP). Normal examination showing patent and nondilated common bile and pancreatic ducts.

cholangiopancreaticography (MRCP) uses the intrinsic differential T2 contrast between the fluid in the biliary tree and adjacent organs to generate a cholangiogram without requiring gadolinium (Fig. 3.43). Although contrast is not necessary for detection of ductal stones, it use improves the visualization of cholangitis and pancreaticobiliary tumors (Fig. 3.44). The exogenous administration of secretin improves the visualization of pancreatic ducts at MRCP because of an enlargement of the pancreatic duct system and an increase of the fluid content within the lumen of the pancreatic ducts, responsible of an increase

of MR signal. **ERCP** is a relatively invasive procedure with a 4% risk of major complication such as acute pancreatitis and involves endoscopic cannulation of the ampulla and injection of contrast into the common bile duct (Fig. 3.45). Additionally, a sphincterotomy with endobiliary stent placement may be performed. Currently, the main indication for ERCP is removal of common bile duct stones. The diagnostic role of ERCP has lessened with the advent of MRCP.

Pancreas

Pancreatic cyst follow-up protocol. With the increased the use of CT and MRI, the management of patients with an incidentally detected pancreatic cyst is a significant clinical challenge as to which of the thousands of detected cysts are innocuous and which are potentially malignant (Fig. 3.46). Pancreatic cysts may be intraductal mucinous neoplasms, mucinous cystic neoplasms, serous cystadenomas, or one of several types of nonneoplastic cysts. Mucinous (intraductal mucinous or mucinous cystic) neoplasms have malignant potential and should be distinguished from serous lesions (serous cystadenomas) that are nearly always benign. Advanced imaging including endoscopic US with cyst fluid analysis and cytology is necessary to confirm the type of cyst and determine the risk of malignancy.

In 2015, the American Gastroenterology Association, with multidisciplinary consensus, issued the following management guidelines:

1. Follow-up should be obtained based on the patient's overall medical condition and the guidelines that apply to asymptomatic patients without family history of pancreatic cancer. If the patient is symptomatic, referral to a pancreatic specialist may be warranted.
2. If **pancreatic cysts <2 cm** with no main duct dilation or solid nodule – follow-up is recommended in 1 year with MRI/MRCP. If there is no interval change, subsequent follow-up with MRI/MRCP is recommended every 2 years to establish stability.
3. For patients with **pancreatic cysts > or = to 2 cm** or lesions less than 2 cm with a solid nodule and/or main duct dilation or concerning rate of increase in size during follow-up – referral to a pancreatic specialist (gastroenterologist with pancreatic specialization or pancreatic surgeon) is recommended for further management. If patients have prior negative cytology on endoscopic US with fine needle aspirate, annual follow-up MRI/MRCP is recommended.

Chronic pancreatitis is the result of prolonged inflammation characterized by irreversible morphologic damage, including atrophy, and fibrosis of the pancreas. Functional damage to the pancreas is evident by diabetes and malabsorption. Multiple pancreatic calcifications which occur late in the disease process are seen on plain film and CT and are a diagnostic feature of chronic pancreatitis as is dilatation

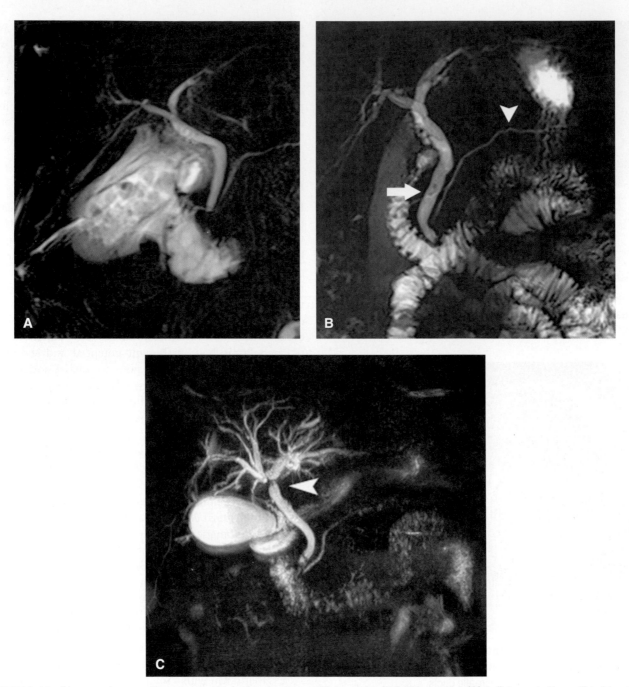

FIGURE 3.44. Abnormal magnetic resonance cholangiopancreaticography (MRCP) showing **(A)** gallstones in the gallbladder; **(B)** gallstones in the common duct (*arrow*); and **(C)** cholangiocarcinoma at the confluence of the right and left main main bile ducts (Klatskin tumor) (*arrowhead*).

of the pancreatic duct, which may be seen on US, MRCP, or CT (Fig. 3.47 and 3.48).

Pancreatic carcinoma. Ductal adenocarcinoma accounts for 90% of all pancreatic tumors, most of which arise in the pancreatic head. Only 20% of patients are candidates for surgery at the time of diagnosis. Accurate staging, on which treatment is based, is dependent on the quality of imaging. Contrast CT is the main imaging modality with the first scan obtained during the pancreatic phase (40 seconds after commencement of contrast injection) and the second scan during the portal venous phase (80 seconds). The CT appearance of pancreatic carcinoma is a poorly defined hypodense mass best seen during the pancreatic phase of CT. Additional findings include dilatation of the common duct for tumors in the pancreatic head and the upstream pancreatic duct. Findings which impact **resectability**

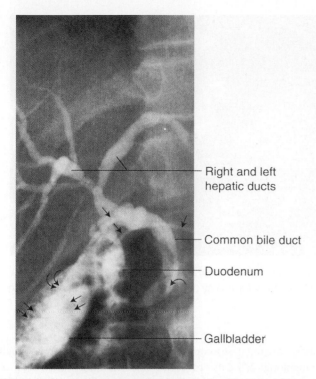

Right and left
hepatic ducts

Common bile duct

Duodenum

Gallbladder

FIGURE 3.45. **Endoscopic retrograde cholangiopancreatography (ERCP)** is a relatively invasive procedure. Cholelithiasis and choledocholithiasis. The gallbladder is filled with calculi (*double straight arrows*), and there is a large calculus in the distal common bile duct (*single curved arrow*). A nasobiliary drain (*single straight arrows*) is in place with the tip (*double curved arrows*) in the gallbladder.

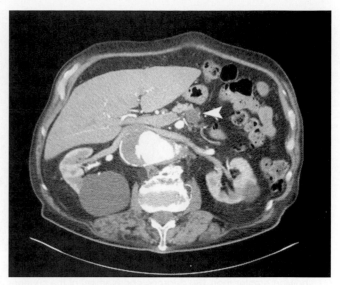

FIGURE 3.46. **Pancreatic cyst.** Axial CT showing a 1.9 cm diameter cyst (*arrowhead*) in the pancreatic body which was diagnosed incidentally during CT for abdominal aortic aneurysm.

include vessel encasement, as defined by obliteration of the normal fat plane between the pancreas and vessel and more than hundred and, more than 180 degrees contact between the tumor and vessel. Lymphatic spread to adjacent nodes also impacts resectability and should be sought on CT. Endoscopic US permits fine-needle aspiration biopsy of pancreatic tumors.

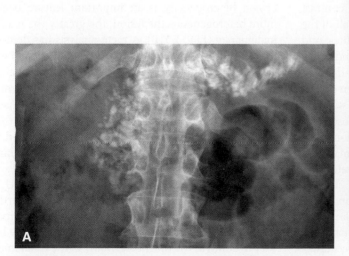

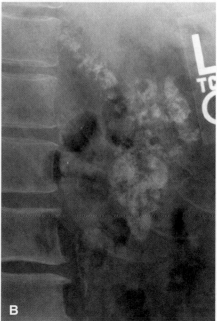

FIGURE 3.47. **Chronic pancreatitis. (A)** Frontal and **(B)** lateral plain abdominal films showing extensive pancreatic calcification.

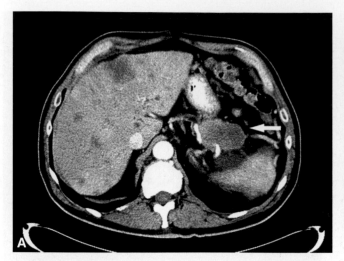 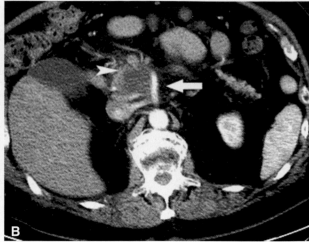

FIGURE 3.48. Pancreatic carcinoma. A: Axial CT showing mass in the pancreatic tail (*arrow*) and several liver metastases. **B:** Axial CT showing greater than 180 degrees encasement of the superior mesenteric artery (*arrow*) by pancreatic cancer (*arrowhead*), making the tumor inoperable.

Urological Tract

Hematuria can be due to a wide variety of causes, including calculi, neoplasms, infection, trauma, and parenchymal renal disease including glomerulonephritis. Renal US may be helpful to exclude renal parenchymal disease in patients with microscopic hematuria and it should be used in patients with suspected glomerular disease. Otherwise, most adults with gross or persistent hematuria require imaging, primarily **CT urography (CTU)**. CTU has largely replaced intravenous urography because of its increased sensitivity and specificity. Typically, the CTU protocol comprises a noncontrast CT scan of the abdomen and pelvis followed by contrast administration with scans obtained during the nephrographic and excretory phases. A **split bolus protocol** may be used in patients under 45 years to reduce radiation dose by eliminating one of the contrast-enhanced scans. This protocol requires injection of half of the IV contrast after the initial noncontrast CT scan. The second half of the IV contrast bolus is injected after a delay of 7 minutes, and the patient is rescanned after a delay of 100 seconds. The second scan provides a combined nephrographic and excretory phase imaging of the urinary tract and has been shown to be of equivalent sensitivity and specificity to the standard three-phase protocol while reducing radiation dose. The CTU protocol allows a greater volume of the abdomen to be covered and allows additional formatting of images in maximum intensity projection (MIP), multiplanar reformats (MPR), and volume rendering (Fig. 3.49).

MRI and CT have similar accuracy in detection and characterization of most renal lesions. However, MRI lacks the sensitivity of CT for the detection of calculi. Transitional cell carcinomas of the collecting system may be missed because of their size and location. Retrograde pyelography which involves injection of contrast into the collecting system via a catheter placed during cystoscopy may be necessary to diagnose small transitional cell cancers (Fig. 3.50). The noncontrast scan of the CTU has replaced radiographic plain films (KUB) as the initial modality for investigation of hematuria as it is more sensitive and specific for the diagnosis of stones and renal calcification as 20% of calculi are not radiopaque on plain films.

Renal Masses

Most renal masses are benign cysts, the prevalence of which increases with age. Incidental renal masses are a common problem in imaging as cysts can be seen in as many as 40% of patients on CT. The **Bosniak classification** system uses CT to grade cystic renal lesions I-IV on imaging features with a higher likelihood of malignancy in the higher classes (Table 3.15). The Bosniak system emphasizes contrast enhancement pattern, and morphology rather than lesion size. Lesion heterogeneity is an important feature because the more heterogeneous the lesion, the greater the likelihood of malignancy (Fig. 3.51B). A meta-analysis has demonstrated that the Bosniak system is 90% sensitive and 65% specific for detecting malignancy. Because cystic renal malignancies are generally indolent, less aggressive management may be appropriate and recent American Urological Association guidelines recommend active surveillance rather than intervention when the risk of intervention or risk of death outweigh the benefit of treatment, especially for Bosniak 3 and 4 lesions, if less than 2 cm in size.

Any homogeneous mass greater than 20 HU but less than 70 HU on NCCT requires IV contrast for further evaluation, and contrast enhancement defined as an increase of 20 HU ≥ is suspicious for carcinoma. Biopsy may be necessary to confirm the diagnosis. Many of the renal masses that are too small to characterize (less than 1.5 cm) on noncontrast CT are either benign or insignificant.

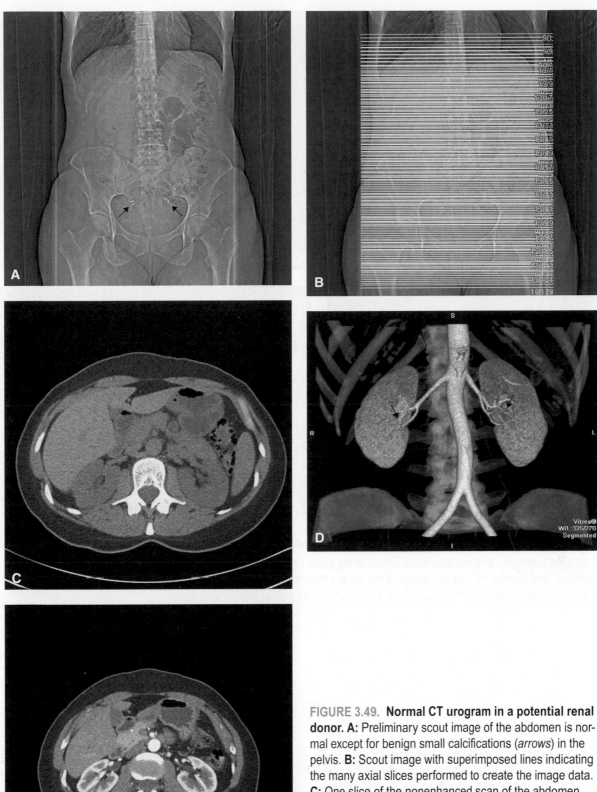

FIGURE 3.49. Normal CT urogram in a potential renal donor. A: Preliminary scout image of the abdomen is normal except for benign small calcifications (*arrows*) in the pelvis. **B:** Scout image with superimposed lines indicating the many axial slices performed to create the image data. **C:** One slice of the nonenhanced scan of the abdomen before administration of contrast. No abnormalities of the kidneys or other areas are noted. **D:** Coronal CT images after contrast administration shows aorta, single bilateral renal arteries (*arrows*), and normal size kidneys. **E:** Axial scan early after contrast demonstrates well demarcation of the renal cortex and medulla.

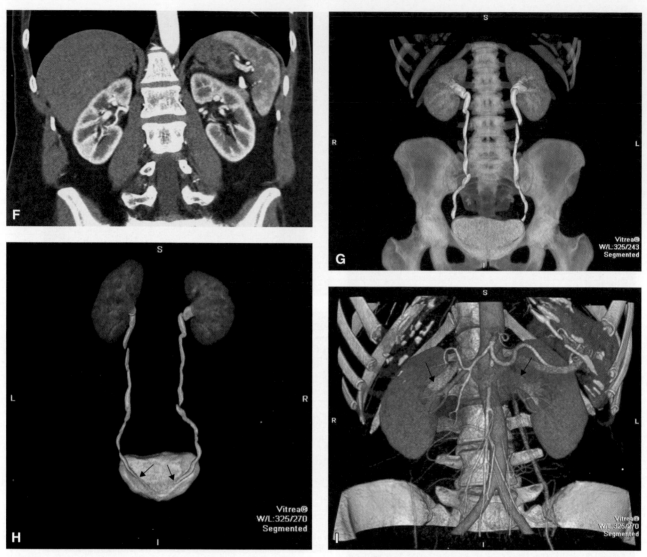

FIGURE 3.49. *(Continued)* **F:** Coronal reconstruction at the same time as **(E)**. **G:** Later reconstructed coronal image showing normal kidneys, ureters, and bladder. **H:** Coronal image of the urinary tract viewed from posterior, showing entry of the ureters into the bladder *(arrows)*. **I:** Later coronal image showing both renal veins *(arrows)* as well as arterial structures.

Renal cell carcinoma usually enhances with contrast and may invade venous structures in up to 10% of cases, with tumor thrombus extending from the renal veins to the main renal vein, IVC, and right atrium (Fig. 3.52). Venous invasion is a poor prognostic sign even in the absence of metastatic disease, with long-term survival rates of 60% or less. Accurate staging is important not only from a prognostic standpoint but for surgical planning as tumor thrombus extension into the right atrium requires cardiac bypass, increasing the morbidity and mortality of the resection procedure.

If a renal mass contains **fat** (region of interest measuring less than -10 HU) and is without calcification, the diagnosis is **angiomyolipoma (AML)** (Fig. 3.53). If these are solitary and under 4 cm in size, no further workup is necessary but patients may benefit from imaging surveillance to document lack of growth. For AML's over 4 cm in size or those with hematuria, flank pain or perilesional hemorrhage, treatment in the form of arterial embolization is recommended. For patients with multiple AMLs, diagnostic workup for tuberous sclerosis is recommended. If a renal mass contains fat and calcification, then renal cell carcinoma is suspected and further imaging with contrast CT and MRI is recommended.

Vesicoureteral reflux describes the reflux of urine in a retrograde fashion into the ureters and is usually confined to childhood where it may predispose to urinary tract infection. Reflux is diagnosed on a voiding cystourethrogram (VCU), in which contrast medium is introduced via a urethral catheter into the bladder. Fluoroscopy is used to

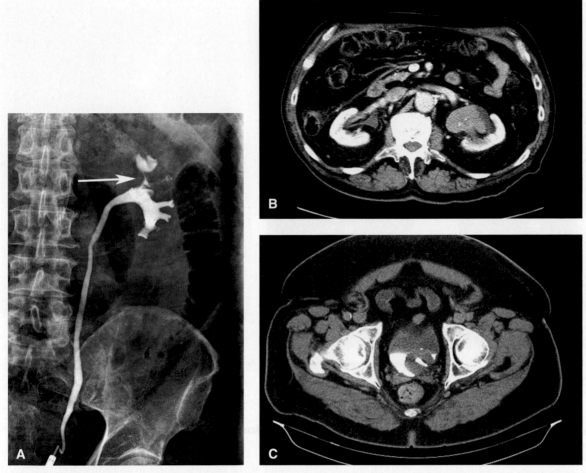

FIGURE 3.50. Transitional cell carcinoma in different patients. **A:** Left retrograde pyelogram showing a filling defect in the upper pole collecting system (*arrow*). **B:** Axial CT showing a large soft tissue mass occupying much of the left renal collecting system. **C:** Delayed image of a CT urogram showing a filling defect in the bladder.

TABLE 3.15	Bosniak Classification of Renal Cystic Masses	
Classification	**Imaging Features**	**Follow-Up/Treatment**
I	Attenuation −10 to 20 HU. Imperceptibly thin wall. No septa. No calcifications	None
II	Attenuation −10 to 20 HU. May have few thin septa which minimally enhance	None
II F	Multiple septa with smooth thickening with or without mural calcification. Also, nonenhancing hyperattenuating cysts greater than 3 cm	Follow-up
III	Irregular or thickened walls or septa with measurable enhancement	Resection
IV	Discrete enhancing nodule components	Resection

After Ward RD, Remer EM. Cystic renal masses: an imaging update. *Eur J Radiol.* 2018;99:103-110.

detect and quantify vesicoureteral reflux (Fig. 3.54). At the completion of the study, the patient voids again under fluoroscopy to allow diagnosis of urethral abnormalities, which may cause bladder obstruction and secondary vesicoureteral reflux.

Cystography and retrograde urethrography are performed to detect bladder or urethral extravasation in patients with pelvic trauma. Direct injection of contrast material into the bladder or ureter (retrograde pyelogram) is of value when a detailed view of a portion of the ureter or pelvicalyceal system is necessary. It is done in conjunction with cystoscopy and ureteroscopy.

Adrenal Gland

The widespread use of imaging has led to increased detection of incidental adrenal lesions which occur in 5% of

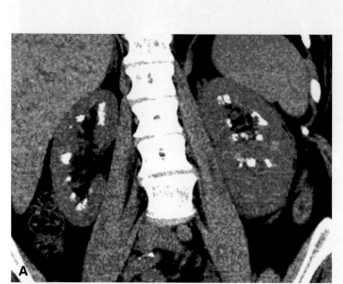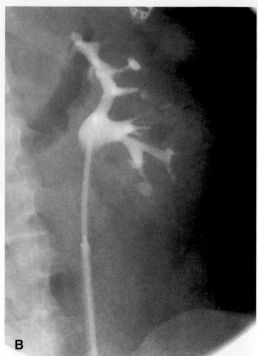

FIGURE 3.51. Nephrocalcinosis. A: Noncontrast coronal CT shows multiple calcific opacities in the renal medulla. **B:** Retrograde pyelogram confirm the location of these opacities.

all abdominal CT examinations. In patients scanned for known malignancy, the incidence of adrenal nodules is over 10%, but only a third of these are metastatic. On NCCT, findings that are suspicious for malignancy include size (>4 cm), irregular margins, heterogeneous appearance, and growth in size. Adrenal adenomas enhance rapidly on CT following injection of contrast and show a rapid loss or "washout" of contrast. Malignant adrenal lesions usually show a slower washout of contrast than adenomas. If the patient is rescanned 15-minute after contrast administration, an absolute percentage contrast washout of 60% or higher has an accuracy of almost 90% for the diagnosis of an adenoma. Most adrenal adenomas are nonfunctioning. The clinical presentation of functioning tumors of the adrenal gland depends on the hormone secreted (Tables 3.16 and 3.17).

Adrenal vein sampling is recommended in patients with primary hyperaldosteronism (hypertension and hypokalemia) to determine which adrenal gland is producing excessive aldosterone as imaging (CT or MRI) is only 50% sensitive for the detection of adrenal adenoma. Primary hyperaldosteronism may also be due to bilateral adrenal hyperplasia in which case aldosterone levels from both adrenal glands are equivalent. **Pheochromocytomas** are usually large (greater than 4 cm). They should not be biopsied because of the risk of hypertensive crisis. Malignant tumors of the adrenal gland include metastasis (Fig. 3.55), adrenocortical carcinoma, and lymphoma.

Abdominal Aorta

CTA is the preferred modality for imaging the abdominal aorta because of its availability and speed. Although **abdominal aortic aneurysm (AAA)** rupture may be diagnosed on noncontrast CT, IV contrast is necessary for evaluation and measurement of the aneurysm lumen before elective endovascular repair (EVAR). Pre-EVAR relevant imaging information includes the maximum aortic diameter, length, and morphology of the aneurysm neck, vessel diameter at the proximal (aortic) and distal (aortic or iliac) fixation sites, and patency of the iliac and femoral vessels for access. In patients, who are post EVAR, delayed CT imaging is necessary for detection of endoleaks (see Chapter 12).

The normal diameter of the abdominal aorta varies depending on age, sex, and body habitus. In most patients, an abdominal aortic diameter of greater than 3 cm is regarded as aneurysmal (Fig. 3.56). By location, 90% of AAA are infrarenal (begin below the renal arteries), 5% are juxtarenal (begin at the level of the renal arteries), and 5% are suprarenal. The mortality rate for ruptured abdominal aortic aneurysm is over 80%, making it one of the most fatal surgical conditions. The risk of rupture depends on aneurysm size. The average risk of rupture in male patients with 5.0-cm to 5.9-cm AAA is 1.0% per year, in female patients with 5.0-cm to 5.9-cm AAA is 3.9% per year, in male patients with 6.0-cm or greater AAA was 14.1% per year, and in female patients with 6.0-cm or greater AAA was 22.3% per year.

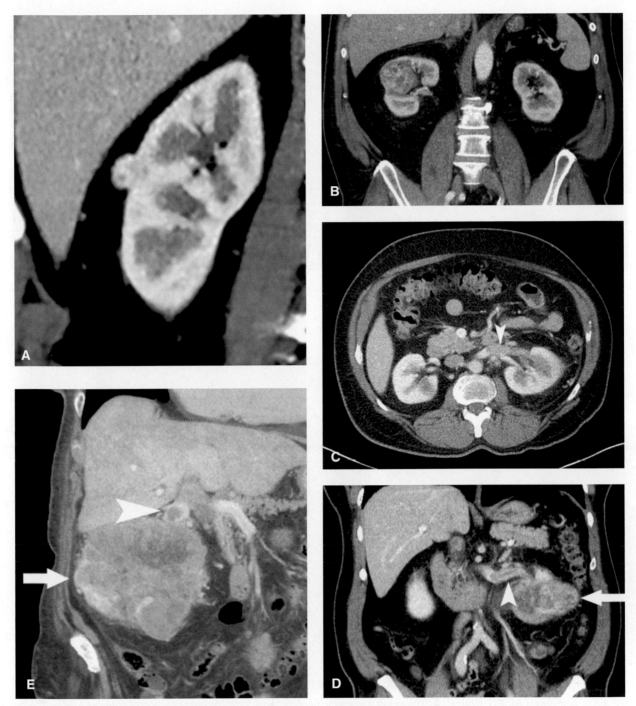

FIGURE 3.52. **Renal cell carcinoma. A:** Small exophytic renal mass (biopsy proven carcinoma). **B:** Large exophytic renal mass. **C-E:** Renal vein thrombosis due to tumor extension (*arrowheads*) due to carcinoma (*arrows*).

Currently, elective repair is recommended in men with an asymptomatic AAA greater than 5.5 cm in diameter or one that expands more than 0.5 cm within a six-month period. In women, repair of AAAs greater than 5 cm is recommended as the risk of rupture is greater in women than men. Repair should also be considered for people with AAAs that are greater than twice the size of a normal portion of the aorta.

Screening ultrasound for AAA is recommended by the US Preventative Task Force in men between 65 and 75 years who have ever smoked and in individuals of age 60 years or older who have a family history of AAA. Although the risk of AAA is much lower in women than men, the risk of rupture in women is higher than in men, and some advocate that one-time screening for women with risk factors is worthwhile.

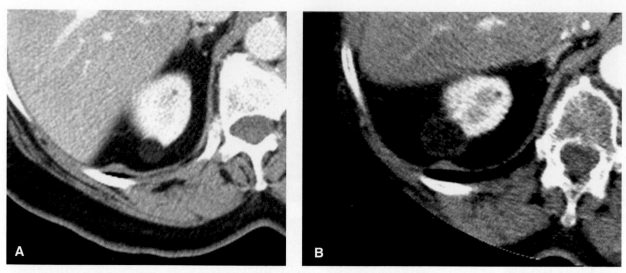

FIGURE 3.53. **Renal angiomyolipoma. A and B:** Axial CT scans 5 years apart show an increase in size of the fat-containing tumor.

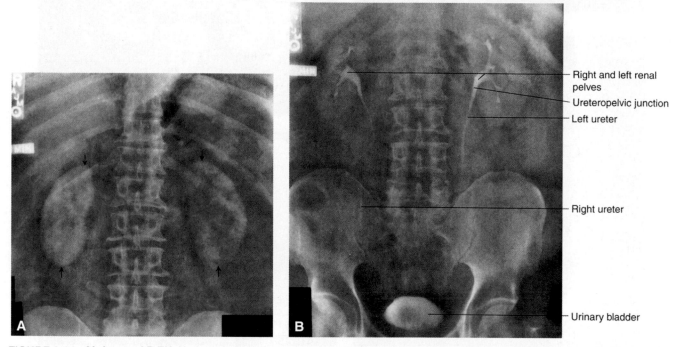

FIGURE 3.54. **Abdomen AP EU.** Normal. **A:** These are symmetric nephrograms 1 minute post injection of contrast media. The renal outlines (*arrows*) are clearly defined owing to the presence of the contrast media within the kidneys. **B:** Note that it is possible to see the calyces, infundibula, renal pelves, portions of ureters, and urinary bladder on this 15-minute radiograph.

A **penetrating atherosclerotic ulcer** (PAU) extends to the media of the aortic wall. PAU may resolve, or progress to an intramural hematoma, dissection, pseudoaneurysm, or aortic rupture. Isolated **abdominal aortic dissection** is rare compared with dissection of the thoracic aorta. Most isolated abdominal aortic dissections occur infrarenally and may not involve the mesenteric or renal arteries. On CT, an intimal flap divides the aorta into true and false lumens, of which the true lumen is typically smaller and enhances more rapidly than the false lumen. An **intramural hematoma** is due to rupture of the vasa vasorum in the aortic medial layer and resembles an early-stage aortic dissection. IMH appears as an eccentric crescent-shaped

TABLE 3.16	Clinical Syndromes Caused by Functioning Adrenal Adenomas
Clinical Syndrome	**Hormone Production**
Conns	Primary hyperaldosteronism
Cushing	Primary hypercortisolism
Pheochromocytoma	Catecholamines
Adrenal carcinoma	Cushing syndrome in association with the virilization or feminization

TABLE 3.17	Causes of an Acute Abdomen by Abdominal Quadrant
Right Upper Quadrant	**Left Upper Quadrant**
Cholecystitis	Peptic Ulcer
Cholangitis	Bowel perforation
Hepatitis	Splenic infarction
Right Lower Quadrant	**Left Lower Quadrant**
Appendicitis	Diverticulitis
Diverticulitis	Ureteral calculus
Inflammatory bowel disease	Colitis
Ureteral calculus	

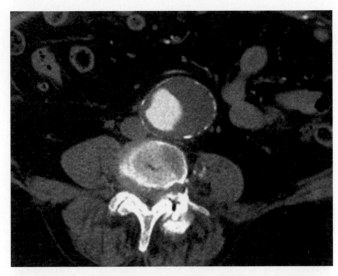

FIGURE 3.56. Abdominal aortic aneurysm. Axial CT shows a 6 cm nonruptured infrarenal abdominal aortic aneurysm with intraluminal thrombus.

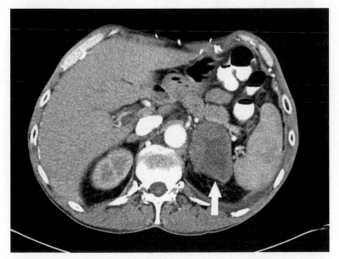

FIGURE 3.55. Adrenal metastasis. Axial CT shows a markedly enlarged left adrenal gland (*arrow*) due to a metastasis from lung cancer.

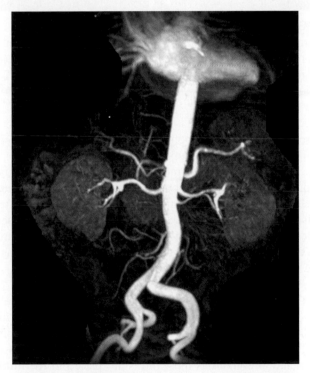

FIGURE 3.57. MR angiogram. Normal aortoiliac system.

hematoma in the aortic wall, best seen as a smoothly contoured hyperattenuation abnormality on noncontrast images. IMH may resolve, stabilize, or progress to aortic dissection.

MRA may also be used to image the aorta, from valve to bifurcation in addition to imaging of the iliac system and lower limb runoffs (Fig. 3.57).

Inferior Vena Cava

Congenital IVC variants, include absence, duplication, left-sided location, azygous or hemiazygous continuation, and web formation. **Duplication** of the IVC occurs in less than 1% of the population, but it is an important diagnosis to make in patients undergoing IVC filter placement to

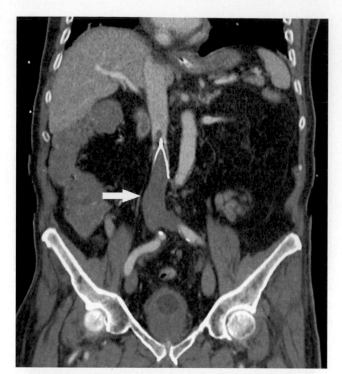

FIGURE 3.58. IVC thrombosis. Coronal reformat CT shows thrombosis of the infrarenal IVC (*arrow*). Note the difference in density of the contrast enhanced blood above the IVC filter due to renal vein inflow compared with the thrombus below the IVC filter.

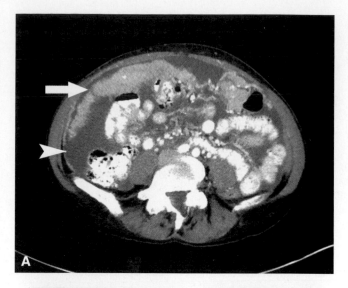

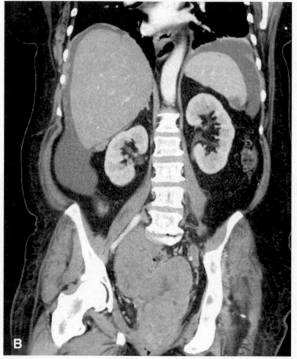

FIGURE 3.59. Peritoneal metastases. A: Axial CT of the lower abdomen showing soft tissue omental caking (*arrow*) and ascites (*arrowhead*) due to metastatic disease. **B:** Coronal reformat CT shows ascites, and a pelvic soft tissue mass.

prevent pulmonary embolism. A second IVC filter is necessary in patients with a duplicated IVC.

MRI with contrast is more reliable than CT for evaluation of IVC tumor thrombus. When using CT, an imaging delay of 90 seconds post injection of contrast allows better visualization of the IVC. US including Doppler may be used for IVC imaging although visualization of the infrahepatic IVC may be limited because of bowel gas. Doppler US may be used to evaluate IVC flow.

IVC thrombosis is a well-recognized complication of IVC filter placement, occurring at a rate of approximately 1% of patients per annum (Fig. 3.58). Patients present with bilateral lower extremity edema and well-developed venous collaterals may be apparent on imaging. Renal vein flow is typically preserved as most filters are placed in the infrarenal IVC. The complication of IVC thrombosis has contributed to increased utilization of temporary IVC filters, which may be retrieved when the risk of PE is reduced (see Chapter 12).

Peritoneal Cavity/Retroperitoneal Space

The **peritoneal cavity** is a potential space between the parietal peritoneum and visceral peritoneum and normally only contains a small volume of peritoneal fluid. The space acts as a route of spread for metastatic disease

(Fig. 3.59). The **retroperitoneal space (retroperitoneum)** is a potential space behind the peritoneum. Structures in this "space" include the aorta, IVC, kidney, ureter, adrenal, pancreas, second, third, and fourth parts of the duodenum, and the ascending and descending colon as they have peritoneum on their anterior side. Other contents include lymph nodes which when enlarged may compress and obstruct other structures in the retroperitoneum (Fig. 3.60).

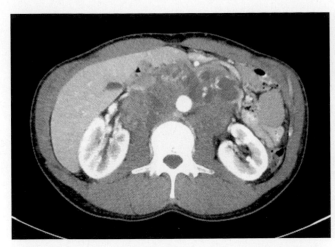

FIGURE 3.60. Retroperitoneal lymphadenopathy. Axial CT showing extensive retroperitoneal lymphadenopathy encasing the aorta.

ACUTE ABDOMEN

The clinical condition of acute abdomen can be defined as sudden onset (less than 24 hours) of localized or generalized abdominal pain usually prompting the patient to seek medical help. Cross-sectional imaging (US, CT, MRI) plays a crucial role in the management of patients with acute abdominal pain. Contrast-enhanced CT (CECT) of the abdomen and pelvis is the examination of choice because of its ability to provide a global perspective, reduced acquisition time, potential use of multiple phases of contrast enhancement, and image reconstructions.

The diagnostic yield of CT for causes of abdominal pain approaches 50% and an unsuspected diagnosis may be found in over one quarter of patients. Coronal and sagittal CT reformats should be routinely reviewed to facilitate accurate radiologic diagnosis. US is frequently the first imaging modality used in pregnant patients with an acute abdomen. MRI without contrast should follow US in the imaging of pregnant patients but is inferior to CT in the diagnosis of renal calculi. Despite longer acquisition times, MRI is also useful in the diagnosis of acute bowel disorders and gynecological emergencies such as ovarian hemorrhage, ectopic pregnancy, tumor rupture, torsion, hemorrhage, infarction, and pelvic inflammatory disease. In practice, the feasibility of US or MRI for acute abdominal pain will rely on institutional expertise, availability, and adoption of protocols that are aimed at rapid acquisition and multiorgan assessment.

About one-third of patients with an acute abdomen never have a diagnosis established, one-third have appendicitis, and one-third have some other disorder such as acute cholecystitis, SBO, pancreatitis, renal colic, perforated peptic ulcer, cancer, and diverticulitis. In the elderly the most common diagnoses are SBO, diverticulitis, abdominal aortic aneurysm rupture and dissection, bowel ischemia, appendicitis, and colonic obstruction. The typical signs of abdominal sepsis may be absent in a neutropenic patient, delaying diagnosis and resulting in a high mortality rate. As a many as 75% of patients after colorectal surgery with clinical suspicion for an infection will have a fluid collection, but only those collections in proximity to the site of surgery are likely to be an infected collection.

Except when bowel perforation or postoperative anastomotic leaks are suspected, oral contrast is not given to patients with an acute abdomen before CT because of the associated delay in scan acquisition and questionable diagnostic benefit.

Right Lower Quadrant Pain

In patients with RLQ pain with fever and leukocytosis, the differential diagnosis includes **acute appendicitis**, mesenteric adenitis, right-sided diverticulitis, and IBD. CECT of abdomen and pelvis is usually appropriate to evaluate for suspected appendicitis in adults. In patients who are pregnant, noncontrast MRI or US are recommended with the latter modality preferred for children with suspected appendicitis. Acute appendicitis is the most common nonobstetric surgical emergency in pregnant patients, complications of which include premature labor and fetal and maternal death following appendiceal perforation. The fetal loss rate exceeds 30% in patients with ruptured appendicitis.

The role of US as the primary modality for the diagnosis of acute appendicitis is disappointing because the technique is operator dependent and the nonvisualization rate of the appendix is as high as 27% even in expert hands (Fig. 3.61). Limitations of US include inability to image beyond bowel gas and reduced sensitivity in obese patients. The abnormal appendix is seen as a noncompressible tubular structure larger than 6 mm on US with decreased or absent flow on Doppler US in gangrenous appendicitis (Fig. 3.62A-C). The MRI appearance of acute appendicitis includes a dilated appendix, with wall thickness of greater than 2 mm and T2 hyperintense fluid intraluminally and in the adjacent periappendiceal fat (Fig. 3.62D).

The CT appearance of acute appendicitis depends on the degree of inflammation with mild cases showing a distended appendix up to 6 mm in diameter and minimal associated fat stranding. In more severe cases, circumferential wall thickening of the appendix with contrast enhancement and an appendiceal luminal diameter of up to 15 mm, with associated inflammatory fat stranding is seen. The presence of an abscess or extraluminal air may indicate the presence of appendiceal perforation (Fig. 3.63).

Acute exacerbation of **Crohn's disease** may present as right lower quadrant pain because of its predilection to affect the terminal ileum. CT or MR (preferred in younger patients) typically show mucosal enhancement and mural thickening with possible complications of fistula and abscess formation.

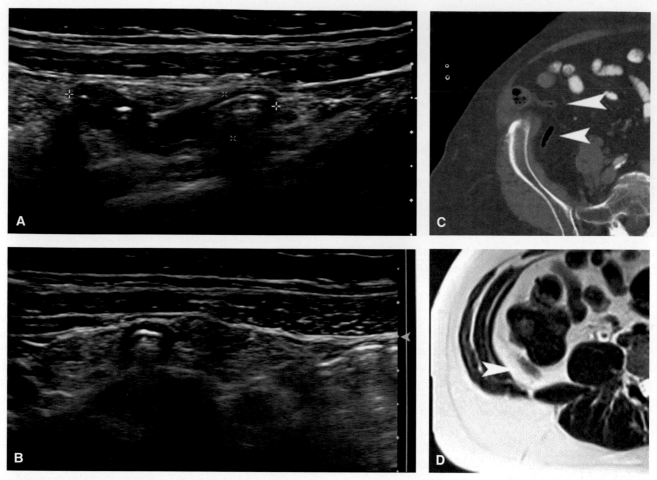

FIGURE 3.61. Normal appendix. A and B: Longitudinal and transverse ultrasound views showing a normal appendix without wall thickening or focal fluid collection. **C:** Axial CT shows a normal appendix (*arrowheads*). **D:** Axial MRI shows a normal appendix (*arrowhead*).

Right Upper Quadrant Pain

US is the first choice of initial investigation for biliary symptoms or right upper quadrant abdominal pain because it is very accurate at diagnosing or excluding gallstones (Fig. 3.64A and B). Most cases of **acute cholecystitis** are due to stone impaction in the cystic duct causing gallbladder distention. A positive scintigraphic Murphy sign in the presence of gallstones has a very high positive predictive value for the diagnosis of acute cholecystitis. Diffuse gallbladder wall thickening (greater than 3 mm) is seen in most patients with acute cholecystitis but is also found in other conditions including ascites, chronic liver disease, and heart failure. If US is negative, CECT is appropriate and useful for the diagnosis of complications such as gallbladder gangrene, gas formation, intraluminal hemorrhage, and perforation (Fig. 3.64C). However, the sensitivity of CT for the detection of gallstones is *less* than US because it is dependent on the different density of the gallstone relative to bile. **Chronic cholecystitis** is invariably associated with the presence of gallstones

which cause the gallbladder wall to become thickened and fibrotic. On CT, there may be absence of adjacent liver parenchymal hyperemia and pericholecystic inflammatory change, with nonvisualization of gallstones. Plain films are of limited value because only 20% of gallstones are radiopaque. The role of hepatobiliary scintigraphy is discussed in Chapter 10. **Acute acalculous cholecystitis (AAC)** accounts for 10% of all cases of acute cholecystitis and occurs more commonly in patients who are critically ill (Fig. 3.65). The risk factors for developing AAC include biliary stasis, cystic duct obstruction, and sepsis. Hepatic scintigraphy is of limited value with a false-positive rate of up to 40% in patients with AAC. Gallbladder gangrene and perforation are two serious complications of acute cholecystitis. Lack of gallbladder wall contrast enhancement on CT is seen in gangrene which may progress to perforation and a focal fluid collection in the gallbladder bed or the development of free intraperitoneal fluid. **Emphysematous cholecystitis** appears as intramural gas on CT (Fig. 3.66).

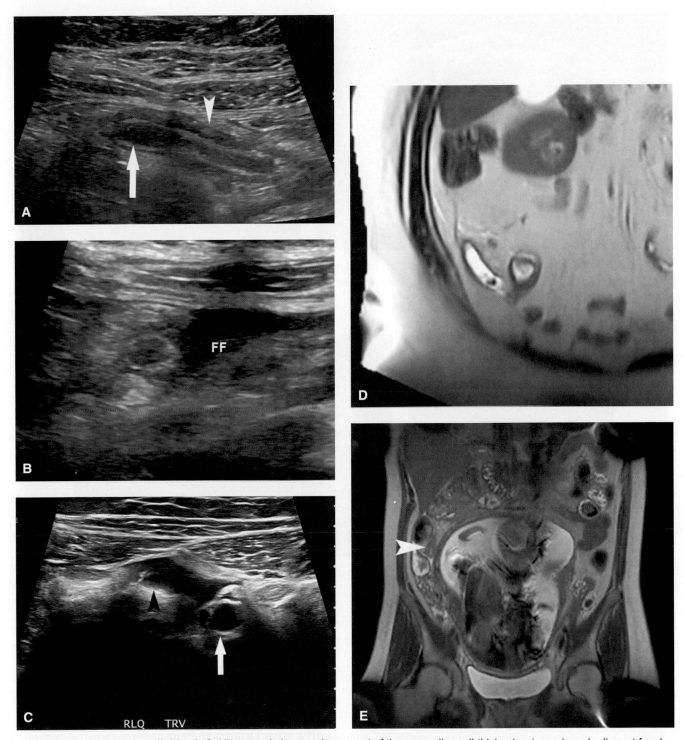

FIGURE 3.62. Acute appendicitis. A-C: Ultrasound shows enlargement of the appendix, wall thickening (*arrow*), and adjacent focal fluid (FF and *arrowheads*). **D:** MRI shows enlargement of the appendix with adjacent fluid. **E:** MRI showing an inflamed appendix (*arrowhead*) in a pregnant patient. Note relatively high position of appendix during pregnancy.

Percutaneous cholecystostomy is the treatment of choice in most patients with acute cholecystitis, allowing gallbladder decompression and resolution of inflammation, leading to a safer and less complicated interval cholecystectomy after 6 weeks.

Choledocholithiasis

Most bile duct stones have migrated from the gallbladder through a patent cystic duct and may present as biliary colic, acute pancreatitis, or cholangitis. MRCP, which is a

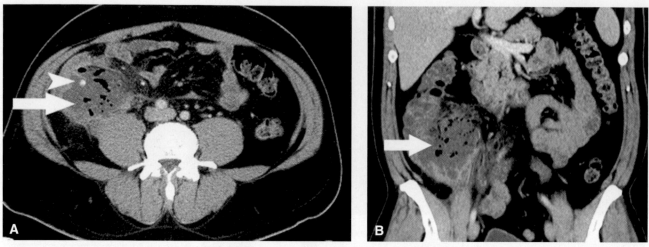

FIGURE 3.63. Appendiceal abscess. A and B: Axial and coronal reformatted CT shows a well-defined abscess (*arrows*) in the right lower quadrant secondary to appendicitis. Note the appendicolith (*arrowhead*).

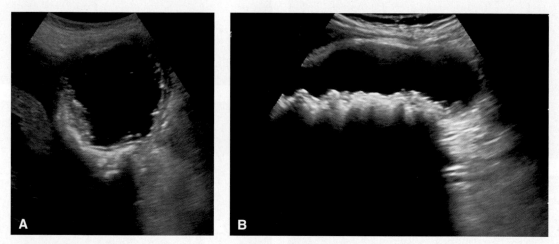

FIGURE 3.64. Acute cholecystitis. A and B: Ultrasound shows multiple gallstones with echogenic shadowing and a thickened gallbladder wall consistent with cholecystitis.

heavily weighted T2-weighted, thin slice MR examination, allows accurate diagnosis of choledocholithiasis, in which stones appear as well defined low signal intensity filling defects (Fig. 3.44B). In cholangitis, periportal inflammation is seen in the intra- and extrahepatic ductal system on MRCP. ERCP or percutaneous transhepatic cholangiography and drainage (PTCD) are necessary to decompress the obstructed common duct.

Liver diseases such as acute hepatitis, hepatic abscess, hepatic tumors which bleed, portal vein thrombosis, and Budd–Chiari syndrome may present with right upper quadrant pain. Before the widespread availability of antibiotics, seeding of the liver via the portal vein from appendicitis or diverticulitis was the most common cause of hepatic abscess. Currently, the biliary tract (cholecystitis) is the most common source of liver abscess. Both

US and CT are sensitive tests for detecting liver abscess (Fig. 3.67).

Acute appendicitis may present as right **upper** quadrant pain during pregnancy or in patients with a retro cecal appendix.

Left Lower Quadrant Pain

The most common cause of left lower quadrant pain in adults is **diverticulitis** which occurs in up to 25% of patients with diverticulosis. The role of imaging, preferably CECT of the abdomen and pelvis, is to confirm the diagnosis of diverticulitis, evaluate the extent of disease, and detect possible complications such as abscesses, fistulas, obstruction, or perforation, before deciding on appropriate conservative, interventional, or surgical treatment. In general, oral contrast is not given as it is of limited diagnostic benefit in

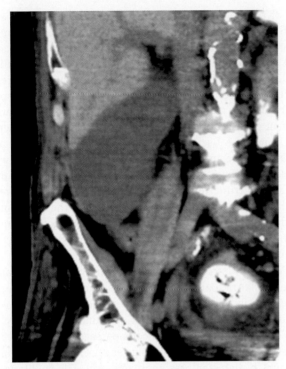

FIGURE 3.65. **Acute a calculus cholecystitis.** Coronal reformat. CT shows a distended gallbladder without stones.

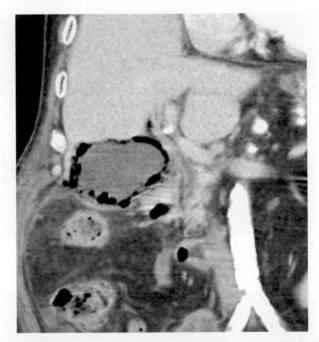

FIGURE 3.66. **Acute emphysematous cholecystitis.** Coronal reformat. CT shows intramural gas in the gallbladder wall.

patients with abdominal pain. In patients with diverticulitis, rectal contrast may have a limited role in the diagnosis of perforation. CT findings of diverticulitis include bowel wall thickening (greater than 3 mm in colonic inflammation and diverticulosis (Fig. 3.68). The presence of an abscess, free air or free fluid should be sought as percutaneous drainage or surgery may be indicated (Fig. 3.69 and 3.70). Other complications of diverticulitis include bowel obstruction and fistula formation. The differential diagnosis

of perforated diverticulitis includes perforated colon cancer, which should be excluded once inflammation resolves.

Renal Calculi

Renal calculi affect approximately 1 in 11 people in the United States, and ureteric colic accounts for approximately 1% of all hospital admissions. Current recommendations from the American College of Radiology (ACR) and the American Urological Association are for a low-dose noncontrast CT (NCCT) CT stone protocol of the abdomen and pelvis in patients presenting with suspected renal calculi. The

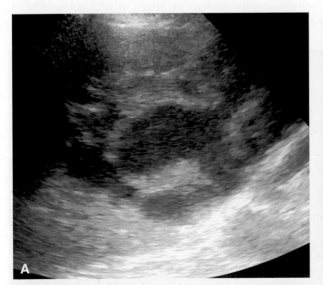

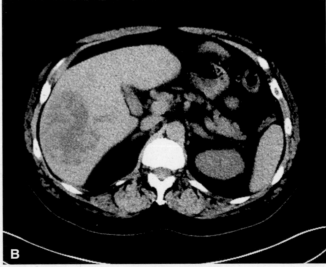

FIGURE 3.67. **Liver abscess. A:** Ultrasound of the liver shows a regular poorly defined hypoechoic mass consistent with abscess. **B:** Axial CT shows a large heterogeneous hypodense mass.

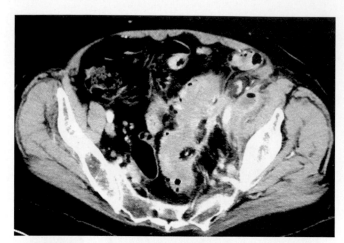

FIGURE 3.68. Diverticulitis. Axial CT shows diffuse inflamed sigmoid colon and a small associated diverticular abscess.

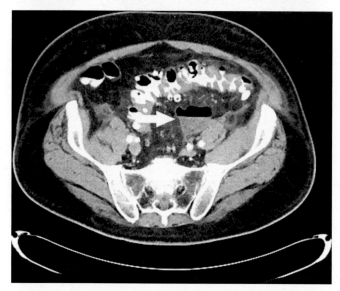

FIGURE 3.69. Diverticular abscess. Axial CT shows a large left lower quadrant fluid collection (*arrow*) with a fluid level.

use of IV contrast is not recommended except in patients with unilateral renal enlargement with risk factors for renal infarction or vein thrombosis, renal mass or complicated cyst, or unexplained hematuria. The use of plain films (KUB) are of limited value in patients with suspected renal calculi because of their relatively low sensitivity and specificity and are reserved for surgical planning, confirmation of stent placement, and follow-up of calculi posttreatment.

US may be used for detection of hydronephrosis and should be the initial modality in pregnant women with flank pain. Physiologic right hydronephrosis may occur in the second trimester due to obstruction of the distal ureter by the gravid uterus. MRI should be used in the first trimester during organogenesis and CT during the second trimester because of its higher sensitivity than MRI for detecting calculi.

While CT stone protocol and intravenous urography have similar radiation doses, CT has a higher detection rate for calculi in the distal ureter. An added benefit of CT was the detection of significant additional findings.

The likelihood of spontaneous passage of a ureteral calculus is related to both stone size and location. Most stones ≤4 mm in diameter pass spontaneously. The spontaneous passage rate of a stone in diameter ≥5 mm falls progressively with increasing size. Calculi often lodge at one of three narrow locations of the ureter: (1) the ureteropelvic junction, (2) the level of the common iliac artery and vein, and (3) the ureterovesical junction. Proximal ureteral stones are less likely to pass spontaneously.

Imaging is not necessary to diagnose **acute pyelonephritis** and should be reserved for patients who do not demonstrate clinical improvement after 72 hours of antibiotic treatment. Imaging is recommended in specific patient groups who are at increased risk of disease progression including diabetics, pregnancy, elderly, immunocompromised, or those with a congenital, GU abnormality. CTU consists of a noncontrast scan followed

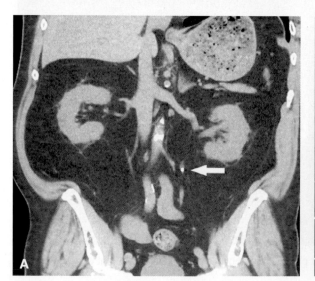
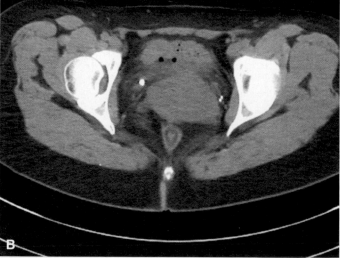

FIGURE 3.70. Ureteral calculi in different patients. **A:** Coronal CT showing a calculus in the left mid ureter (*arrow*). **B:** Axial CT shows a distal right ureteral calculus and left pelvic venous phlebolith.

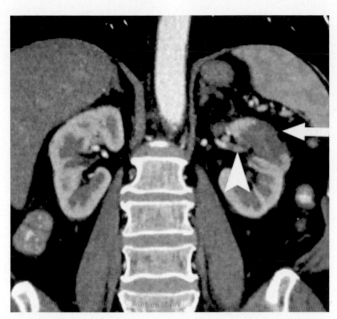

FIGURE 3.71. Renal infarct. Coronal CT shows a wedge perfusion defect in the upper pole of the left kidney (*arrow*) secondary to thrombus in a renal artery branch (*arrowhead*).

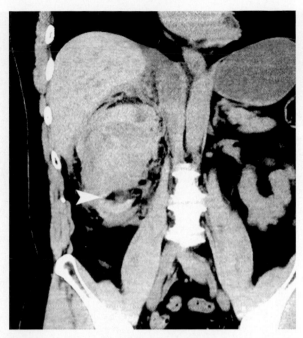

FIGURE 3.72. Renal angiomyolipoma. Coronal reformat CT shows a large right renal hematoma due to lower pole angiomyolipoma (*arrowhead*).

by a scan 90 seconds after injection of IV contrast when there is uniform enhancement of the renal parenchyma (nephrographic phase). A third scan is performed during the excretory phase for visualization of the collecting systems, ureters, and bladder. A split dose protocol is preferred in younger patients to reduce the radiation dose (see workup of hematuria). CT findings of acute pyelonephritis include a delayed or striated nephrogram, renal enlargement, urothelial enhancement, and inflammatory changes in perirenal fascia. US is usually normal in acute pyelonephritis and may be used to exclude obstruction. If both infection and obstruction (**pyonephrosis**) are present, prompt decompression by either percutaneous nephrostomy or ureteral stent is recommended.

Acute renal infarction presents as sudden onset, flank pain, the most common cause of which is an embolism from a cardiac source. CT urography may show an occluded renal artery or branch with wedge-shaped infarct (Fig. 3.71). The differential diagnosis includes acute pyelonephritis in which the CT shows perinephric inflammation and urothelial enhancement. Prompt catheter-directed thrombolysis of the occluded artery may restore flow and preserve renal function. **Renal vein thrombosis** may occur secondary to tumor extension or in hypercoagulable states such as nephrotic syndrome. The onset of symptoms may be subacute. CT findings include an enlarged kidney with edema of the renal sinus and perinephric fact. Tumor thrombus typically enhances and distends the renal vein (Fig. 3.52C-E)

In patients with **spontaneous renal hemorrhage**, CT urography is the study of choice with acute hemorrhage seen on the noncontrast scan and contrast extravasation present on the arterial phase. Spontaneous hemorrhage is most commonly due to a renal mass such as renal cell carcinoma or an angiomyolipoma (AML), a benign renal tumor in which elastin poor aneurysms may develop and grow (Fig. 3.72). When an AML is greater than 4 cm, the risk of spontaneous hemorrhage is over 50% and an aneurysm diameter of greater than 5 mm is a positive predictor of subsequent hemorrhage. Most patients with small AMLs should undergo CT surveillance with selective embolization indicated in patients with large AMLs.

Inflammatory Bowel Disease and Acute Infectious Enterocolitides

Contrast CT is the modality of choice because of its ability to detect unsuspected abnormalities including complications in contrast to plain films which have limited sensitivity and specificity. The causes of an acute abdomen in patients with **IBD** (UC, Crohn's disease) include severe colitis and mesenteric venous thrombosis. The CT findings of severe colitis include nodular or asymmetric fold thickening, submucosal edema, and edema of the pericolonic soft tissue. If the colonic lumen is greater than 6 cm in diameter, it is regarded to be a **megacolon**, in the presence of colitis (Fig. 3.73; Table 3.18). Use of the adjective "toxic" to describe a megacolon should be reserved based on the clinical findings and is not an appropriate radiological diagnosis. Patients with IBD are hypercoagulable with a complication of acute mesenteric vein thrombosis occurring in less than 1%. CT findings include small bowel wall thickening, mucosal hyperenhancement, and submucosal edema. Two

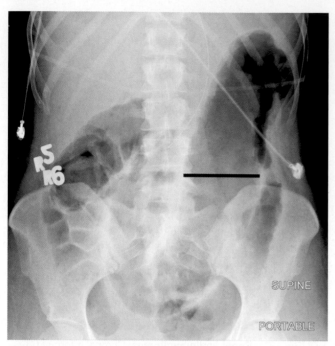

FIGURE 3.73. Megacolon. Supine abdominal film showing a dilated (8 cm) transverse colon (*black line*).

TABLE 3.18	Causes of a Megacolon

Ulcerative colitis
Crohn's disease
Infection—Pseudomembranous colitis
Ischemia

The term "toxic megacolon" should only be used in the appropriate clinical setting.

complications specific to Crohn's disease are SBO and penetrating disease. SBO is usually caused by stenotic disease or adhesions rising from prior surgery. The development of sinus tracts, fistulae, abscess formation, and rarely free perforation are collectively known as penetrating disease, a hallmark of Crohn's disease. Interestingly, small bowel perforation occurs more commonly than colonic perforation in Crohn's disease and is often from a single site.

Infectious enterocolitides. Patients with infectious colitis rarely present with an acute abdomen, and do not require imaging. Nonspecific findings on CT include wall thickening and homogeneous hyperenhancement with soft tissue stranding and edema (Fig. 3.74). Patients with *Clostridium difficile* colitis may be clinically toxic and develop a megacolon in addition to the previously described finding of wall thickening. Pneumatosis may occur with loss of mucosal integrity but does not imply ischemia.

Neutropenic colitis (typhlitis) affects the cecum and terminal ileum in patients who are neutropenic post

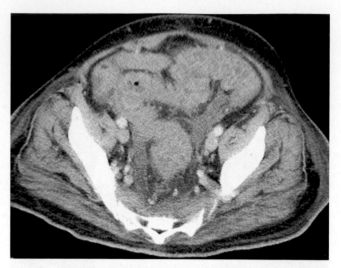

FIGURE 3.74. Pseudomembranous colitis. Axial CT showing a diffuse inflamed colon, the differential diagnosis which includes infection, ischemia, and diverticular disease. *Clostridium difficile* was isolated.

chemotherapy. CT findings of wall thickening and adjacent soft tissue stranding are similar to those found in *C. diff.* colitis.

Acute Pancreatitis

Acute pancreatitis consists of a local inflammation of the gland and exaggerated systemic inflammatory response to the pancreatic injury which may result in organ failure. Alcohol abuse and gallstones are the two most common causes of acute pancreatitis. Most cases of acute pancreatitis are mild with severe complications including organ failure, occurring in up to 20%. The **Revised Atlanta Classification of Acute Pancreatitis (2012)** distinguishes between an early (within the first week) and a late (after the first week) phase of the disease. During the early phase, the severity is determined by the presence of organ failure secondary to a systemic inflammatory response syndrome (SIRS) rather than the development of local complications. The late phase only occurs in patients with moderately severe or severe pancreatitis as patients with mild pancreatitis do not develop organ failure, or local complications.

Typically, imaging in acute pancreatitis is generally not indicated within the first few days of presentation, as complications such as necrosis are rarely seen before 5 to 7 days and initial management is dictated by scoring systems assessing clinical severity. Acute pancreatitis may be classified on the basis of the presence or absence of necrosis on CECT. A dual-phase CT, in which the patient is imaged at 40 seconds (arterial phase) and at 80 seconds (portal venous phase) after injection of IV contrast, is used to diagnose complications. Under the revised Atlanta classification, the generic terms of abscess, phlegmon, and "fluid collection" are no longer used. In interstitial

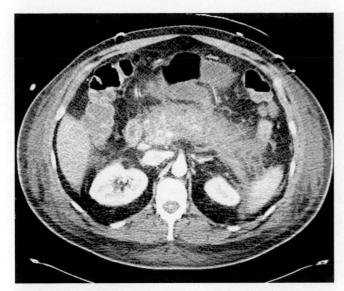

FIGURE 3.75. Acute pancreatitis. Axial CT with contrast shows diffuse inflamed pancreas without necrosis.

edematous pancreatitis (IEP) which accounts for 90% of cases, the gland enhances without necrosis and peripancreatic inflammation is seen. (Fig. 3.75) Complications of IEP include acute peripancreatic fluid collections (APFC) and pseudocysts. A pseudocyst contains pancreatic juice, has a well-defined wall, and usually develops after 4 weeks (Fig. 3.76). Pseudocysts do not contain necrotic debris and are of homogeneously high signal intensity on T2-weighted images on MRI. In necrotizing pancreatitis, CT shows variable areas of acute necrotic collections, walled off necrosis

or postnecrosectomy pseudocyst. The lack of gas in a collection does not exclude infection. MRI is more sensitive than CT for detecting hemorrhage and for diagnosing a fistula between fluid collections in the pancreatic duct. MRI allows distinction between a pseudocyst which has a uniform hyperintense signal on T2-weighted images, from necrotic collections which are heterogeneous and contain regions of relative T2 hypointensity and occasionally T1 hyperintensity from blood products and fat lobules.

Bowel Obstruction

Small bowel obstruction (SBO) and large bowel obstruction (LBO) account for almost 1/5 cases of acute abdomen in adults. The causes of bowel obstruction vary depending on location. Table 3.3. Carcinoma of the colon accounts for over half of LBO cases in adults. Adhesions and hernias cause LBO less frequently than SBO because of the characteristically fixed nature of the colon and its larger caliber. CT accurately detects both the site and cause of obstruction in most patients. Complications of obstruction such as ischemia, perforation, and pneumatosis are also readily detectable on CT. On plain film, the bowel is usually dilated proximal to the obstruction, depending on the competence of the ileocecal valve. However plain films are only moderately sensitive in the diagnosis of SBO and are poor in the diagnosis of closed-loop, ischemic, or strangling obstruction.

Adhesions are the most common cause of SBO, the incidence of which has increased in recent years due to the increasing number of laparotomies performed. While adhesions are not directly seen on CT, the abrupt transition from

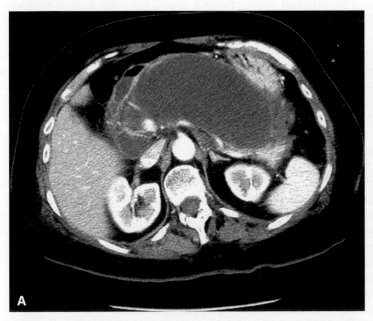

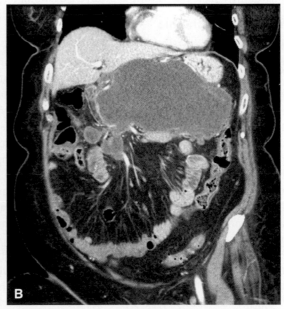

FIGURE 3.76. Pancreatic pseudocyst. A: Axial and **B:** Coronal CT with contrast showing a large well-defined uniformly low cyst 6 weeks after an episode of acute pancreatitis.

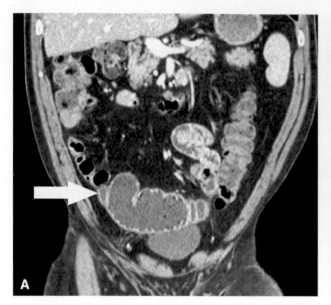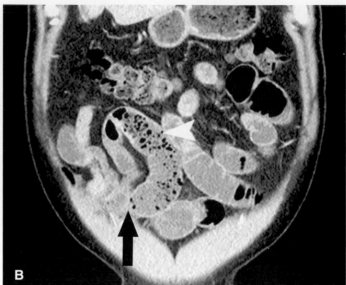

FIGURE 3.77. Small bowel obstruction. A: Coronal reformat CT shows a dilated loop of small bowel proximal to a transition point (*arrow*), beyond which the bowel is of normal caliber. **B:** In a different patient, the transition point (*arrow*) marks the site of obstruction due to adhesions. Intraluminal gas—"feces sign" (*arrowhead*)—is seen in the dilated small bowel proximal to the site of obstruction in the right lower quadrant.

dilated to non-dilated small bowel occurs at the site of the obstruction. The small bowel feces sign may be seen proximal to the obstruction (Fig. 3.77).

In patients with partial or intermittent SBO, oral contrast may add functional information to CECT. However, oral contrast should not be used if high-grade SBO is suspected, as the contrast will not reach the site of obstruction, will not add to diagnostic accuracy, and can lead to complications, particularly vomiting. MRI is more appropriate in younger patients who have had multiple prior CT examinations.

Mesenteric Ischemia

Mesenteric ischemia may be acute or chronic depending on the duration of onset and status of underlying arteries. Arterial emboli from a cardiac source are the most common causes of acute mesenteric ischemia in which patients present with sudden onset of abdominal pain. Older patients may have preexisting atherosclerotic stenoses in the mesenteric circulation (celiac, superior and inferior mesenteric arteries) and more typically present with chronic symptoms of postprandial pain and weight loss. Treatment of ischemia due to proximal stenosis is possible with endovascular stent placement (Fig. 3.78). Bowel infarction causes intramural gas (pneumatosis) and portal vein gas which is an ominous sign (Fig. 3.79). Rarely, systemic vasculitides such as polyarteritis nodosa and SLE may cause distal mesenteric ischemia. Less common forms of mesenteric ischemia include **venous ischemia**, which is more common in patients with a history of hypercoagulability and IBD (Fig. 3.80). **Nonocclusive mesenteric ischemia** (NOMI) occurs most commonly in

elderly patients as a result of low cardiac output and dehydration. Another population at risk of NOMI are end-stage renal disease patients on hemodialysis. These patients are known to have atherosclerotic disease, the effect of which is exaggerated by hypotension, which may occur transiently during hemodialysis.

Abdominal Aortic Aneurysm Rupture

The mortality rate for ruptured abdominal aortic aneurysm is over 80% making it one of the most fatal surgical conditions. The risk of rupture depends on aneurysm size. In male patients with 6.0-cm or greater AAA, the rate of rupture is 14.1% per year, and in female patients with 6.0-cm or greater AAA, it is 22.3% per year. Patients typically present with nonspecific features such as abdominal or back pain and hypotension so a high index of suspicion is necessary. While NCCT is adequate to diagnose an acute aneurysm rupture, CECT allows better delineation of the aneurysm and visualization of visceral vessels (Fig. 3.81; Table 3.19). CTA of the abdomen and pelvis is necessary if endovascular repair (EVAR) is planned for measurement of proximal and distal fixation sites and to determine patency of both common femoral arteries for access. However, the availability of emergent EVAR for ruptured AAA varies between institutions and includes the placement of an aorto-uniliac stent graft and femoral to femoral artery bypass graft.

Retroperitoneum and Abdominal Wall

Patients receiving anticoagulation are at increased risk of bleeding. Two common sites of bleeding, presenting

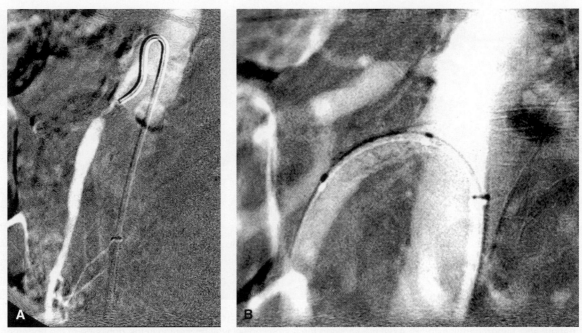

FIGURE 3.78. **Mesenteric ischemia. A:** Selective angiography of the superior mesenteric artery (SMA) shows a greater than 80% proximal stenosis in a patient with weight loss and postprandial angina. **B:** Stenting of proximal SMA stenosis with markedly improved flow.

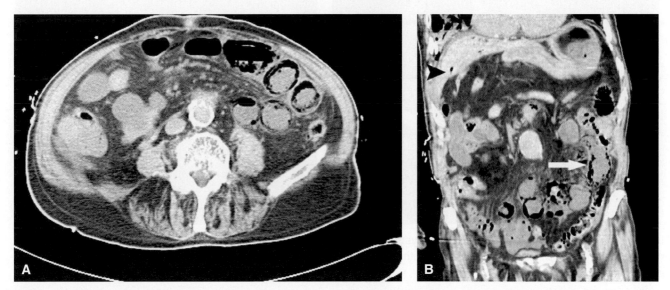

FIGURE 3.79. **Mesenteric infarction. A:** Axial and **B:** coronal CT showing extensive pneumatosis intestinalis (intramural gas) (*arrow*) with gas in the portal venous system (*arrowhead*).

as an acute abdomen, are the retroperitoneum and the rectus muscle in the anterior abdominal wall (Fig. 3.82). Embolization with coils of the lumbar arteries and inferior epigastric artery, respectively, is the appropriate treatment if there is a significant hematoma.

Necrotizing fasciitis is a severe infection that develops suddenly and spreads rapidly, occurring most commonly in the limbs and perineum (Fig. 3.83). Most cases are due to more than one bacteria, and treatment includes emergent surgical debridement and antibiotics.

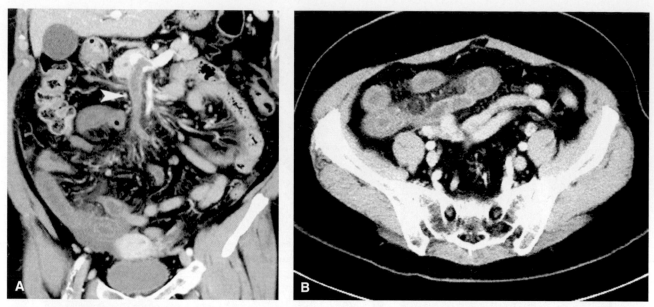

FIGURE 3.80. Mesenteric venous thrombosis. A: Coronal CT showing extensive thrombosis of the superior mesenteric vein (*arrowhead*) in a patient with hypercoagulability. **B:** Axial CT showing focal small bowel wall thickening in the right side of the abdomen and normal-appearing bowel in the left abdomen.

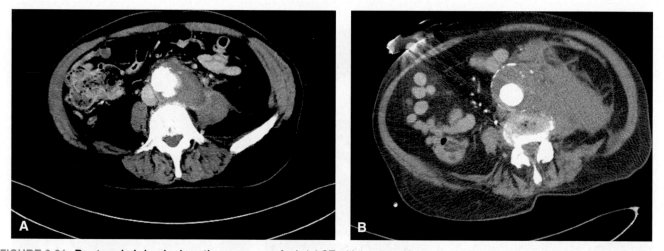

FIGURE 3.81. Ruptured abdominal aortic aneurysm. A: Axial CT with contrast shows an aortic aneurysm with retroperitoneal leak extending to the left. **B:** Different patient, axial CT with contrast showing a large left retroperitoneal hematoma due to a leaking abdominal aortic aneurysm.

TABLE 3.19	CT Findings of Rupture or Impending Rupture of Abdominal Aortic Aneurysm
Primary	**Secondary**
Retroperitoneal hematoma	Hyperattenuating present sign
Contrast extravasation	Focal discontinuity of intimal calcification
Perianeurysmal stranding	

Modified from Rakita D, Newatia A, Hines JJ, Siegel DN, Friedman B. Spectrum of CT findings in rupture and impending rupture of abdominal aortic aneurysms. *Radiographics.* 2007;27(2):497-507.

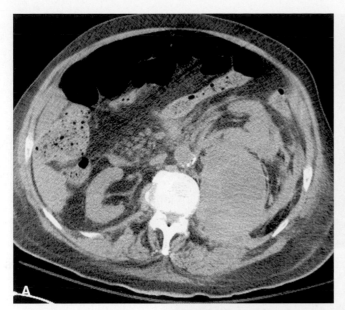

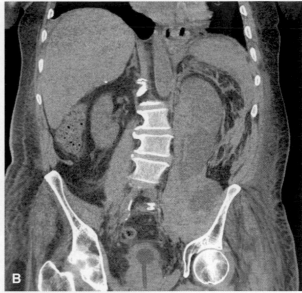

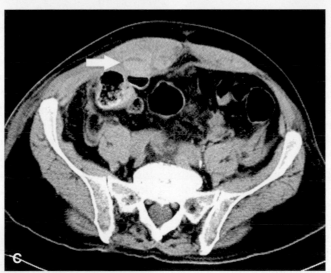

FIGURE 3.82. Retroperitoneal and rectus sheath hematoma. A and B: Axial and coronal CT showing a large left retroperitoneal hematoma in an anticoagulated patient. **C:** Axial CT showing a rectus sheath hematoma (*arrow*) in the anterior abdominal wall in an anticoagulated patient.

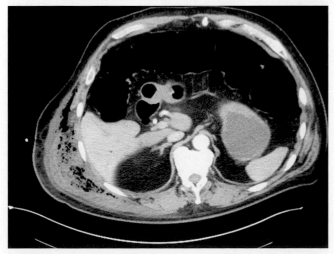

FIGURE 3.83. Necrotizing fasciitis. Axial CT showing subcutaneous gas and inflammation in the right lower chest wall.

TRAUMA

Blunt Trauma

Abdominal trauma can be divided into **blunt** and **penetrating** injuries with penetrating injuries further divided into stab and gunshot wounds. The patient's hemodynamic status is the primary initial focus of evaluation as most hemodynamically **unstable** patients with abdominal trauma will require emergent surgical management, while many hemodynamically **stable** patients can be managed nonoperatively.

Unstable patients (those with unresponsive profound hypotension despite resuscitation) should have an immediate bedside focused abdominal sonography for trauma **(FAST)** that evaluates the dependent intraperitoneal sites where blood can accumulate which includes the hepatorenal space (Morison pouch), splenorenal space, suprapubic region (bladder and pouch of Douglas), and the

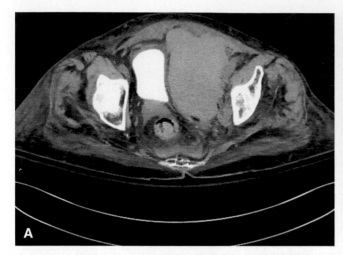
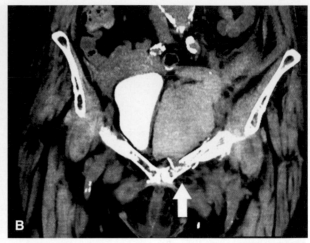

FIGURE 3.84. Pelvic fracture and hematoma. A: Axial and **B:** coronal CT showing a left pelvic fracture (*arrow*) and associated hematoma.

pericardium. A positive FAST suggests that intra-abdominal bleeding is the source of hypotension. Unstable patients with hemoperitoneum on US and no sign of hemopericardium or another immediately treatable cause of hypotension such as pneumothorax should proceed to immediate laparotomy. A negative FAST in a hypotensive patient may indicate bleeding elsewhere, such as the retroperitoneum or associated with a pelvic fracture (Fig. 3.84). Additionally, US is not sensitive for spleen and liver lacerations or for bowel injury.

Unstable patients do not belong in radiology departments and unstable patients should not be long in radiology departments. With the advent of multidetector CT, a CT scan of the head and neck, chest, abdomen and pelvis can be performed in less than 60 seconds and is feasible and justifiable in unstable patients if performed and interpreted rapidly by a well-organized trauma team and if there is no delay in time-critical interventions such as emergent surgery or angiography with embolization. On the other hand, one should resist the temptation to obtain "one more imaging test" as these patients require immediate surgery. If unstable patients are not responding to resuscitation and if they have clear clinical or suspected evidence of abdominal injury, they should go immediately to the operating room.

In a **stable** patient, CECT abdomen and pelvis with portal venous phase images for optimal visualization of visceral bleeding is recommended (Figs. 3.85 and 3.86). Dependingon the nature and mechanism of injury, CT of the chest with contrast can be incorporated into this examination. The liver is the most commonly injured organ in blunt abdominal trauma and the second most commonly injured organ (after bowel) in penetrating abdominal trauma. Stable patients with injuries of the **liver or spleen** and intraperitoneal blood may be managed conservatively with close observation only. While the CT-based grading systems for liver or spleen contusion, lacerations, and

avulsions are useful for describing the nature and extent of organ injury, the decision on which patients need surgery or other interventions such as arterial embolization depends on their clinical status. Abdominal US has a lower sensitivity than CT for the detection of abdominal injury, and a negative US examination is insufficient evidence on which to discharge patients home following abdominal trauma.

Conservative management of **renal trauma** is usually appropriate for a contusion or minor laceration. Renal angiography with possible embolization is indicated if there is bleeding on CT, an enlarging hematoma, or a major laceration or avulsion. (Fig. 3.87). Patients with gross hematuria

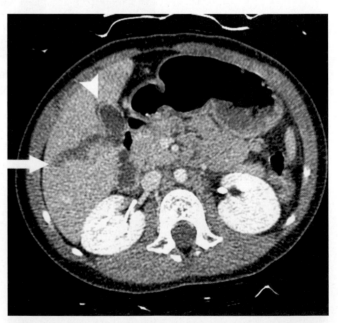

FIGURE 3.85. Liver laceration. Blunt trauma. Axial CT showing a liver laceration (*arrow*) and free fluid in the gallbladder fossa (*arrowhead*).

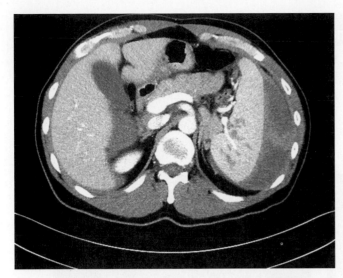

FIGURE 3.86. **Splenic laceration.** Blunt trauma. Axial CT showing a perisplenic hematoma due to a splenic laceration.

and pelvic fracture require a CT cystogram using dilute iodinated contrast infused via an indwelling Foley catheter to exclude bladder rupture. High-grade blunt and penetrating kidney injuries managed nonoperatively are associated with 11.1% and 20.0% complication rates, respectively, identified on follow-up CT, usually in 8 to 10 days so routine CT follow-up may not be justified in all patients (Table 3.20).

Signs of pancreatic injury on CT include peripancreatic fluid (nonspecific), fluid between the pancreatic parenchyma and splenic vein (specific) and direct visualization of pancreatic contusion or laceration. The serum amylase and lipase levels are often normal within the first 3 to 6 hours following trauma.

Penetrating Trauma

Abdominal gunshot wounds, due to their higher kinetic energy, are associated with higher mortality rates than

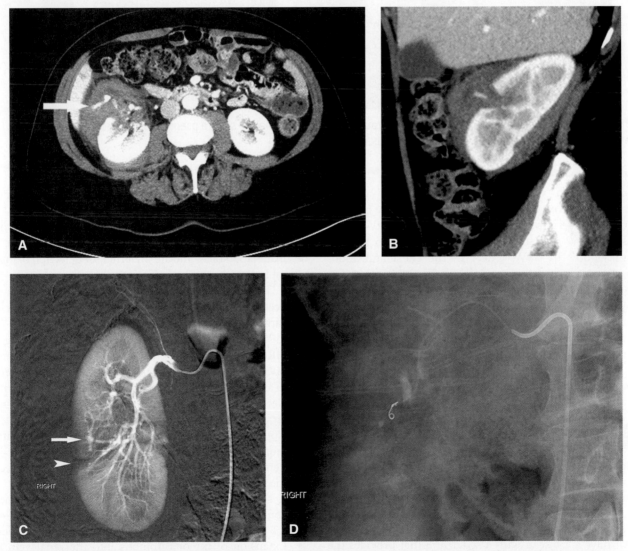

FIGURE 3.87. **Renal laceration.** Blunt trauma. **A and B:** Axial and sagittal CT shows a right renal laceration with associated pseudoaneurysm (*arrow*). **C:** Selective right renal angiogram shows a distal arterial pseudoaneurysm (*arrow*) due to a parenchymal laceration (*arrowhead*). **D:** Embolization of right artery distal pseudoaneurysm with coils.

TABLE 3.20	Complications of Renal Trauma	
Early		**Late**
Urinoma		Hydronephrosis
Pseudoaneurysm		AV fistula
Fistula		Hypertension
Hypertension		Ureteral stricture

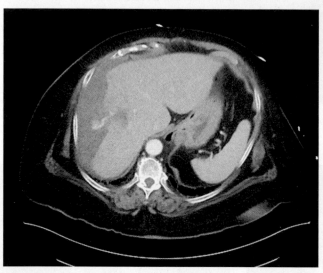 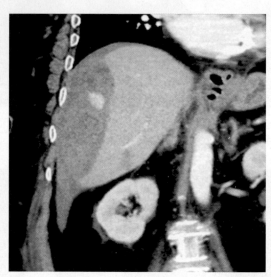

FIGURE 3.88. Liver laceration due to penetrating trauma. Axial and coronal CT show a pseudoaneurysm and large perihepatic hematoma which was successfully treated with coil embolization.

abdominal stab wounds. Abdominal aortic injuries caused by **penetrating trauma**, most commonly gunshot wounds (GSW), are associated with a mortality rate in excess of 50%. CT scout films can be used to localize foreign bodies in GSW. CECT of the chest and abdomen is recommended, especially if the entry wound is below intermammary line in stab wounds and almost always with GSW. Consider triple-phase contrast CT (noncontrast, scan at 40 seconds for arterial extravasation and scan at 80 seconds for venous extravasation in the upper abdomen) and consider adding a fourth phase (5–10 minutes delay) if the kidney and ureter are in the injury trajectory (Fig. 3.88).

KEY POINTS

- Plain films are mainly used to detect calcific and other opacities and bowel gas patterns.
- The main differential diagnoses for too much bowel gas is adynamic ileus and bowel obstruction.
- Many patients being investigated for an acute abdomen will have a CT scan with a scout film that provides the same information as a radiographic plain film.

- Upright or decubitus plain films are optimal for the demonstration of free intraperitoneal air.
- Upper and lower GI barium series may be single or double contrast. Double contrast examinations involve the insufflation of air and are preferred for detection of mucosal lesions.
- CTE and MRE of the tests of choice in patients with suspected Crohn's disease as SBFT does not reliably exclude early Crohn's disease.
- MRI accurately stages rectal carcinoma by imaging the MRF and measuring the circumferential resection margin. MRI can be repeated after neoadjuvant chemoradiotherapy to assess the treatment response and for surgical planning.
- Not every patient who has a CT scan with contrast requires a noncontrast scan beforehand.
- Not every patient who has a CT scan with contrast requires delayed imaging.
- Renal US and CT urography are the main tests used in the workup of hematuria.
- A split bolus CTU protocol may be used in patients younger 45 years to reduce radiation dose.
- CT is superior to MRI for the detection of renal calculi.
- Extension of tumor thrombus into the renal vein is a poor prognostic feature.

- Most adrenal adenomas are nonfunctioning and can be characterized by measuring contrast washout on delayed CT scans.
- For abdominal aortic aneurysms of similar size, women have a relatively higher risk of rupture than men.
- In the management of unstable trauma patients, imaging should be focused and expedited as these patients require emergent surgery.

Further Readings

General Reference

1. Gore R, Levine M, eds. *Textbook of Gastrointestinal Radiology*. Elsevier; 2015.

Imaging During Pregnancy

1. Bahouth SM, Wong VK, Kampalath RV, et al. US findings of first-trimester pregnancy radiographics fundamentals | online presentation. *Radiographics*. 2018;38:2193-2194. doi:10.1148/rg.2018180065.
2. Shur J, Bottomley C, Walton K, et al. Imaging of acute abdominal pain in the third trimester of pregnancy. *BMJ*. 2018;361:10. doi:1136/bmj.k2511.

Acute Pancreatitis

1. Banks PA, Bollen TL, Dervenis C, et al. Classification of acute pancreatitis—2012: revision of the Atlanta classification and definitions by international consensus. *Gut*. 2013;62:102-111. doi:10.1136/gutjnl-2012-302779.
2. Vege SS, Ziring B, Jain R, et al. American gastroenterological association institute guideline on the diagnosis and management of asymptomatic neoplastic pancreatic cysts. *Gastroenterology*. 2015;148:819-822; quize 812-813. doi:10.1053/j.gastro.2015.01.015.

Adrenal Masses

1. Boland GWL, Blake MA, Hahn PF, et al. Incidental adrenal lesions: principles, techniques, and algorithms for imaging characterization. *Radiology*. 2008;249:756-775. doi:10.1148/radiol.2493070976.

Non Alcoholic Fatty Liver Disease

1. Byrne CD, Patel J, Scorletti E, et al. Tests for diagnosing and monitoring non-alcoholic fatty liver disease in adults. *BMJ*. 2018;362:10. doi:1136/bmj.k2734.
2. Kennedy P, Wagner M, Castéra L, et al. Quantitative elastography methods in liver disease: current evidence and future directions. *Radiology*. 2018;286:738-763. doi:10.1148/radiol.2018170601.

Renal Masses

1. Herts BR, Silverman SG, Hindman NM, et al. Management of the incidental renal mass on CT: a white paper of the ACR Incidental Findings Committee. *J Am Coll Radiol*. 2018;15:264-273. doi:10.1016/j.jacr.2017.04.028.
2. Ward RD, Remer EM. Cystic renal masses: an imaging update. *Eur J Radiol*. 2018;99:103-110. doi:10.1016/j.ejrad.2017.12.015.

Staging of Rectal Carcinoma

1. Horvat N, Rocha CCT, Oliveira BC, et al. Mri of rectal cancer: tumor staging, imaging techniques, and management. *Radiographics*. 2019;39:367-387. doi:10.1148/rg.2019180114.

CT Protocols

1. Johnson PT, Bello JA, Chatfield MB, et al. New ACR choosing wisely recommendations: judicious use of multiphase abdominal CT protocols. *J Am Coll Radiol*. 2019;16:56-60. doi:10.1016/j.jacr.2018.07.026.

Questions

1. True or False: Squamous carcinoma account over 90% of all cases of esophageal malignancies.

2. True or False: Barrett esophagus is a risk factor for the development of squamous esophageal carcinoma.

3. True or False: Adrenal vein sampling is used for the investigation of pheochromocytoma.

4. True or False: The severity of acute pancreatitis in the early phase is determined by the development of local complications rather than the presence of organ failure secondary to a systemic inflammatory response syndrome.

5. True or False: "Toxic" megacolon can be reliably diagnosed on plain films.

6. True or False: Most gallstones are radiopaque on plain films.

7. True or False: 20% of all renal calculi are not radiopaque on plain films.

8. True or False: The presence of pneumatosis implies bowel infarction and is always an ominous sign.

9. True or False: US and MRI are the preferred modalities for investigation of acute appendicitis in pregnancy.

10. True or False: CT and MRI have equivalent accuracy in the detection of renal calculi.

CHAPTER 4

Pelvic Imaging, Including Obstetric Ultrasound

Carolyn Donaldson, MD • Thomas A. Farrell, MB, BCh

Imaging of the pelvis uses three modalities US, CT, and MRI, in that order of frequency. US is the most frequently used when gynecologic pathology is suspected. CT is more commonly performed when GI or GU pathology is suspected and MRI is usually performed for further evaluation of a complex finding on US or CT. MRI also plays an important role in the pregnant patient when US is limited by the enlarged uterus, for example, in the setting of suspected acute appendicitis.

SCROTAL IMAGING

Ultrasound is the modality of choice for evaluation of the scrotum. Common indications for scrotal US include palpable mass or pain. In patients with a palpable **scrotal mass**, US allows the important distinction between intra- and extratesticular masses. Extratesticular masses are overwhelmingly benign. When a mass is intratesticular, the key question is whether the mass is cystic or solid. Cystic testicular masses are overwhelmingly benign and solid testicular masses are malignant until proven otherwise (Fig. 4.1).

The most common cause of a palpable scrotal mass is an **epididymal cyst** or spermatocele which develops from obstruction of the ejaculatory duct. They are usually small (<1 cm) but can become quite large (Fig. 4.2). Intratesticular cystic masses are usually tunica albuginea cysts (Fig. 4.3). Hydroceles are the most common extratesticular cause of scrotal enlargement. They can occur after scrotal inflammation or as an extension of ascites through a patent processes vaginalis.

In the setting of acute scrotal **pain**, Doppler US is helpful to evaluate for hyperemia which can also be seen with infection (such as epididymitis) versus lack of flow or ischemia (in the setting of testicular torsion). **Epididymitis** is the most common cause of scrotal pain and swelling. Imaging includes an enlarged hyperemic epididymis. **Epididymo-orchitis** results from a more prolonged infection and appears as an enlarged hyperemic epididymis and with associated orchitis (Figs. 4.4 and 4.5).

Varicoceles are a common cause of scrotal pain, enlargement, or palpable mass. Primary varicoceles result from incompetent valves in the internal spermatic vein, and they

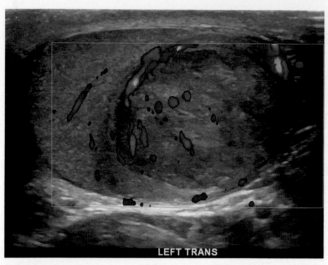

FIGURE 4.1. **Testicular neoplasm.** Ultrasound shows a solid vascular testicular mass.

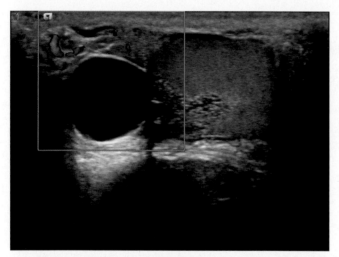

FIGURE 4.2. **Epididymal cyst.** Ultrasound shows an extratesticular cyst.

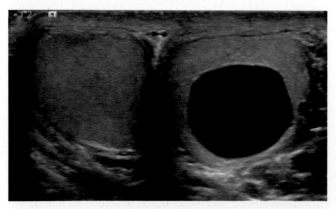

FIGURE 4.3. **Tunica albuginea cyst.** Ultrasound shows an intratesticular cyst.

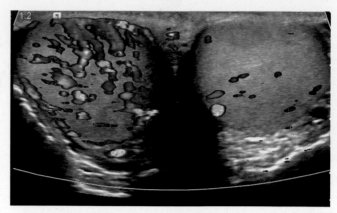

FIGURE 4.4. **Orchitis.** Color Doppler shows increased flow in the right testis and normal vascularity in the left testis.

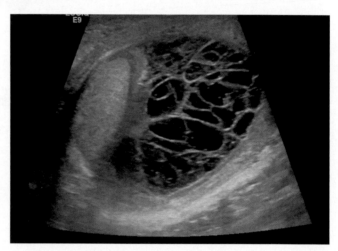

FIGURE 4.5. **Scrotal abscess.** Ultrasound shows a loculated fluid collection surrounding the testis.

are bilateral in 70% of cases, but when unilateral, they are more commonly left sided. A unilateral right-side varicocele should prompt a search for a retroperitoneal process such as a mass or occlusion of the inferior vena cava that causes obstruction of the right internal spermatic vein (Fig. 4.6).

Testicular torsion is a surgical emergency because if detorsion is performed within 4 hours, salvage of the testis is possible. If torsion is missed, the testicle infarcts and becomes necrotic. Doppler evaluation plays a critical role as lack of flow in the testis allows a confident diagnosis of torsion. Reduced flow can be seen in the setting of early torsion. With delayed or missed torsion, the testis is enlarged, heterogeneous with surrounding reactive hyperemia (Figs. 4.7 and 4.8).

Microlithiasis occurs in a small percentage of normal males and may be present in up to 20% of men with subfertility. Microlithiasis can be subtle with only a few punctate nonshadowing echogenic foci or marked with innumerable calcifications as seen in image. It is usually asymptomatic and nonprogressive. There is a questionable association between testicular cancer and microlithiasis (Fig. 4.9).

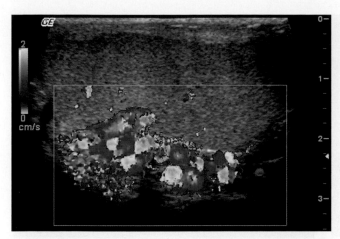

FIGURE 4.6. **Varicocele.** Color Doppler shows increased flow in the venous plexus.

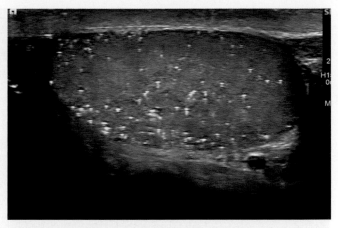

FIGURE 4.9. **Testicular microlithiasis.** Ultrasound shows multiple small hyperechoic foci.

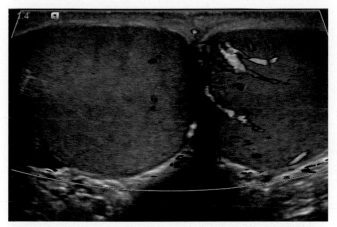

FIGURE 4.7. **Testicular torsion.** Color Doppler shows no flow in the right testis and comparatively normal flow in the left testis.

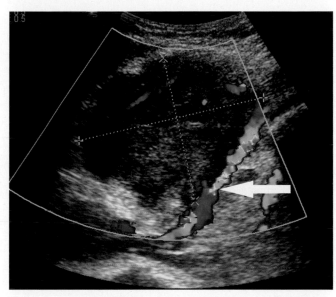

FIGURE 4.10. **Lymphadenopathy.** Color Doppler shows extensive adenopathy with compression of the adjacent right external iliac artery (*arrow*).

Groin masses such as **lymphadenopathy** can be confidently diagnosed on US (Fig. 4.10). **Inguinal hernias** may present as a groin mass and typically contain bowel and fat. Bowel containing hernias often demonstrate peristalsis. Herniation may be limited to the groin or extend into the scrotum (Fig. 4.11A and B). Ultrasound may identify an undescended testicle in the left inguinal canal (Fig. 4.12).

GYNECOLOGIC IMAGING

Pain from gynecologic, urologic, or gastrointestinal causes is the most common indication for pelvic imaging in both the outpatient and ER settings. Ultrasound is the initial imaging of modality of choice for suspected gynecologic or obstetrical complications. CT is more helpful when gastrointestinal or urinary tract pathology is likely. MR is rarely used in the

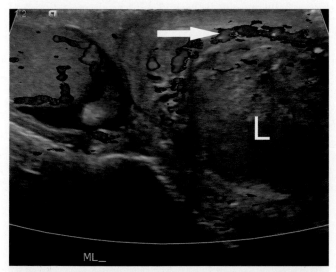

FIGURE 4.8. **Missed testicular torsion.** Color Doppler shows hyperemia circumferentially but no flow in the left testis (*arrow*).

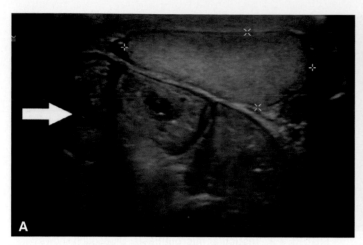
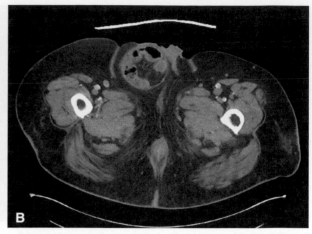

FIGURE 4.11. **Inguinal hernia containing bowel. A:** Ultrasound shows bowel (*arrow*) within the inguinal hernia. **B:** CT shows bowel within the inguinal hernia.

emergent setting except to exclude appendicitis during pregnancy. MR also plays a very important role in the nonemergent setting for evaluating complex pelvic masses.

Pelvic pain in premenopausal females is most commonly due to physiologic ovarian cysts. Ruptured ovarian cysts are usually self-limiting but can cause significant pain and hemoperitoneum requiring surgery. The most common cause for acute pelvic pain is a **hemorrhagic corpus luteal cyst**. A corpus luteum develops following rupture of a dominant follicle. On ultrasound, a hemorrhagic corpus luteal cyst appears complex often mimicking a solid mass (Fig. 4.13). Color Doppler may be used to distinguish a cystic from a solid mass as the latter demonstrates vascularity, but a hemorrhagic cyst will not have vascularity. A unique feature of hemorrhagic corpus luteum cyst is the abundant peripheral vascularity as it is metabolically active and may show uptake on PET scanning which can result in a false-positive study.

Ovarian torsion (OT) most commonly occurs in teens and young adults. The typical clinical presentation is acute pelvic pain and occasionally nausea and vomiting. In this setting, it can be difficult to determine if symptoms are GI or gynecologic in origin. Patients with right-sided symptoms may initially undergo evaluation for acute appendicitis. OT usually occurs in the presence of a mass (most commonly a cyst or dermoid) which acts as a fulcrum. The ovary will be enlarged and edematous (Fig. 4.14A). The ovary contains small peripheral follicles with a distinct appearance, the "follicular ring sign" on ultrasound (Fig. 4.14B). Ovarian blood flow can persist with torsion, and therefore, the Doppler US evaluation can be misleading. Torsion is rare in patients with endometriosis due to pelvic scarring. OT can be a very difficult diagnosis to make even in the setting of an experienced imager.

Ectopic pregnancy (EP) occurs when the embryo implants outside the uterus. It is the most common cause of death among women during the first trimester. Patients present with abdominal pain and/or vaginal bleeding, although less than 50% of patients have both symptoms. EP typically presents between 5 and 6 weeks gestation, and most (95%) are tubal in location.

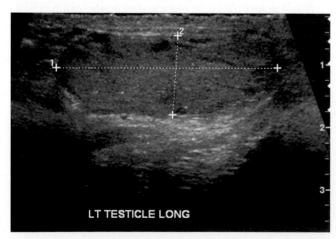

FIGURE 4.12. **Undescended testicle.** Ultrasound shows undescended testicle in the inguinal canal.

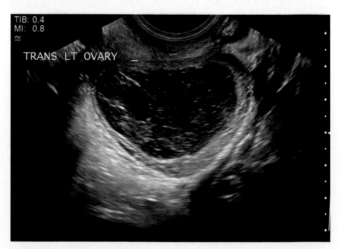

FIGURE 4.13. **Hemorrhagic corpus luteal cyst.** Transvaginal ultrasound shows a well-defined hemorrhagic cyst.

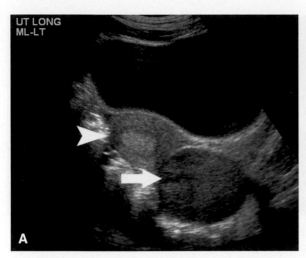
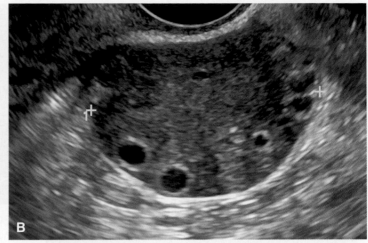

FIGURE 4.14. **Ovarian torsion.** Ultrasound shows an edematous ovary (*arrow*), which is larger than the adjacent uterus (*arrowhead*).

While the threshold of 1,500 IU/m β-hCG when an intrauterine pregnancy should be visible on transvaginal ultrasound is the subject of debate, the presence of an adnexal mass in the absence of an intrauterine pregnancy on transvaginal sonography increases the likelihood of an EP 100-fold. The likelihood of an EP decreases when there are no adnexal abnormalities on transvaginal sonography.

Imaging findings of EP are variable. The presence of an intrauterine gestation is felt to exclude an EP in patients who are not on fertility treatment. Most commonly, the US findings are sequelae of a tubal rupture including free pelvic fluid (hemoperitoneum) and a complex adnexal "mass" due to clot formation (Figs. 4.15 and 4.16). The size of the adnexal mass determines subsequent management. Rarely, an extrauterine gestation will be visible on US, but if seen, it is imperative to check for cardiac activity as a live EP requires emergent laparoscopy or laparotomy, as it can cause hypovolemic shock. A nonviable EP may be treated with nonsurgical techniques including methotrexate.

Ovarian masses can present with acute symptoms due to enlarging size, rupture, or even torsion. Dermoids, endometriomas, hydrosalpinx, and enlarged nonfunctioning ovarian cysts have classic imaging findings based on their composition. **Dermoids** can be confidently diagnosed when a pelvic mass contains fat and/or calcification. On US, fat appears very echogenic and causes "dirty shadowing" (Fig. 4.17). Calcification causes dense shadowing on US. Calcification on CT is very bright due to its high density compared with fat which measures negative in Hounsfield units and is similar in density to the subcutaneous fat (Figs. 4.18 and 4.19). **Endometriomas** in the ovary result from an endometrial implant undergoing cyclical bleeding resulting in a homogeneous lesion with low level echoes and no internal vascularity. Endometriomas can be complex or atypical. Such mass warrants further imaging with MRI to exclude malignancy.

Hydrosalpinx appears as a convoluted fluid-filled fallopian tube folded on itself (Fig. 4.20). Identification of an

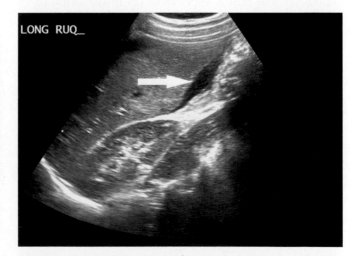

FIGURE 4.15. **Ectopic pregnancy.** Ultrasound shows free fluid (FF) superiorly. No intrauterine gestational sac is seen. *Arrow* denotes the normal endometrium.

FIGURE 4.16. **Ectopic pregnancy.** Ultrasound of the right upper quadrant shows free (intraperitoneal) fluid in the hepatorenal fossa (Morison pouch) (*arrow*).

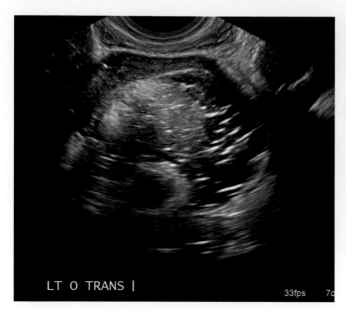

FIGURE 4.17. Ovarian dermoid. Ultrasound shows an ovarian mass with calcification and fat. The short echogenic lines represent hair.

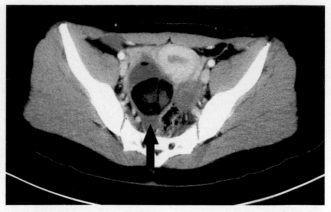

FIGURE 4.19. Ovarian dermoid. Axial CT shows a dermoid containing fat (*arrow*).

adjacent ovary allows for a confident diagnosis of hydrosalpinx. In **tubo-ovarian abscess** the ipsilateral ovary is not seen and there is an adnexal thick-walled complex cystic mass with tubal structure and surrounding peritoneal thickening and stranding (Figs. 4.20 and 4.21).

Endometriosis occurs when ectopic endometrial tissue that undergoes cyclical bleeding (menses) results in trapped blood in the ovary (endometrioma), tube (hematosalpinx), and the serosal surfaces of bladder and bowel. There is a spectrum of imaging findings in endometriosis ranging from normal to bilateral adnexal masses, hematosalpinx, and adhesions of bowel and bladder. On US, endometriomas contain homogenous low-level echoes and no internal vascularity (Fig. 4.22). MRI is useful in evaluating atypical endometriomas and is superior to US in the detection of

deep tissue endometriosis. MRI is very specific for detection of blood products with increased signal on T1 weighted imaging. Endometriomas demonstrate a characteristic T2 shading (Figs. 4.23 and 4.24).

Uterine Fibroids

Fibroids (myomata) are benign uterine tumors that may present as mass(es), abnormal bleeding, and complications during pregnancy including premature delivery and obstruction of the birth canal resulting in C-section delivery. They are present in approximately 1/3 of women of childbearing age and may enlarge with time and usually regress in the postmenopausal patient.

Fibroids are classified by their location. Intramural myomas are the most common and located in the uterine muscular wall. Submucosal myomas abut or extend into the endometrium and typically cause abnormal bleeding. Endometrial intracavity myomas may cause infertility (Fig. 4.25). Subserosal or pedunculated myomas may cause bladder or bowel symptoms.

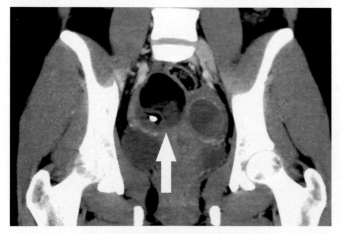

FIGURE 4.18. Ovarian dermoid. Coronal CT shows a dermoid containing fat and calcium (*arrow*).

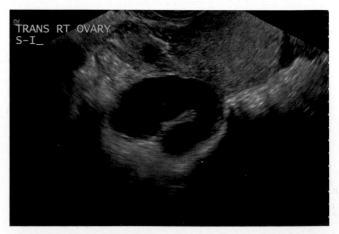

FIGURE 4.20. Hydrosalpinx. Ultrasound shows a dilated and torturous, fluid-filled fallopian tube.

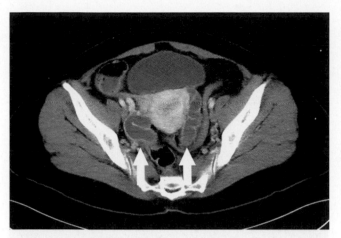

FIGURE 4.21. Pelvic inflammatory disease. CT shows bilateral hydrosalpinx (*arrows*).

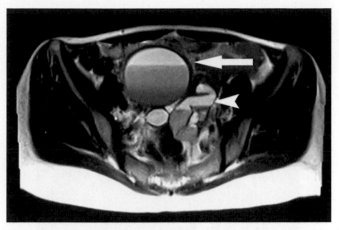

FIGURE 4.24. Endometrioma on MRI with characteristic T2 shading (*arrow*) and fallopian tube endometriosis (*arrowhead*).

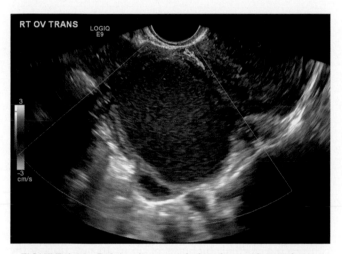

FIGURE 4.22. Pelvic ultrasound showing endometrioma.

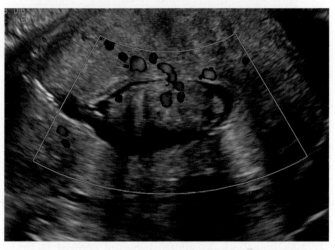

FIGURE 4.25. Intracavitary fibroid on ultrasound.

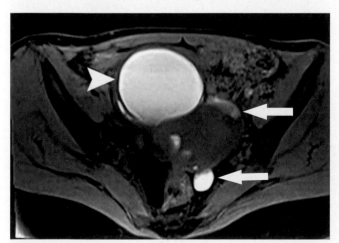

FIGURE 4.23. Endometriosis implants on the serosal surface of the uterus (*arrows*) and endometrioma (*arrowhead*) on pelvic MRI.

The imaging features of fibroids are variable depending on composition. Most fibroids contain disorganized muscular and fibrous tissue which appears heterogeneous and hypoechoic on US (Fig. 4.25). Calcification within fibroids is common particularly older women. Fibroids often cause scan lines or shadowing bands that allow for more specific diagnosis. On MR, fibroids are typically low signal on T1 and T2 weighted imaging. The differential diagnosis includes adenomyosis (Fig. 4.26). Fibroids can degenerate, hemorrhage, or necrose resulting in a cystic appearance. Uterine fibroid embolization (UFE) is a minimally invasive treatment in which arterial embolization of fibroids cause infarction and atrophy. About 5% of patients develop premature ovarian failure following UFE due to nontarget embolization of ovaries (Fig. 4.27A and B. Fibroid MRI before and after UFE).

Gynecologic malignancy can present with abnormal menstrual bleeding or postmenopausal bleeding, pain in addition to abdominal distension or palpable mass on examination. The most common imaging feature of malignancy is

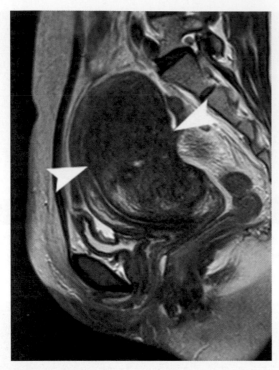

FIGURE 4.26. **Adenomyosis.** Sagittal MRI showing an increase in the size of the junctional zone posteriorly between the *arrowheads.*

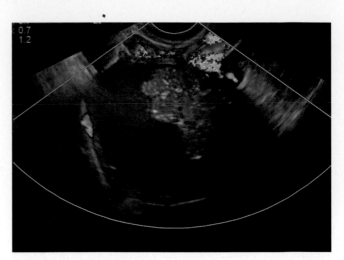

FIGURE 4.28. **Ovarian carcinoma.** Pelvic ultrasound showing a partially solid ovarian mass.

a cystic mass with solid components demonstrating internal vascularity (Fig. 4.28). In patients with gynecologic malignancy, multiple imaging modalities including CT and MR are often used for accurate staging and treatment planning (Fig. 4.29). Ascites in the presence of pelvic masses is highly suggestive of malignancy (Fig. 4.30). Features less suspicious for malignancy are septations including nodular or thickened septations. Preoperative imaging of an adnexal mass

plays a role in determining who should operate. If a mass demonstrates features of a classically benign mass, it is often removed by a gynecologist, whereas for a mass demonstrating suspicious features or features typical of malignancy, surgery is usually performed by a gynecologic oncologist.

MR plays an invaluable role for evaluating complex mass seen on ultrasound. While the classic endometrioma is homogeneous with low-level echoes, larger endometriomas are often complex. Fibrinous material within an endometrioma can coalesce and appear solid. MR allows for superior soft tissue visualization to distinguish between benign and malignant disease.

The **endometrial thickness** varies throughout the menstrual cycle; it is thinnest during the menstrual phase and can reach a normal thickness of up to 16 mm during the secretory phase. Pelvic ultrasound is useful in the diagnostic

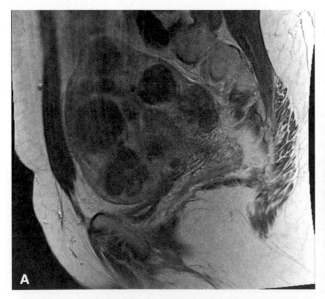

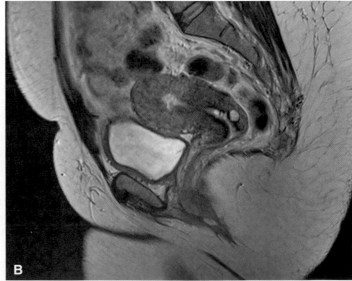

FIGURE 4.27. **Fibroids. A:** Sagittal MRI showing multiple fibroids. **B:** Note reduction size of fibroids post uterine fibroid embolization.

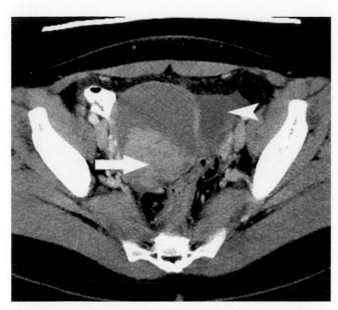

FIGURE 4.29. **Ovarian carcinoma.** CT showing a partially solid ovarian mass (*arrow*) displacing the bladder (*arrowhead*) to the left.

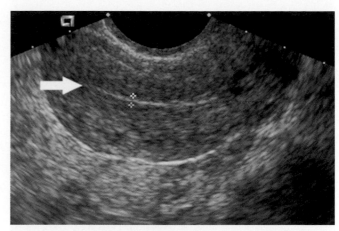

FIGURE 4.31. **Normal endometrial stripe.** Transvaginal ultrasound showing a 2 mm endometrial stripe (*arrow*).

workup of postmenopausal bleeding including identification of normal endometrial stripe (Fig. 4.31). Features suspicious for malignancy include endometrial thickening, cystic changes, a polypoid mass in the endometrial cavity, and complex endometrial fluid (Fig. 4.32).

Molar Pregnancy

A hydatidiform mole or molar pregnancy is a rare complication of pregnancy characterized by the abnormal growth of gestational trophoblasts, cells which normally develop into the placenta. It is considered a premalignant condition and requires evacuation of the pregnancy to prevent the development of malignancy. There are two types of molar pregnancy, **complete and partial**. A partial mole may have a coexisting fetus or fetal parts and is associated with early miscarriage. The placental tissue becomes edematous with cystic change. A molar pregnancy may occur in the setting of twins with a normal coexisting twin. The serum beta hCG is very elevated in molar pregnancy and can be followed following evacuation of a molar pregnancy to exclude persistent or invasive gestational trophoblast disease (Fig. 4.33).

Infertility

Congenital uterine anomalies occur in up to 3% of women and may be asymptomatic. They result from abnormal embryonic development of the Mullerian ducts. As many as one quarter of women with a second trimester

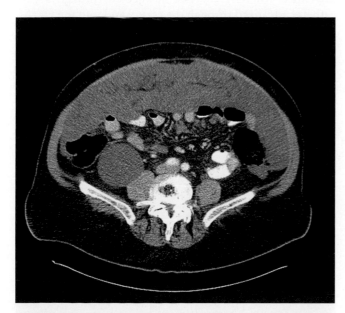

FIGURE 4.30. **Ascites and omental caking.** CT pelvis showing extensive omental caking and ascites, secondary to ovarian carcinoma (right pelvic cyst).

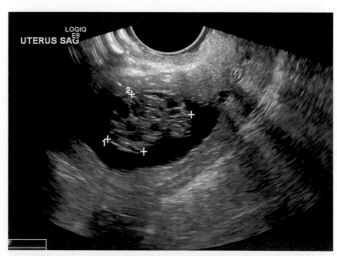

FIGURE 4.32. **Endometrial carcinoma.** Ultrasound showing a cystic endometrial mass.

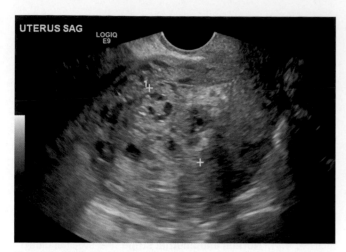

FIGURE 4.33. **Gestational trophoblast disease.** Transvaginal ultrasound showing thickening of the endometrium with cystic change (*crosshairs*).

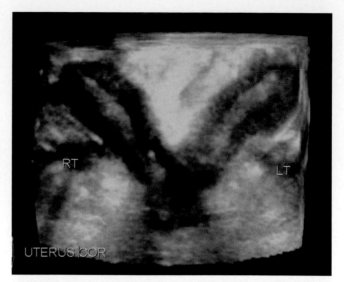

FIGURE 4.35. **Bicornuate uterus.** 3-D ultrasound showing right and left moieties of a bicornuate uterus.

miscarriage have uterine anomalies. The most common and only treatable uterine anomaly is a **septated uterus** (Fig. 4.34). Surgical resection of the uterine septum is usually performed hysteroscopically and significantly reduces future pregnancy loss. **3-D US** allows coronal visualization of the uterus and is an alternative to MR for imaging anomalies. The uterine fundus is heart shaped in a bicornuate uterus but is smooth in a septated uterus (Fig. 4.35). 3-D US also allows for measurement of the septum for surgical planning. Associated renal anomalies are frequently found in the setting of uterine anomalies. The classic association is renal agenesis in the setting of a unicornuate uterus. The absent kidney and atrophic or absent uterine horn will be on the same side.

If **polycystic ovary morphology** (PCOM) is present with specific biochemical derangements, it can manifest as **polycystic Ovary Syndrome (PCOS)**, which accounts for 80% of anovulatory subfertility cases. Polycystic ovary morphology is traditionally defined as 12 or more follicles of 2 to 9 mm and/or an ovarian volume of 10 mL or greater, per the Rotterdam Diagnostic Criteria (2003) (Fig. 4.36). The ovaries in PCOS have increased stroma due to the increased androgen. However, recent studies have proposed that the threshold of 12 follicles per ovary may no longer be valid and recommend measuring anti-Müllerian hormone level in its place where a level >35 pmol/L supports a diagnosis of PCOS.

Hysterosalpingogram (HSG) is a widely performed procedure for evaluation of tubal patency in women with infertility, whereby contrast is injected through a thin catheter advanced through the cervix and into the uterus. If the fallopian tubes are patent, contrast will spill into the peritoneal cavity (Fig. 4.37). Occlusion of fallopian

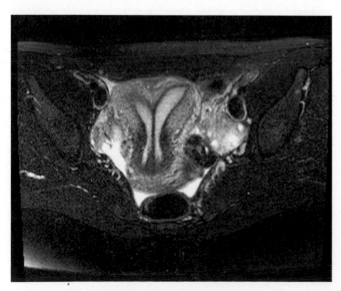

FIGURE 4.34. **Septate uterus.**

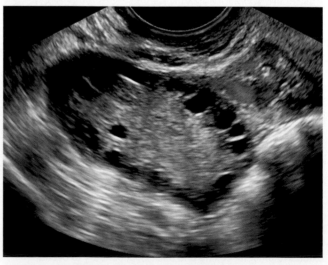

FIGURE 4.36. **Polycystic ovary morphology.** Ultrasound showing more than 12 small peripheral follicles.

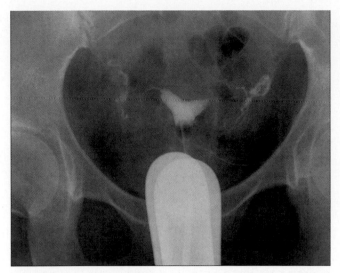

FIGURE 4.37. Normal hysterosalpingogram. Note the normal flow of contrast into the peritoneal cavity.

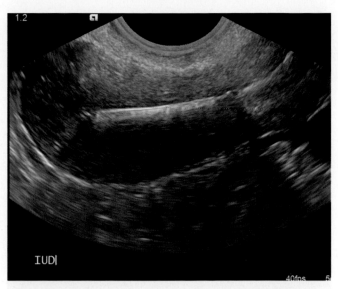

FIGURE 4.39. Normal intrauterine devices (IUD) position. Ultrasound shows the linear echogenicity of the IUD in the endometrial cavity.

tubes may be due to pelvic inflammatory disease or a foreign body (Fig. 4.38). HSG also allows for evaluation of uterine anomalies and endometrial masses. MRI and 3D ultrasound can provide the same information without radiation and with less discomfort.

Intrauterine devices (IUDs). There has been a resurgence in the use of IUDs in the United States with a 75% increase in use between 2008 and 2012. IUD surveillance or "missing" IUD string is a common indication for US scanning which can readily confirm the presence of an IUD (Fig. 4.39). Nonvisualization of an IUD requires further workup. While nonvisualization is usually due to an expelled IUD, plain film of the abdomen is recommended to exclude a perforated IUD located in the peritoneal cavity. 3-D US is also helpful for IUD localization.

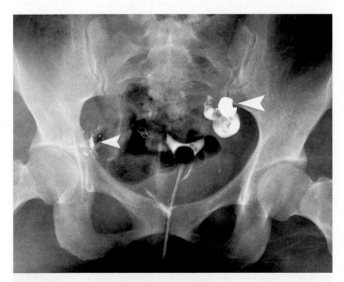

FIGURE 4.38. Abnormal hysterosalpingogram. Note occlusion of the fallopian tubes secondary to bullet fragments (*arrowheads*).

Complications of IUD usually occur at the time of placement and include uterine perforation and malposition.

OBSTETRICAL IMAGING

Ultrasound is the primary modality for imaging during pregnancy. US is frequently performed in the first trimester for accurate dating of a pregnancy. Emergently, first trimester US is done in patients with pain to exclude an EP and to establish fetal viability. With few exceptions, ultrasound should not be used to diagnose an uncomplicated pregnancy.

Transvaginal ultrasound findings diagnostic of pregnancy failure include a crown to rump length of greater than 7 mm with no heartbeat and a mean sac diameter of greater than 25 mm in the absence of an embryo. Guidelines for fetal viability are listed in Ref. 1. The yolk sac is visible by 5 weeks, and an embryo and cardiac activity are visible by approximately 6 weeks. Fetal cardiac activity is documented with M-mode ultrasound (Fig. 4.40). Normal first trimester anatomy is seen in Figure 4.41.

A "threatened abortion," defined as vaginal bleeding in early pregnancy, is the most common indication for US in the first trimester. This occurs in approximately one quarter of all pregnancies, half of whom go on to miscarriage. Fetal viability depends on imaging a heartbeat or fetal movement on ultrasound (Fig. 4.42). Other possible ultrasound findings include a blighted ovum (most have chromosomal abnormalities), missed abortion, or an incomplete abortion.

Fetal surveys are usually performed with US at 20 weeks and include biometric parameters to assess fetal age and growth by measuring biparietal diameter (BPD), head circumference (HC), abdominal circumference (AC), and femur length (FL). Evaluation of the amniotic fluid volume is an important component of the US examination (Table

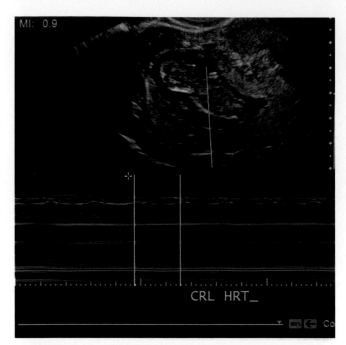

FIGURE 4.40. **Normal obstetric ultrasound** with fetal cardiac activity.

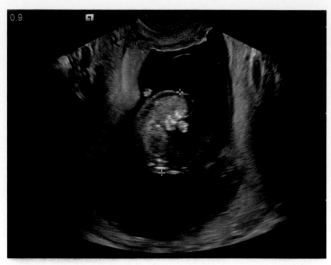

FIGURE 4.42. **Nonviable first trimester pregnancy with hydropic embryo.** Note a small rim of fluid surrounding the embryo.

4.1). MRI is increasingly being used to evaluate fetal anomalies when visualization with US is limited as in the setting of oligohydramnios.

Neural tube defects (NTD) occur in less than 1:1,000 pregnancies and include spina bifida, anencephaly, occult spinal dysraphism, and encephalocele. US imaging of the fetal cranium and spine allow for detection of NTD with considerable accuracy (Figs. 4.43-4.45).

Imaging of the Pregnant Patient With an Acute Abdomen

Ultrasound is the first-line imaging modality for evaluation of the pregnant patient with abdominal pain. CT

TABLE 4.1	Causes of Abnormal Amniotic Fluid Volumes	
Oligohydramnios (Pool <2 cm)	**Polyhydramnios (>8 cm)**
Renal agenesis	Maternal diabetes
Premature rupture of membranes	Fetal anomaly (check for fetal hydrops)
Intrauterine growth restriction (IUGR)	

scans are rarely performed during pregnancy because of the radiation risk to the fetus. The ACR recommends MRI as a useful problem-solving tool in the evaluation of abdominal and pelvic pain during pregnancy, particularly in suspected acute appendicitis where the appendix will be dilated, fluid filled and surrounded by inflammatory changes (Fig. 4.46). Renal stones

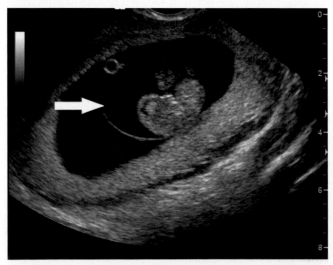

FIGURE 4.41. **Normal fetal ultrasound** showing an amniotic sac (*arrow*).

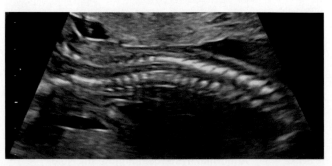

FIGURE 4.43. **Normal neonatal spine.** Ultrasound showing parallel orientation of fetal spine.

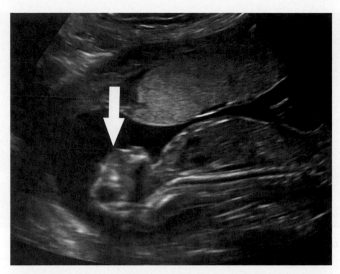

FIGURE 4.44. **Anencephaly.** No fetal cranium is present. Note the lack of fetal tissue above the eye (*arrow*).

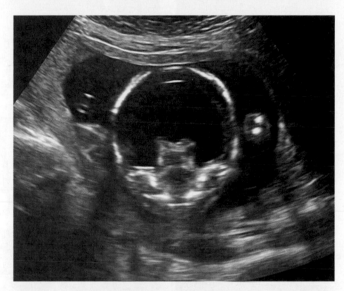

FIGURE 4.45. **Holoprosencephaly.** Ultrasound showing fusion of the thalami and a monoventricle.

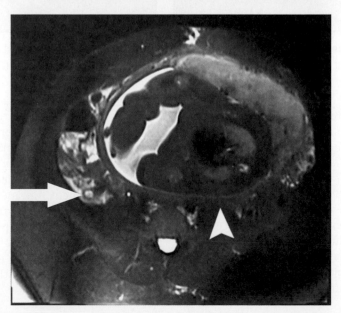

FIGURE 4.46. **Acute appendicitis in pregnancy.** MRI shows acute inflammation the right lower quadrant consistent with acute appendicitis (*arrow*). Note the gravid uterus (*arrowhead*).

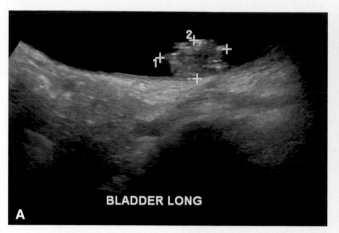

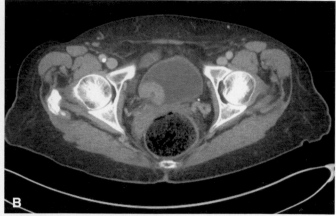

FIGURE 4.47. **Bladder carcinoma. A:** Ultrasound and **B:** CT showing a soft tissue bladder mass.

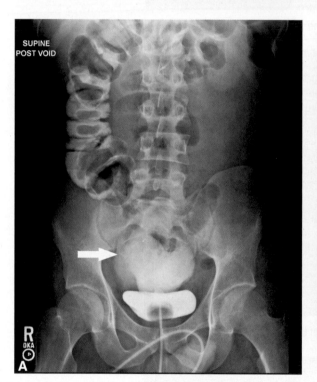

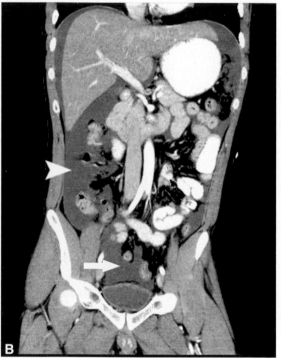

FIGURE 4.48. **Intraperitoneal bladder rupture. A:** Plain film showing intraperitoneal leak of contrast (*arrow*) from the bladder. **B:** Coronal CT in a different patient showing intraperitoneal free fluid (*arrow*) extending up the right paracolic gutter (*arrowhead*).

particularly small stones are not well visualized on MRI, and renal stone disease is the most common indication for CT scanning in pregnancy.

BLADDER IMAGING

The bladder is well suited to imaging with US and CT. Postvoid imaging of the bladder is often performed to evaluate for increased residual volume particularly in patients with benign prostatic hyperplasia (BPH). The bladder wall will be thickened in bladder outlet obstruction seen commonly with BPH and less commonly neurogenic bladder.

Soft tissue masses may represent bladder carcinoma (Fig. 4.47A and B). **Bladder rupture** due to trauma can be intraperitoneal or extraperitoneal. Extraperitoneal rupture is more commonly associated with pelvic fractures and is usually treated conservatively with Foley catheter placement. Intraperitoneal rupture occurs after blunt trauma to a very distended bladder and is treated surgically (Fig. 4.48). **Emphysematous cystitis** results from infection due to a gas-forming organism and is seen in immunocompromised patients including diabetics (Fig. 4.49). It can occur with or without pyelonephritis.

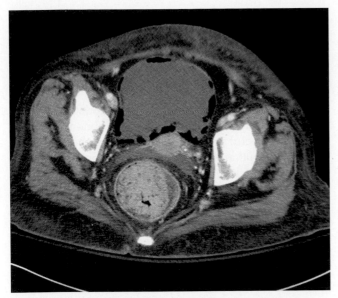

FIGURE 4.49. **Emphysematous cystitis.** CT shows diffuse intramural gas in the bladder.

PROSTATE IMAGING

Prostate cancer is a spectrum of disease, ranging from indolent small low-grade tumors that may be managed expectantly to larger and aggressive tumors requiring a combination of surgery, chemotherapy, or radiation.

Modalities commonly used to evaluate prostate cancer include transrectal ultrasound (TRUS), MRI, CT, and bone scintigraphy. CT and bone scintigraphy are used primarily to evaluate metastatic disease. TRUS is most commonly used by urologists to localize the prostate (not for tumor localization) prior to a 6 core needle sectoral biopsy but is subject to substantial sampling error resulting in false-negative biopsies and undergrading of tumors. Multiplanar **MRI** with diffusion weighted imaging **(DWI)** is a more accurate technique than TRUS which increases the detection rate for clinically significant cancers (Figs. 4 50 and 4.51). The recent introduction of MRI-targeted biopsy of prostate lesions will have a higher diagnostic yield than TRUS.

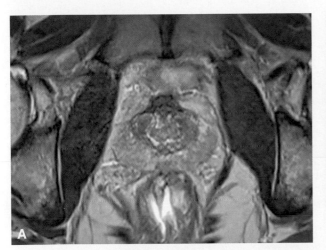

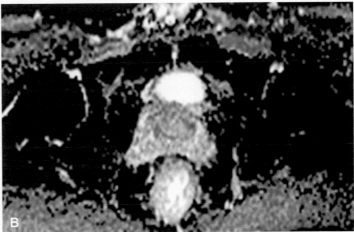

FIGURE 4.50. **Normal prostate MRI. A:** Axial T2WI and **B:** diffusion weighted images.

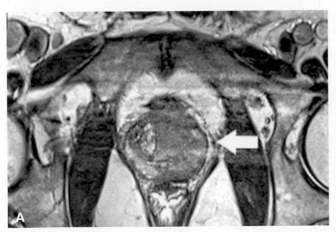

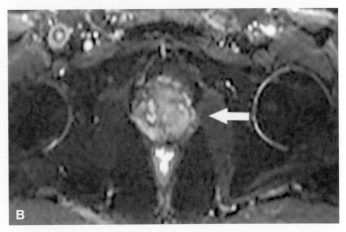

FIGURE 4.51. **Prostate carcinoma. A:** Axial T2WI and **B:** diffusion weighted images. Extensive replacement of the peripheral left lobe with carcinoma.

KEY POINTS

- Ultrasound and MRI are the dominant modalities for imaging of the pelvis.
- Testicular torsion is a surgical emergency in which Doppler evaluation plays a critical role as lack of flow in the testis allows a confident diagnosis of torsion.
- The most common cause of acute pelvic pain in premenopausal females is a hemorrhagic corpus luteal cyst.
- Ectopic pregnancy is the most common cause of maternal mortality in the first trimester typically presenting between 5 and 6 weeks gestation.
- Dermoids can be confidently diagnosed when a pelvic mass contains fat and/or calcification.

- The serum beta hCG is very elevated in molar pregnancy and can be followed following evacuation of a molar pregnancy to exclude persistent or invasive gestational trophoblast disease.
- Polycystic ovary syndrome accounts for 80% of anovulatory subfertility cases.
- Ultrasound is the first-line imaging modality for evaluation of the pregnant patient with abdominal pain. MRI is a useful problem-solving tool in the evaluation of abdominal and pelvic pain during pregnancy, particularly in suspected acute appendicitis.

Reference

1. Doubilet P, Benson C, Bourne T, Blaivas M. for the Society of Radiologists in Ultrasound Multispecialty Panel on Early First Trimester Diagnosis of Miscarriage and Exclusion of a Viable Intrauterine Pregnancy. Diagnostic criteria for nonviable pregnancy early in the first trimester. *N Engl J Med.* 2013;369:1443-1451.

Questions

1. True or False: Most extratesticular scrotal masses are malignant.

2. True or False: Most ectopic pregnancies occur in the uterine fundus.

3. True or False: Regarding varicoceles, the left gonadal vein arises from the inferior vena cava (IVC) and the right gonadal vein arises from the right renal vein.

4. True or False: Acute appendicitis during pregnancy may present as right upper quadrant pain.

5. All of the following are risk factors for ectopic pregnancy except
   a. Pelvic inflammatory disease
   b. Previous tubal surgery
   c. In vitro fertilization
   d. Previous termination of pregnancy

6. True or False: Office based transrectal ultrasound is used to target the biopsy of prostate tumors.

7. True or False: The most specific imaging features of malignancy in an adnexal lesion are solid elements without internal vascularity.

8. True or False: Corpus luteal cysts are characterized by intense peripheral vascularity on color Doppler ultrasound.

9. True or False: Pregnant patients with an IUD have an increased risk of pregnancy related adverse outcomes.

10. True or False: CT is more sensitive than US in the detection of retrocecal appendix.

CHAPTER 5

Pediatric Imaging

Ethan A. Smith, MD • Wilbur L. Smith, MD

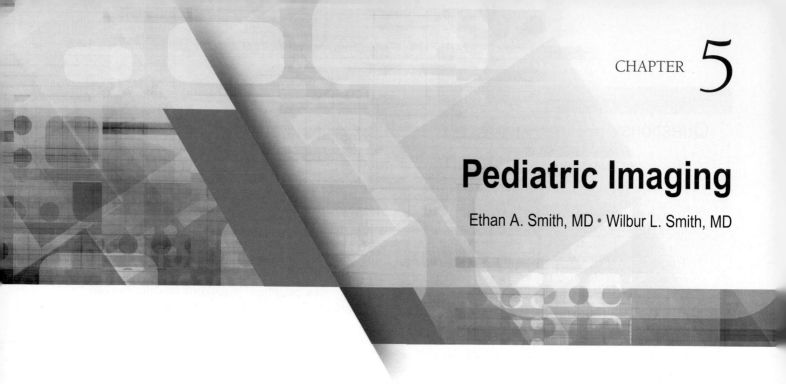

Ask any pediatrician and they will tell you: Children are not just little adults. Sure, the body parts (hearts, eyes, noses) are the same, but the fact that children are constantly growing and changing subjects them to different diseases as well as different radiographic appearances. As children evolve from neonates to adult-sized adolescents, the changing proportions and appearances of the various structures can lead to misinterpretation of normal and abnormal findings.

The classic illustrative example of this is concept is the **thymus**, that ubiquitous but often misinterpreted anterior mediastinal "mass" seen on chest radiographs in young children (Fig. 5.1). This organ, important in the immune response, usually becomes inconspicuous on radiographs by the age of 5 years or so; however, its appearance and size are both extremely variable. It is not uncommon to find thymic tissue on chest computed tomography (CT) scans in patients up to 20 years of age (Fig. 5.2). The thymus is a living piece of tissue that changes its configuration in a number of ways. In response to stress, it may shrink; after the stress has abated, it may grow (so-called "thymic rebound"). When indented by

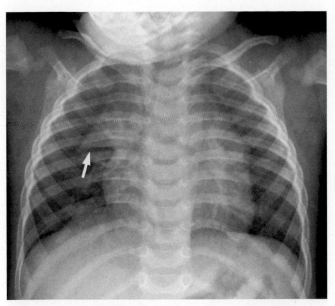

FIGURE 5.1. Normal thymus. The triangular opacity (*arrow*) arising from the mediastinum in this healthy 3-month-old is a typical appearance of the normal thymus. The triangular shape is sometimes referred to as the "sail sign."

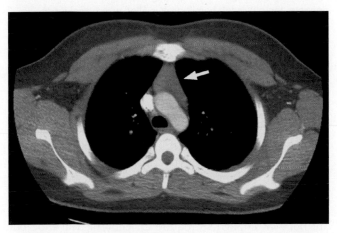

FIGURE 5.2. Normal thymus. This 17-year-old boy had a CT scan of the chest as routine follow-up for a prior history of cancer. The triangular soft tissue in the anterior mediastinum (*arrow*) represents normal residual thymus.

the ribs, it may form a wavy border; in pathologic conditions, such as a pneumomediastinum, it may even be displaced superiorly and laterally. With this variability in mind, the first rule in looking at children's radiographs is to consider normal variation before inventing pathology that is not real (Fig. 5.3).

As a general rule, congenital abnormalities are much more likely to present as clinical problems in neonates and younger children than they are in adults. To put it another way, if a patient gets to adulthood without a congenital anomaly bothering them, it is unlikely to cause clinical problems (i.e., it may just be a normal variant

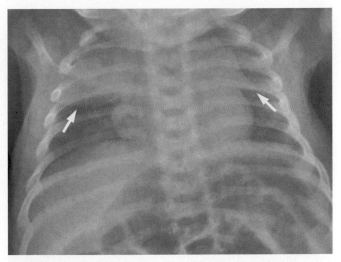

FIGURE 5.3. Normal thymus. The large soft tissue structure (*arrows*) in the superior and anterior mediastinum of this 1-month-old is all due to normal thymus. If you call anything in the anterior superior mediastinum of a neonate normal thymus, you will be right 99% of the time.

as opposed to a true disease). When presented with an abnormal abdominal radiograph in a neonate, a congenital anomaly is extremely likely; in a 4-year-old, it is somewhat likely; and in a 15-year-old, it is less likely. If you play the odds, in an 80-year-old you probably should not even think of a congenital abnormality as the cause of an acute abdomen. Having said this, everyone will be able to find the unusual case of a congenital defect causing grief to an 80-year-old, but remember that it is the zebra, not the horse!

In this chapter, we will discuss some of the most common radiographic diagnoses in children, first neonates and infants, then the older children. The intent is not to be comprehensive; rather, this is intended to show practical imaging approaches to common diagnoses.

CHEST: NEONATE AND INFANT

The newborn chest radiograph is a complex study with a substantial number of differences from that of an adult (Fig. 5.4). Along with the potential confusion caused by the normal variability of the thymus come a variety of other factors that can make newborn chest radiographs difficult to interpret. The respiratory rate of a neonate is quite fast compared with an adult, and a neonate cannot be expected to suspend respirations during imaging; therefore, radiographs are often inadvertently obtained in expiration, resulting in lower lung volumes, crowding of normal structures, and even patchy atelectasis. The small size of the neonatal chest also makes things more difficult because even normal structures are very close together and are often difficult to distinguish clearly from adjacent structures.

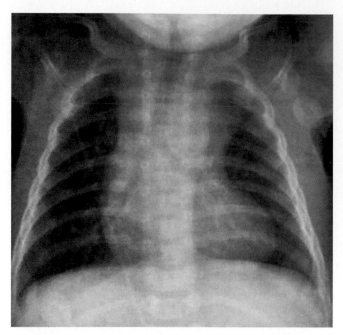

FIGURE 5.4. Normal chest radiograph of a neonate. Notice that due to the small size of the chest, the heart looks relatively prominent.

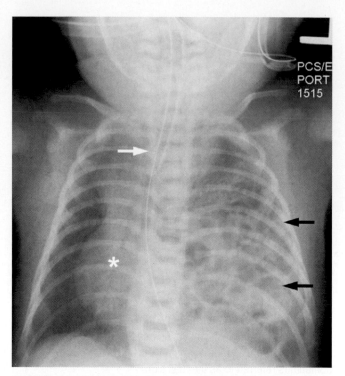

FIGURE 5.5. Congenital diaphragmatic hernia. In this neonate, the entire left hemithorax is filled with bowel loops, some of which contain bowel gas (*black arrows*). Notice how the mass effect from the bowel loops pushes the heart (*asterisk*) and mediastinal structures (*white arrow*) toward the right, away from the side of the hernia.

Neonatal and infant chest diseases can be roughly divided into two categories: medical and surgical conditions. Medical conditions are usually diffuse processes and require medical management. Surgical diseases can be defined as anything that needs prompt intervention. By this definition, for example, a tension pneumothorax needing treatment with a chest tube is a surgical disease. In assessing a newborn's chest radiograph when surgical disease is suspected, you must take two steps. First, identify which side is abnormal (most surgical conditions are unilateral). Second, determine the direction of shift of the mediastinum. Mediastinal shift is best determined by looking at the trachea, but the position of the heart and thymus can also be secondary clues. As a general rule, surgical conditions will displace the mediastinum *away* from the abnormal side. For example, in the instance of a diaphragmatic hernia (a condition owing to an in utero defect that allows the abdominal contents to protrude into the chest), the heart and mediastinum are clearly shifted away from the side of the hernia by the mass of the protruding bowel (Fig. 5.5).

Medical Diseases

Transient Tachypnea

All neonates have to change from an intrauterine environment where their lungs were fluid filled to one where they are breathing air. This transformation, which must occur within moments of birth, involves a complex interaction of the pulmonary lymphatics, capillary vessels, and chest compression (from normal passage through the birth canal). This normal process is not always smooth. In fact, many babies, if not all, have some very short-lived tachypnea in the first minute or two after being born, owing to the variability of clearing their normal in utero lung fluid.

However, in some otherwise normal infants, the clearance of fetal fluid causes clinically significant respiratory distress and even mild hypoxia. In general, these infants are not sick enough to require an endotracheal tube but may require supplemental oxygen or other support. This condition, called "transient tachypnea of the newborn" (TTN), improves rapidly and resolves 24 hours after birth. Radiographs obtained in an infant with TTN will show linear interstitial opacities, streaky opacities, and small (bilateral) pleural effusions, all reflecting the normal movement of fetal fluid from the alveoli into the interstitium and lymphatics. The lung volumes will usually be normal (Fig. 5.6). If follow-up radiographs are obtained, they are typically normal by 24 hours after birth. One confounding problem is that **neonatal pneumonia**, a much more serious condition, can also present with respiratory distress and similar radiographic findings to transient tachypnea (interstitial and streaky opacities). In this situation, the neonatologist may be forced to treat for pneumonia even if they suspect they are dealing with TTN because the potential consequences of an untreated pneumonia can be dire. Other, less

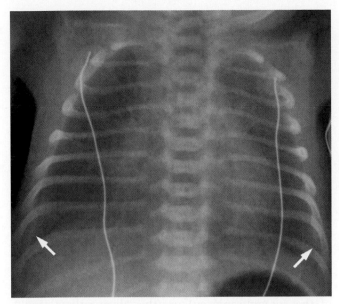

FIGURE 5.6. Respiratory distress syndrome. Full-term baby born by cesarean section with respiratory distress immediately after birth. The streaky perihilar opacities and small bilateral pleural effusions (*arrows*) are typical of transient tachypnea of the newborn. Notice that the patient is not sick enough to require an endotracheal tube.

common conditions could also present with a similar radiographic picture, including congenital lymphatic abnormalities and congenital heart disease. One radiographic clue that you may be dealing with pneumonia as opposed to TTN would be the presence of a **unilateral pleural effusion** (Fig. 5.7).

Respiratory Distress Syndrome (aka Surfactant Deficiency)

Previously known as "hyaline membrane disease," this process is seen almost exclusively in **preterm infants** (except in rare instances of congenital causes). Respiratory distress syndrome (RDS) occurs as a result of deficient surfactant, the lipid-based molecule that helps to keep alveoli open by lowering the alveolar surface tension. Surfactant is produced by the type II alveolar cells and does not begin to be made in sufficient quantities until well into the third trimester. If there is insufficient surfactant, the result is diffuse alveolar collapse leading to poor oxygen exchange, decreased lung compliance and respiratory compromise. Clinical information is quite helpful in the diagnosis, as these babies will be preterm and have significant respiratory distress shortly after birth, almost uniformly requiring mechanical ventilation. The radiographic appearance of RDS is secondary to diffuse microatelectasis and has **four key features: (1) low lung volumes, (2) granular opacities, (3) air bronchograms, and (4) uniform distribution throughout both lungs** (Fig. 5.8). A potential fifth sign, although less specific, is the presence of an endotracheal tube indicating that the infant is experiencing severe respiratory distress. Pleural effusions are uncommon in RDS. With the introduction of a synthetic surfactant, the prognosis for these babies has improved tremendously. The drug is administered as an aerosol through an endotracheal tube or at bronchoscopy. The patient is moved (rolled) around

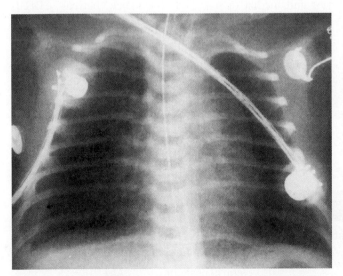

FIGURE 5.7. Neonatal pneumonia. A very ill newborn with a streaky pattern in both lungs and a large unilateral right pleural effusion. The unilateral pleural effusion (*arrow*) is suspicious for pneumonia. This pattern is typical of group B streptococcal infection in a neonate.

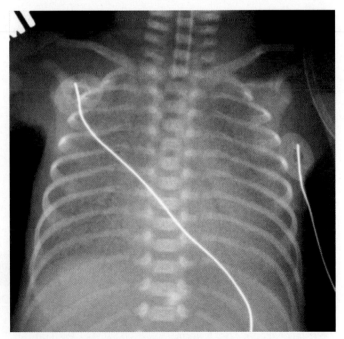

FIGURE 5.8. Respiratory distress syndrome. Extremely premature infant born at 24 weeks of gestational age. Note the low lung volumes, granular opacities, air bronchograms, and uniform distribution. The presence of the endotracheal tube tells you that this baby is critically ill.

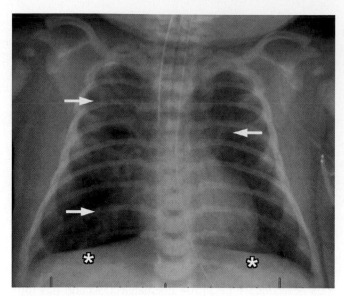

FIGURE 5.9. Meconium aspiration. Neonate born at 41 weeks of gestational age requiring intubation. The lungs are hyperinflated, evidenced by flattening of the diaphragm (*asterisks*). The patchy airspace opacities (*arrows*) likely represent areas of atelectasis.

in order to distribute the surfactant throughout the lungs. Occasionally, in recently treated infants, you may see partial clearing with residual opacities and air bronchograms at the lung bases, representing areas where the drug has not yet distributed.

Meconium Aspiration

Meconium aspiration is a disease seen in term or postterm infants and occurs if the baby passes meconium while still in utero. The sticky, tenacious meconium can then be aspirated into the lungs and cause plugging and obstruction of the small airways. Postnatally, this leads to a combination of air trapping (areas of lung where air can get in but cannot get out) and atelectasis (collapsed areas where no air can get in). These infants often have significant respiratory distress soon after birth, often requiring intubation and mechanical ventilation. Chest radiographs will demonstrate **hyperinflated** lungs with coarse and patchy bilateral airspace opacities, intermixed with areas

of relative hyperlucency secondary to air trapping (Fig. 5.9). Hyperinflation can lead to alveolar rupture and pneumothorax.

A review of the radiographic features of neonatal medical lung diseases is presented in Table 5.1.

Surgical Diseases

Pneumothorax

Although pneumothorax is rare in healthy babies, neonates and infants that require mechanical ventilation (secondary to medical processes such as RDS or meconium aspiration) or have underdeveloped lungs (hypoplasia) for other reasons are at a relatively high risk (Fig. 5.10). Remember that most neonatal chest radiographs are obtained supine, so the nice, clear apical pneumothorax and pleural edge you see in an adult may be absent. **Signs of a pneumothorax** in a supine baby include **asymmetric hyperlucency of an entire hemithorax, deepening of the costophrenic sulcus (the "deep sulcus sign"), and sharply defined cardiac or diaphragmatic borders (secondary to these structures being outlined by air).** Remember to always look for signs of tension—if you see the mediastinal structures being shifted away, or if you see an asymmetrically flattened diaphragm, you should be concerned for a tension pneumothorax which needs prompt intervention.

Congenital Diaphragmatic Hernia

A congenital defect in the diaphragm is termed a congenital diaphragmatic hernia (CDH). If the diaphragm does not develop properly and a defect remains, bowel and abdominal contents can herniate through the hole and into the chest. The most common location for the defect is posterior and medial (a so-called "Bochdalek" hernia). CDH is more common on the left (owing to the liver beneath the right hemidiaphragm). CDH has varying degrees of severity, depending on how big the defect in the diaphragm is and how much abdominal contents herniate through it, because the more abdominal contents there are in the chest, the less room there is for normal lung to develop. **Lung hypoplasia** and resultant respiratory and circulatory problems that come with it are the main cause of mortality in these patients. The radiographic appearance varies with the patient's age. In the immediate neonatal period, the bowel loops in the chest

TABLE 5.1	Neonatal Medical Lung Diseases			
	Transient Tachypnea	**Respiratory Distress Syndrome**	**Meconium Aspiration**	**Neonatal Pneumonia**
Gestational age	Term	Preterm	Term or postterm	Any
Lung volumes	Normal	Low	High	Any
Opacities	Streaky	Diffuse, granular	Patchy	Any
Pleural effusions	Yes(bilateral)	No	No	+/−
Endotracheal tube	No	Yes	Yes	+/−

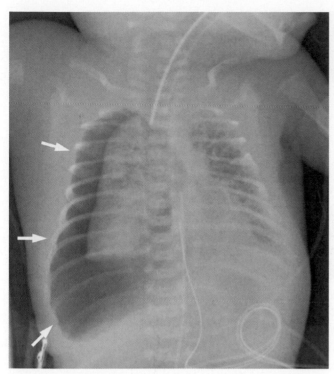

FIGURE 5.10. Tension pneumothorax. This premature neonate was on a ventilator due to severe respiratory distress syndrome and developed a large right pneumothorax (*arrows*) and required an emergent chest tube. Notice that the right lung maintains a relatively normal shape despite the pneumothorax. This is due to the abnormal stiffness of the lung tissue because of the underlying lung disease.

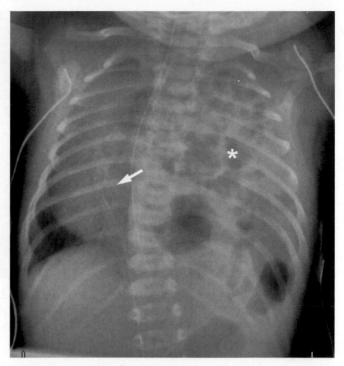

FIGURE 5.11. Congenital diaphragmatic hernia. Another neonate with bowel loops filling the left hemithorax (*asterisk*) and shift of the heart and mediastinal structures to the right (*arrow*). The left lung is severely hypoplastic.

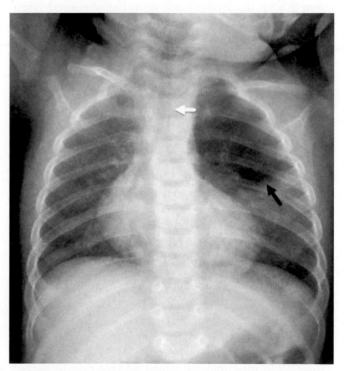

FIGURE 5.12. Congenital lobar hyperinflation. The left upper lobe is enlarged and is more lucent than surrounding lung due to air trapping (*black arrow*). There is mild shift of the trachea (*white arrow*) and other mediastinal structures away from the abnormal left upper lobe.

will be filled with fluid, giving the appearance of a soft tissue mass. Hours to days later, as gas progresses through the bowel loops, multiple lucent gas-filled bowel loops will be present. Owing to the mass effect from the herniated abdominal contents, the mediastinal structures are almost always displaced toward the opposite side of the chest (see Figs. 5.5 and 5.11).

Congenital Lung Lesions

Other congenital lung masses occur infrequently but are worth a brief mention here. The first is **congenital lobar hyperinflation** (CLH). This entity, formerly known as "congenital lobar emphysema," is caused by an abnormal airway that causes a one-way valve. Essentially, air can get in to the affected segment of the lung, but it cannot get back out. This causes progressive hyperinflation of a portion of the lung, most commonly the left upper lobe. On radiographs, you will see a hyperlucent area with associated mass effect, pushing structures away from the abnormal hyperinflated segment. In the immediate neonatal period, the affected lung is filled with fluid and may be opaque, but as the fluid absorbs and more air gets trapped, it will soon become hyperlucent (Fig. 5.12).

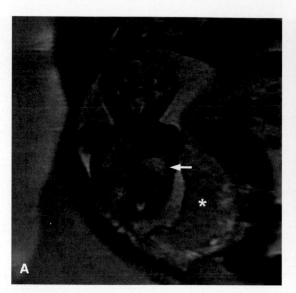
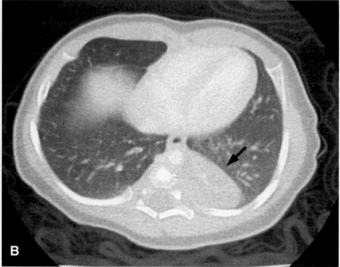

FIGURE 5.13. Pulmonary sequestration. A: Fetal MRI obtained before birth, demonstrating an area of abnormal high signal (*light gray*) in the lower aspect of the left chest (*arrow*). Note the normal placenta (*asterisk*). **B:** A CT scan of the same patient obtained after birth demonstrates a rounded soft tissue mass in the left lower lobe (*arrow*) which was a pulmonary sequestration.

The second congenital lung lesion worth mentioning is the spectrum of lesions that includes both **congenital pulmonary airway malformation (CPAM) and pulmonary sequestration**. Both of these entities involve abnormal development of a section of lung, which may or may not connect with the airways and often has abnormal vascularity. In general, these lesions show up as solid masses on chest radiographs, although CPAM may occasionally be predominantly made up of air-filled cysts. Many of these lesions are identified prenatally on either ultrasound or MRI (Fig. 5.13). Both of these lesions are usually surgically resected due to a risk of recurrent infections and a small risk of future malignancy.

Esophageal Atresia

Our discussion so far has focused mostly on lung disease, but of course there are other organs in the pediatric chest, including the heart and the esophagus. Esophageal abnormalities that are of importance in children are usually related to esophageal atresia. The most common form of **esophageal atresia** is a blind-ending proximal esophagus with a fistula extending from the trachea or left main stem bronchus to the distal esophagus. Inhaled air travels through the fistula and into the rest of the GI tract; therefore, the initial films can look superficially normal, with normal-appearing gas-filled loops of bowel in the abdomen. Clinicians become alert to this condition when the neonate chokes on feedings and the pediatrician cannot pass a nasogastric (NG) tube into the stomach. This also provides a clue on the chest radiographs, as the NG tube will be seen within the pouch (Fig. 5.14).

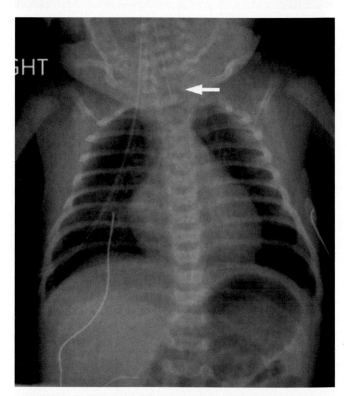

FIGURE 5.14. Esophageal atresia with tracheoesophageal fistula. This baby choked on her first feeds, and the pediatrician was unable to pass a nasogastric tube. Note the tip of the nasogastric tube overlying the neck (*arrow*). The findings are consistent with esophageal atresia. There is bowel gas present, indicating the presence of a fistula between the trachea and the distal portion of the esophagus.

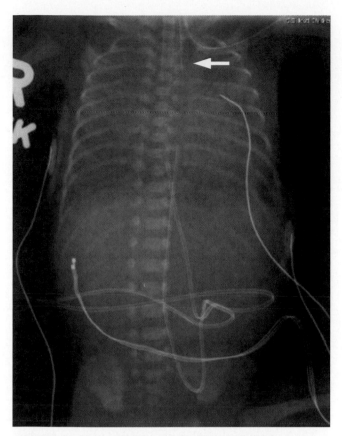

FIGURE 5.15. **Esophageal atresia without a fistula.** A premature neonate that could not tolerate feeds. The NG tube is stuck in the cervical esophagus (*arrow*). There is no bowel gas, consistent with esophageal atresia without a distal fistula. Notice that this baby also has uniform, granular opacities throughout both lungs, typical of respiratory distress syndrome secondary to prematurity.

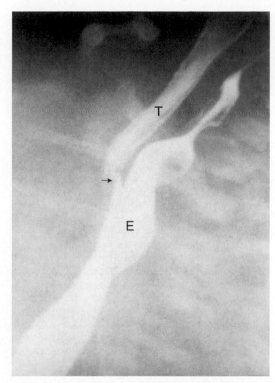

FIGURE 5.16. **H-type tracheoesophageal fistula.** A barium esophagram on a baby with recurrent pneumonia shows a connection between the esophagus (*E*) and the trachea (*T*), a so-called H-type tracheoesophageal fistula (*arrow*). This abnormality can sometimes be extremely difficult to detect.

There are two less prevalent but still frequent variants of esophageal abnormalities. The first is **esophageal atresia without a tracheoesophageal fistula**, in which case the abdomen will be completely gasless (Fig. 5.15). The second variant is **tracheoesophageal fistula without esophageal atresia**. This so-called H-type fistula can be more difficult to diagnose. Unlike with esophageal atresia, an NG tube can pass into the stomach, so the diagnosis is not readily apparent to the clinician. The child may present weeks or even years later with frequent pneumonias because each time the child eats, some of the material goes into the lung. Whenever you have an infant or young child with frequent and recurrent pneumonia, this entity should be considered. An esophagram with careful true lateral positioning can confirm the diagnosis (Fig. 5.16).

ABDOMEN: NEONATE AND INFANT

Abdominal radiographs of neonates are very different from those of adults, whereas radiographs of older children and teenagers begin to have a lot of similarities with adults. Abdominal films of neonates are different because of a number of physiologic factors. First and foremost, **neonates swallow a tremendous amount of air** during their relatively inefficient breathing and eating. It is, therefore, not at all unusual to find many loops of gas-filled small bowel on the plain film of a normal neonate (Fig. 5.17), whereas in an adult or older child it is unusual to see so much small bowel gas (Fig. 5.18). In fact, it is usually abnormal and ominous to see a gasless abdomen in a neonate (Fig. 5.19)! All of this air in the small bowel makes the interpretation of the films difficult as far as determining bowel distention. The best rule to remember is that the bowel loops of a normal neonate are thin walled and lie in close proximity to each other. The appearance of thick-walled bowel or marked separation of the bowel loops suggests an abnormal intra-abdominal process (Fig. 5.20).

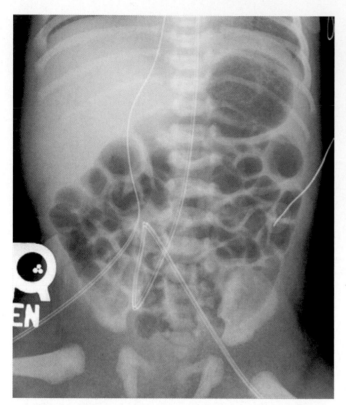

FIGURE 5.17. Normal bowel gas pattern in a neonate. While there are multiple gas-filled loops of small bowel, notice that all of the bowel loops are thin walled and are close together, not separated.

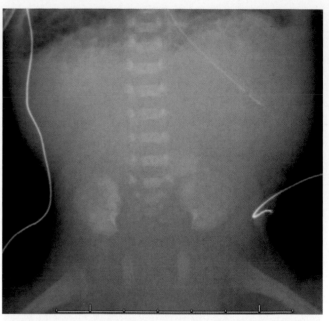

FIGURE 5.19. Necrotizing enterocolitis. Completely gasless abdomen in a critically ill infant with necrotizing enterocolitis. Babies typically have at least some bowel gas, so seeing a gasless abdomen is almost always an ominous sign.

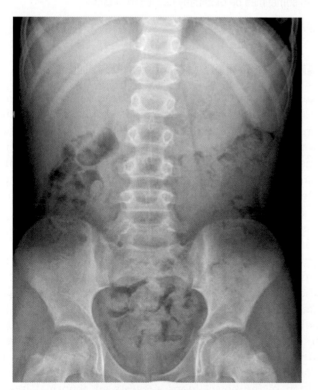

FIGURE 5.18. Normal bowel gas pattern in an 8-year-old boy. Compared with the neonate in Figure 5.17, there is much less small bowel gas. Some gas is present within the normal caliber colon, and the haustral pattern of the colon is clearly visible.

The haustra of the colon are variable in their development and do not become prominent until about 6 months of age. For this reason, trying to differentiate large from small bowel on the plain radiographs of a neonate's abdomen is usually unreliable. This makes the determination of whether there is rectal gas or not even more critical. The vast majority of newborns will have gas all the way through their GI tract 24 hours after birth. If there is any doubt as to whether a child has bowel gas through to the rectum, the *prone* cross-table lateral film is invaluable in making this distinction (Fig. 5.21). Remember that on a supine image (which almost all neonatal abdominal radiographs are), the rectum is posterior (or dependent), whereas air collects in nondependent structures. By turning the patient prone, the rectum now becomes nondependent, so if bowel gas can get there (i.e., there is no obstruction), it will!

A quick mention of the **umbilicus** is in order. This necessary structure and the accessories attached to it make for sometimes confusing shadows on abdominal films of neonates. Many an unsuspecting physician has called an umbilical clamp a bone or a foreign body (Fig. 5.22). The umbilicus itself protrudes much farther in a neonate than in an adult. Any coin-shaped soft tissue density lesion in the lower midabdomen of a neonate should probably be considered the umbilical remnant until proven otherwise. A good clue is that, owing to the air surrounding the protruding umbilical stump, the edges of the umbilicus are very sharply defined, particularly the inferior edge.

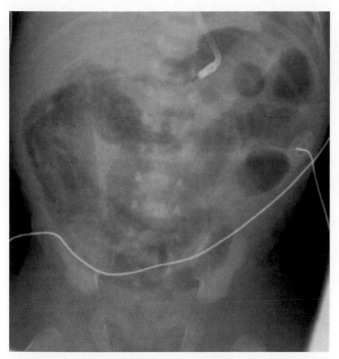

FIGURE 5.20. Necrotizing enterocolitis. This is a very abnormal bowel gas pattern in another infant with necrotizing enterocolitis. Notice how the bowel loops look separated from each other. This appearance is due to thickening of the bowel walls and probably also from some free fluid within the abdomen. The linear lucencies in the bowel in the right side of the abdomen represent gas inside the bowel wall or pneumatosis, another sign that this baby is critically ill.

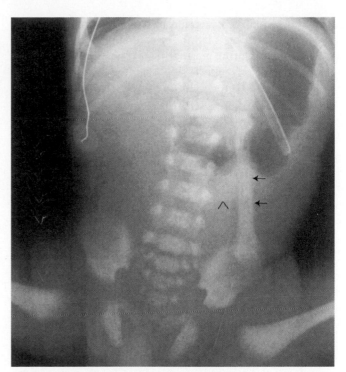

FIGURE 5.22. Normal bowel gas pattern. A newborn infant who has just begun to swallow air. Note the nasogastric tube in place in the stomach. The oblong structure to the left of the spine (*arrows*) almost looks like a bone of some sort; however, it is clearly attached to the umbilical stump (*arrowhead*) and in fact represents an umbilical cord clamp.

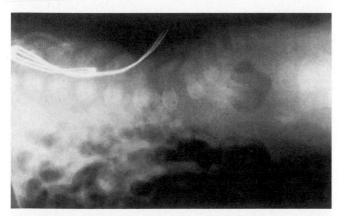

FIGURE 5.21. Technique for detecting rectal gas. A prone cross-table lateral view of the abdomen can often be helpful in showing whether or not gas is present in the rectum.

Neonate

The most common indication for abdominal imaging in the immediate neonatal period is the concern for **intestinal obstruction**. Clinically, the infant will present with feeding intolerance, often with progressive abdominal distention and sometimes with failure to pass meconium. In this setting, abdominal radiographs are commonly obtained and demonstrate variable degrees of gaseous distention of the bowel. The savvy physician can use the appearance of the abdominal radiograph to occasionally make a definitive diagnosis, but more often the bowel gas pattern acts as a guide to what imaging test should be done next. If there are only a few dilated loops of bowel confined to the upper abdomen, a more proximal obstruction should be suspected and an **upper gastrointestinal contrast swallow and meal** should be performed. However, if there are multiple loops of dilated bowel throughout the abdomen, the higher-yield diagnostic test will be a **fluoroscopic contrast enema**. Occasionally things are not this clear, and both tests need to be done.

Atresias

In a neonate, the most common cause of bowel obstruction is **bowel atresia**. Atresia occurs owing to a number of complex intrauterine processes, usually with the final common pathway of compromise of vascular supply to the wall of the bowel. Often, the affected segment completely disappears and all that is left is a wedge-shaped defect in the mesentery. The exception to this is **duodenal atresia**, which is caused by a failure of recanalization of the duodenal lumen. During normal development, the lumen of the duodenum is temporarily obliterated by an ingrowth of cells. If these cells then fail to regress, the lumen remains closed and causes an obstruction.

Radiographs of bowel atresias vary according to the level at which the atresia occurs; however, they have common features. First, there is usually no gas distal to the level of the atresia. Second, the bowel proximal to the atresia is disproportionately dilated. Beyond that, it is just a matter of looking at the radiograph to try to guess how far down the bowel you can go before you encounter the atresia. As a general rule, remember that the duodenal bulb is located in the right upper quadrant of the abdomen; therefore, if you have a dilated stomach and loop only a single dilated loop in the right upper quadrant, duodenal atresia is likely (the so-called "double bubble sign") (Fig. 5.23). The jejunum is predominantly in the upper abdomen and predominantly on the left side, whereas the ileum is in the right lower quadrant. If you see many dilated bowel loops and particularly large loops to the right of the spine, it is probably an ileal atresia, whereas if the loops are confined to the upper abdomen and predominantly to the left, it is probably jejunal atresia (Fig. 5.24). These are 70:30 rules, so do not get too

preoccupied with them. An upper GI or contrast enema can be helpful to confirm the diagnosis (Fig. 5.25). Remember, the important thing is to recognize the obstruction and to think about the diagnosis of atresia—from there, it is the surgeon's job to run the bowel and find the exact location.

Microcolon

Microcolon should be considered in a neonate with a distal bowel obstruction. The diagnosis of microcolon is made by doing a contrast enema. The appearance is just what you would expect, a tiny colon (Fig. 5.26). The typical microcolon is diffusely small, although there are variants where only the more distal portions of the colon are "micro." A microcolon is small because it is essentially an unused colon. This occurs because the normal secretions, mucus and cells that get excreted into the fetal GI tract (the stuff that becomes meconium), cannot get into the colon because of an obstruction, commonly in the distal or terminal ileum. The colon remains small because it does not need to grow in order to accommodate the developing bulk of meconium. This is why microcolon typically occurs with more distal obstruction—the more proximal the obstruction, the longer the normal GI tract between the obstruction and the colon and therefore the more mucus and material there is to get to

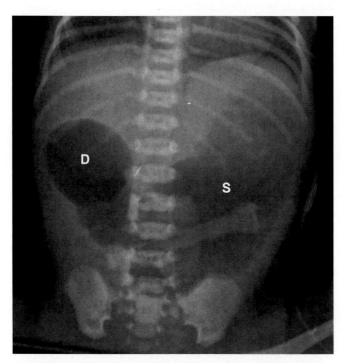

FIGURE 5.23. **Duodenal atresia.** This newborn had marked abdominal distention shortly after birth. The abdominal radiograph demonstrates a dilated stomach (S) and duodenal bulb (D), but no distal bowel gas. This is the classic "double bubble sign" and is diagnostic of duodenal atresia.

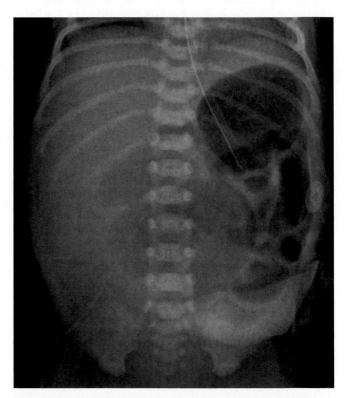

FIGURE 5.24. **Jejunal atresia.** This neonate also presented with abdominal distention shortly after birth. Compared with the baby in Figure 5.23, there are more dilated loops of bowel, suggesting the obstruction is more distal. At surgery this baby was found to have a jejunal atresia.

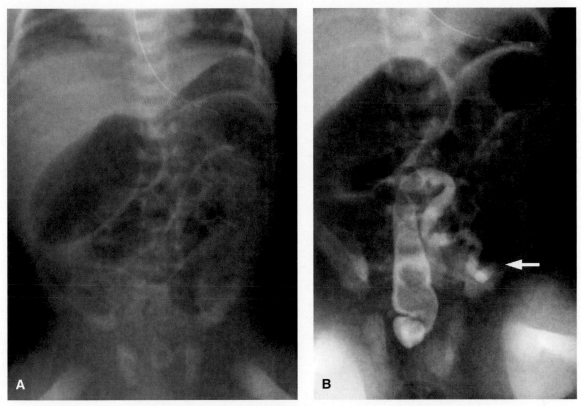

FIGURE 5.25. **Colonic atresia.** Another neonate with abdominal distention. **A:** Initial abdominal radiographs demonstrate multiple dilated loops of bowel. Owing to the concern for a distal obstruction, a contrast enema was performed. **B:** The contrast enema shows a small caliber colon which abruptly ends (*arrow*), consistent with a colonic atresia.

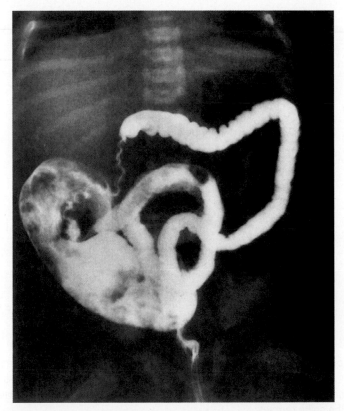

FIGURE 5.26. **Microcolon.** A contrast enema demonstrating a very small colon (microcolon) leading to a very dilated ileum distended with multiple filling defects. The filling defects are impacted meconium, which gives *meconium ileus* its name. Remember that a microcolon is a sign of a distal obstruction or a diffusely abnormal colon.

the colon and stimulate its normal development. The classic cause of a microcolon is **meconium ileus**. This condition is seen in patients with cystic fibrosis. Owing to abnormal GI tract secretions, these patients have abnormally thickened meconium which then gets stuck in the terminal ileum, causing an obstruction and resulting in a microcolon. Ileal atresia is another cause of distal obstruction that results in a microcolon. Finally, other processes such as Hirschsprung disease (absent colonic ganglion cells) can also rarely cause a microcolon, but for slightly different reasons. In summary, a microcolon is a radiographic finding that indicates an unused or diffusely abnormal colon.

Infant

There are a few very important diagnoses that occur early on in life, but not necessarily in the immediate newborn period. Two examples of this type of process are malrotation with midgut volvulus and pyloric stenosis. While both occur as a result of a congenital abnormality, the presentation may (in the case of midgut volvulus) or does (in the case of pyloric stenosis) occur outside of the immediate neonatal period.

Malrotation With Midgut Volvulus

Malrotation is a congenital abnormality of fixation of the bowel and mesentery. In and of itself, having an abnormally rotated bowel is not a direct threat to the patient.

However, the anatomic consequence of malrotation puts the patient at risk for midgut volvulus, a catastrophic and potentially lethal event. Remember that the fetal bowel forms about the axis of the superior mesenteric artery and that during the first trimester the bowel herniates out of the body for a short period of time and then returns to the abdominal cavity. If, on return, the bowel does not rotate appropriately, it fixes in abnormal positions. This error in fixation of the bowel sets the scene for the bowel to twist around its abnormal mesenteric attachments, causing midgut volvulus. Not only does this twisting cause a bowel obstruction, but because the bowel twists about the superior mesenteric artery and vein, vascular compromise and ischemia occurs. If the bowel is not untwisted, the gut will die, leaving the child a nutritional cripple. This is truly a surgical emergency and should be considered whenever you have an abnormal film suggesting obstruction as well as the presence of bilious vomiting in a young child. Although malrotation is discussed with the neonatal and infant abdominal diseases, be aware that it can present at any time in life. The majority of malrotation patients who develop midgut volvulus do so within the first year of life; however, older children and adults can occasionally have malrotation-related problems. The diagnostic test of choice in suspected malrotation is an emergent upper GI study (Fig. 5.27). In malrotation with midgut volvulus, the upper GI study will demonstrate a duodenal

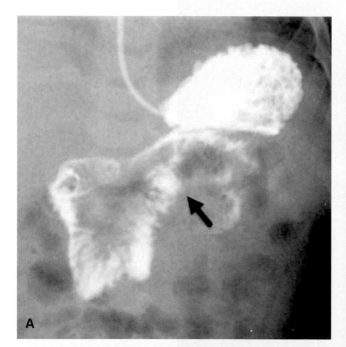
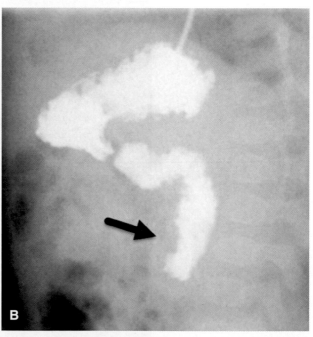

FIGURE 5.27. Normal upper GI contrast examination, demonstrating the normal appearance of the duodenum, with a normal position of the ligament of Treitz. **A:** On the frontal view, the C-loop of the duodenum should descend, cross the midline, and then ascend back up to the same level of the duodenal bulb, representing the ligament of Treitz (*arrow*). **B:** On the lateral view, the duodenum is located posteriorly, just in front of the spine (*arrow*).

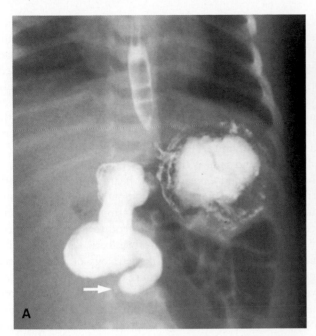

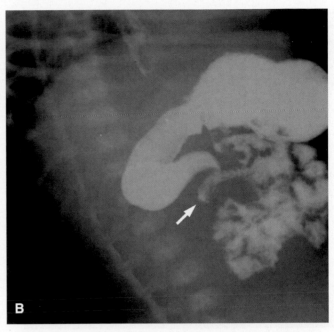

FIGURE 5.28. Malrotation and midgut volvulus. A: A 10-day-old baby presented with vomiting. An upper GI examination was performed, demonstrating obstruction of the duodenum (*arrow*). The duodenum also appears to have a somewhat spiral or twisted appearance. **B:** This 9-day-old baby presented with bilious emesis. The upper GI examination demonstrates spiraling of duodenum consistent with volvulus (*arrow*). Note that some contrast does get through the twist, and the bowel is not completely obstructed. Regardless, this still represents a surgical emergency due to the associated twisting of the mesenteric vasculature and risk of bowel ischemia.

obstruction, usually involving the second to third portion of the duodenum (Fig. 5.28). If there is an incomplete obstruction, the upper GI will show an abnormal course of the duodenum, occasionally with a "corkscrew"-type appearance.

Pyloric Stenosis

Pyloric stenosis is a relatively common intra-abdominal condition in infants (typically about 4–6 weeks old). Pyloric stenosis is not a true congenital anomaly; instead, it is due to hypertrophy of the pyloric muscle induced by a heritable error in metabolism. Pyloric stenosis does not present right after birth because it takes some time for the pyloric muscle to hypertrophy to a sufficient degree to obstruct gastric outflow. The disease is more common in males and classically presents with nonbilious vomiting and weight loss. The plain abdominal radiograph may show a dilated stomach (Fig. 5.29). Upper GI will show fixed elongation and thickening of the pyloric channel and the narrowing of that channel. Ultrasound has replaced upper GI in the diagnosis of pyloric stenosis for several reasons, including the lack of ionizing radiation and the anatomic detail provided that assists in surgical planning. With ultrasound, the pyloric channel appears elongated (over 14 mm) and the wall will be circumferentially thickened (over 3 mm) (Fig. 5.30). Often, the stomach will be filled with debris. Real-time imaging may demonstrate an obstruction of flow through the pylorus; however, even if some material gets through the pylorus, that does not exclude pyloric stenosis.

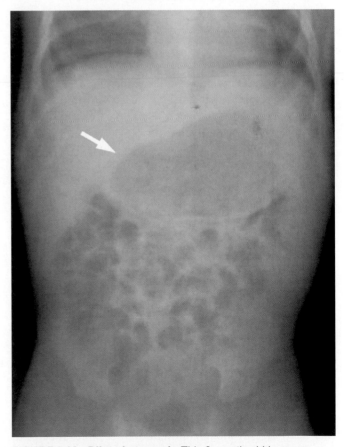

FIGURE 5.29. Dilated stomach. This 2-month-old boy presented with nonbilious emesis. The abdominal radiograph demonstrates a dilated stomach (*arrow*). The remainder of the bowel gas pattern is normal.

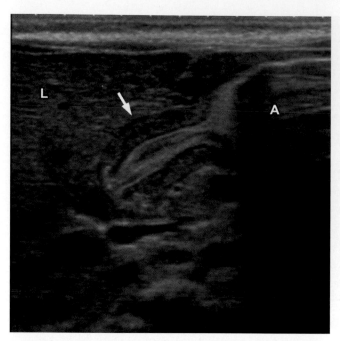

FIGURE 5.30. **Pyloric stenosis.** An ultrasound performed on the same patient as in Figure 5.29. This longitudinal image of the pylorus shows a thickened, elongated pylorus consistent with pyloric stenosis (*arrow*). The left lobe of the liver is seen in the upper left corner of the image (*L*). The gastric antrum is located immediately to the right of the abnormal pylorus (*A*).

CHEST: OLDER CHILDREN

As children get older, their chest radiographs gradually become more and more like adults. Older children are more able to cooperate with breath-holding instructions, so you are more likely to see a nice, inspiratory image. They are also often able to stand or sit up, so standard upright PA and lateral chest radiographs are more frequently obtained. However, there are still several important differences between children and adults, both in terms of anatomy of the chest and pathologic processes that occur. In the following section, we will look at some common conditions that occur in older children (remember: for a pediatric radiologist, older means over about 6 months of age), focusing on processes that are more specific to children as opposed to adults.

Congenital Heart Disease

Serious congenital heart disease has a prevalence of approximately 1 per 1,000 live-born infants and, therefore, is a disease that you will likely encounter if you care for children.

Although radiography is valuable for screening for congenital heart disease, it is often difficult to make a specific diagnosis based on the radiographic appearance alone. Several principles are very important. The **first rule** is that heart size in infants and children is more difficult to estimate than that in adults. The rule of thumb of 50%

cardiothoracic ratio is not valid in children. When you are looking for cardiomegaly in a child, you need to be sure that you are not looking at thymus, that the film has been taken on a good breath, and that lateral views are used. If the heart protrudes significantly beyond the visible airway on lateral view, the heart is usually enlarged. If, on an anteroposterior view, the heart appears large whereas on the lateral view it is normal, then you are usually dealing with a deceiving thymus (Fig. 5.31).

The **second rule** is that children can have very serious heart disease and a normal-sized heart. This is particularly true in conditions in which blood flow to the lungs is insufficient because of right-to-left shunting. As a general rule, children's hearts, being resilient, tend to dilate owing to a volume rather than a pressure overload. Conditions that cause right-to-left shunting, like tetralogy of Fallot, do not give you an enlarged heart because the volume of blood traversing the heart is actually diminished. A truly cyanotic neonate with a normal chest film (including heart size) often has some variant of tetralogy of Fallot (Figs. 5.32 and 5.33).

Rule number **three** is that if you think that the pulmonary vascularity is increased in a patient suspected for congenital heart disease, you are probably right; however, if you think it is decreased, you are probably wrong. An enlarged heart and increased vascularity in an older child who is not cyanotic usually mean some form of left-to-right shunt such as a ventricular septal defect (Fig. 5.34).

Rule number **four** is applicable to neonates. In utero, very little blood goes through the pulmonary artery circuit. To understand this, think about physiology. In utero, the baby is not breathing air; therefore, there is no need for blood to bring oxygen to the baby from the lungs. Immediately following birth, the baby breathes air and the situation changes dramatically. It takes some time for the pulmonary arterial flow to reach more balanced levels of blood flow through the lungs. All neonates, therefore, have a relative state of pulmonary hypertension. Early on, lesions that should have increased pulmonary vascularity, such as transposition of the great vessels or left-to-right shunts, may not manifest on radiographs (Fig. 5.35).

With those rules to consider, it is possible to set out a systematic approach to looking at the chest radiograph of a newborn with congenital heart disease. First, see whether the heart is enlarged and whether you can determine which chamber is enlarged. Next, determine whether the vascularity is normal or increased, keeping in mind that the younger the baby is, the less confident you can be to find increased vascularity. Finally, you need to talk to your clinical colleagues and find out whether the baby is truly cyanotic, as defined by arterial oxygen saturation of less than 80% with a normal arterial CO_2 saturation. With those pieces of information you can use Figures 5.36 and 5.37 and make a rough estimate as to what type of congenital heart disease the baby may have.

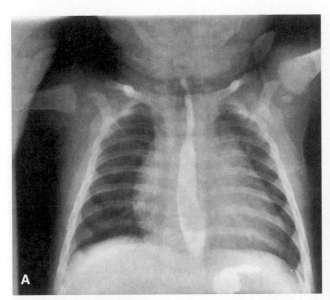
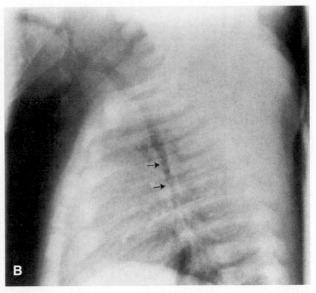

FIGURE 5.31. **Normal heart size. A:** This child's heart measures over 60% of the transverse diameter of the chest on the radiograph. In an adult, this would be a large heart; however, this is a normal child with a large thymus simulating cardiomegaly. **B:** Note that on the lateral view, the heart does not protrude posterior to the airway (*arrows*).

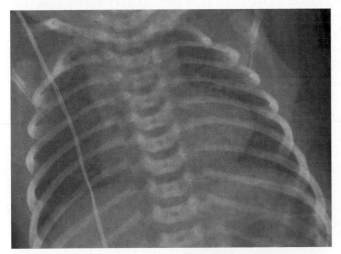

FIGURE 5.32. **Tetralogy of Fallot.** This cyanotic infant has tetralogy of Fallot (TOF). The cardiac size is normal, but the heart has an upturned apex, a finding that can be seen with TOF. The pulmonary vascularity is normal to decreased.

Infections

The most common indication for chest imaging in older children is to investigate for possible infection. Children get pneumonia just like adults, and the manifestations on chest radiographs are similar in most cases. However, owing to the less developed architecture of the pediatric lung, children also occasionally develop what is called a "**round pneumonia**," which is a bacterial pneumonia that appears round and can look like a mass on a chest radiograph (Fig. 5.38). Awareness of round pneumonia is important,

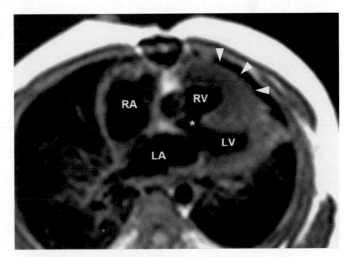

FIGURE 5.33. **Tetralogy of Fallot.** A different baby with tetralogy of Fallot (TOF). This is an axial image from a cardiac MR, obtained with a technique called "black blood imaging" in which the blood looks black and the soft tissues are gray. In this image, you can see the majority of the findings of TOF, including a ventricular septal defect (*asterisk*), hypertrophy of the muscle of the right ventricle (*arrowheads*), and overlap of the left ventricular outflow tract and the right ventricle. There was also stenosis of the pulmonary outflow tract, and the pulmonary arteries were diminutive (not shown). LA, left atrium; LV, left ventricle; RA, right atrium; RV, right ventricle.

because the child may only need antibiotics and possibly a follow-up chest radiograph after treatment, as opposed to a much more extensive (and invasive) workup to evaluate a suspected mass. The small size of the pediatric airways

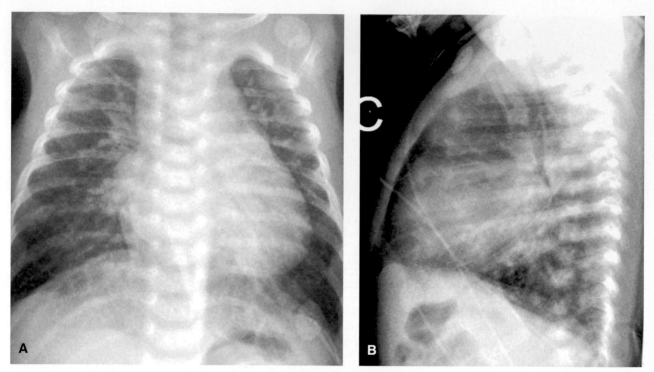

FIGURE 5.34. **Ventricular septal defect** AP **(A)** and lateral **(B)** radiographs of a 2-month-old infant with respiratory distress when feeding, but no evidence of cyanosis, show markedly increased pulmonary vascularity and a mildly enlarged heart. These findings in an acyanotic child are characteristic of a congenital left-to-right shunt. The most common left-to-right shunt is a ventricular septal defect.

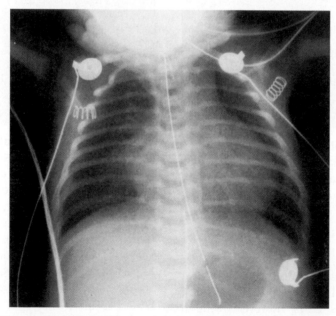

FIGURE 5.35. **Transposition of the great arteries.** This very cyanotic patient has a chest radiograph showing a mildly enlarged heart, narrow superior mediastinum, and pulmonary vascularity that is slightly, but not dramatically, increased. The patient is a 3-day-old infant with transposition of the great arteries; the vascularity is going through the transition between very high vascular resistance in utero to the lower vascular resistance of an air-breathing baby. Over the course of subsequent days, the vascular resistance will drop further and the lungs will become flooded.

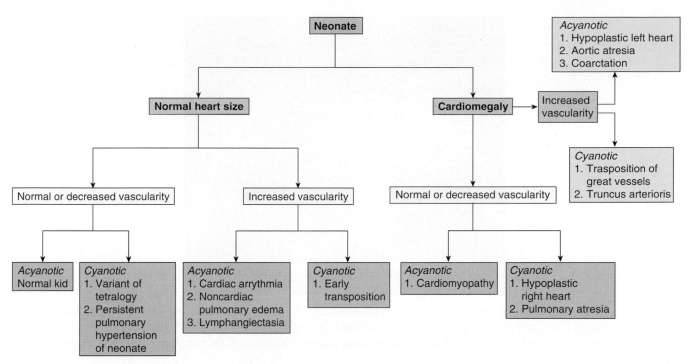

FIGURE 5.36. **Algorithm for neonates with suspected heart disease.**

also makes children more susceptible to viral processes such as respiratory syncytial virus (RSV). Typically, RSV and other viruses cause airway inflammation which then shows up clinically with wheezing, along with infectious symptoms such as fever. Radiographs will demonstrate peribronchial thickening (circumferential wall thickening of small airways), streaky opacities (from subsegmental atelectasis), and hyperinflation due to mild air trapping (Fig. 5.39). Occasionally the radiographs will be normal, which is fine. The whole point of getting a chest radiograph

of these children is to exclude a bacterial pneumonia that may require antibiotics for treatment. Supportive treatment is generally adequate, although rarely causes of RSV can cause critical illness.

Cystic Fibrosis

Cystic fibrosis, the most prevalent lethal genetic disease among the Caucasian population, begins with recurrent pneumonias but also has a number of features that allow a specific diagnosis from chest radiographs. The lungs are

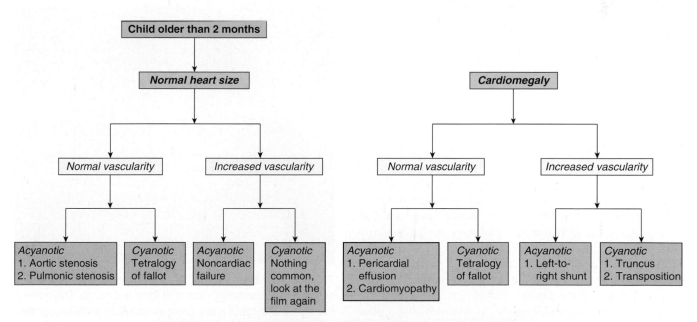

FIGURE 5.37. **Algorithm for older children with suspected heart disease.**

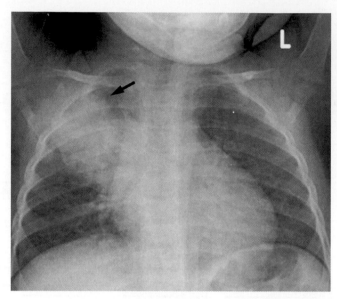

FIGURE 5.38. **Pneumonia.** This 20-month-old presented to the emergency department with cough and fever. The chest radiograph shows a focal opacity in the right upper lobe with a somewhat well-defined and rounded margin (*arrow*). The radiographs and the clinical picture were consistent with a round pneumonia, and the patient was treated with antibiotics. On follow-up imaging, the opacity completely resolved.

usually hyperexpanded because of the blockage of many of the smaller airways by mucous plugs. The mucus-filled bronchi manifest on radiographs as branching opacities, often in the periphery of the lungs. The hilar structures may be prominent, due to the combination of the inflamed lymph nodes and pulmonary artery enlargement resulting from pulmonary hypertension (due to lung damage and chronic hypoxia). The last common finding of cystic fibrosis is that of peribronchial cuffing or thickening of the walls of the bronchus, due to the intense inflammatory change induced by the disease. Ongoing damage leads to irreversible dilation of the airways, a finding known as bronchiectasis (Fig. 5.40). None of these signs are pathognomonic for cystic fibrosis; however, all of these signs taken in combination make the likelihood of this disease very high.

Foreign Bodies

Young children explore their environment with their mouths. As a child crawls around a room, they are constantly putting things in their mouth, testing which things are edible, how things feel, and how they taste. Even older children tend to still manifest this behavior, often putting things in their mouths as part of a nervous habit or for no reason at all. Older children with autism spectrum disorders and some development problems are particularly susceptible to this behavior. Foreign bodies can be either **swallowed or aspirated** and can cause a variety of clinical manifestations and radiographic appearances (Figs. 5.41 and 5.42). Some foreign bodies (such as coins) are radiopaque, and thus the diagnosis is relatively easy. Other foreign bodies, such as organic materials and plastic, do

not show up on radiographs, which makes the diagnosis more challenging. In these cases, one has to look for secondary signs of a foreign body such as air trapping (for an airway foreign body) or soft tissue swelling (for an esophageal foreign body) (Fig. 5.43). There are some tricks you can do to investigate a suspected foreign body; for example, obtaining inspiratory–expiratory views or decubitus views in order to accentuate air trapping. Two types of ingested

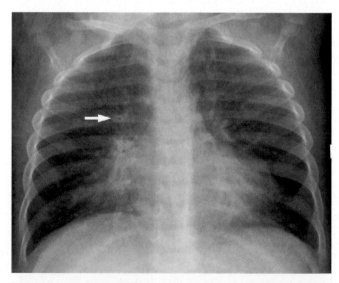

FIGURE 5.39. **Bronchiolitis.** A 22-month-old boy who presented to the emergency room with fever and cough. This patient has typical findings of a viral process, including perihilar opacities and peribronchial thickening or cuffing (*arrow*).

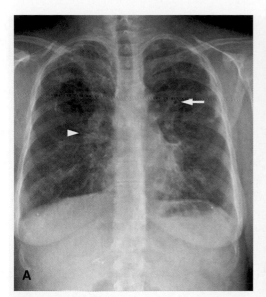
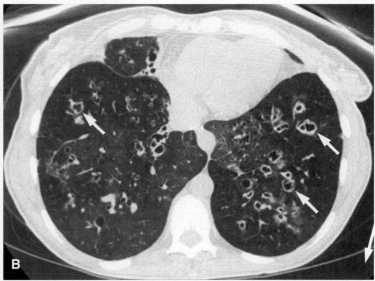

FIGURE 5.40. **Cystic fibrosis.** This 17-year-old girl has cystic fibrosis. **A:** Frontal chest radiograph demonstrates bilateral perihilar opacities. The bronchi appear mildly dilated (*arrow*). The hila are also prominent (*arrowhead*), either due to enlarged lymph nodes or due to big pulmonary arteries related to pulmonary hypertension. **B:** CT image in the same patient demonstrating thickened, dilated bronchi (*arrows*).

foreign bodies warrant specific mention. Button batteries, if ingested, can cause a caustic reaction in the esophagus or stomach and are important to recognize in order to facilitate their prompt removal. Button batteries appear as a disc-shaped metallic foreign body with a beveled edge. Ingestion of multiple magnets is also important to recognize. The magnets can attract each other while in the stomach or bowel and may cause bowel obstruction or bowel wall necrosis. The ingestion of multiple magnets may require surgical intervention.

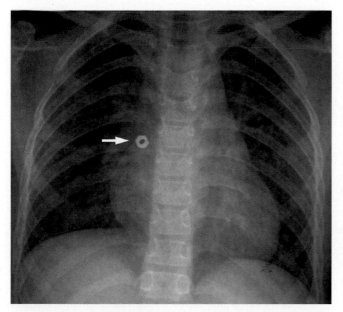

FIGURE 5.41. **Inhaled foreign body.** A 12-year-old accidentally aspirated a nut (as in "nuts and bolts"), and it became lodged in his right main bronchus (*arrow*). Bronchoscopy was required to remove the foreign body.

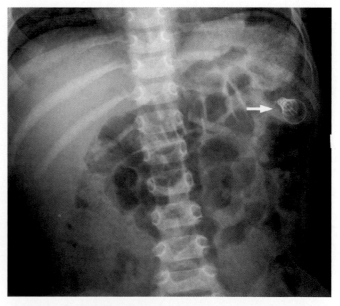

FIGURE 5.42. **Swallowed foreign body.** An abdominal radiograph from a 3-year-old girl who swallowed a small light bulb from the family Christmas tree (*arrow*).

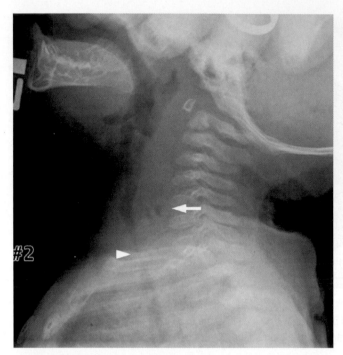

FIGURE 5.43. Swallowed foreign body. This 11-month-old boy presented with stridor. A lateral radiograph of the neck demonstrates soft tissue swelling and soft tissue gas (*arrow*). Notice the focal narrowing of the trachea at the same level (*arrowhead*). After further investigation, it was discovered that the patient's 4-year-old brother had been feeding the patient pistachio nuts, and one had become lodged in his esophagus, causing an inflammatory reaction. Remember to always consider a foreign body in your differential diagnosis in children.

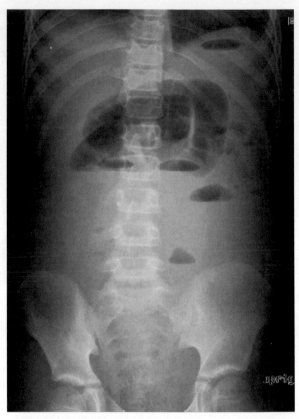

FIGURE 5.44. Intestinal obstruction. A 7-year-old girl with abdominal pain. The upright abdominal radiograph shows multiple dilated loops of small bowel with air–fluid levels, consistent with an obstruction. In this case, the patient turned out to have a congenital internal hernia that caused the obstruction.

ABDOMEN: OLDER CHILDREN

Abdominal diseases in older children are less likely to be due to congenital abnormalities and more likely to be an acquired process. One of the most common causes of abdominal pain in children is **viral gastroenteritis**, which does not usually require imaging for diagnosis. Another relatively common cause of abdominal pain in children is **constipation**, which also does not usually require imaging for management. However, children do frequently have more serious causes of abdominal pain, and imaging can play a critical role in the diagnosis and management of these patients. For example, there is an increasing prevalence of inflammatory bowel disease in pediatric patients, for which imaging is an important component of the diagnosis. For this section, we will focus on a few common conditions in which imaging plays a key role in the diagnosis and that may require relatively prompt intervention.

Obstruction

Bowel obstruction in children is relatively uncommon. Depending on the level of the obstruction, abdominal radiographs will generally show multiple dilated loops of bowel with air–fluid levels on upright or decubitus views (Fig. 5.44). Determining the underlying cause of the obstruction is important. Common causes of pediatric bowel obstruction are relatively few and can be remembered with the mnemonic **"AIM" (really AAIIMM): A, adhesions, appendicitis; I, intussusception, inguinal hernia; M, malrotation, Meckel diverticulum**. The differential diagnosis can be further refined based on the patient's age and clinical history. For example, appendicitis is relatively rare in children younger than 2 years, so if you have a toddler with an obstruction that "A" is less likely. Intussusception would be unlikely in a 17-year-old, so you can throw out that "I." If there is no history of prior surgery, adhesions are unlikely, so there goes another "A." Using this technique, you can usually get the differential diagnosis down to a reasonable list of two or three entities.

Intussusception

Intussusception, a disease in which one segment of bowel telescopes into a more distal segment, has its peak prevalence between the ages of 6 months and 2 years. The bowel is constantly in motion because of normal peristaltic activity. If an inflamed lymph node or some other structure

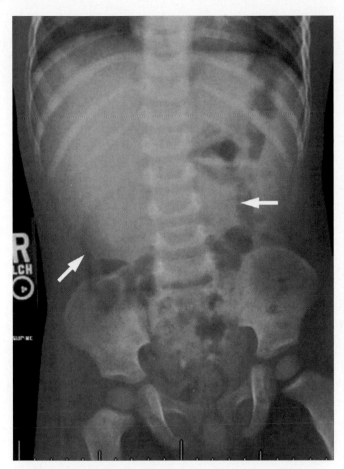

FIGURE 5.45. Intussusception. This 2-year-old presented to his pediatrician with intermittent abdominal pain and one episode of bloody stools. The abdominal radiograph shows a soft tissue mass in the right upper quadrant (*arrows*), suspected to represent an intussusception.

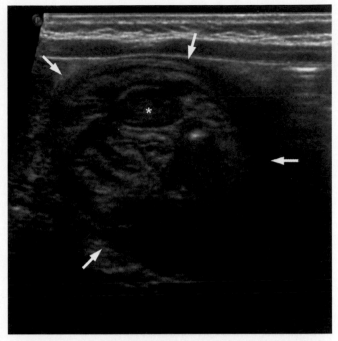

FIGURE 5.46. Intussusception. Abdominal ultrasound in the same patient as in Figure 5.45. There is a round structure in the right upper quadrant with concentric layers, consistent with an intussusception (*arrows*). Notice the oval-shaped gray structures (*asterisk*). These are mesenteric lymph nodes that have been pulled in with the intussusceptum. The lighter gray ("hyperechoic") material centrally represents mesenteric fat which has also been pulled into the intussusception.

alters this peristaltic activity, such that one segment of bowel begins to be propelled at a differential rate, this can lead to prolapse of one segment (intussusceptum) into the next contiguous portion of bowel (intussuscipiens). The prolapsed segment becomes edematous and swells because the blood supply is compromised. This compounds the problem and leads to further extension of the intussusception. The most common anatomic area involved in intussusception is the **terminal ileum**, and most intussusceptions are ileocecal.

Radiology plays a key role in the diagnosis as the clinical presentation can vary from classic findings (abdominal pain, bloody stools) to nonspecific (somnolence, lethargy, poor feeding). Plain radiographs often show evidence of partial bowel obstruction, and the intussusceptum may be visible as a rounded soft tissue density near the point of obstruction (Fig. 5.45). The diagnosis is usually confirmed by ultrasound (Fig. 5.46). Increasingly, ultrasound is being used as the first-line test in suspected intussusception. Rarely a diagnostic enema is performed. Radiology often plays both

a diagnostic and a therapeutic role in intussusception. Up to 80% of intussusceptions can be nonoperatively reduced using either an air enema or a contrast enema. With an air enema, the radiologist fills the colon with air and uses the resultant pressure to "push" the intussusceptum back to its normal location, all the while closely monitoring the pressure in the colon to prevent a perforation.

Appendicitis

Appendicitis is the most common surgical condition in children. Imaging of appendicitis in children is somewhat different than in adults, as there is a greater focus placed on ultrasound. Although CT has excellent sensitivity and specificity in the diagnosis of appendicitis, the use of ionizing radiation and the relatively common (but nonspecific) chief complaint of right lower quadrant pain in children make CT suboptimal as a first-line test. Therefore, great effort has been made to optimize focused right lower quadrant **ultrasound** to evaluate the appendix in children. In the setting of acute appendicitis, ultrasound may show a dilated appendix (usually greater than 6 mm), a thickened appendiceal wall, an appendicolith, periappendiceal inflammation (thickened, echogenic fat), and, in cases of perforation, abscesses. Ultrasound is a great test if the appendix can be

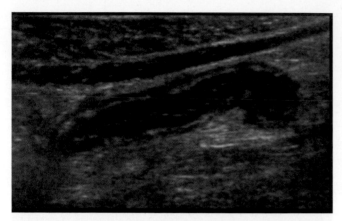

FIGURE 5.47. Acute appendicitis. Focused right lower quadrant ultrasound in a 6-year-old who presented to the emergency department with fever and abdominal pain. The tubular structure in the middle of the image represents the dilated appendix, consistent with acute appendicitis.

found, whether normal or abnormal (Fig. 5.47). However, the location of appendix is somewhat variable and sometimes you just cannot find it, while other times the appendix is obscured by bowel gas (which the ultrasound waves cannot penetrate). In these cases, you have to turn the case back over to the ED physician or surgeon—if they are concerned enough based on clinical findings, they may take the patient to the OR anyway. If there is still confusion, an additional test, usually a CT, may be needed (MRI is also emerging as a second-line test) (Fig. 5.48).

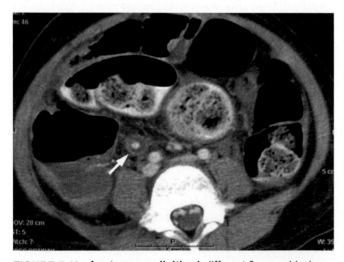

FIGURE 5.48. Acute appendicitis. A different 6-year-old who also presented with abdominal pain and fever. This axial CT image demonstrates a dilated appendix in the right lower quadrant (*arrow*). The higher attenuation structure within the appendix represents an appendicolith. The findings are consistent with acute appendicitis.

ONCOLOGY

Fortunately, cancer is relatively rare in children. The most common childhood malignancy is leukemia which is not usually diagnosed by imaging (although rarely the radiologist may make the diagnosis based on changes in the bones or kidneys). Solid tumors in children are also rare, although if your practice includes children you may come across one or two over the course of your career. Localizing the site of origin of the tumor is critical. Combining the location of the tumor with a few of the imaging characteristics, occasionally a relatively definitive diagnosis can be made based on the imaging alone.

Mediastinum

The differential diagnosis of mediastinal masses is based on location. The mediastinum is divided into four sections; anterior, middle, posterior, and superior. The location of a mediastinal mass can usually be determined by what it is doing to adjacent structures. The anterior mediastinum is defined as part of the mediastinum visible in front of the airway and heart on the lateral view, and the posterior mediastinum is defined as that portion of the mediastinum just posterior to the anterior edge of the vertebral bodies on the lateral view. Everything else is the middle mediastinal compartment (Fig. 5.49). The whole trick is telling these compartments apart and there are a few clues.

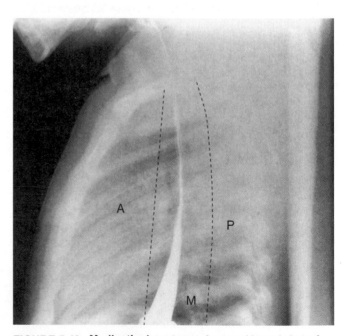

FIGURE 5.49. Mediastinal anatomy. A normal lateral view of the chest with barium in the esophagus delineates the boundaries of the anterior (*A*), middle (*M*), and posterior (*P*) mediastinum. When you consider mediastinal masses, it is important to divide the mediastinum into these components, as it will help you refine your differential diagnosis for the mass.

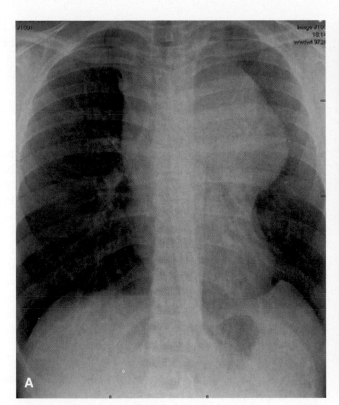

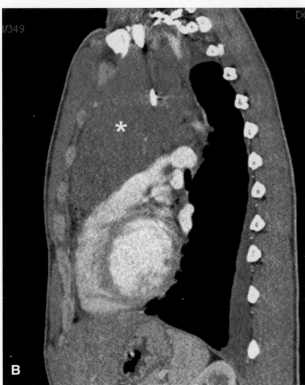

FIGURE 5.50. **Anterior mediastinal mass. A:** The frontal radiograph demonstrates a mediastinal opacity that stops at the level of the left clavicle (the "clavicle cutoff sign"). Notice that the left lung apex can still be seen above the mass. **B:** A sagittal CT image in the same patient showing the anterior location of the mass (*asterisk*).

- **Clavicle cutoff sign:** The anterior chest is anatomically lower than the posterior chest, so if a mass stops at the inferior margin of the clavicle on the PA chest radiograph, it has to be in the anterior mediastinum (Fig. 5.50).
- **Hilum overlay sign:** Structures in the far anterior mediastinum overlie the vessels at the lung hilum; therefore, the vessels are usually seen through these structures (Fig. 5.51).
- **Posterior rib effacement:** Posterior mediastinal masses frequently spread the posterior ribs; therefore, distortion or asymmetry of the posterior ribs is a good sign that the mass is posterior (Fig. 5.52).
- **Airway distortion sign:** Masses that distort the esophagus or compress the airways are almost surely middle mediastinum (Fig. 5.53).

Once you have applied these rules and decided in which compartment to look, the pathologic processes tend to categorize themselves fairly easily. Anterior mediastinal masses are almost always lymphoma or thymus related with the occasional thyroid mass or teratoma. An Aunt Minnie applies here: If the anterior mediastinal mass contains calcium or fat, always go for teratoma. Middle mediastinal masses are generally either lymph nodes or anomalous vessels related to the aortic arch. Esophageal and bronchial duplications are less frequent but also occur in the middle mediastinum. Posterior mediastinum masses are neurogenic in origin (including neuroblastoma). When confronted with

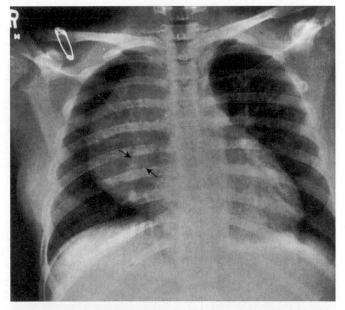

FIGURE 5.51. **Anterior mediastinal mass.** Note that the descending branch of the right pulmonary artery (*arrows*) is clearly visible through the mass, documenting that the tumor is not in the same plane as the vessel; otherwise, the silhouette sign would prevent the vessel from being visible. This is called the "hilum overlay sign" where masses out of the plane of the hilum allow the hilar structures to be visualized.

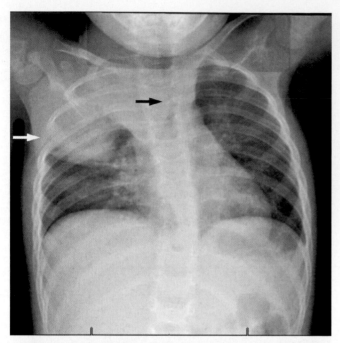

FIGURE 5.52. Posterior mediastinum mass. This 2-year-old boy presented with Horner syndrome. The chest radiograph shows a mass at the right apex. Notice how the right posterior ribs are being spread apart (*white arrow*). This tells you that the mass is located in the posterior mediastinum, in this case a posterior mediastinal neuroblastoma. The mass is so large that it also extends to the middle mediastinum and causes some displacement of the trachea (*black arrow*).

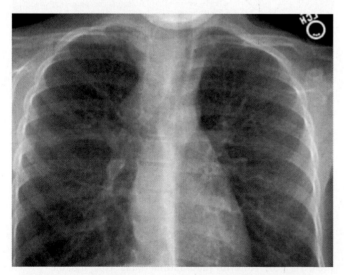

FIGURE 5.53. Middle mediastinal mass. A 14-year-old boy with newly diagnosed lymphoma. Notice how the trachea is displaced to the left, indicating that the mass is located within the middle mediastinum. The differential diagnosis for a middle mediastinal mass includes enlarged lymph nodes, abnormal vasculature, or a congenital lesion like an esophageal duplication cyst.

a suspected pediatric mediastinal mass, the first rule is to place it in the proper compartment; thereafter, it is a matter of pursuing the differential diagnosis.

Neuroblastoma

Neuroblastoma is one of the most common solid malignancies in young children. The tumor arises from immature neural crest cells along the path of the sympathetic nervous system. The typical location for neuroblastoma is the **adrenal glands**, but the tumor can arise anywhere along the sympathetic chain. On imaging, the tumor presents as a solid mass. Calcifications are present in up to 50% of cases. Another characteristic feature is that neuroblastoma tends to surround vascular structures without occluding them, whereas most other masses just push the vessels out of the way and compress them (Fig. 5.54). Lymphoma can also surround vessels, so this finding is not 100% specific. Neuroblastoma commonly metastasizes to the bones and to the liver, but only rarely goes to the lungs (which can help differentiate neuroblastoma from Wilms tumor in some cases).

Wilms Tumor

The most common renal mass in a young child is a Wilms tumor. Owing to their retroperitoneal location, these masses can often grow quite large before they are found. Imaging will show a large, heterogeneous mass arising from the kidney. One clue to the renal origin of the mass is "claw sign," a claw-shaped rim of renal tissue surrounding a portion of the mass, almost like it was holding the mass in a lobster claw (Fig. 5.55). Wilms tumors commonly metastasize to the lungs and liver and have also been known to invade the renal vein, sometimes going all the way up into the inferior vena cava and right atrium. Metastases to the bone is a relatively uncommon finding in Wilms tumor, which may be an important clue to differentiate it from neuroblastoma and other much more rare renal tumors. There is a differential diagnosis, but in a young child, the other renal masses are so much less common, it is probably fair to say a solid renal mass is a Wilms tumor until proven otherwise.

Hepatoblastoma

Although much less common than neuroblastoma or Wilms tumor, hepatoblastoma is a rare tumor that arises from the liver in younger children. There is an increased incidence of this tumor in formerly premature infants. Clinically, hepatoblastoma presents as a palpable right upper quadrant mass in a young child. On imaging, the tumor will be heterogeneous in appearance and can invade the portal vein and other vascular structures (Fig. 5.56). Metastases are relatively uncommon at presentation, but when they are present, they are usually to the lung. One clue to the diagnosis is that the serum alpha-fetoprotein (AFP) will be elevated. The differential diagnosis includes hepatocellular carcinoma, although this is usually seen in much older children with underlying liver disease.

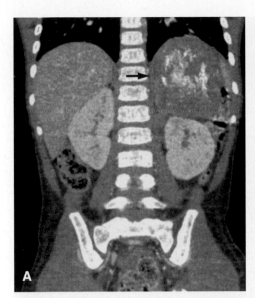 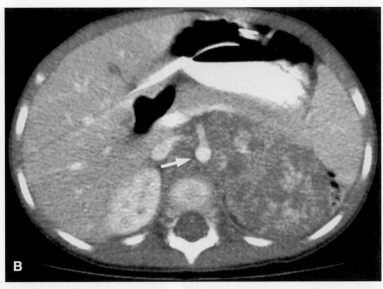

FIGURE 5.54. **Neuroblastoma.** An 18-month-old girl who presented with abdominal pain. An ultrasound (not shown) was suspicious for a mass above the left kidney, so a CT was performed. **A:** Coronal CT image demonstrating a left suprarenal mass with multiple calcifications (*arrow*), consistent with neuroblastoma. **B:** Notice how the abnormal soft tissue surrounds the aorta (*arrow*) but does not narrow or occlude it. This is typical of either neuroblastoma (which this child had) or lymphoma.

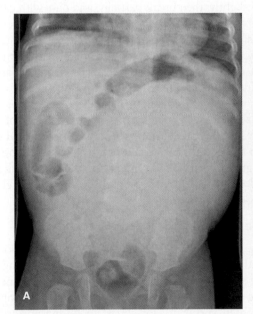 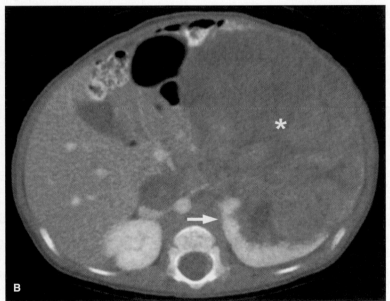

FIGURE 5.55. **Wilms tumor. A:** All of the bowel gas is displaced superiorly and to the right on this abdominal radiograph, indicating there is a large mass in the left side of the abdomen. If you look closely, you will see there are lung nodules at the left lung base consistent with metastasis. **B:** An axial CT image in the same patient demonstrating a large mass (*asterisk*) in the left side of the abdomen surrounded by a "claw" of residual, normally enhancing left kidney (*arrow*).

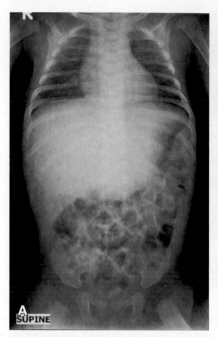
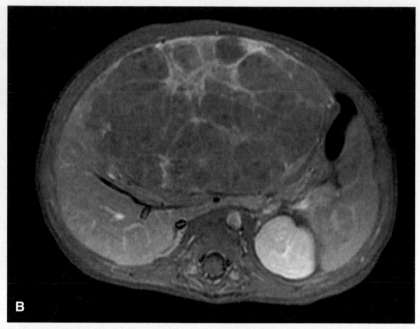

FIGURE 5.56. Hepatoblastoma. This is a former premature baby who presented with an abdominal mass at 18 mo of age. **A:** On this radiograph, the bowel gas is pushed inferiorly and to the left, indicating a mass in the right upper quadrant. **B:** An axial contrast-enhanced MR image of the same patient showing a large, heterogeneous mass arising from the liver.

SKELETON

Like the rest of a child's body, the pediatric skeleton is a growing and changing entity. The child's skeleton has to be rigid enough to support the body and facilitate movement, while at the same time being flexible enough to allow for growth. Long bones (bones of the extremities) grow primarily through a process called "**endochondral ossification**," through which longitudinal growth occurs at the physis (or growth plate) (Fig. 5.57). Most long bones have two growth plates, one proximal and one distal. Some bones, such as the metacarpals, only have one growth plate. During endochondral ossification, cartilage cells within the growth plate undergo a programmed sequence of proliferation, hypertrophy, apoptosis (cell death), and mineralization, the end result of which is formation of new bone and increased bone length. A different process, called "**membranous ossification**," contributes to bone circumference as well as to the growth of some of the flat bones, such as those in the skull. Bone growth can be abnormal because of congenital problems (such as achondroplasia), trauma (if the growth plate is injured), or metabolic abnormalities preventing the normal mineralization of new bone (such as rickets).

Fractures

Children's bones are more pliable than those of an adult. As such, a child's bones can bend slightly before they break, or they can break only partially. It is analogous to the difference between breaking a piece of chalk and breaking a piece of celery. If you try to bend a piece of chalk (adult bone), it will not bend, but rather it will break across its whole width;

however, if you try to break a piece of celery (pediatric bone), it will bend slightly, then break partially, and only with continued force will it break all the way across. Fractures in pediatric bones are a spectrum, ranging from bending deformities (where no actual fracture is apparent) to complete fractures. In between are buckle fractures (*aka* torus fractures) and greenstick fractures (*aka* incomplete fractures) (Fig. 5.58).

Another unique consideration in pediatric fractures is the potential for involvement of the growth plate or physis. Fractures at the ends of the bones have the potential to extend into the growth plates and can have consequences on further growth (Fig. 5.59). The Salter–Harris classification is used to describe the location of the fracture in relation to the growth plate (Fig 6.26).

Nonaccidental Injury

Child abuse, or nonaccidental injury (NAI), is a serious public health problem. Most abused children are younger than 1 year at the time of presentation, with the peak incidence being around 4 months of age. Certain skeletal injuries have a high specificity for abuse, including posterior rib fractures and metaphyseal corner fractures (Figs. 5.60 and 5.61). Other fractures are less specific but also occur, including long bone fractures and skull fractures. In reality, any fracture in a young child, and especially in a nonambulatory child, without an adequate explanation should raise the concern for abuse and should be investigated. If abuse is suspected, a standard skeletal survey should be performed and the proper authorities (such as the local child protective services agency) should be notified.

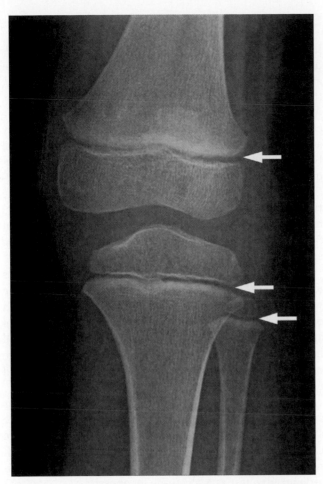

FIGURE 5.57. **Normal knee** radiograph in a 4-year-old girl. The lucent areas (*arrows*) represent the nonossified cartilage of the physis (or growth plate).

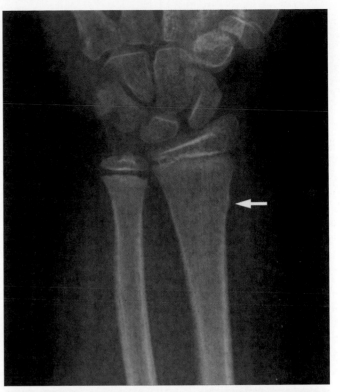

FIGURE 5.58. **Torus fracture.** This child fell on an outstretched hand while playing. Notice how the cortex of the distal radius appears to be buckled (*arrow*). This is a typical buckle fracture, an injury that occurs in children due to the relative plasticity of growing bones compared with the more stiff bones of adults.

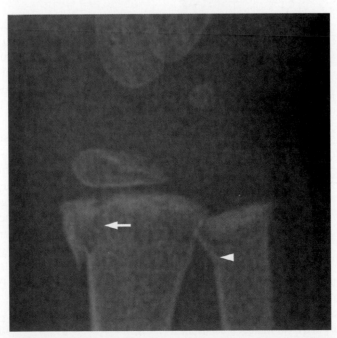

FIGURE 5.59. **Salter–Harris type II fracture.** Another child who presented to the emergency department after a fall. There is a linear lucency that extends from the metaphysis into the growth plate, consistent with a Salter–Harris type II fracture (*arrow*). Note that there is also a buckle fracture of the distal ulna (*arrowhead*).

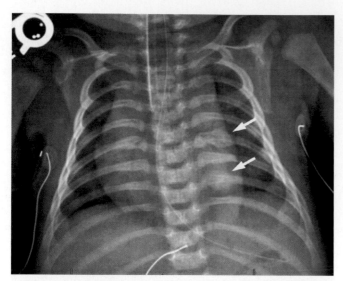

FIGURE 5.60. Nonaccidental injury. This 3-month-old boy was brought into the emergency department with lethargy and respiratory distress. A chest radiograph was obtained, demonstrating multiple healing posterior rib fractures (*arrows*). On further investigation, the child was found to have been abused by his mother's boyfriend.

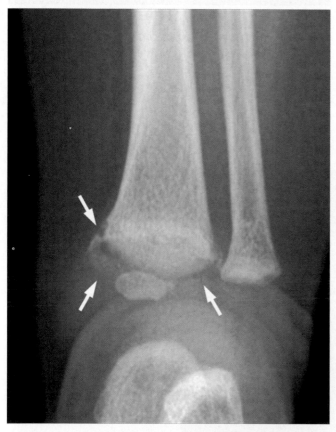

FIGURE 5.61. Nonaccidental injury. Metaphyseal corner fracture (or "bucket-handle fracture") (*arrows*). This type of fracture has high specificity for nonaccidental trauma (child abuse). Remember that any fracture or injury in a child without a sufficient explanation should be further investigated for possible abuse.

SUMMARY

In this chapter, we have discussed the radiographs of children with particular emphasis on those conditions that are common and unique to pediatrics. As in any imaging, there will always be exceptions, but a few rules are key. Always remember the thymus as a deceiver in evaluating chest films in children, particularly younger children. Any anterior mediastinal mass is thymus, thymus, and thymus! Neonatal medical and surgical chest disease can be frequently differentiated by remembering the rules of mediastinal shift and unilateral abnormality. If you apply the rules of looking at congenital heart disease and mediastinal masses, you should be able to get into the ballpark about 80% of the time for making an accurate diagnosis of the correct lesion.

In the abdomen, remember that it is normal for neonates to have considerable gas in their small bowel. As long as the walls are thin and the bowel loops are approximating each other, do not worry. Also remember that up to 6 months of age, it is extremely difficult to tell large bowel from small bowel, and guesses as to whether a loop represents large or small bowel on plain film are exactly that—educated estimates.

The pediatric skeleton is growing and changing and as such may respond differently to trauma, including buckle and incomplete fractures. Trauma through the growth plate can, but does not always, affect future growth. Finally, remember that child abuse does occur and treat every pediatric imaging test as a screening for abuse!

KEY POINTS

Chest

- In some babies, in utero lung fluid takes more than a few minutes to clear, resulting in TTN. This appears on radiographs as pleural effusions and streaky densities. TTN should resolve within the first 24 hours after birth.
- TTN is indistinguishable on radiographs from early neonatal pneumonia.
- The best clue to diagnosing congestive heart failure in babies is a radiograph displaying abnormal pulmonary vascularity and cardiomegaly. If the heart protrudes significantly beyond the visible airway on a lateral radiograph, the heart is generally enlarged.
- RDS displays four characteristic radiographic features: diffuse granularity, uniform disease, air bronchograms, and a relatively small lung volume.
- Generally, surgical conditions are unilateral and will displace the mediastinum away from the more abnormal side.
- Radiographic features of cystic fibrosis include hyperexpanded lungs, mucoid impactions, very prominent hila, and peribronchial cuffing.

Abdomen

- Babies typically have a lot of bowel gas, and it is difficult to differentiate large from small bowel by plain film.
- Neonates and infants usually have congenital anomalies or atresias; slightly older children have manifestations of either congenital anomalies or heritable anomalies such as pyloric stenosis and malrotation.
- In children older than 6 months, intussusception and appendicitis are the major clinical entities.
- Wilms tumor and neuroblastoma are the two most common solid malignancies in children.
- In looking at abdominal films of children, remember that your odds are much better in diagnosing an unusual manifestation of a common disease (such as appendicitis) than in diagnosing a common manifestation of a rare disease.

Skeleton

- Pediatric bones are growing and changing, so normal variants are very common.
- Younger children have relatively pliable bones, so bending fractures, including buckle fractures and incomplete (greenstick) fractures happen frequently.
- Use the Salter–Harris classification when describing fractures that involve the growth plate.
- Some fractures have a high specificity for child abuse (posterior rib fractures, metaphyseal corner fractures), but all fractures without a satisfactory explanation should raise your suspicion.

Questions

1. An infant is born at 26 weeks of gestational age and rapidly develops significant respiratory distress requiring intubation. A chest radiograph is obtained, demonstrating uniform granular opacities throughout both lungs and low lung volumes. What is the most likely diagnosis?
   a. Transient tachypnea of the newborn
   b. Meconium aspiration
   c. Congenital heart disease with pulmonary edema
   d. Respiratory distress syndrome

2. True or False: The presence of small bowel gas on abdominal radiographs in a 3-day-old is abnormal and indicates a bowel obstruction.

3. A 3-month-old child presents with respiratory distress and feeding difficulties. A chest radiograph demonstrates diffusely increased pulmonary vascularity and a mildly enlarged heart. Which of the following is the most likely diagnosis?
   a. Ventricular septal defect
   b. Atrial septal defect
   c. Cystic fibrosis
   d. Viral pneumonia

4. An infant presents to the emergency department with a 2-hour history of bilious emesis. What is the most appropriate radiologic test?
   a. Chest radiograph
   b. Abdominal ultrasound to evaluate for pyloric stenosis
   c. Upper gastrointestinal series
   d. Abdominal CT

5. True or False: An ultrasound is ordered on a 2-month-old male patient with projectile vomiting. During the ultrasound, the pyloric channel appears thickened (4 mm) and elongated (20 mm). These findings are consistent with pyloric stenosis.

6. A 14-month-old presents to the emergency department with wheezing, fever, and cough. A viral process is suspected clinically. What findings would you expect to see on chest radiographs?

   a. Low lung volumes, dilated bronchi, focal airspace opacities
   b. A rounded opacity with well-defined borders
   c. Hyperinflated lungs, peribronchial thickening, and streaky opacities
   d. Enlarged heart and increased pulmonary vascularity

7. A 10-month-old child presents with stridor and respiratory distress, and the parents suspect the child may have aspirated one of their sibling's small plastic toys. Unfortunately, the suspected toy is plastic, so it will not be expected to be radiopaque. What diagnostic imaging test could you perform?
   a. Airway ultrasound
   b. Decubitus chest radiographs to look for air trapping
   c. CT
   d. MRI

8. You see a focal opacity on a frontal chest radiograph of a 2-year-old. The opacity causes spreading of the adjacent ribs. What is the most likely location of the mass?
   a. Within the lung parenchyma
   b. Anterior mediastinum
   c. Middle mediastinum
   d. Posterior mediastinum

9. True or False: Calcification within a mass excludes a diagnosis of neuroblastoma.

10. A 2-month-old boy is brought in to the pediatrician's office because of leg swelling. A radiograph is obtained which demonstrates a displaced femur fracture. The patient's mother states that she does not recall any specific injury. What is the appropriate next step?
    a. Obtain a complete skeletal survey and contact the child protective agency to investigate for possible abuse
    b. Obtain a follow-up radiograph in 2 weeks to confirm the fracture
    c. Check the patient's vitamin D levels
    d. Council the patient's mother on accident prevention

CHAPTER 6

Musculoskeletal Imaging

Nicholas Florence, MD • Stephen Thomas, MD •
Thomas A. Farrell, MB, BCh

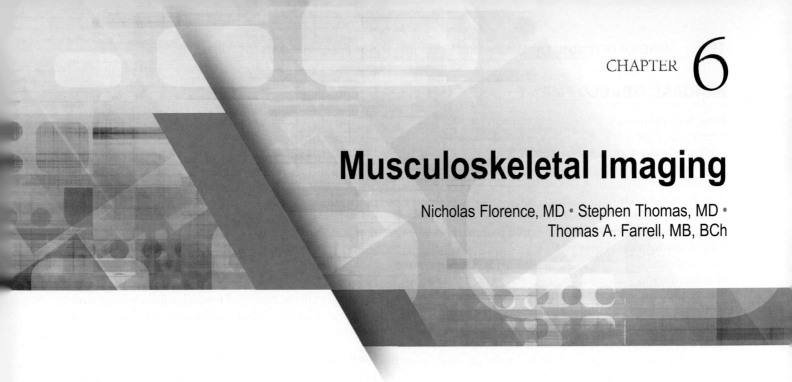

The key concept of pattern recognition prevails when imaging the musculoskeletal system (bones, joints, and associated soft tissues). Despite advances in computed tomography (CT), magnetic resonance imaging (MRI), and nuclear medicine, plain films (radiography) are the mainstay of musculoskeletal imaging and much of this chapter is devoted to their interpretation. The following three tenets of MSK imaging will be reiterated: (1) Obtaining two orthogonal views are imperative when diagnosing or excluding fractures. (2) In patients with arthritis, the distribution of affected joints, the presence of juxta-articular erosions, and osteoporosis are helpful in making a diagnosis. (3) The differential diagnosis of bone lesions can be narrowed down depending on the patient's age (skeletal maturity), the number of lesions, their location, and the nature of their margins.

NORMAL DEVELOPMENT

Bone formation occurs by either **intramembranous** (transformation of mesenchymal tissue) or **endochondral** (conversion of an intermediate cartilage form) methods or by both. Many flat bones, such as the skull, pelvis, clavicle, and mandible, develop by intramembranous bone formation. Both methods of ossification occur in the extremities, spine, and pelvis. With endochondral ossification, cartilage is replaced by bone initiated at specific sites called **centers of ossification**. These centers of ossification appear in such a predictable order that they are used for estimation of bone age and skeletal maturity (Table 6.1). The cartilage between the centers of ossification is called the growth plate or **physis**. Eventually, the centers of ossification fuse across the physis. Understanding this concept is important in the evaluation of fractures in children as a small bone adjacent to a joint may be incorrectly assumed to be an ossification center when it is, in fact, a fracture.

Bone components such as physis, epiphysis, metaphysis, and diaphysis are demonstrated in Figure 6.1A. The physis (physeal or epiphyseal plate) is the growth plate as bone formation occurs here. The epiphysis is the end of a long bone and contains a secondary ossification center. In children, the physis is mostly cartilage appearing radiolucent and it is the weakest part of a growing bone and most susceptible to injury. The diaphysis (bone shaft, primary ossification center) is the long, thin center of a long bone, and the metaphysis is located between the diaphysis and the physis. The term apophysis is confusing and merely refers to a secondary ossification center that does not articulate

with another bone. Apophyses contribute to bone contour, but not overall length (as an epiphysis does) (see Fig. 6.55).

Joints develop between the ends of bones and are necessary for articulation. There are three types of joints: **synchondrosis, symphysis, and synovial joints.** A **synchondrosis** has hyaline cartilage between the ends of bones and is not mobile. There are few permanent synchondroses in the adult skeleton, one of which is the first sternocostal joint. **Symphysis** joints contain fibrocartilage and allow minimal motion. Examples include the pubic symphysis and the intervertebral symphyses, where vertebral bodies are joined by intervertebral disks. **Synovial** joints, for example, the shoulder and the knee, compromise a majority of the joints in the body and have a hyaline cartilage surface and synovial lining, which produces fluid to lubricate these movable joints.

Radiographic Terminology

Anteroposterior (AP) radiographs are named by the direction the x-ray beam as it travels through the body part, assuming the person is in the standard anatomic position (the arms at the sides with palms facing forward). In a typical hand radiograph the hand is placed with palm down on the radiographic plate and the x-ray beam enters through the posterior (dorsal) side of the hand to reach the plate, which makes it a posteroanterior (PA) radiograph (Fig. 6.1A-C). The foot, however, when radiographed with the plantar surface (sole of the foot) on the radiographic plate is an AP orientation. This is somewhat of a misnomer since the dorsal surface of the foot is really the cephalic surface of the foot in anatomic position. The **AP and lateral views** constitute the standard projections for most bone plain films with additional oblique views if necessary.

A checklist to evaluate upper and lower extremity images is recommended (Table 6.2).

Nomenclature: Upper Extremity

The proper terminology for each digit and the numbering system for the metacarpals are displayed in Figure 6.1B. It is this author's preference to name the individual digits of the hand. Beginning on the radial side of the hand, the thumb is always the thumb and not the first finger. Next is the index finger (not the second finger and not the first finger as some say there are four fingers and a thumb). Following are the long finger (not the third), the ring finger (not the fourth), and the small or little finger (not the fifth).

Metacarpals (Fig. 6.1B) are numbered with the thumb articulating with the first metacarpal, the index finger with the second metacarpal, and so on. As a general rule, each hand digit has three phalanges except the thumb, which has only two. The phalanges are named proximal, middle, and distal. The joint between the proximal phalanx and the metacarpal is the metacarpophalangeal (MCP) joint (Fig. 6.1B). The joint between the proximal and middle

TABLE 6.1	Average Age of Appearance of Major Ossification Centers
Ossification Center	**Average Age (Girls Earlier Than Boys)**
Head of humerus	2 wk
Head of femur	4 mo
Distal radius	1 y
Patella	4 y
Elbow	
Capitellum	3 y
Radial head	5 y
Medial epicondyle	6 y
Trochlea	8 y
Lateral epicondyle	10 y
Olecranon	11 y
Acromion	13 y
Coracoid process of scapula	14 y
Ischial tuberosity	15 y
Inner margin clavicle	19 y

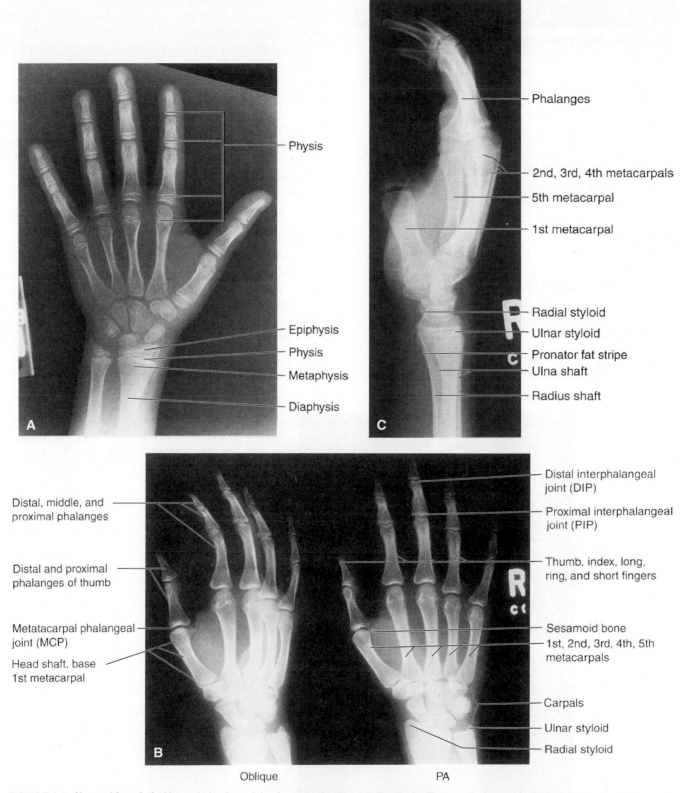

FIGURE 6.1. Normal hand. A: Normal physis, epiphysis, metaphysis, and diaphysis. The cartilaginous physis is lucent on a radiograph. **B:** Right-hand oblique and posteroanterior (PA) radiographs. **C:** Right-hand lateral radiograph.

TABLE 6.2 Checklist for Radiographs

Each Bone Should Be Evaluated for
Density
Anomaly
Fracture
Destruction
New bone formation
Masses
Foreign body

Each Joint Should Be Evaluated for
Articular surface smoothness
Symmetry
Fracture
Dislocation
Arthritis
Calcification

Soft Tissues Should Be Evaluated for
Swelling
Ulcers
Calcifications
Masses
Foreign bodies

phalanges is the proximal interphalangeal (PIP) joint. The joint between the distal and middle phalanges is the distal interphalangeal (DIP) joint.

The thumb, with only two phalanges, has one interphalangeal (IP) joint. The distal-most part of the metacarpals and the phalanges is the head, whereas the proximal parts are the bases. The central aspects of these bones are the shafts. These relationships are well visualized on standard PA, lateral, and oblique radiographic views of the hand and wrist (Fig. 6.2). In addition to the standard views, a "ball catcher" view of the hand and wrist is useful in patients with arthritis.

Standard elbow and forearm radiographs consist of AP and lateral views (Figs. 6.3 and 6.4), but external rotation oblique views of the elbow may be necessary for better visualization of the radial head (Fig. 6.40C). Radiographs of the humerus usually consist of AP (Fig. 6.5A) and lateral views. Generally, an AP radiograph is obtained to evaluate the shoulder (Fig. 6.5B) and can be supplemented by either an axillary or lateral or scapular Y view. Other views of the shoulder include the axial view (from top to bottom) and the Grashey view (AP glenoid view) in which the patient is rotated 30 to 45 degrees toward the affected shoulder and the humeral head is internally rotated to eliminate overlap

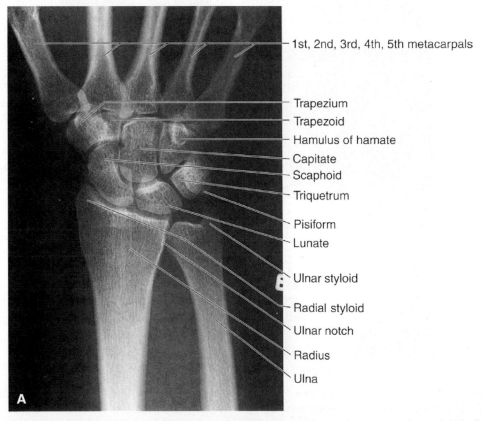

1st, 2nd, 3rd, 4th, 5th metacarpals

Trapezium
Trapezoid
Hamulus of hamate
Capitate
Scaphoid
Triquetrum

Pisiform
Lunate

Ulnar styloid

Radial styloid
Ulnar notch
Radius
Ulna

FIGURE 6.2. Normal wrist. A: PA, **B:** oblique, and **C:** lateral radiographs. Notice that the tip of the radial styloid is distal to the tip of the ulnar styloid and the radius articulates distally with the scaphoid and lunate carpals and laterally with the ulna (ulnar or sigmoid notch). The distal radial articular surface slopes toward the ulna and anteriorly (palmar). The distal ulna articulates with the radius laterally and wrist fibrocartilage distally. The ulna does not articulate directly with a carpal.

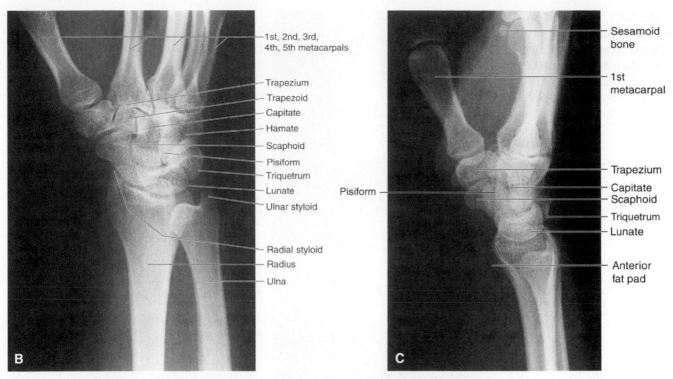

B

— 1st, 2nd, 3rd, 4th, 5th metacarpals

— Trapezium
— Trapezoid
— Capitate
— Hamate
— Scaphoid
— Pisiform
— Triquetrum
— Lunate
— Ulnar styloid

— Radial styloid
— Radius
— Ulna

C

— Sesamoid bone

— 1st metacarpal

Pisiform —

— Trapezium
— Capitate
— Scaphoid
— Triquetrum
— Lunate

— Anterior fat pad

FIGURE 6.2. *(Continued)*

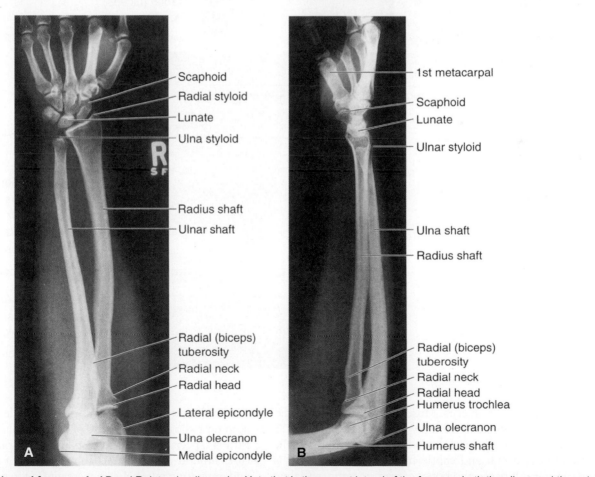

A

— Scaphoid
— Radial styloid
— Lunate
— Ulna styloid

— Radius shaft
— Ulnar shaft

— Radial (biceps) tuberosity
— Radial neck
— Radial head
— Lateral epicondyle
— Ulna olecranon
— Medial epicondyle

B

— 1st metacarpal
— Scaphoid
— Lunate
— Ulnar styloid

— Ulna shaft
— Radius shaft

— Radial (biceps) tuberosity
— Radial neck
— Radial head
— Humerus trochlea
— Ulna olecranon
— Humerus shaft

FIGURE 6.3. Normal forearm. A: AP and **B:** lateral radiographs. Note that in the correct lateral of the forearm, both the elbow and the wrist are in the lateral position. The distal radius is large and the proximal radius is small, whereas the distal ulna is small and the proximal ulna is large. The radius is far more important than the ulna in the wrist joint, whereas the ulna is more important in the elbow joint than the radius.

FIGURE 6.4. Normal elbow. A:
AP and **B:** lateral radiographs. The
elbow is usually flexed 90 degrees
to minimize the appearance of the
anterior and posterior fat pads. The
dotted line on **(B)** indicates the ulna
coronoid process.

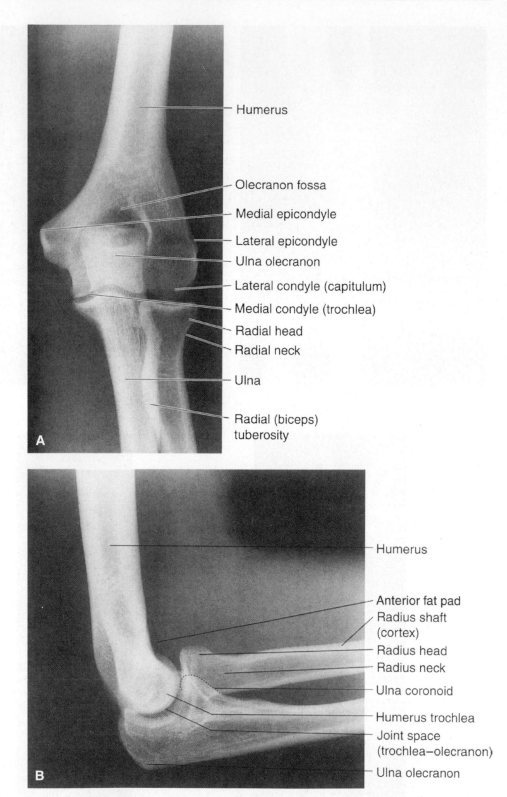

A
- Humerus
- Olecranon fossa
- Medial epicondyle
- Lateral epicondyle
- Ulna olecranon
- Lateral condyle (capitulum)
- Medial condyle (trochlea)
- Radial head
- Radial neck
- Ulna
- Radial (biceps) tuberosity

B
- Humerus
- Anterior fat pad
- Radius shaft (cortex)
- Radius head
- Radius neck
- Ulna coronoid
- Humerus trochlea
- Joint space (trochlea–olecranon)
- Ulna olecranon

of the glenoid and humerus. Musculoskeletal anatomy and disease is well demonstrated by both CT and MRI. CT imaging is especially useful for fine bone detail and the evaluation of occult and subtle fractures, whereas MRI is superior for soft tissue and bone marrow imaging, revealing edema caused by bone contusions or subtle fractures not seen on radiographs. Because of its multiplanar capability, MRI is especially helpful in displaying the soft tissue structures around joints such as shoulder rotator cuff anatomy and evaluating internal derangement (Fig. 6.6).

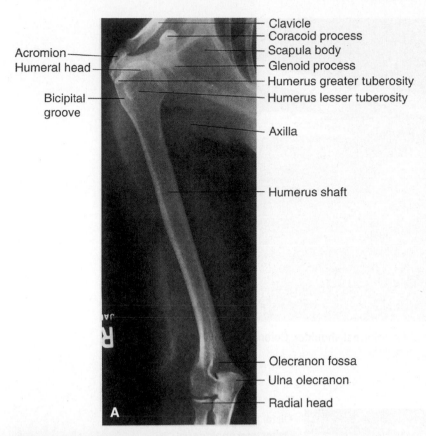

Acromion
Humeral head

Bicipital groove

Clavicle
Coracoid process
Scapula body
Glenoid process
Humerus greater tuberosity
Humerus lesser tuberosity

Axilla

Humerus shaft

Olecranon fossa
Ulna olecranon
Radial head

A

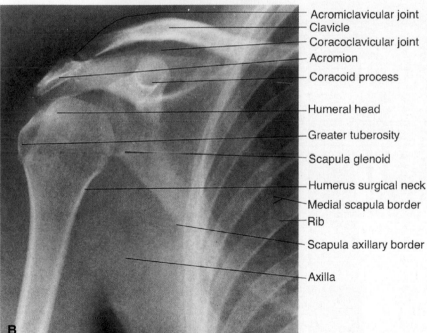

Acromiclavicular joint
Clavicle
Coracoclavicular joint
Acromion
Coracoid process

Humeral head

Greater tuberosity

Scapula glenoid

Humerus surgical neck
Medial scapula border
Rib
Scapula axillary border

Axilla

B

FIGURE 6.5. Normal humerus. A: AP radiograph with external rotation of the humerus. The right elbow is in an oblique position. **B:** Right shoulder AP radiograph with external rotation of the humerus. Note the prominence of the greater tuberosity.

Nomenclature: Lower Extremity

The standard views of the **foot** are AP, lateral, and oblique (Fig. 6.7). We refer to the big toe or great toe as the first toe and the remaining toes are numbered ending with the little or the fifth toe. Similarly, the metatarsals are numbered sequentially with the great toe articulating with the first metatarsal, the second toe articulating with the second metatarsal, and so forth. The ankle is usually imaged by AP, lateral, and either oblique or mortise view (a 10-degree internally rotated view) radiographs (Fig. 6.8). MRI may be

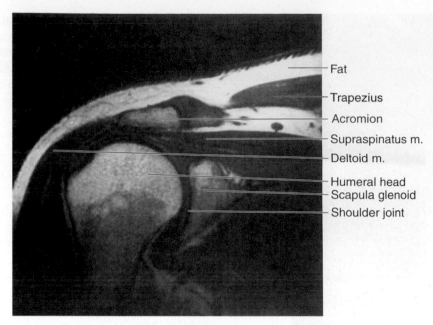

FIGURE 6.6. **Normal shoulder.** Coronal T1 MRI.

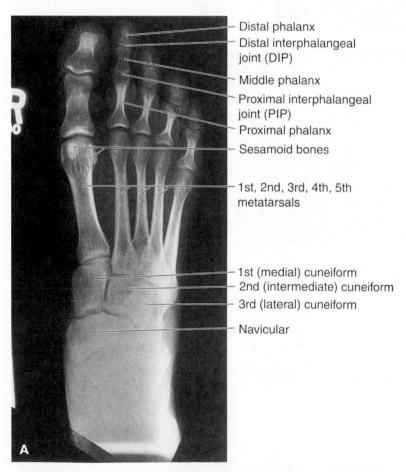

FIGURE 6.7. **Normal foot. A:** AP, **B:** oblique, and **C:** lateral radiographs.

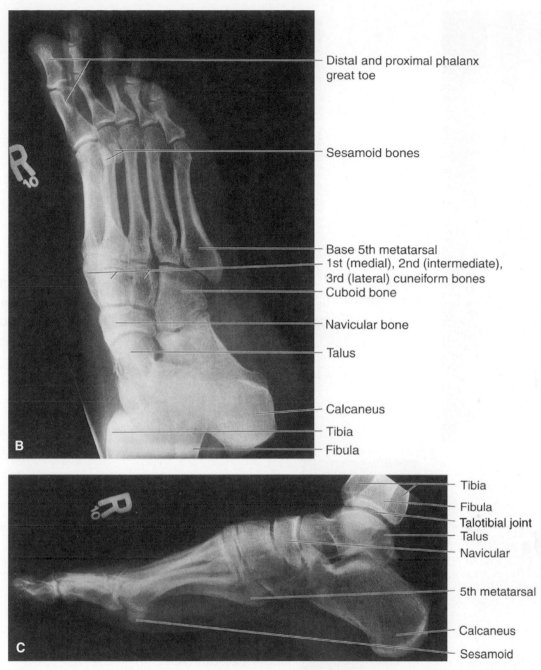

Distal and proximal phalanx great toe

Sesamoid bones

Base 5th metatarsal
1st (medial), 2nd (intermediate), 3rd (lateral) cuneiform bones
Cuboid bone

Navicular bone

Talus

Calcaneus

Tibia

Fibula

Tibia

Fibula

Talotibial joint

Talus

Navicular

5th metatarsal

Calcaneus

Sesamoid

FIGURE 6.7. *(Continued)*

used to image the ankle to detect soft tissue injury (Fig. 6.9). Radiographs of the tibia and fibula usually consist of AP and lateral views (Fig. 6.10).

Routine **knee** radiographs consist of AP and lateral views and they may be supplemented by AP standing radiographs (Fig. 6.11A-C) and sunrise or oblique views for evaluation of the three compartments that compose the knee joint. A cross-table lateral view of the knee is necessary to detect lipohemarthrosis (layering fat and fluid in the joint space)

as a secondary sign of an occult fracture (Fig. 6.11D). Axial, coronal, and sagittal MR images of the knee are useful for evaluation of the nonosseous structures, including the medial and lateral menisci, articular cartilage, ligaments, tendons, and muscles (Fig. 6.12).

The **femur and the hip joint** are imaged in AP and lateral views (Fig. 6.13). An AP view of the pelvis is useful for comparing both hips. A cross-table lateral view of the hip may be necessary in trauma (Fig. 6.75B).

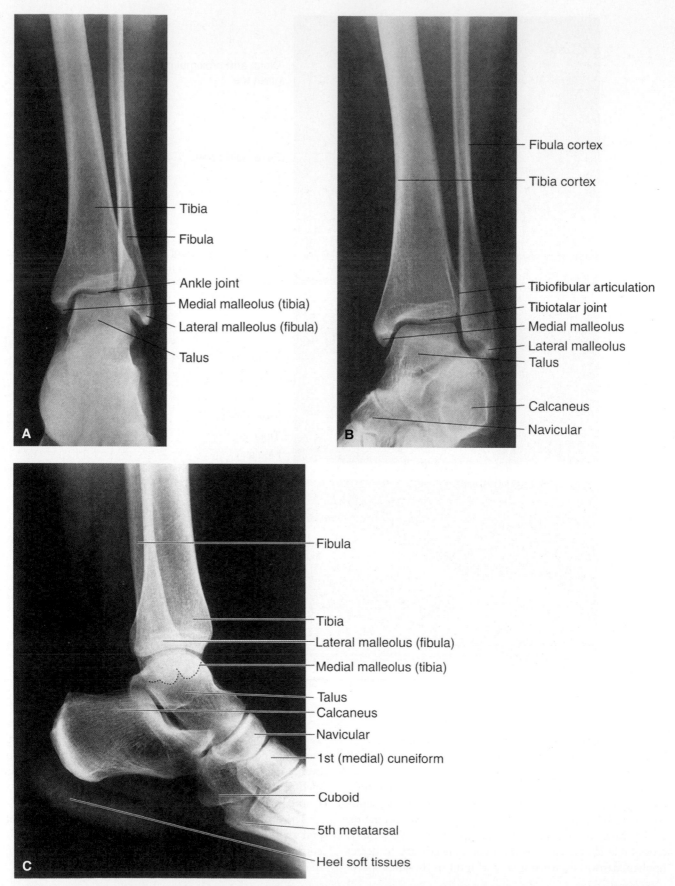

FIGURE 6.8. Normal ankle. A: AP, **B:** oblique/mortise, and **C:** lateral radiographs. The mortise view allows improved visualization of the distal tibiofibular articulation.

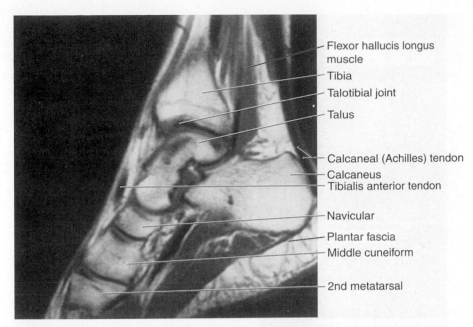

Flexor hallucis longus muscle
Tibia
Talotibial joint
Talus

Calcaneal (Achilles) tendon
Calcaneus
Tibialis anterior tendon

Navicular

Plantar fascia
Middle cuneiform

2nd metatarsal

FIGURE 6.9. Normal ankle. Sagittal T1 MRI. Note that the calcaneal (Achilles) tendon is homogeneously low (*black*) signal.

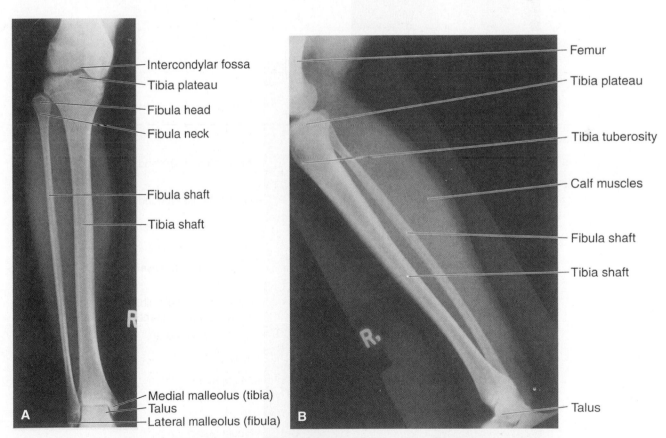

Intercondylar fossa
Tibia plateau
Fibula head
Fibula neck

Fibula shaft
Tibia shaft

Medial malleolus (tibia)
Talus
Lateral malleolus (fibula)

Femur
Tibia plateau

Tibia tuberosity

Calf muscles

Fibula shaft

Tibia shaft

Talus

FIGURE 6.10. Normal tibia and fibula. A: AP and **B:** lateral radiographs.

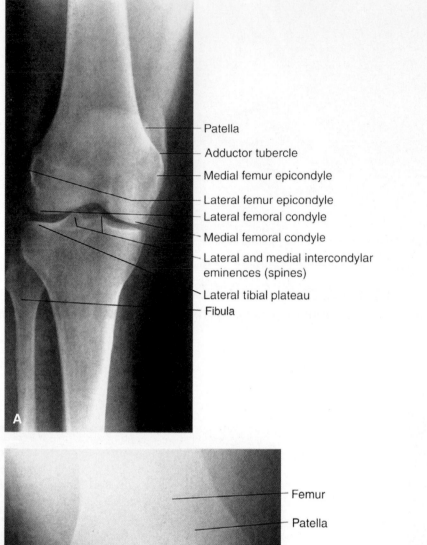

Patella

Adductor tubercle

Medial femur epicondyle

Lateral femur epicondyle

Lateral femoral condyle

Medial femoral condyle

Lateral and medial intercondylar eminences (spines)

Lateral tibial plateau

Fibula

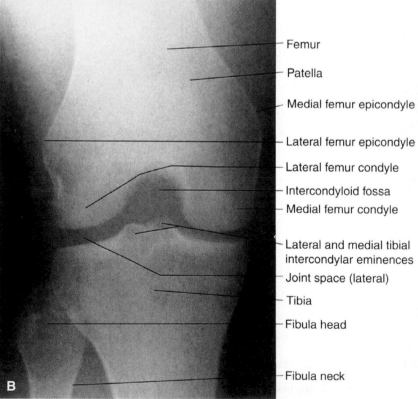

Femur

Patella

Medial femur epicondyle

Lateral femur epicondyle

Lateral femur condyle

Intercondyloid fossa

Medial femur condyle

Lateral and medial tibial intercondylar eminences

Joint space (lateral)

Tibia

Fibula head

Fibula neck

FIGURE 6.11. **Knee. A:** AP, **B:** AP standing, and **C:** lateral normal radiographs. **D:** Cross-table lateral showing a lipohemarthrosis, indicating an underlying fracture.

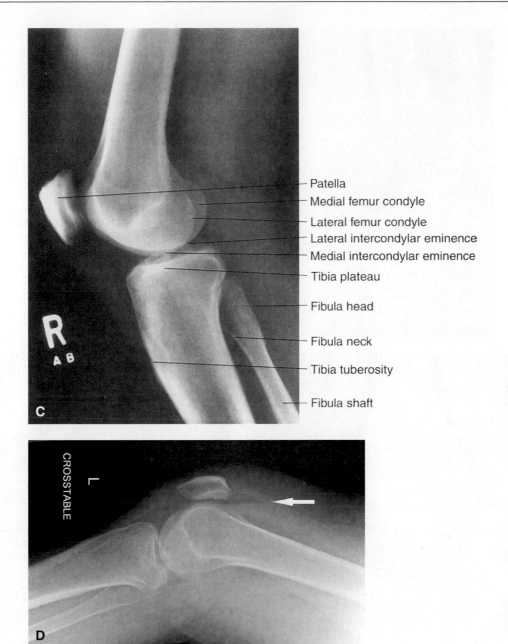

Patella
Medial femur condyle
Lateral femur condyle
Lateral intercondylar eminence
Medial intercondylar eminence
Tibia plateau
Fibula head
Fibula neck
Tibia tuberosity
Fibula shaft

FIGURE 6.11. *(Continued)*

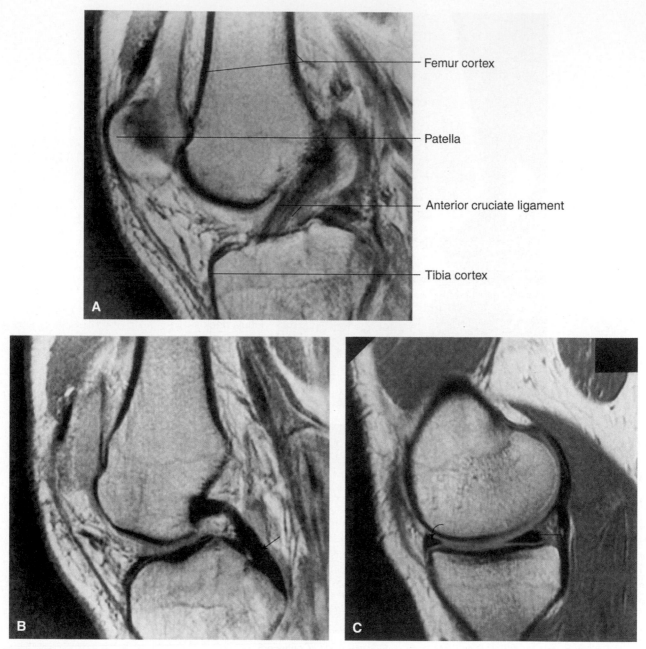

Femur cortex

Patella

Anterior cruciate ligament

Tibia cortex

FIGURE 6.12. Normal knee. A: Proton-dense sagittal MRI showing the anterior cruciate ligament. **B:** Proton-dense sagittal MRI showing the normal posterior cruciate ligament. The posterior cruciate ligament (*arrow*) is more homogeneous and has a lower-intensity signal (*blacker*) than the anterior cruciate ligament. **C:** Proton-dense medial-sagittal MRI showing a normal posterior horn (*straight arrow*) and anterior horn (*curved arrow*) of the medial meniscus.

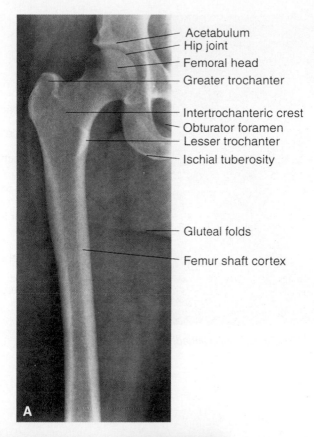

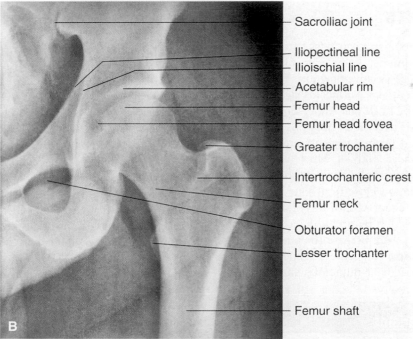

FIGURE 6.13. **Normal hip. A:** Hip and proximal femur AP radiograph. **B:** Left hip AP.

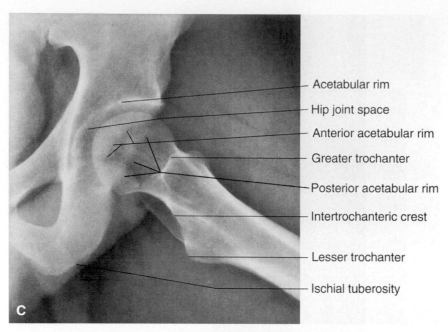

- Acetabular rim
- Hip joint space
- Anterior acetabular rim
- Greater trochanter
- Posterior acetabular rim
- Intertrochanteric crest
- Lesser trochanter
- Ischial tuberosity

FIGURE 6.13. *(Continued)* **C:** Frog-leg lateral radiographs.

NORMAL VARIANTS

There are many normal bone and soft tissue variants that resemble pathologic conditions, knowledge of which is important in avoiding a false-positive diagnosis (Table 6.3). The reader is referred to an *Atlas of Normal Roentgen Variants That May Simulate Disease* by Keats and Anderson now in its 9th edition, which contains over 5,600 images.

Commonly encountered normal variants are sesamoid bones and accessory ossicles both of which are usually small, well corticated, ovoid or nodular, may be bipartite or multipartite, and are found close to a bone or a joint. **Sesamoid bones** usually occur within a tendon and act as pulleys, diminishing friction by providing a surface for tendons to slide over. They also increase the tendon's ability to transmit and sometimes alter the direction of muscular forces. Sesamoids occur at numerous sites and are commonly found in the plantar aspect of the foot near the head of the first metatarsal (Fig. 6.55) and in the palmar aspect of the hand near the head of the first and sometimes other metacarpals (Fig. 6.1B), where they are actually located in the volar plate rather than in a tendon. The patella is the largest sesamoid bone in the body, forming in quadriceps tendon and attached to the patellar tendon. Thus, the quadriceps group of muscles becomes hypertrophied to compensate for increased work following the removal of the patella. Calcification of sesamoid bones is one of the important features of pubertal growth, which occurs earlier in females than in males. A bipartite or multipartite patella (Fig. 6.14E-G) develops when one or more of the patellar ossification centers fail to fuse with the main patellar body producing a patella with two or more sections.

Ossicles are another common normal variant. They are small, supernumerary bones that commonly derive from unfused primary or secondary ossification centers and are found next to and usually named after the neighboring bone (Fig. 6.14D). One example of an **epiphyseal variant** is a prominent distal right radial epiphyseal spur (Fig. 6.14H), which may be mistaken for a fracture. The presence of a well-corticated edge is evidence against a recent fracture and occurs in all the previously described variants.

TABLE 6.3 Normal Variants
Sesamoid bones (located within a tendon, e.g., the patella)
Ossicles (extra small bones)
Supernumerary epiphyses
Coalitions/fusions
Bone islands

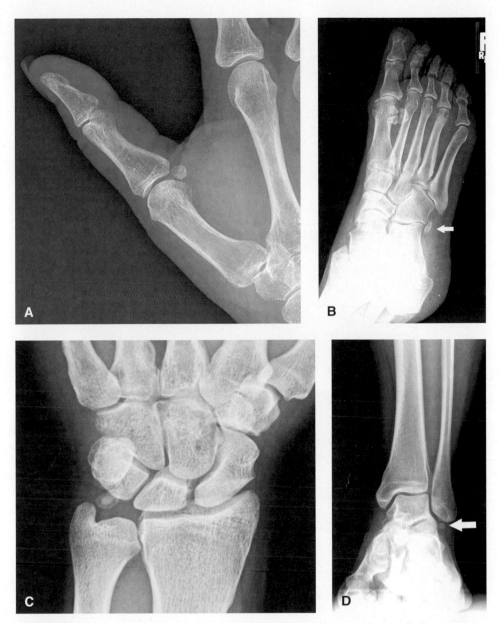

FIGURE 6.14. **Normal variants. A:** Sesamoid at the metacarpophalangeal joint of the right thumb. **B:** The os peroneum (*arrow*) is in the cuboid tunnel near the calcaneocuboid joint. Displacement is an indirect sign of a peroneus longus tendon tear. The hallucal sesamoids are always present at the plantar aspect of the first metatarsal head. **C:** The lunula is an accessory ossicle between the triquetrum and the triangular fibrocartilage complex (TFCC). **D:** The os fibulare (*arrow*) is seen at the tip of the lateral malleolus.

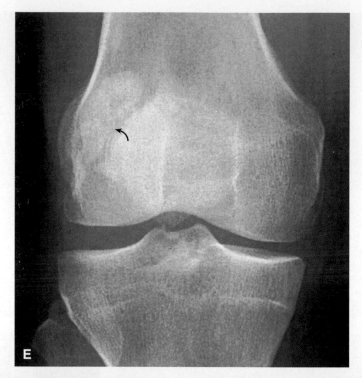

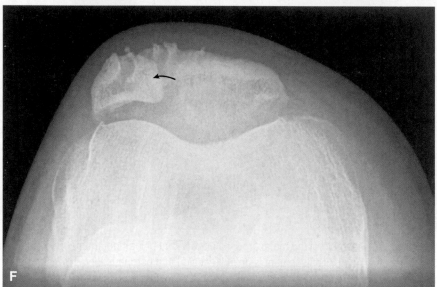

FIGURE 6.14. *(Continued)* **E and F:** AP and tangential views showing a bipartite patella *(curved arrows)*.

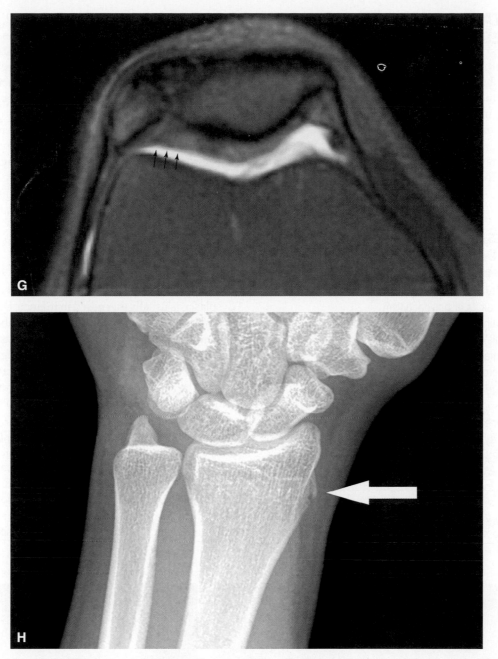

FIGURE 6.14. *(Continued)* **G:** MRI shows continuous cartilage over the ossification center of the patella *(arrows)*, differentiating it from a fracture. **H:** Wrist AP radiograph showing a distal radial epiphyseal spur *(arrow)*.

CONGENITAL AND DEVELOPMENTAL ANOMALIES

Common congenital bone anomalies are listed in Table 6.4 and examples shown in Figures 6.15-6.20. **Coalition** is a failure of segmentation of bones during fetal development, resulting in fusion, which may be bony or fibrous. Common locations of coalition are the lunate and triquetrum in the wrist (see Fig. 6.15) and bridging of the calcaneus and navicular or the calcaneus and talus in the foot (see Fig. 6.16).

TABLE 6.4	Common Congenital and Acquired Bone Anomalies

Upper Extremity
Supernumerary digits or polydactylism
Missing bones (fingers, radius)
Coalition (carpals)
Large digits or macrodactyly
Supracondylar process (humerus)

Lower Extremity
Polydactylism
Coalition (calcaneus with talus or navicular)
Developmental dysplasia of the hip
Legg–Calvé–Perthes disease (avascular necrosis)
Talipes equinovarus (club foot)
Pes planus (flat foot)

Generalized
Osteogenesis imperfecta
Achondroplasia

Osteogenesis imperfecta is a congenital, non–sex-linked, hereditary abnormality of primary defects in collagen synthesis, causing deficient bone matrix. These patients have fragile bones (Fig. 6.20) that fracture easily and are often deformed. Common radiographic findings include gracile (thin), overtubulated bones, multiple fractures, and pseudoarthroses due to nonunion (failure of healing) of fractures of the long bones with subsequent joint-like motion between the fragments. Osteogenesis imperfecta is in the differential diagnosis of nonaccidental injury (NAI) in children. **Achondroplasia** is a hereditary autosomal-dominant anomaly often caused by spontaneous mutation and is the most common cause of (rhizomelic) short-limb dwarfism. Only bones formed by endochondral ossification are affected (Fig. 6.21). Bones formed by membranous ossification are not affected, allowing normal development of the skull vault.

Developmental dysplasia of the hip (DDH), formerly known as congenital dislocation of the hip or congenital hip dysplasia, is usually diagnosed in infancy. DDH is an *acquired* disorder of the hip joint, resulting in an abnormal acetabulum and femoral head owing to displacement of the femoral head deforming the acetabular cartilage (Fig. 6.22). The femoral head usually displaces superiorly but can displace posteriorly. The acetabulum becomes shallow and the angle of the femoral neck between the femoral head and shaft is widened.

Two frequently confused hip diseases in children are **slipped capital femoral epiphysis (SCFE)** and **Legg–Calvé–Perthes disease** (Table 6.5). SCFE (Fig. 6.23) typically occurs in overweight adolescent males and is associated with groin, thigh, or knee pain, and a limp. It is typically idiopathic with anterosuperior displacement of the metaphysis, while the epiphysis remains in the acetabulum. Rare causes include trauma, endocrine disorders, renal failure, or radiation therapy.

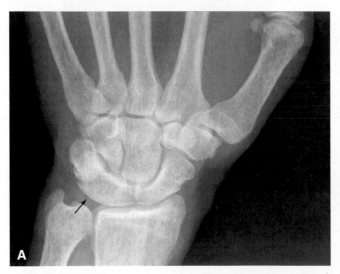
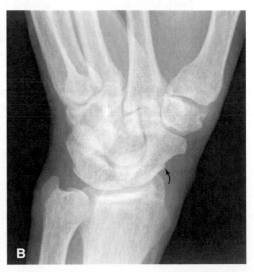

FIGURE 6.15. Congenital fusion. A: Left wrist PA and **B:** oblique radiographs. There is coalition of the lunate and triquetrum (*straight arrow*) and a prominent scaphoid tubercle (*curved arrow*). This tubercle should not be confused with a fracture. Compare with the normal carpals in Figure 6.2.

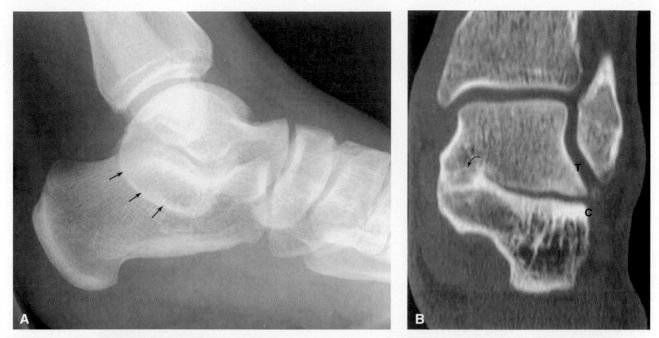

FIGURE 6.16. **Bridging. A:** Lateral radiograph of the left ankle, **B:** coronal CT image. There is a prominent C on the radiograph (*arrows*). Compare with the normal lateral in Figure 6.8. The CT image show bone bridging (*curved arrow*) between the talus (T) and calcaneus (C).

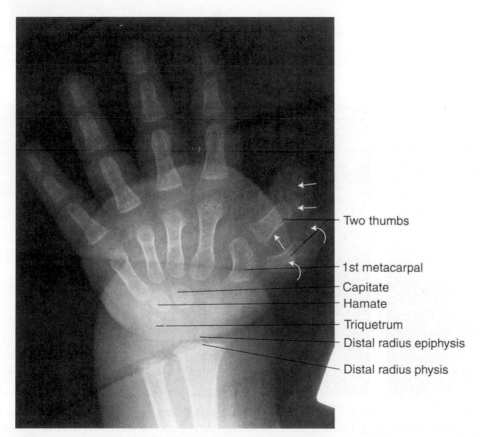

Two thumbs

1st metacarpal

Capitate

Hamate

Triquetrum

Distal radius epiphysis

Distal radius physis

FIGURE 6.17. **Polydactylism.** Left-hand PA radiograph (child). There are two thumbs and one first metacarpal. One thumb has three phalanges (*straight arrows*) and the other thumb has two phalanges (*curved arrows*).

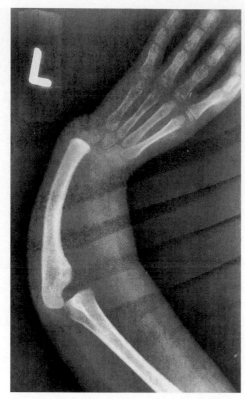

FIGURE 6.18. **Congenital absence of the radius, first meta-carpal, and thumb.**

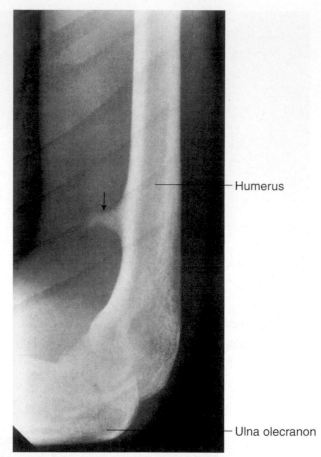

FIGURE 6.19. **Supracondylar process or spur (*arrow*).** It is usually located in the anteromedial aspect of the distal humerus.

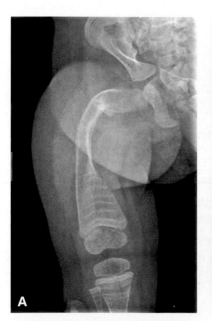

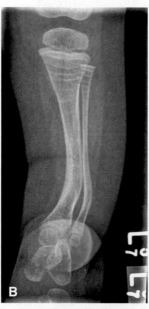

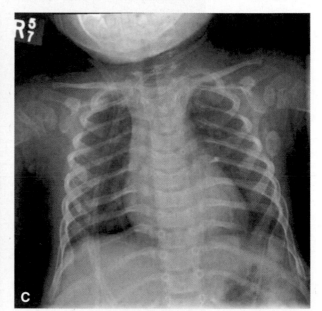

FIGURE 6.20. **Osteogenesis imperfecta. A:** Right femur AP radiograph. There is a severe bowing deformity of the femur and multiple growth arrest lines proximal to the physis. **B:** Left tibia and fibula radiograph. In this same patient there is also a severe bowing deformity and growth arrest lines involving the left tibia and fibula. **C:** Ribs AP radiograph. The ribs are "gracile" (or thin) in appearance with multiple healed fractures bilaterally.

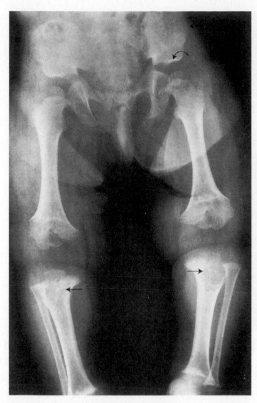

FIGURE 6.21. **Achondroplasia.** Right hemipelvis and right lower extremity AP radiograph. The proximal long bones are shorter and wider than normal, especially the proximal tibia (*straight arrows*). The iliac bone is rounded and the acetabulum is flat (*curved arrow*).

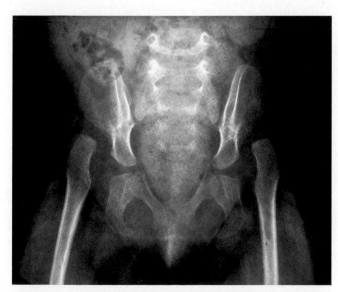

FIGURE 6.22. **Developmental dysplasia of both hips.** Pelvis AP radiograph in a young child. The acetabulum is poorly formed and the bilateral femurs are directed superolaterally and outside the socket of the acetabulum.

TABLE 6.5	Comparison of Slipped Capital Femoral Epiphysis (SCFE) and Legg–Calvé–Perthes Disease (LCP)	
Feature	SCFE	LCP
Age	Adolescence	4–10 y
Gender	Boys more than girls (usually overweight)	Boys more than girls
Etiology	Unknown (usually during growth spurt)	Unknown
Symptoms	Hip and/or knee pain	Hip or knee pain and limping
Radiographic	Epiphysis slips posterior, medial, and inferior to the femoral neck. Early onset arthritis in adulthood	Flat and sclerotic epiphysis. Wide, slightly flattened femoral head with similarly shaped acetabulum in adulthood

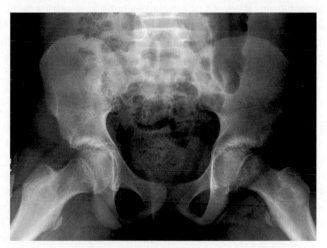

FIGURE 6.23. **Slipped capital femoral epiphysis (SCFE).** Pelvis AP radiograph with widening of the left capital femoral physis and superolateral displacement of the femoral neck with respect to the head. Compare this with the normally aligned femoral head and neck on the right.

The radiographic findings show the epiphyseal slipping or displacing posteriorly and medially. The proximal epiphysis becomes widened. Patients with unstable SCFE have a much greater risk of osteonecrosis. Mild cases may go undetected and present as early onset osteoarthritis.

Legg–Calvé–Perthes disease (Fig. 6.24A) is an osteochondrosis (an aseptic ischemic necrosis of a normal epiphysis) that typically occurs in boys between 3 and 10 years of age who present with hip pain and a limp. The hip pain may be referred to the ipsilateral knee. Radiographic findings vary but include increased density of the femoral capital

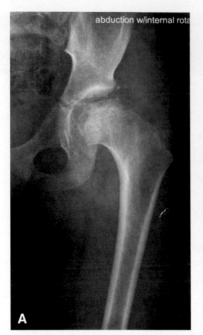
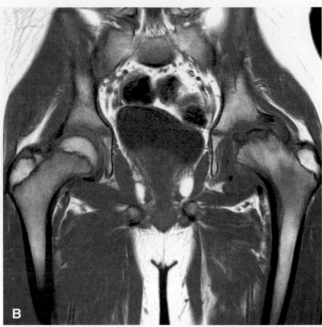

FIGURE 6.24. Legg–Calvé–Perthes disease. A: Left femur AP radiograph. The left femoral head is collapsed, and the head and superior neck are irregular in contour. There is patchy sclerosis of the femoral head. This is consistent with advanced avascular necrosis of the femoral head. There is a differential diagnosis for avascular necrosis, but in this case, the diagnosis was Legg–Calvé–Perthes disease. **B:** Pelvis T1-weighted coronal MR image. Avascular necrosis (AVN) of the left hip. AVN initially appears as a curvilinear area of low signal intensity on T1-weighted images and corresponding high signal intensity on T2-weighted images, commonly within the femoral head. As it progresses, there is collapse and loss of the normal hemispherical shape of the femoral head, as seen in the left hip of this patient.

epiphysis, femoral head flattening (also referred to as "coxa plana" deformity), rarefaction (bone demineralization) of the metaphysis, and medial joint space narrowing.

Osteonecrosis (formally known as avascular necrosis) can occur in any bone and has many possible causes in addition to those listed in Table 6.6. The typical findings of osteonecrosis are sclerotic bone changes on one side of a joint that may progress to fracture, fragmentation, and collapse. MRI (Fig. 6.24B) is useful for the early diagnosis of osteonecrosis, allowing initiation of treatment prior to radiographic changes. MRI is also useful in detecting complications such as early onset of arthritis.

TABLE 6.6 Common Causes of Osteonecrosis
Steroids (endogenous or exogenous) and anti-inflammatory drugs
Trauma including fractures and dislocations
Sickle-cell anemia
Hemophilia (synovitis and elevated intra-articular pressure)
Alcohol
Systemic lupus erythematosus
Renal transplant
Infection
Pancreatitis

TRAUMA

Fractures and Dislocations

A fracture is defined as a cortical discontinuity. Because a fracture or dislocation may be visible on only one view, we routinely obtain at least two orthogonal views (AP and lateral) of a bone or joint. One should never accept just one radiographic view of a bone or joint when excluding a fracture. At risk of repeating ourselves: **ONE VIEW IS NO VIEW.** Additional radiographic views such as obliques, cross-table laterals, and swimmer's view for the C-spine may be necessary and your friendly radiology technologist is a useful resource. A bone bruise is an injury of the bone marrow indicating edema, bleeding, or trabecular bone fractures and is seen as a marrow signal change on MRI.

When there is suspicion of a fracture and the radiographs are normal, clinical judgment is needed and a protocol should be followed. In many circumstances the injury can be immobilized for 7 to 10 days after which repeat radiographs may reveal a fracture. Other clinical scenarios such as hip or pelvic fractures in the elderly may warrant a prompt CT or MRI depending on availability, if the initial radiographs do not demonstrate a fracture. Similarly, CT may be used to diagnose cervical spine fractures or dislocations and are often used to better define fractures in many locations prior to treatment.

Another useful rule for imaging fractures is that paired bones such as the radius and ulna rarely have an isolated fracture; look closely for an associated fracture or a dislocation of the other bone at its proximal or distal joint. Structures that function as a ring, such as the pelvis, the mandible (with the facial bones), or the bones surrounding the ankle joint, also usually fracture in more than one location.

Missed Fractures

Failure to diagnose is the most common error alleged in medical malpractice lawsuits against radiologists, and extremity fractures are the second most frequently missed diagnosis after breast cancer. Early diagnosis may prevent inherent complications such as nonunion, malunion, premature osteoarthritis, and avascular osteonecrosis. Most fractures that are missed on radiographs are the result of errors in perception and many of these misses occur in predictable locations where the radiographic anatomy is complex. Subtle fractures account for one-third of these errors and radiographically occult fractures account for another third. While occult fractures present no radiographic findings, radiographically subtle fractures are easily overlooked on initial radiographs.

The subtle nature of some foot fractures and the associated complex anatomy may result in an increased propensity to missed fractures at this site. The mechanism of injury may also be helpful to locate the potential fracture (Table 6.7).

Fracture Terminology

Many terms applied to fractures are necessarily descriptive and quite specific (Fig. 6.25A and B). Examples of straightforward common terms for describing fractures include the following:

- **Simple:** There are two significant fracture fragments.
- **Complex or comminuted:** The fracture has more than two fragments.

Tiny bone fragments are not considered fracture fragments if they are clinically irrelevant. One criterion is to determine if a major tendon or ligament is attached or if the bone piece is large enough to secure with a screw, then they are comminuted fractures.

- **Compound or open fracture:** The skin is not intact near the fracture. This occurs when one or more of the bone fragments or a penetrating foreign body penetrates the skin. There is an increased risk of infection.
- **Orientation of the fracture line:** spiral, transverse, longitudinal, or oblique.
- **Orientation of the distal fracture fragment with respect to the more proximal** bone of origin: nondisplaced, displaced, impacted, foreshortened/overriding, distracted, or angulated.

Additional descriptive fracture terms (Fig. 6.25C) that are not quite so obvious include the following:

- **Avulsion** fractures occur at the site of a tendon attachment. The tendon and muscle remain intact while the bone gives way (avulses) at the site of the tendon attachment to the bone.
- **Torus** describes the convex molding/projection located at the base of a classical column. A torus fracture usually appears as a minimal bump or buckle on the cortex without a classic visible fracture line because a child's bones are more elastic and able to bend (Fig. 6.25C). When the bone is subject to greater force, an incomplete or **greenstick** fracture (Fig. 6.25C) may occur, so named because a "green" or freshly cut stick will not break through when bent as a dried one will.

When describing the position of **displaced** fractures, the distal fragment is described relative to the proximal fragment. This means that if the distal part of the fracture is displaced toward the midline of the body, it is displaced medially. One may substitute medial with volar, dorsal, radial, ulnar, or any other appropriate direction of displacement. The same concept may be used to describe fracture **angulation**. Unfortunately, much confusion can be created by the nomenclatures for fracture angulation. A fracture described as medially angulated by one nomenclature (using the position of the distal fragment) may be described as laterally angulated by another nomenclature (using the fracture apex). You can see where confusion may arise! A preferred nomenclature uses the word "apex" of the angle created by the fracture fragments as the key. If the apex of the fracture fragments points laterally, the fracture is described as "apex lateral" (Fig. 6.25D). **Varus and valgus** angulation are other common terms to describe angulation and are also illustrated. A **varus** deformity is an inward angulation (medial angulation, that is, toward the body's midline) of the distal segment of a bone or joint. The opposite of varus is called **valgus**. The terms varus and valgus always refer to the direction that the distal segment of the joint points.

The **Salter–Harris** classification (Fig. 6.26) is used to describe fractures around a physis in children in whom fusion has not occurred. There are five basic types (I-V) based on the nature and location of the fracture in relation

TABLE 6.7	**Occult and Subtle Fractures by Location and Mechanism of Injury**		
Type	**High Energy**	**Fatigue**	**Insufficiency**
Mechanism	Direct trauma	Repetitive Stress	Weakened Bone
Locations	Tibial plateau	Fibula	Sacrum
	Posterior acetabulum	Metatarsal	Proximal femur
	Scaphoid	Anterior tibia	
	Triquetrum	Femoral neck	

After Jarraya M, Hayashi D, Roemer FW, et al. Radiographically occult and subtle fractures: a pictorial review. *Radiol Res Pract.* 2013;2013. doi:10.1155/2013/370169.

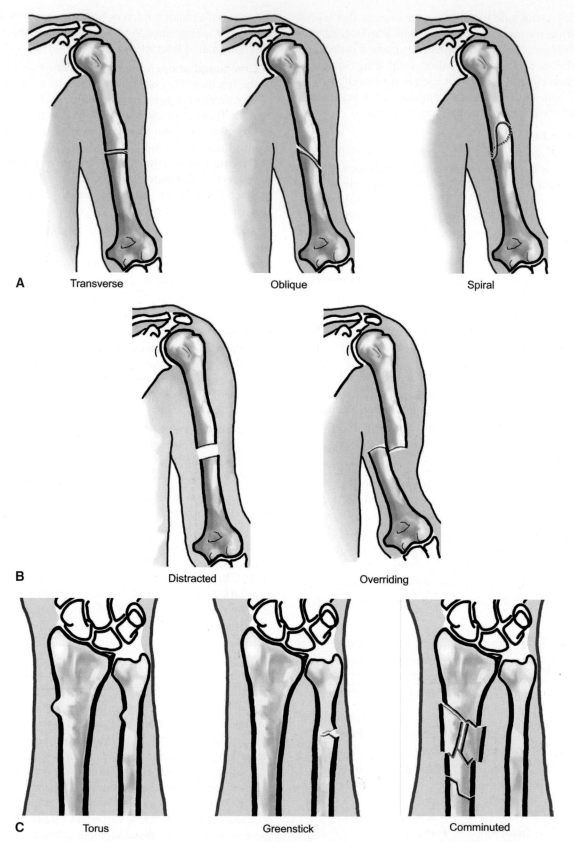

FIGURE 6.25. Fracture terminology. A-C: Common descriptive terms for fractures which are not simple.

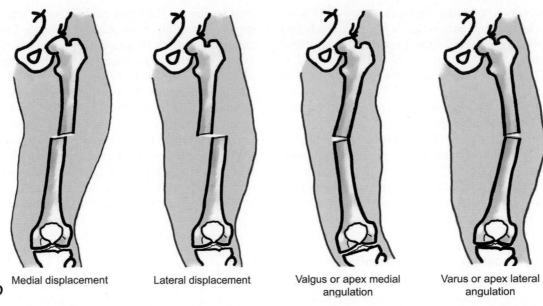

Medial displacement   Lateral displacement   Valgus or apex medial angulation   Varus or apex lateral angulation

D

FIGURE 6.25. *(Continued)* **D:** Illustrations of the nomenclature used to describe fracture displacement and angulation. (Illustration by CBoles Art.)

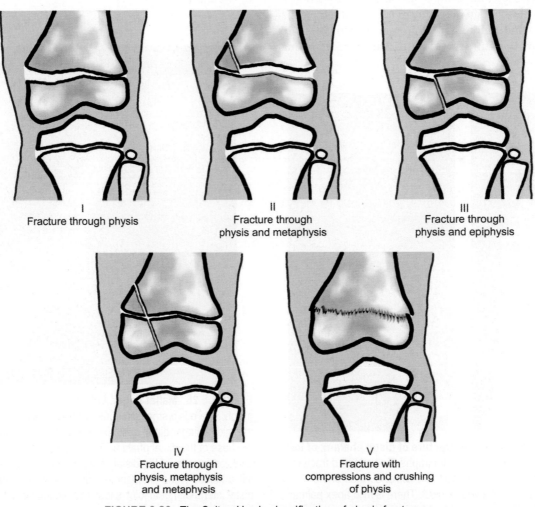

I
Fracture through physis

II
Fracture through physis and metaphysis

III
Fracture through physis and epiphysis

IV
Fracture through physis, metaphysis and metaphysis

V
Fracture with compressions and crushing of physis

FIGURE 6.26. The Salter–Harris classification of physis fractures.

to the physis, which represents the weakest point in a bone. The higher the grade of Salter–Harris fracture, the higher the risk of premature fusion of the growth plate and subsequent deformity.

Type I: The fracture involves only the physis. SCFE is an example of a type I fracture.

Type II: This is the most common type and the fracture involves the physis and metaphysis.

Type III: The fracture involves the physis and epiphysis.

Type IV: The fracture involves the physis, metaphysis, and epiphysis.

Type V: The fracture results in compression of the physis. While rare, type V has a high risk of the physis fusing as the fracture heals. As a result, the bone stops growing prematurely.

Fractures by Location: Upper Extremity

Upper extremity fractures may result from a wide variety of activities including a **f**all **on an o**utstretched **h**and (**FOOSH**). Standard view radiographs (AP and lateral) are the exams of choice. Subtle fractures can occur in any bone and are most commonly missed in the phalanges of the hand (Fig. 6.27). **Mallet injuries** include bony avulsion at the insertion of the extensor mechanism of the finger to the distal interphalangeal joint. Indications for surgery include involvement of more than one-third of the articular surface, palmar

displacement of the distal phalanx, or an interfragmentary gap of >3 mm (Fig. 6.28). Almost all upper extremity joints are susceptible to dislocation or subluxation (Fig. 6.29). Fractures of the fifth metacarpal often result from punching a solid object (Fig. 6.30). Fractures occur at the thumb at the base of the proximal phalanx (Fig. 6.31) and the base of metatarsal (Fig. 6.32). A **scaphoid** fracture may not be visualized on the standard views, and additional "scaphoid views" are obtained in which the wrist is angulated toward the ulna so that the scaphoid is visualized longitudinally (Fig. 6.33A). If clinical suspicion of a scaphoid fracture remains in the presence of normal radiographs, repeat radiographs at 7 to 10 days are recommended. Most scaphoid fractures occur transversely at the waist and if not recognized promptly, they may result in osteonecrosis of the less vascular proximal aspect of the bone leading to collapse and arthritis (Fig. 6.33B-F). Another carpal injury that should not be missed for the feared potential complication of injury to the ulnar nerve as it passes through the underlying Guyton canal is fracture of the **hook of the hamate**. A "carpal tunnel view" can be obtained with the wrist in hyperflexion to remove the overlying anatomy from the incident x-ray beam (Fig. 6.34A and B).

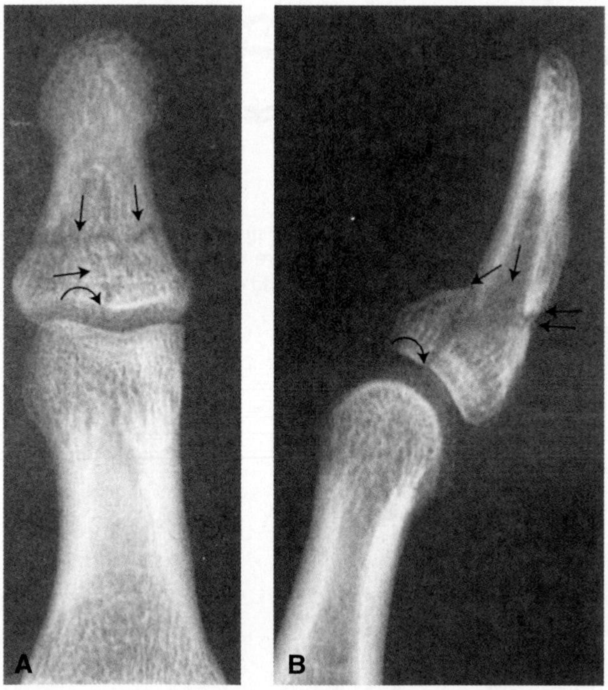

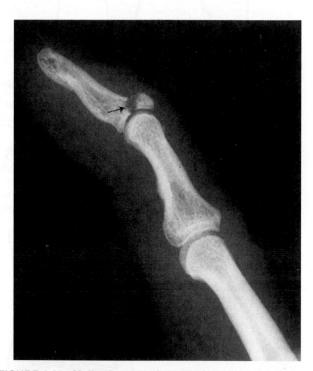

FIGURE 6.28. Mallet finger. Left middle finger lateral radiograph. There is a small osseous fragment dorsal to the base of the middle finger distal phalanx (*arrow*) with clear donor site at the base of the distal phalanx. This is consistent with a displaced avulsion fracture of the distal phalanx with the avulsed fragment still attached to the extensor tendon. The ability to extend at the distal interphalangeal joint is lost and the joint is subsequently held in flexion.

FIGURE 6.27. Comminuted fracture of distal phalanx of left thumb. A: PA and **B:** lateral radiographs. Comminuted fracture (*straight arrows*) that extends to the articular surface of the interphalangeal joint (*curved arrows*). There is mild apex palmar angulation at the fracture site (*double arrows*).

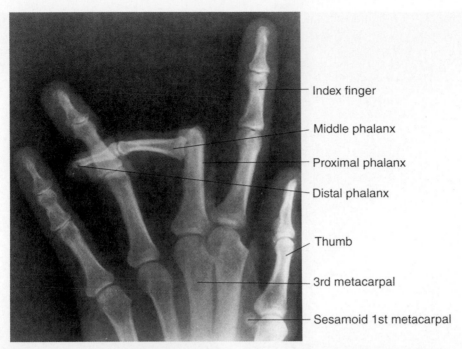

Index finger

Middle phalanx

Proximal phalanx

Distal phalanx

Thumb

3rd metacarpal

Sesamoid 1st metacarpal

FIGURE 6.29. Dislocation at the proximal interphalangeal (PIP) joint of the left long finger. Left-hand PA radiograph. The middle and distal phalanges are completely dislocated relative to the proximal phalanx. There are no fractures.

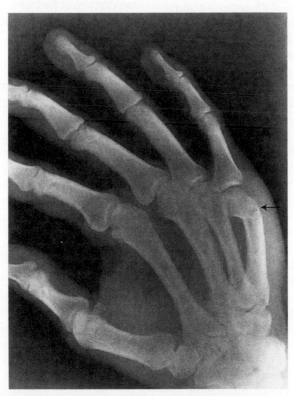

FIGURE 6.30. Boxer fracture. Right hand oblique radiograph. The apex dorsal angulated fracture (*arrow*) is through the neck of the right fifth metacarpal. It commonly occurs from punching a hard object with greatest impact on the fifth metacarpophalangeal joint.

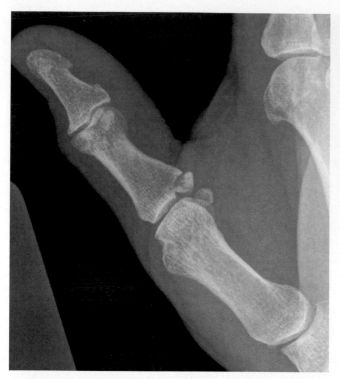

FIGURE 6.31. Gamekeeper's fracture. Right thumb oblique radiograph. There is a small fracture fragment at the ulnar base of the proximal phalanx of the thumb (*arrow*). This occurs through stress on the ulnar collateral ligament, causing an avulsion of the bone at its distal attachment on the base of the proximal phalanx. Historically, this was a common injury for gamekeepers, who repetitively wrung the necks of rabbits. Now it occurs when skiers suffer an injury where their gripped pole becomes planted against their forward motion. A complication is the Stener lesion, where the adductor pollicis tendon becomes trapped between the ulnar collateral ligament and the metacarpophalangeal joint.

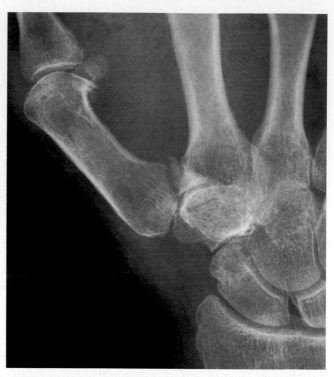

FIGURE 6.32. Bennett fracture. Left thumb oblique radiograph. There is an obliquely oriented fracture at the base of the first metacarpal with intra-articular extension and mild dorsolateral displacement of the distal fragment (*arrow*). This is the most common fracture of the thumb, occurring when axial loading causes forced abduction of the carpometacarpal joint. A Rolando fracture has three components.

While young adults typically fracture the scaphoid, children and older adults are more likely to fracture the distal radius and ulna following a FOOSH (Fig. 6.35A-C). One such common fracture in older adults is called a **Colles fracture** (Fig. 6.36A and B). For patients with suspected distal radius fractures, a three-view examination of the wrist usually includes a posteroanterior (PA), a lateral, and a 45-degree semipronated oblique view. When the initial radiographs are equivocal, **CT** is used to exclude or confirm suspected wrist fractures. In patients with intra-articular fractures, CT allows improved visualization of articular fracture fragment displacement, depression, and comminution compared with conventional radiographs. Indications for surgery include the presence of a coronally oriented distal radial fracture line, fragment depression, or more than three articular fracture fragments. **MR arthrography** is recommended for suspected tendon and ligament trauma of the wrist including tears of the scapholunate ligament, which may affect surgical treatment (Fig. 6.35D and E).

Elbow fractures (Figs. 6.37-6.40) and **dislocations** (Fig. 6.41) can occur after a fall directly on the elbow or on an extended arm or hand. In general, children are more likely to have a supracondylar fracture of the distal humerus and adults may fracture the radial head. Dislocations of the elbow are named for the direction the radius and ulna dislocate relative to the humerus. When the radius and ulna dislocate posterior to the humerus, it is a posterior dislocation. Some elbow fractures may be difficult or impossible to directly visualize on radiographs and a useful secondary sign of a fracture in this location is the **"fat pad"** sign, in which the normally invisible **posterior fat pad** is displaced posteriorly from the olecranon fossa by an elbow joint effusion and becomes visible as a triangular or linear lucency posterior to the distal humerus. The **anterior fat pad**, which is normally visible, may become more prominent or elevated, a finding commonly referred to as the "sail sign" for its resemblance to the spinnaker sail of a sailboat (Fig. 6.40B). Fractures and dislocations of the elbow may compress the brachial artery as it runs behind the distal humerus. In children the radiographic anatomy of the elbow is complicated by the presence or absence of multiple ossification centers.

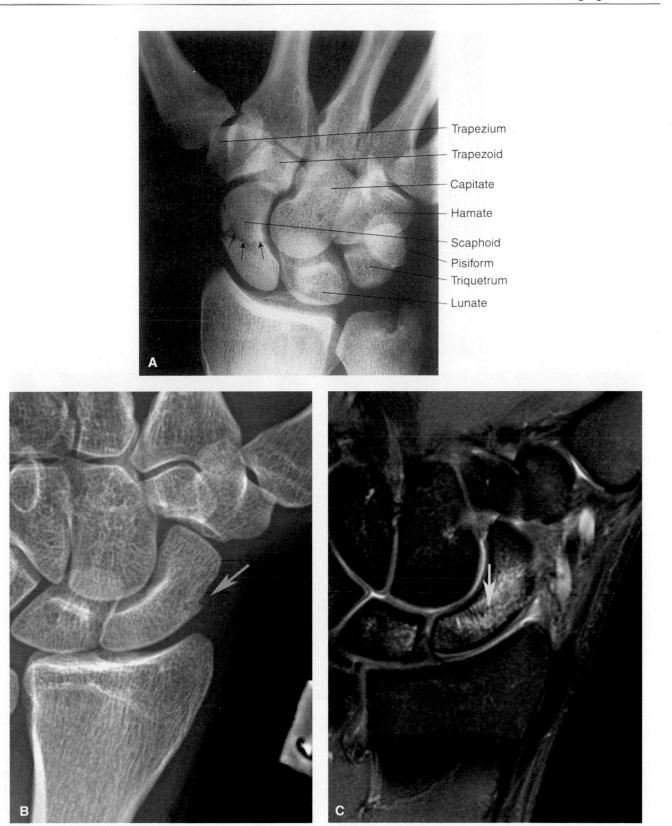

FIGURE 6.33. Scaphoid fracture. A: Right wrist PA radiograph. Nondisplaced fracture of the scaphoid waist (*arrows*). **B:** PA oblique radiograph of the scaphoid. A prominent scaphoid tubercle is seen (*arrow*) and obliteration of normal fat next to the bone, but no definite fracture is seen. **C:** Fat-suppressed T2-weighted MRI of the scaphoid reveals edema and a fracture line (*arrow*), which does not extend through the medial margin consistent with an incomplete fracture.

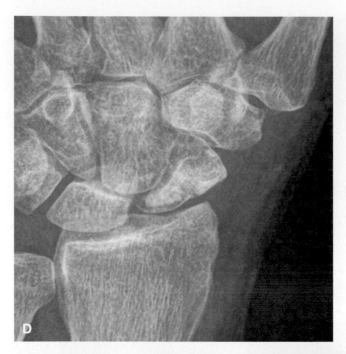

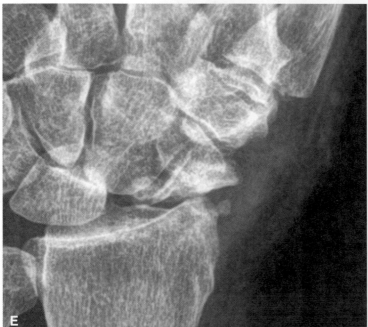

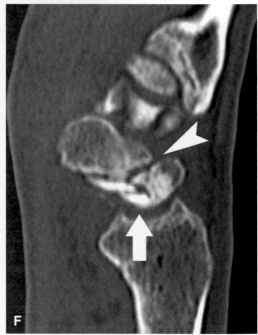

FIGURE 6.33. *(Continued)* **D and E:** Radiographs showing necrosis and collapse of the scaphoid as result of fracture nonunion. **F:** CT showing sclerosis secondary to nonunion (*arrowhead*). Note the tip of an internal fixation screw (*arrow*).

When in doubt about an elbow fracture or dislocation, **imaging the noninvolved elbow** may be useful for comparison (see Fig. 6.41A and B).

Soft tissue injuries of the elbow are difficult to evaluate on radiographs. Although a biceps tendon tear may be obvious clinically owing to the bulge of a retracted muscle (Fig. 6.42A), MRI can demonstrate how far the tendon is retracted and the degree of the structural integrity of the torn tendon (Fig. 6.42B). MRI is also used to assess tendons and

ligaments of the elbow, particularly in sports injuries, such as baseball pitchers, in whom the ulnar collateral ligament is commonly injured (Fig. 6.43A and B).

Shoulder

In the elderly, FOOSH may result in a fracture of the surgical neck of the humerus (Fig. 6.44), whereas in children a similar fracture can occur through the physis of the proximal humerus (Fig. 6.45).

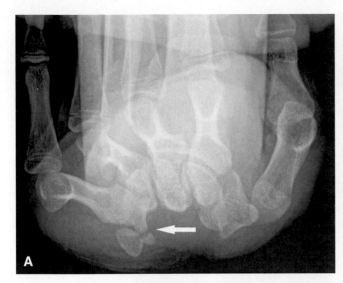
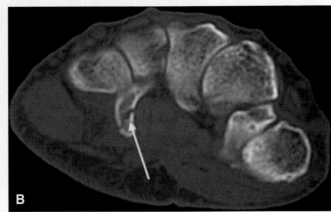

FIGURE 6.34. Hook of hamate fracture. A: "Carpal tunnel view" radiograph of the wrist. There is a subtle linear lucency through the hook of the hamate, representing a nondisplaced fracture (*arrow*). This fracture would be difficult or impossible to see on other views because of overlying anatomy. **B:** Axial CT at the level of the hamate more clearly demonstrates the same fracture (*arrow*).

Dislocation of the shoulder: In the more commonly occurring **anterior dislocation** of the shoulder, the humeral head displaces medial and inferior to the glenoid cavity on an AP radiograph, and sometimes an impaction fracture of the greater tuberosity, referred to as a Hill–Sachs deformity, may result or the greater tuberosity may fracture completely (Fig. 6.46A-C). Milder degrees of anterior shoulder dislocation or subluxation may be missed on a single anterior view and an axillary or scapular Y view should be obtained. (Fig. 6.46E). In the less common **posterior dislocation**, the glenohumeral joint can be slightly widened on an AP view, but often alignment may appear normal on this view (Fig. 6.47A). The fixed internal rotation of the humeral head on the AP view in posterior dislocation is described as **the lightbulb sign**. Again, an axillary view (Fig. 6.47B) may be necessary for confirmation. CT is useful to diagnose fractures and occasionally a missed dislocation (Fig. 6.47E).

The **rotator cuff** is composed of four muscles (and their tendons): the supraspinatus, infraspinatus, tears minor, and subscapularis that act to stabilize the shoulder. The four tendons converge to form a rotator cuff tendon, which combined with the joint capsule, the coracohumeral ligament and glenohumeral ligament inserted to the humeral tuberosities. **Shoulder instability** occurs when the capsule, ligaments, or labrum becomes stretched, torn, or detached, allowing the humeral head to move either completely or partially out of the socket. The supraspinatus is most commonly involved in rotator cuff tears. Radiographs should be the initial imaging study performed in patients with shoulder pain (Fig. 6.48). Tendinosis and full-thickness tears of the rotator cuff tendons can be reliably diagnosed using MRI (Fig. 6.49). Apart from the diagnosis and treatment of

adhesive capsulitis, contrast arthrography with iodinated contrast (Fig. 6.50) has largely been replaced with CT and MR arthrography, the latter of which are especially helpful for evaluating tears of the glenoid labrum (Fig. 6.51). CT may be useful for further evaluation of a humeral head, humeral neck, glenoid rim fractures in patients with repeated dislocations or chronic instability. The major limitation of CT arthrography is its poor sensitivity for bursal tears because they do not fill with contrast material injected into the glenohumeral joint. If there is concern for associated vascular injury or compromise, a CTA of the upper extremity should be obtained. Ultrasound can also be used to assess the rotator cuff but requires an experienced sonographer and interpreter (Fig. 6.52).

Scapula

Fractures of the scapula are rare and usually result from a high-force injury as in motor vehicle accidents (Fig. 6.53). CT is useful to determine whether the fracture involves the glenoid or the suprascapular notch through which the nerve to the supraspinatus and infraspinatus muscle travels.

Clavicle

Fractures of the clavicle are relatively common, especially in children (Fig. 6.54). The most common site for clavicle fractures is at the junction of the middle and distal thirds.

Lower Extremity

Lower extremity injuries are common reasons for presentation to the ER, but not all patients with foot and ankle injuries require imaging. The **Ottawa Rules** recommend foot radiographs under certain conditions. When an acute

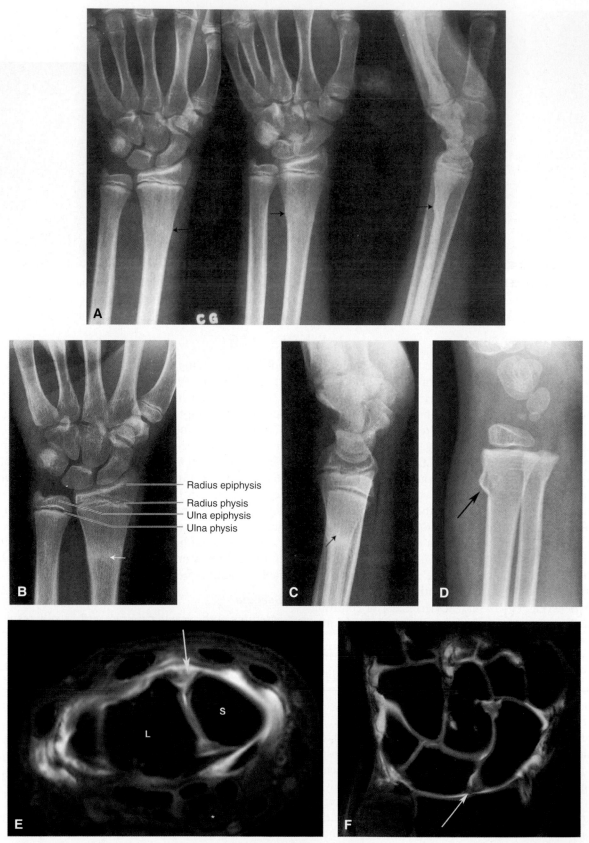

FIGURE 6.35. Distal radial injury. Torus (buckle) fracture of the distal radius. **A-C** (*arrows*): These fractures can be as subtle as a focal relative bulging of the cortex. **B** shows a sclerotic zone consistent with a healing fracture (*arrow*). **D and E: Scapholunate ligament tear.** MR arthrogram. Axial **(D)** and coronal **(E)** fat-suppressed T1-weighted MRI of the right wrist after the injection of gadolinium into the radiocarpal joint. There is a partial tear of the dorsal (posterior) aspect of the scapholunate ligament (*arrow*) allowing contrast (*white*) to enter the midcarpal joint. S, scaphoid; L, lunate; *, median nerve.

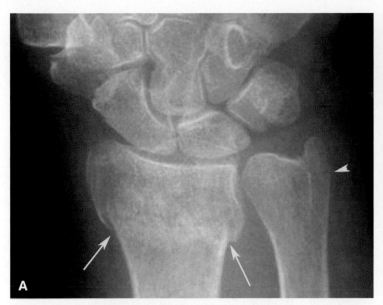
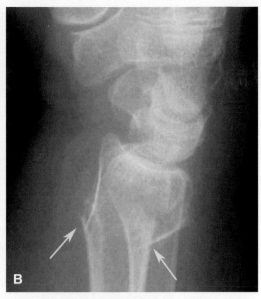

FIGURE 6.36. **Colles fracture. A:** PA, and **B:** Lateral wrist radiographs. There is a fracture of the distal radius (*arrows*) with dorsal angulation, dorsal tilt, and radial deviation. Fracture reduction and cast application is with the distal fragment in palmar flexion and ulnar deviation. Associated fracture of the ulnar styloid process occurs in more than 60% of cases (*arrowhead*).

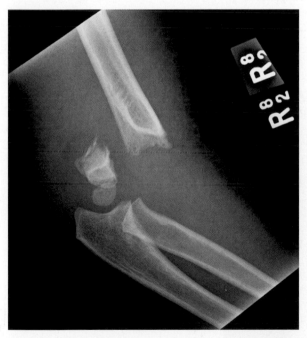

FIGURE 6.37. **Supracondylar fracture of the humerus**. Right elbow lateral radiograph showing a markedly displaced supracondylar fracture.

Lisfranc injury (one or more of the metatarsal bones are displaced from the tarsus) is suspected, the foot should be imaged with a weight-bearing AP view in addition to the standard three-view radiographic study of the foot (AP, oblique, and lateral), looking for abnormal alignment at the first intermetatarsal space.

When evaluating foot radiographs in young patients, note an apophysis (normal variant) at the base (proximal end) of the fifth metatarsal. An apophysis is a growth center (like the epiphysis) that does not contribute to bone length but alters bone contour. It is usually not located in a joint but typically has tendons attached to it. A *lateral* radiolucent line near the base of the fifth metatarsal that runs parallel to the long axis of the metatarsal represents a normal apophysis (see Fig. 6.55C), in contrast to a *transverse* lucent line at the base of the fifth metatarsal represents a fracture (see Fig. 6.55D). The metatarsal shaft is a common location for stress fractures (repetitive trauma in underlying normal bone) (Fig. 6.56).

The hindfoot is composed of two tarsal bones, the talus and the calcaneus. Calcaneal fractures typically occur after a fall from a height or following a motor vehicle accident and are best imaged with CT (Fig. 6.57).

Ankle injuries vary from minor sprains to severe trimalleolar fracture-dislocations (Figs. 6.58-6.61). Standard radiographic views of the ankle (AP and lateral) may be supplemented with an "ankle mortise" view, which is taken with 15 to 25 degrees of internal rotation of the foot to optimize visualization of the medial and lateral joint spaces. If there is clinical suspicion or radiographic evidence of syndesmotic injury, tibia/fibular radiographs should be obtained to exclude a more proximal fibular fracture.[1]

MRI should be done in patients with persistent pain and symptoms of locking, clicking, stiffness, and ankle swelling or if radiographs demonstrate an osteochondral fracture, which appears as a crescent-shaped lucency of the dome of the talus. Many ankle sprain injuries and most ankle

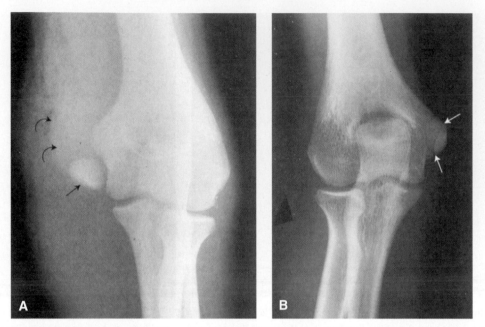

FIGURE 6.38. Avulsion fracture of the medial epicondyle epiphysis. A: Left elbow AP radiograph (*straight arrow*) in a 13-year-old. There is considerable soft tissue prominence (*curved arrows*), probably owing to edema and hemorrhage secondary to the avulsion fracture. Remember that the pronators and flexors of the forearm attach to the medial epicondyle and the extensors and supinators to the lateral epicondyle. **B:** Normal right elbow (*arrows*) AP radiograph for comparison.

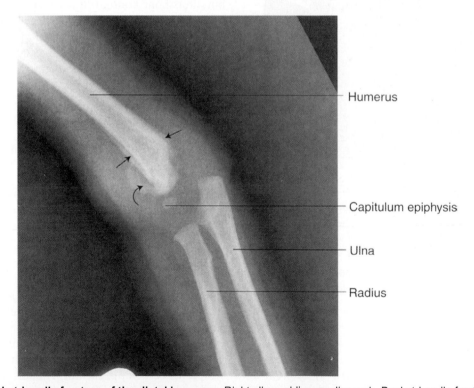

FIGURE 6.39. Bucket-handle fracture of the distal humerus. Right elbow oblique radiograph. Bucket-handle fracture (*curved arrow*) in a 14-month-old child consistent with nonaccidental injury. The *straight arrows* indicate periosteal reaction that occurs as a part of the healing process.

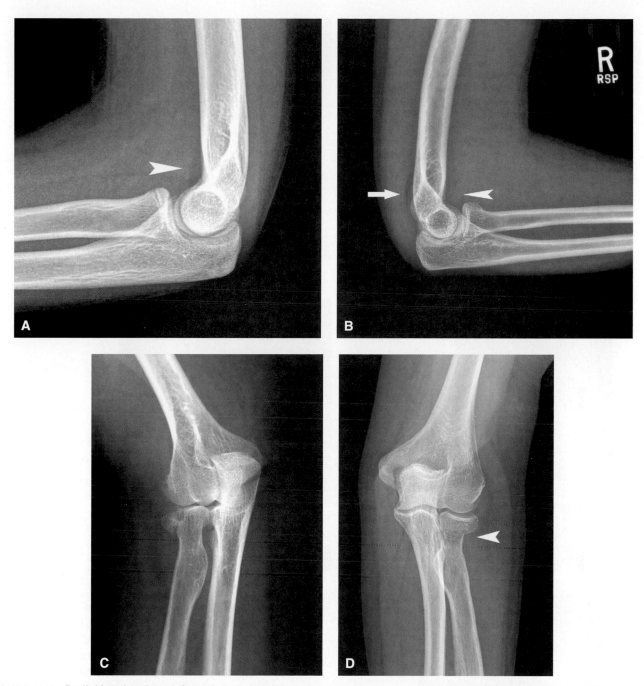

FIGURE 6.40. Radial head and neck fractures. A: Lateral elbow radiograph showing a small elbow joint effusion as manifested by mild elevation of the anterior fat pad (*arrowhead*). **B.** Lateral elbow radiograph showing elevation of the anterior fat pad (*arrowhead*) and, more tellingly, the posterior fat pad (*arrow*), which in children is highly suggestive of a supracondylar fracture and in adults, of a radial head fracture. **C.** Radial head fracture. **D.** Radial neck fracture with focal cortical disruption (*white arrowhead*).

fractures are associated with some degree of cartilage injury, which is not usually visible on radiographs. When a large ankle effusion (>15 mm) is seen on a radiograph but no fracture is visible, CT will demonstrate a fracture in a third of cases. CT with reformats is necessary to evaluate ankle fractures, particularly those involving a joint space. A spiral fracture of the distal tibia is associated with a nondisplaced

fracture of the posterior malleolus of the tibia that may not be demonstrated on radiographs.

The **Ottawa Ankle/Foot Rules** recommend that radiographs of the **foot** should be obtained only if there is pain in the midfoot AND any one of the following: point bone tenderness of the navicular, OR point bone tenderness of the base of the fifth metatarsal, OR inability to bear weight

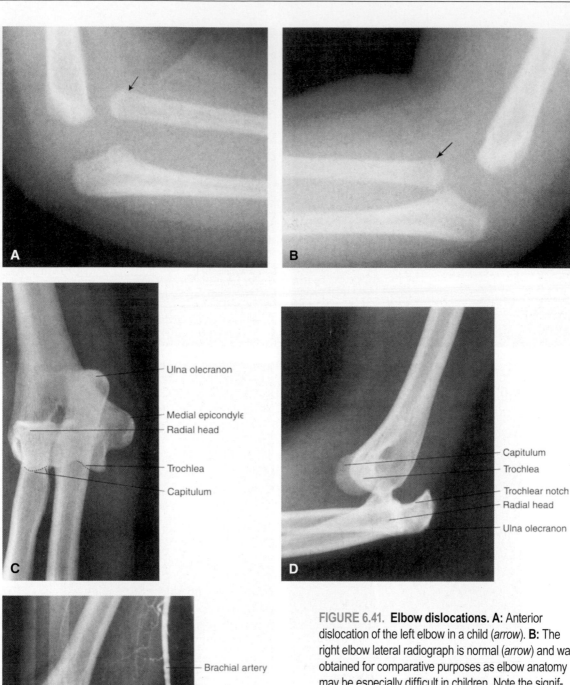

FIGURE 6.41. **Elbow dislocations. A:** Anterior dislocation of the left elbow in a child (*arrow*). **B:** The right elbow lateral radiograph is normal (*arrow*) and was obtained for comparative purposes as elbow anatomy may be especially difficult in children. Note the significant difference in position of the proximal left radius relative to the left humerus compared to the normal right proximal radius relative to the right humerus. **C and D:** Posterior dislocation of the olecranon. This injury can occur from a fall on an outstretched hand and is usually associated with fractures of the coronoid process of the ulna. **E:** Left elbow angiogram following a fracture–anterior dislocation of the left elbow in a different patient. The radius and ulna are dislocated anteriorly relative to the humerus and there is a comminuted fracture of the ulna olecranon (*arrows*). The brachial artery is displaced anteriorly by the dislocation and the associated soft tissue edema and hemorrhage.

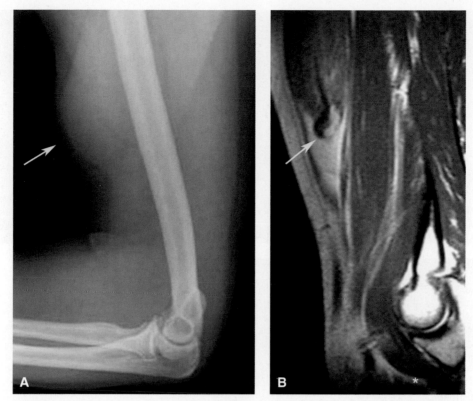

FIGURE 6.42. **Biceps tendon tear.** **A:** Lateral radiograph of the right distal humerus reveals a prominent soft tissue bump (*arrow*). **B:** Sagittal T2-weighted MRI demonstrates the retracted, torn biceps tendon (*arrow*). The level of its normal attachment on the radial tuberosity is marked by an *asterisk* and the amount of retraction can be measured.

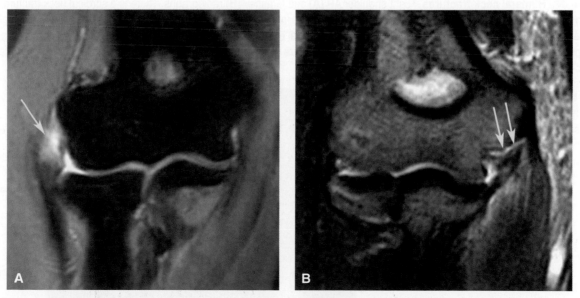

FIGURE 6.43. **A: Common extensor tendon injury:** Coronal elbow MRI shows thickening and increased signal in the common extensor tendon and radial collateral ligament (*arrow*). **B: Ulnar collateral ligament tear**. Right elbow fat-suppressed T1-weighted MR arthrogram coronal image. Contrast can be seen medial to the olecranon, resulting in bright signal in the configuration of a T on its side (*arrows*) that is pathognomonic for an ulnar collateral ligament tear of the elbow. It is a common injury in pitchers, who apply excessive valgus strain on their elbow while pitching.

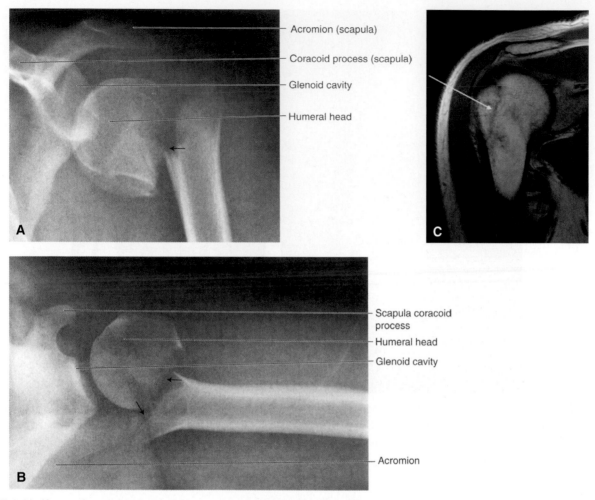

Acromion (scapula)

Coracoid process (scapula)

Glenoid cavity

Humeral head

Scapula coracoid process

Humeral head

Glenoid cavity

Acromion

FIGURE 6.44. Humeral neck fractures. Right shoulder AP **(A)** and Grashey **(B)** radiographs. There is a surgical neck fracture with mild impaction and angulation (*arrows*). This is a common site of fracture in elderly patients during falls on outstretched arms. **(C)** Right shoulder T1-weighted oblique coronal MR image showing linear low signal extending obliquely through the humeral head and neck, indicating a nondisplaced fracture of the greater tuberosity (*arrow*). This fracture was not seen on radiographs, and persistent pain prompted MRI.

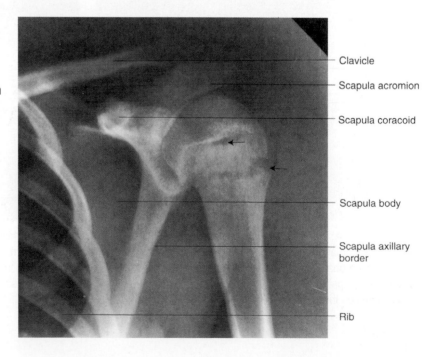

FIGURE 6.45. Salter I fracture (*arrows*) through the proximal physis of the left humerus in a 15-year-old patient. The patient fell on an outstretched arm. The major clue to the presence of a fracture is that the physis width is greater than normal.

Clavicle

Scapula acromion

Scapula coracoid

Scapula body

Scapula axillary border

Rib

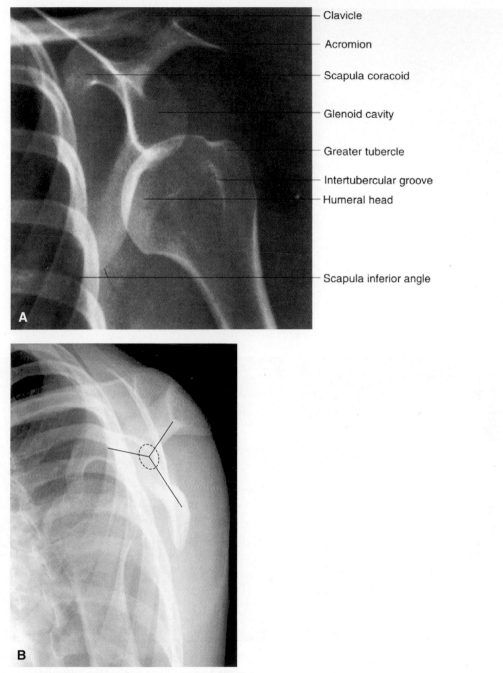

— Clavicle

— Acromion

— Scapula coracoid

— Glenoid cavity

— Greater tubercle

— Intertubercular groove
— Humeral head

— Scapula inferior angle

FIGURE 6.46. Anterior dislocation of the shoulder. Right shoulder AP **(A)** and scapular Y-view **(B)** radiographs. Greater than normal overlap between the humeral head and the glenoid on AP view suggests glenohumeral dislocation, although it is unclear whether this is an anterior (more common) or posterior dislocation. The scapular Y-view confirms anterior dislocation.

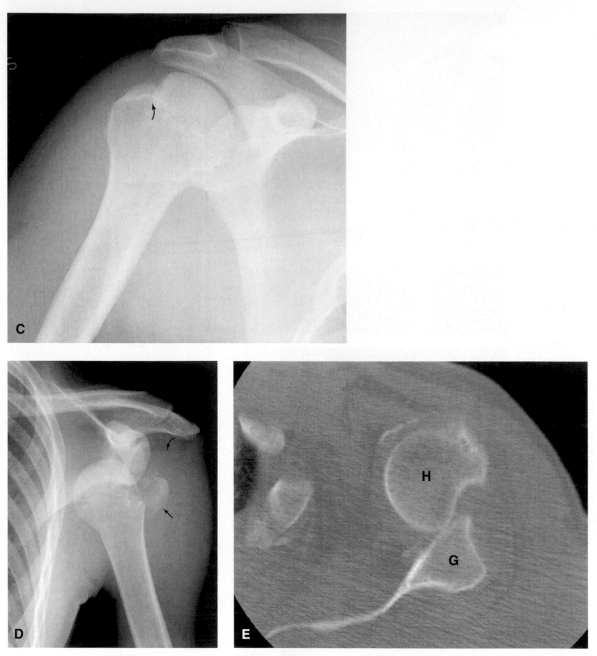

FIGURE 6.46. *(Continued)* **(C)** Flattening of the superolateral humeral head *(arrow)* is consistent with a Hill–Sachs lesion, a result of recurrent anterior dislocations causing impaction fractures of the humeral head against the anteroinferior glenoid. **(D)** There is anterior dislocation of the humeral head with respect to the glenoid with subsequent impaction of the humeral head on the antero-inferior glenoid. The resultant fractures are of the posterolateral humeral head *(arrow)* and anteroinferior glenoid, where there is a small adjacent fracture fragment *(curved arrow)*. These fractures are eponymously known as the "Hill–Sachs lesion" and the "bony Bankart lesion," respectively. **(E)** Right shoulder axial CT. Anterior shoulder dislocation with Hill–Sachs lesion and bony Bankart lesion (H-humerus, G-glenoid).

immediately and in the ER (inability to walk four steps). Radiographs of the **ankle** should be obtained only if there is pain in the malleolar zone AND any one of the following: tenderness along the distal 6 cm of the posterior edge of the tibia or tip of the medial malleolus, OR tenderness along the

distal 6 cm of the posterior edge of the fibula or tip of the lateral malleolus, OR inability to bear weight immediately after the injury and to ambulate for four steps in the ER.[2]

These rules apply to children older than 5 years and to adults, and using these guidelines, the rate of missed

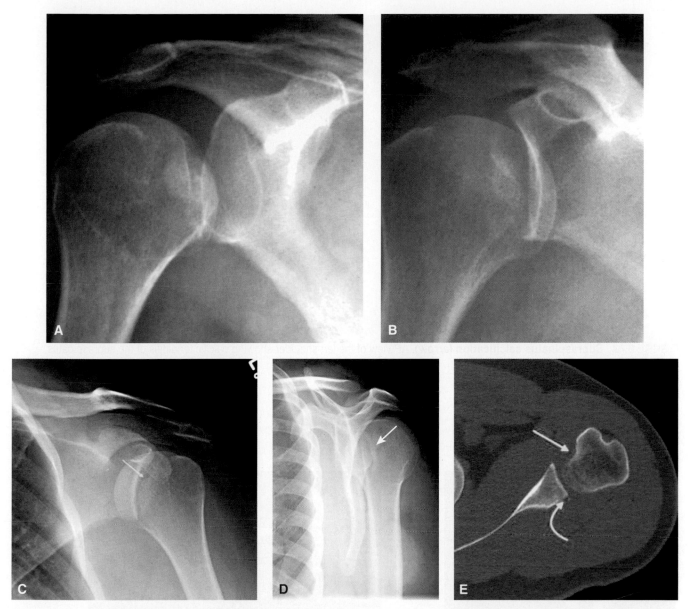

FIGURE 6.47. Posterior dislocation of the shoulder. A: Right shoulder. AP. The posterior dislocation may be overlooked as the shoulder joint may appear normal or slightly widened. **B:** Oblique or Grashey view shows the glenoid cavity tangentially with overlap of the humeral head and glenoid. Normally there should be a distinct space on this view. Left shoulder AP **(C)** and scapular Y-view **(D)** radiographs. On the AP view, the humeral head looks relatively normal in alignment. There is a subtle linear vertical lucency in the medial humeral head (*arrow*), which likely represents an impaction of the humeral head against the posterior glenoid. This is known as the "trough sign." Scapular Y-view clearly shows posterior dislocation of the humerus with respect to the scapula and more clearly demonstrates the "trough sign" (*arrow*). **E:** Left shoulder axial CT. Reverse Hill–Sachs lesion and reverse bony Bankart lesion. Posterior dislocations are (conversely to anterior dislocations) associated with the reverse Hill–Sachs lesions (*arrow*) and reverse bony Bankart lesions (*curved arrow*).

fractures is less than 2%. The Ottawa Ankle/Foot Rules have a greater than 90% **sensitivity** for ruling out fractures but are poor for ruling in fractures (many false positives) with **specificities** of 40% and 80% for ankle and foot fractures, respectively, although the rule is not designed or intended for specific diagnosis. These rules have been prospectively validated in different populations. However, if the patient does

not fit the criteria using the Ottawa rules or is not neurologically intact or has persistent pain a week following trauma, radiographs should be obtained. Other caveats include its use in patients younger than 18 years, in patients with gross malleolar swelling, and those who are intoxicated.

The **Weber classification** is used to describe ankle fractures. **Weber type A** fractures are transversely

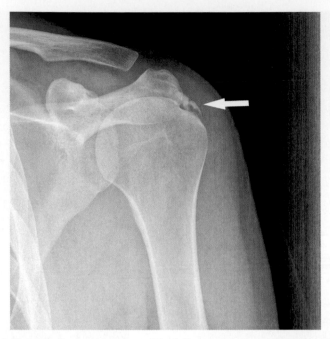

FIGURE 6.48. **Supraspinatus calcification (*arrow*).** AP view of the left shoulder showing calcific tendinitis of the supraspinatus

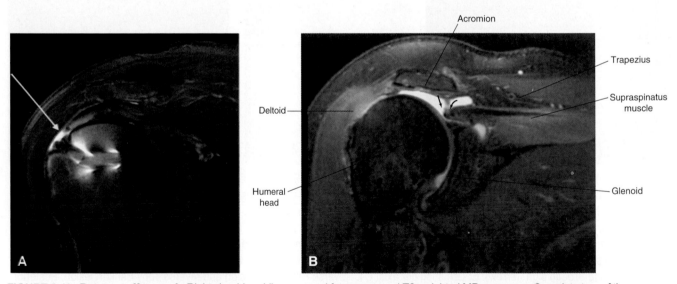

FIGURE 6.49. **Rotator cuff tears. A:** Right shoulder oblique coronal fat-suppressed T2-weighted MR sequence. Complete tear of the supraspinatus tendon. High signal extending from the greater tuberosity to the fibers of the supraspinatus tendon 1 cm proximal to this indicates complete tearing and proximal retraction of the supraspinatus tendon (*arrow*). **B:** The free margin of the torn supraspinatus tendon is indicated by the *curved arrow*. The increased signal (*straight arrow*) represents blood, edema, and synovial fluid at the laceration of the supraspinatus tendon.

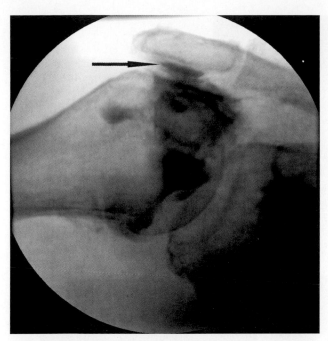

FIGURE 6.50. **Contrast arthrography.** Leakage of contrast into the subacromial bursa (*arrow*) is consistent with a supraspinatus tear.

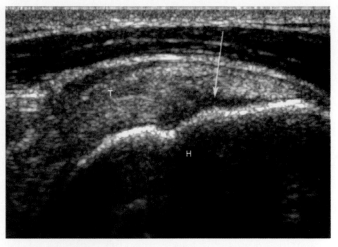

FIGURE 6.52. **Partial supraspinatus tear.** Ultrasound of the supraspinatus tendon insertion shows low echogenicity at the tendon attachment (*arrow*) consistent with a partial tear. The adjacent curved hyperechoic line represents the humeral head (H).

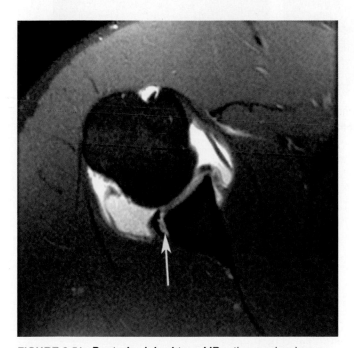

FIGURE 6.51. **Posterior labral tear.** MR arthrography shows contrast between the labrum and its posterior glenoid attachment (*arrow*).

oriented lateral malleolar fractures that occur below the level of the ankle joint (talar dome) and are considered stable as the medial (deltoid) ligaments and the tibiofibular syndesmosis are intact (Fig. 6.58B). If the medial malleolus is also disrupted, a Weber type A fracture may be unstable. **Weber type B** fractures are spiral or oblique fractures through the fibula at the level of the ankle joint (Fig. 6.59A and B). The medial ankle should be closely inspected, as widening of the medial joint space (indicating deltoid ligament tear) or medial malleolar fractures occurs more commonly than in type A fractures and can render the ankle unstable. **Weber type C** injuries are the most serious, as they are always unstable (Fig. 6.59C-E). The fibular fracture line is transverse and above the level of the ankle joint. The tibiofibular syndesmosis is ruptured and there is widening of the distal tibiofibular articulation. Medial malleolar or deltoid ligament injury is also frequently present.

Soft tissue injury: One of the most common injuries of the lower extremity is a **sprained ankle**, which is an injury to a ligament around the ankle varying in severity from a stretching of the ligament to a partial tear to a complete disruption. A common mechanism of ankle injury is twisting, whether by inversion, eversion, internal rotation, or external rotation. In combination with turning, twisting (external rotation) affects the severity of the injury and which structures are involved. Sprains occur with and without associated fractures, and a tiny chip-like fracture at the ligamentous attachment is considered a "sprain equivalent" and is treated more like a sprain than a fracture.

The **Achilles tendon** or calcaneal tendon may be torn following sudden forced plantarflexion (jumping) or forced dorsiflexion (stepping on a curb) of the ankle.

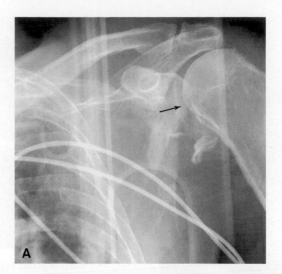

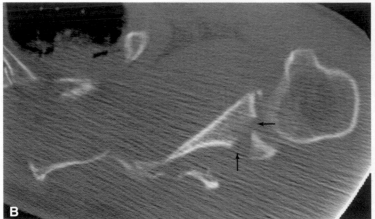

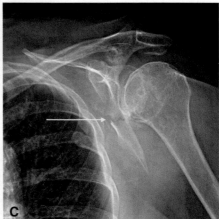

FIGURE 6.53. Scapula fractures. Left scapula AP **(A)** radiograph and **(B)** CT showing scapula fractures involved in the glenoid. Scapular fractures are uncommon and often the result of high impact trauma as in this case (*arrows*). **C:** Fracture involving the inferior scapula (*arrow*).

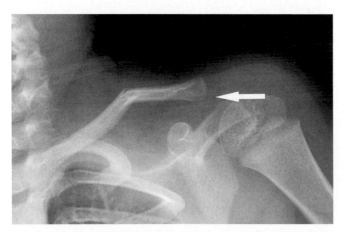

FIGURE 6.54. Clavicle fracture: Left greenstick clavicle fracture with diastasis of the acromioclavicular joint (*arrow*).

When there is a complete tear of the Achilles tendon, physical examination elicits pinpoint tenderness at the site of injury and inability to plantarflex the foot. A lateral radiograph may show a discontinuity of the linear Achilles tendon with associated swelling of the pre-Achilles fat pad. Ultrasound can confirm the presence of a tear or (acute or chronic) tendinopathy. As in many soft tissue injuries, MRI can confirm the presence of inflammation and tear (Fig. 6.62).

Fractures of the tibial and fibular shafts occur in contact sports and skiing.

Nonunion and pseudoarthrosis of mid- and distal tibial fractures may occur because of poor blood flow despite internal fixation to facilitate immobilization (Fig. 6.63). The tibia is also a common site of stress fractures, especially in runners (Fig. 6.64).

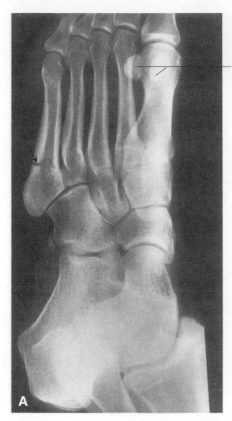

Medial and lateral sesamoids

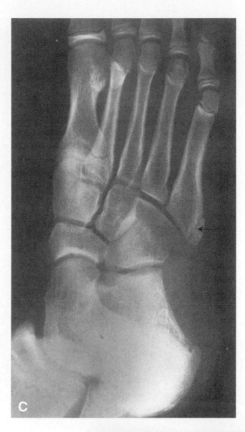

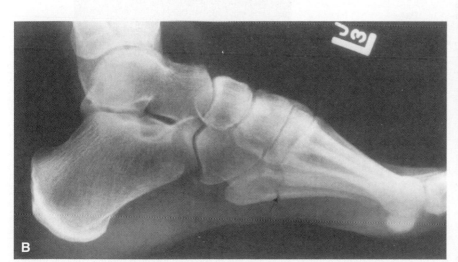

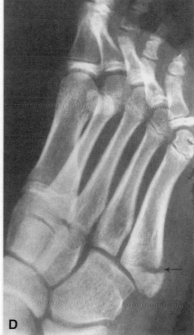

FIGURE 6.55. **Transverse fracture of proximal fifth metatarsal. A and B:** Left foot oblique and lateral radiograph. Nondisplaced transverse fracture of the proximal left fifth metatarsal shaft (*arrow*). This is also known as a "Jones fracture." **C:** Right foot AP radiograph. The **normal apophysis** (*arrow*) at the base of the fifth metatarsal appears as a longitudinal radiolucent or black line and should not be confused with a fracture. **D:** Right foot oblique radiograph. Transverse nondisplaced fracture (*straight arrow*) involving the fifth metatarsal base. This injury usually results from an inversion stress on the peroneus brevis that attaches to the base of the fifth metatarsal. This is also known as a "pseudo-Jones fracture."

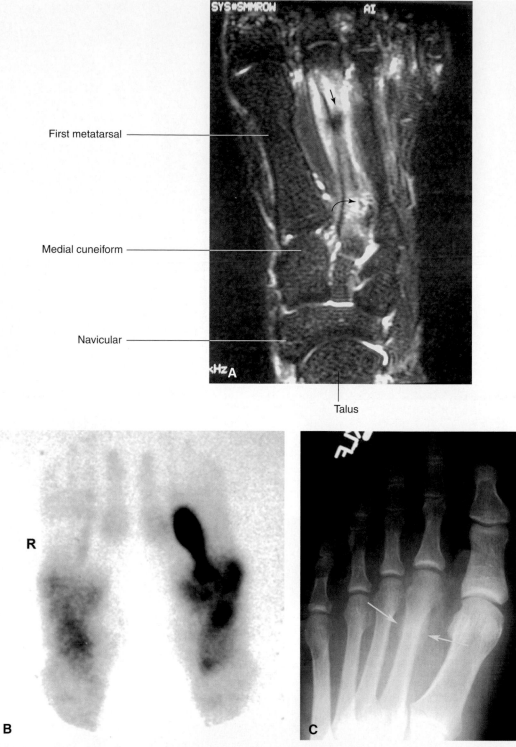

FIGURE 6.56. Metatarsal stress fracture. A: Long-axis fat-suppressed T2-weighted MR of the right foot in a runner. Second metatarsal stress fracture has some callus, which is dark (*straight arrow*), and a large amount of edema in the bone and soft tissues, which is bright (*curved arrow*). Bone scan **(B)** and AP left foot radiograph **(C)** in a similar patient. Callus (*arrows*) is bright on the radiograph. Note the bone scan image is obtained as if looking at the bottom of the patient's feet so the left foot appears opposite to that of the radiograph.

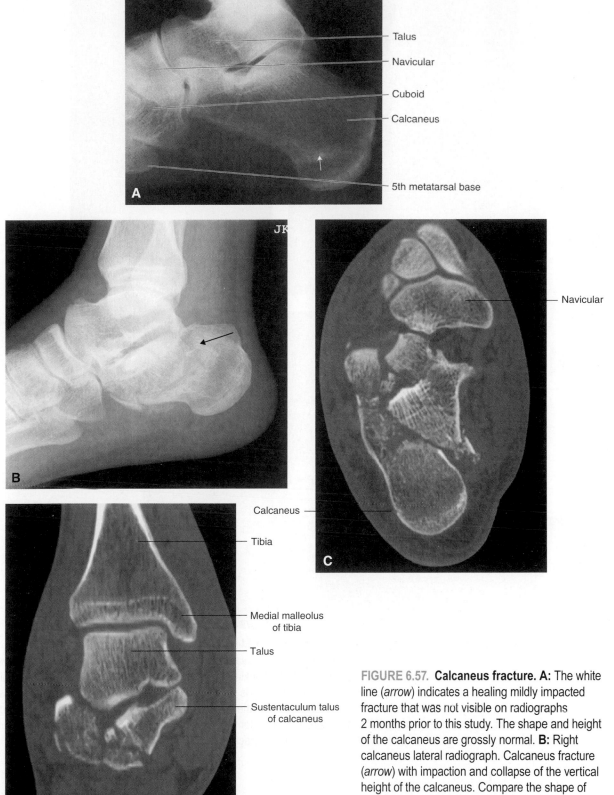

FIGURE 6.57. **Calcaneus fracture. A:** The white line (*arrow*) indicates a healing mildly impacted fracture that was not visible on radiographs 2 months prior to this study. The shape and height of the calcaneus are grossly normal. **B:** Right calcaneus lateral radiograph. Calcaneus fracture (*arrow*) with impaction and collapse of the vertical height of the calcaneus. Compare the shape of the calcaneus in this patient to the calcaneus in **(A)**. Axial **(C)** and coronal reformatted **(D)** CT better demonstrate the extent and comminution of the fracture.

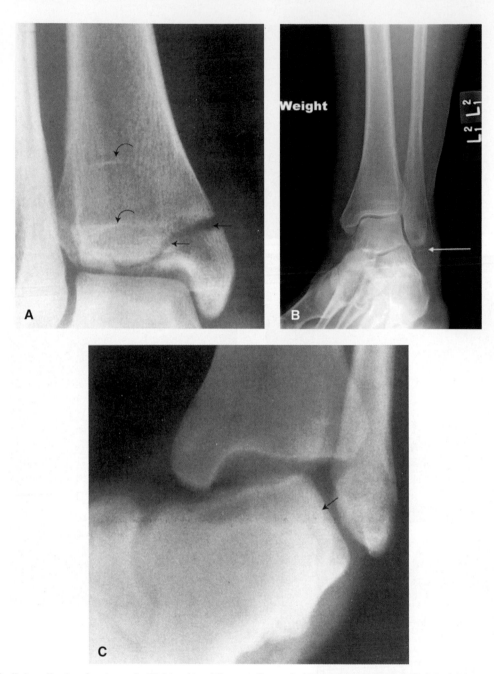

FIGURE 6.58. Medial malleolus fracture. A: Right ankle oblique radiograph. Mildly distracted fracture (*straight arrows*) through the base of the medial malleolus in an adult. The fracture extends onto the articular surface of the distal tibia. The white lines (*curved arrows*) represent previous physis location and arrested growth lines. **B:** Left ankle AP radiograph. **Weber type A fracture.** A small avulsed fracture fragment is seen inferior to the **lateral malleolus** (*arrow*). This is compatible with a Weber type A ankle fracture, which occurs below the level of the ankle joint. These fractures are usually stable, as they are typically not associated with ligamentous injury. **C: Severe ankle sprain.** Left ankle inversion stress AP radiograph. The talus dome is tilted laterally (*arrow*) secondary to disruption of the lateral collateral ligament in an inversion or adduction injury. There are no fractures.

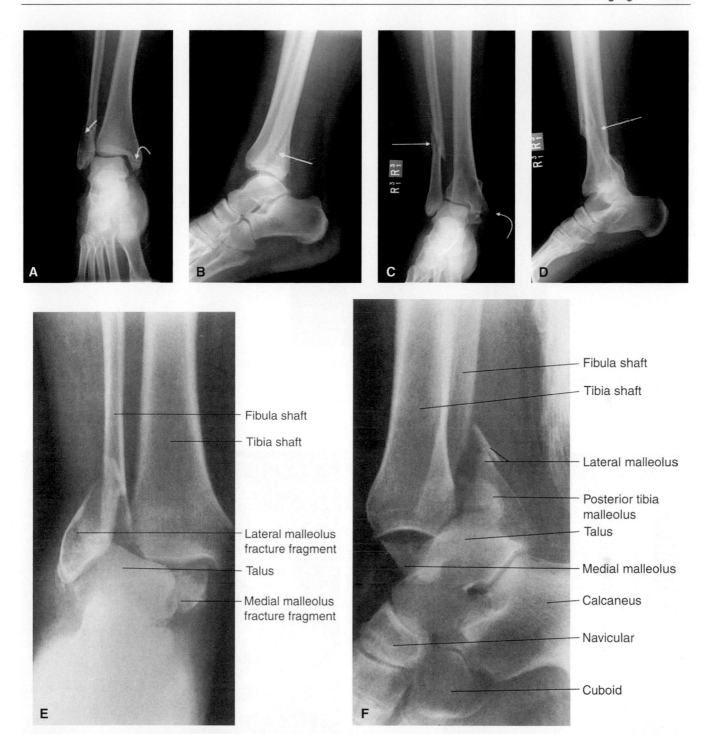

FIGURE 6.59. Weber type B and C fractures. Weber type B: Right ankle AP **(A)** and lateral **(B)** radiographs. There is an obliquely oriented fracture of the fibula (*straight arrow*) at and slightly above the ankle joint. There is also a laterally oriented fracture of the medial malleolus (*curved arrow*). The medial joint space of the ankle mortise is also widened, owing to an injury to the deltoid ligament. This is an unstable ankle joint and will require surgery. **Weber type C fracture:** Right ankle AP **(C)** and lateral **(D)** radiographs. There is a comminuted fracture of the fibula well above the ankle joint (*straight arrow*). There is also a comminuted fracture of the distal tibia (*curved arrow*). There is clear widening of the distal tibiofibular joint, with disruption of the ankle syndesmosis. This is an unstable ankle joint and will require surgery. **Weber type C with displaced trimalleolar fractures and talotibial dislocation.** Right ankle AP **(E)** and lateral **(F)** radiographs. The medial and posterior tibial malleoli fracture fragments and the fibula lateral malleolus fracture fragments are all displaced owing to an eversion injury. The talus is severely displaced laterally and posteriorly relative to the tibia.

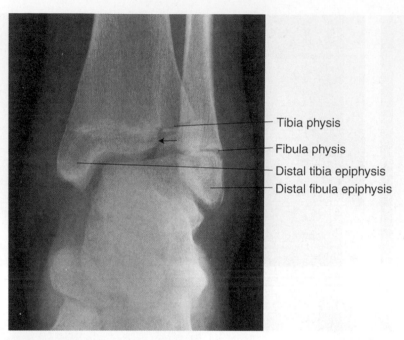

Tibia physis
Fibula physis
Distal tibia epiphysis
Distal fibula epiphysis

FIGURE 6.60. Salter III fracture of the left distal tibia. Left ankle AP radiograph. The fracture line (*arrow*) extends from the physis through the distal tibial epiphysis to the articular surface.

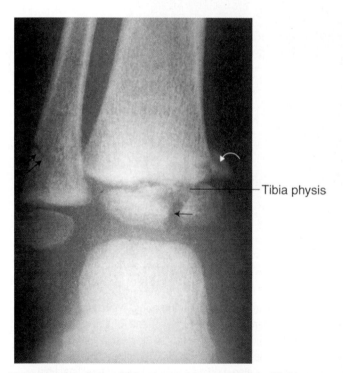

Tibia physis

FIGURE 6.61. Salter IV fracture of the distal tibia. Right ankle AP radiograph. The fracture line (*single straight arrow*) extends from the distal tibial physis through the epiphysis to the tibial articular surface. The fracture also involves the medial tibia metaphysis (*curved arrow*). There is an associated fracture of the distal fibula (*double straight arrows*).

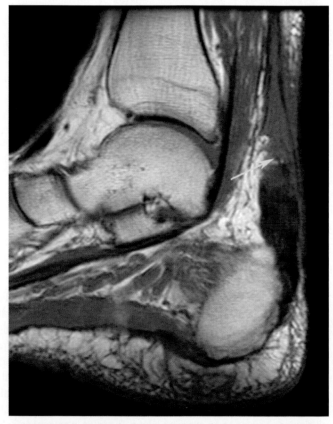

FIGURE 6.62. Achilles tendon tear. Sagittal T1-weighted MR of the ankle. There is thickening and disruption (*arrow*) of the normally uniformly dark Achilles tendon.

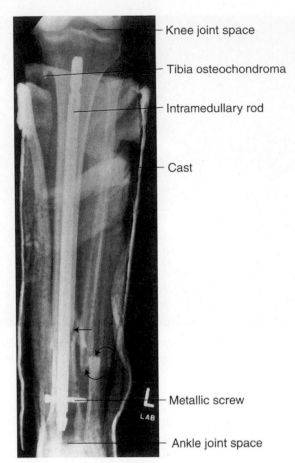

FIGURE 6.63. **Intramedullary rod** for a transverse fracture in the distal one-third of the left tibia (*straight arrow*). There is an offset overriding transverse fracture in the distal one-third of the fibula (*curved arrows*). The fibula is non–weight-bearing, so the displacement is not important to a good functional outcome.

The **Ottawa Knee Rules** recommend radiographs of the knee in patients older than 18 years with acute **knee** injury in the following circumstances: Patients who are of age 55 years or older OR have palpable tenderness over the head of the fibula, or the patella, OR cannot flex the knee to 90 degrees, OR cannot bear weight immediately following the injury and walk in the emergency room for four steps.[3]

Not all fractures of the knee are visible on radiographs. The extent of a tibial plateau fracture may be better evaluated on CT or MRI as this is one of the most common sites of missed fractures (Figs. 6.65 and 6.66). CT estimates the depression of the articular surface and may be helpful in planning of knee surgery (Fig. 6.67). MRI is considered the optimal imaging modality for identifying meniscal, ligament, chondral, and nondisplaced bone injuries around

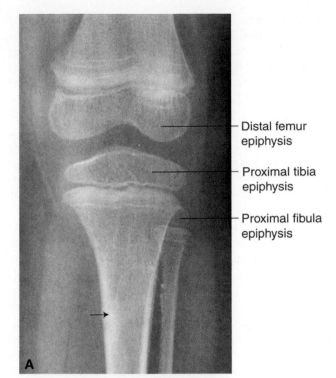

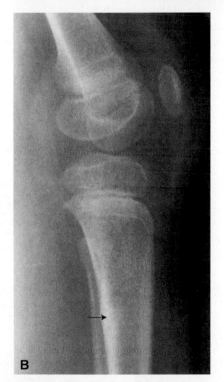

FIGURE 6.64. **Stress fracture.** Left knee AP **(A)** and lateral **(B)** radiographs. A healing stress fracture in this 5-year-old is indicated by the zone of increased density in the posteromedial proximal tibia (*arrows*). The fracture resulted from excessive usage or stress.

the knee. **Knee dislocation** is an orthopedic emergency because of possible nerve or arterial damage. Vascular injury may be found in about 30% of patients following posterior knee dislocation. Although MRI allows visualization of ligaments, tendons, and menisci, CTA of lower extremity is a reliable and noninvasive way of imaging the popliteal artery. The patella may fracture following a fall or blunt trauma (Fig. 6.68).

Osteonecrosis is the result of bone ischemia and may occur in any bone.

Osteonecrosis has several possible causes and the clinical presentations vary with the bone site and size as well as skeletal maturity (Legg–Calvé–Perthes disease, Fig. 6.24). The term **bone infarction** is used when the dead bone is in the diaphysis or metaphysis, whereas **osteonecrosis** describes this process in the epiphysis. **Osteochondritis dissecans** (Fig. 6.69) occurs most frequently along the lateral aspect of the medial femoral condyle in young adults, but it can occur elsewhere in the knee and in other joints including the hip, shoulder, ankle, and elbow. This localized avascular necrosis may occur after a subchondral stress fracture, which results in a necrotic bone fragment that detaches from the donor site and becomes a loose body within the joint. In adults, osteochondritis dissecans occurs on the weight-bearing aspect of the medial femoral condyle and the term **spontaneous osteonecrosis** is often used as these lesions are felt to be due to subchondral ischemia.

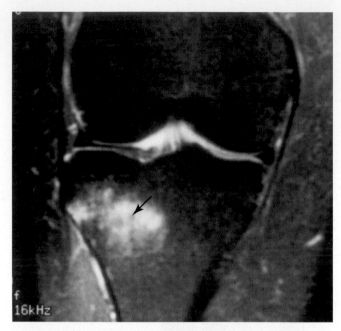

FIGURE 6.66. Insufficiency fracture of the medial tibia. MRI (coronal, inversion recovery) of the right knee shows incomplete fracture line (*arrow*).

Hip fractures are an important cause of morbidity and mortality in the elderly and pose an immense economic burden on the health care system. Hip fractures may be classified as **intracapsular** (femoral head and neck) (Figs. 6.70

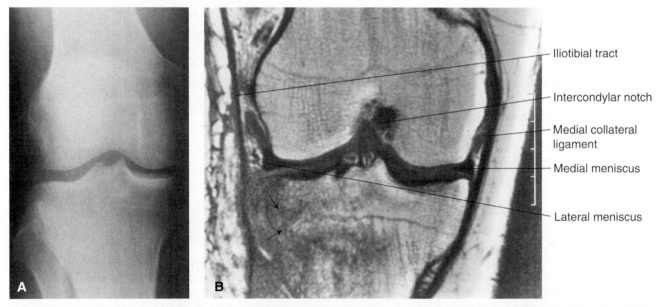

Iliotibial tract

Intercondylar notch

Medial collateral ligament

Medial meniscus

Lateral meniscus

FIGURE 6.65. Occult lateral tibial plateau fracture. A: Right knee AP radiograph. This AP radiograph and a lateral (*not shown*) radiograph obtained following trauma were interpreted as normal. **B:** Right knee coronal T1 MRI. This study was obtained 2 weeks following the initial radiograph in **(A)** because of persistent knee pain and a clinical suspicion of an anterior cruciate ligament injury. The *arrows* indicate an area of low-intensity signal caused by blood and edema replacing the bone marrow fat (*white*) in the tibial plateau fracture. The anterior cruciate ligament was intact. The fracture eventually became apparent on subsequent radiographs.

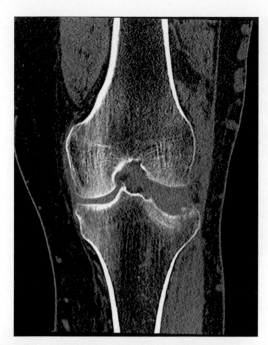

FIGURE 6.67. Lateral tibial plateau fracture. Coronal reformatted CT better evaluates the depression of the articular surface (*straight arrow*) and number and location of fragments.

and 6.71) and **extracapsular** (intertrochanteric and subtrochanteric) (Figs. 6.72 and 6.73). In adults, the femoral head receives its blood supply from two sources, the foveal artery and ascending cervical arteries, of which the latter is the dominant supply. The ascending cervical arteries run parallel to the femoral neck to the femoral head and are at risk of disruption following a fracture of the femoral neck, resulting in osteonecrosis of the femoral head causing nonunion. In contrast, extracapsular fractures have a lower risk of osteonecrosis, but the overall mortality and functional outcome is generally worse with intertrochanteric fractures, which is attributed to comorbidities and postoperative complications. Treatment of subtrochanteric fractures requires the use of rods or nails, which may have a higher rate of failure due to mechanical stress.

Initially an AP view of the pelvis and AP and lateral views of the affected hip should be obtained. If plain radiographs are unrevealing but pain is significant and clinical suspicion is high or the patient is at high risk, a bone scan or MRI can diagnose a fracture (Fig. 6.74). MRI has the advantages of earlier fracture detection and the absence of radiation exposure. It can take up to 72 hours following an injury before diagnostic findings appear on a bone scan.

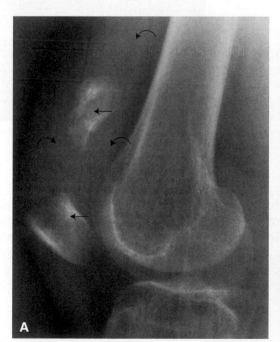
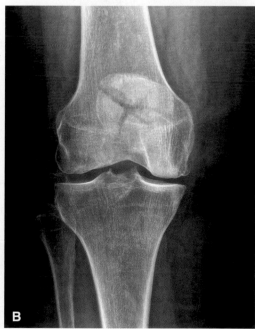

FIGURE 6.68. Patellar fracture. A: Right knee lateral. Mid patella fracture secondary to a motor vehicle accident. There are two distracted fracture fragments (*straight arrows* through the mid patella). The *curved arrows* indicate blood and increased synovial fluid in the supra-, pre-, and retro-patellar spaces of the knee. **B:** AP view.

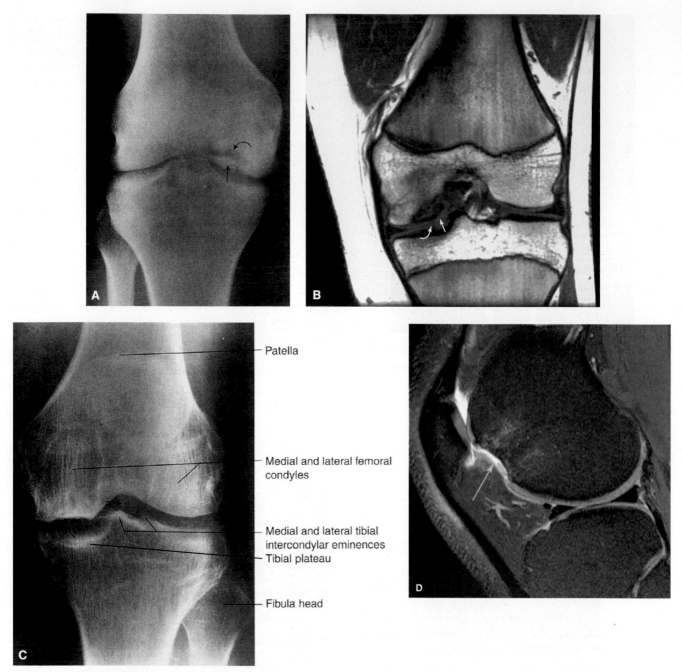

FIGURE 6.69. Osteochondritis dissecans. A: Right knee AP radiograph. The bone fragment (*straight arrow*) is not displaced from the donor site (*curved arrow*) on the lateral aspect of the medial femoral condyle. **B:** Coronal T1-weighted MR right knee in a different patient. The fragment (*straight arrow*) is clearly seen and cartilage covers it (*curved arrow*). **C: Spontaneous osteonecrosis.** Left knee AP radiograph in a different patient. There is a displaced bone fragment or loose body (*straight arrow*) in the joint space. The radiolucent defect surrounded by the sclerotic zone (*curved arrows*) in the weight-bearing portion of the medial femoral condyle is the donor site of the loose body. **D:** Sagittal fat-suppressed T2-weighted MRI. Note the defect in the trochlea (*arrow*). The loose body is in the suprapatellar bursa and not included on this image.

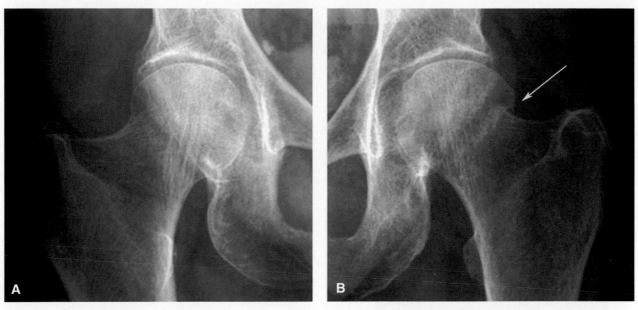

FIGURE 6.70. **Impacted femoral neck fracture.** The right hip **(A)** is normal and makes the impacted left femoral neck fracture (**B**, *arrow*) more apparent.

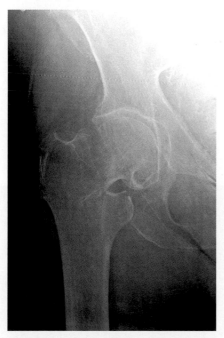

FIGURE 6.71. **Femoral neck fracture.** AP radiograph of right hip shows a femoral neck fracture.

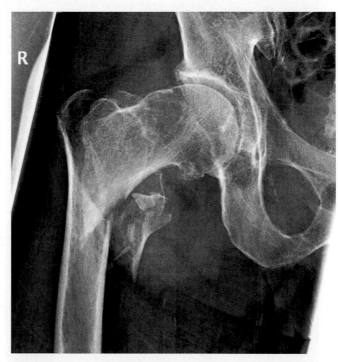

FIGURE 6.72. **Intertrochanteric fracture.** AP radiograph of right hip shows an intertrochanteric fracture.

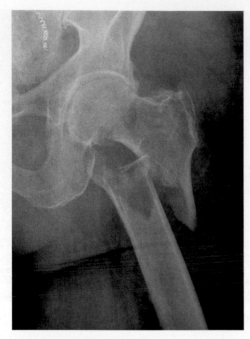

FIGURE 6.73. **Subtrochanteric fracture.** AP radiograph of left hip showing a subtrochanteric fracture.

Radiographs should be obtained for up to 3 years following surgery to screen for the development of **osteonecrosis** particularly in patients with displaced fractures as they are at greatest risk. Confirmation using MRI or bone scan is necessary when osteonecrosis is suspected as changes on plain radiographs do not reliably appear until 6 months after osteonecrosis first develops. MRI is used to assess patients with titanium hardware; whereas those whose fracture fixation hardware is ferromagnetic are better imaged with a bone scan. Femoral shaft fractures generally result in severe pain at the fracture site and the inability to bear weight (Fig. 6.75). Stress fractures may develop in the hip as well, most typically in runners (Fig. 6.76). Dislocations of the hip are not common and require high impact as in MVAs (Fig. 6.77). However, patients with a hip prosthesis may dislocate the prosthetic head with a minimal amount of stress (Fig. 6.78). In contrast to the shoulder, posterior dislocations of the hip are much more frequent than anterior dislocations. Occasionally, dislocations are not visible on a single anterior radiographs and CT is indicated because prompt reduction of hip dislocation is imperative to minimize the likelihood of osteonecrosis of the femoral head. CT is also quite useful in the assessment of complex pelvic

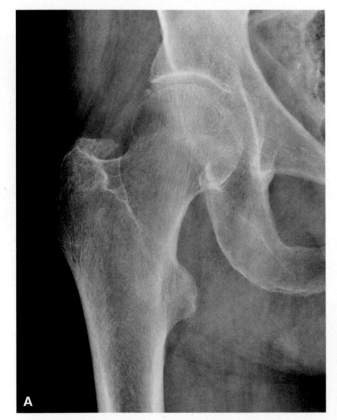

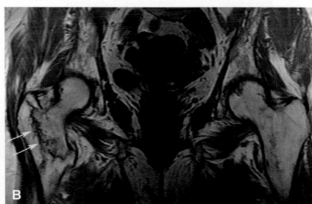

FIGURE 6.74. **Occult hip fracture. A:** Right hip radiograph was interpreted as normal. With persistent clinical suspicion for fracture, an MRI was obtained. **B:** Coronal T1-weighted MR of the pelvis reveals the nondisplaced right intertrochanteric fracture (*arrows*).

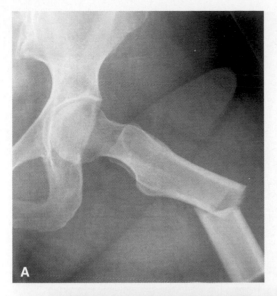

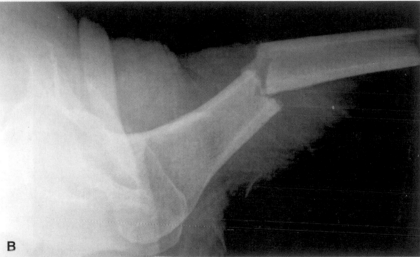

FIGURE 6.75. **Transverse fracture of the femoral shaft.** Left femur frog-leg **(A)** and true **(B)** lateral radiographs showing apex anterior angulation. Displacement is posterior in the frog-leg lateral but was anterior on the true lateral. The patient is supine and the x-ray beam horizontal on the true lateral.

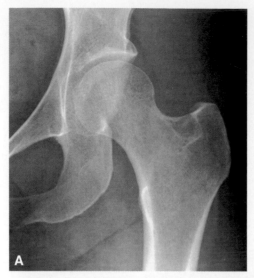

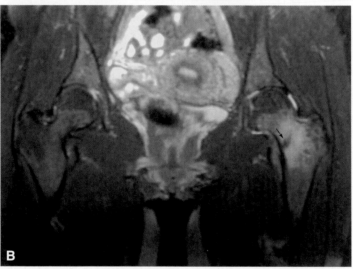

FIGURE 6.76. Femoral neck stress fracture. AP radiograph **(A)** of the left hip was interpreted as normal. This avid runner complained of persistent pain and an MR was obtained. Coronal fat-suppressed T2-weighted image **(B)** demonstrates edema (*white*) around the developing stress fracture (*arrow*). Left untreated, this might well progress to a complete fracture.

FIGURE 6.77. Posterior dislocation of the hip.
Pelvis AP radiograph. The left femoral head is displaced cephalad and lateral relative to the acetabulum (*arrows*). The right hip is normal by comparison.

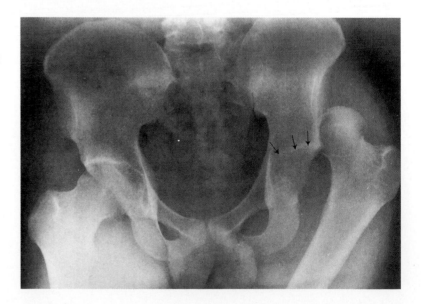

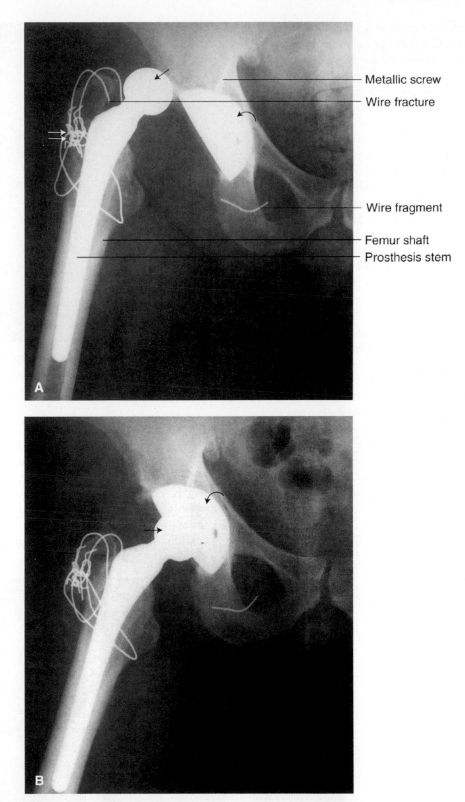

Metallic screw
Wire fracture

Wire fragment

Femur shaft
Prosthesis stem

FIGURE 6.78. Posterior dislocation of the right hip prosthesis head. A: AP radiographs showing the right hip prosthesis (*straight black arrow*) in relation to the acetabular component (*curved arrow*). At least one of the anchoring wires (*white arrows*) is fractured and lies inferior to the prosthesis acetabular component. **B:** Following closed reduction (no surgery) under general anesthesia, the prosthetic head (*arrow*) has been returned to its proper position relative to the acetabular prosthetic component (*curved arrow*).

and acetabular fractures. In cases of pelvic pain or trauma, it is important to assess the integrity of the pelvic ring and obturator foramina. Also of importance are the iliopectineal and ilioischial lines as well as the contour of the acetabular teardrop as evidence of acetabular fractures.

Osteonecrosis unrelated to fracture most commonly affects the femoral heads in which there is ischemia of bone. Predisposing causes include steroid usage and alcohol abuse. Nontraumatic osteonecrosis is bilateral of 70% of cases. AP radiographs of the pelvis and frog-leg lateral views typically show subarticular collapse and should be obtained as the initial study (Fig. 6.79). MRI is the optimal modality for detection of osteonecrosis, the differential diagnosis of which includes transient osteoporosis and subchondral insufficiency fracture. In children, the lack of enhancement or hypoperfusion on postcontrast MRI may be observed. Osteonecrosis involving less than one-third of the femoral head only rarely progresses.

Fracture Healing

Fracture healing depends on many factors including fracture site, type of fracture, degree of displacement, patient age, adequacy of immobilization, nutrition, and absence of infection. Perhaps the most overlooked factor critical for fracture healing is **blood supply**. Although fracture alignment and mobilization may be perfect, the absence of an adequate blood supply prevents successful healing and leads to non- or malunion, for example, femoral neck fractures in the elderly and scaphoid fractures. When a fracture occurs, there usually is an associated hemorrhage into the fracture site with subsequent hematoma formation around and between the fracture fragments. The fibrin in the hematoma serves as a framework for fibroblasts, osteoblasts, and a general inflammatory reaction.

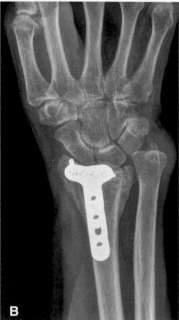

FIGURE 6.79. Osteonecrosis left femoral head. AP view shows flattening and sclerosis of the left femoral head, which has subluxed superiorly. C marks the acetabulum.

Bone matrix or osteoid appears in the repair process after a few days, and this is called **soft callus or provisional callus**, which is not visible on a radiograph. As calcium salts precipitate in the soft callus, new bone grows, and this is called **callus**. As the callus gradually becomes denser, it is visible on a radiograph (Fig. 6.80A). Eventually, the callus becomes solid and bone union is established between the fracture fragments (Fig. 6.80B). As a part of the fracture healing process, some

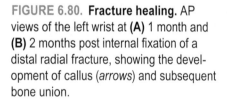

FIGURE 6.80. Fracture healing. AP views of the left wrist at **(A)** 1 month and **(B)** 2 months post internal fixation of a distal radial fracture, showing the development of callus (*arrows*) and subsequent bone union.

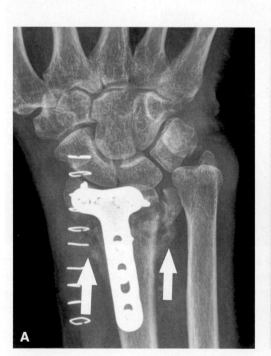

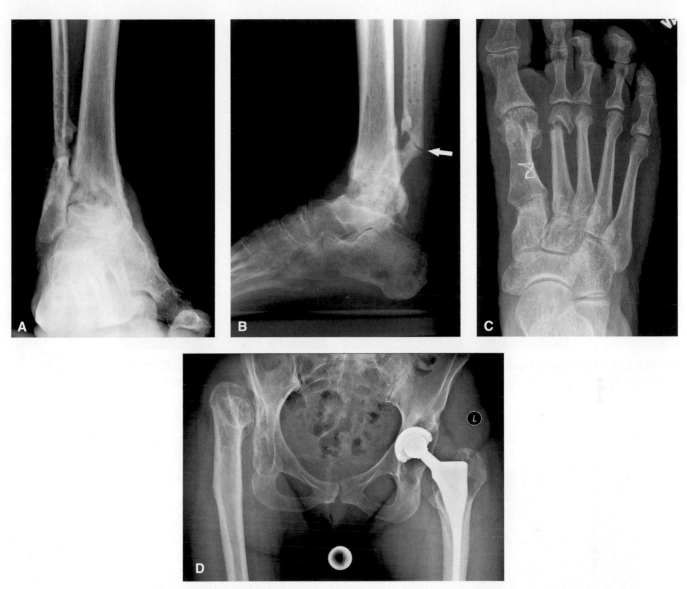

FIGURE 6.81. Fracture nonunion and pseudarthrosis. A and B: Frontal and lateral views of right ankle showing nonunion and subsequent fibular pseudarthrosis (*arrow*). **C:** Nonunion and pseudarthrosis of second metatarsal neck. **D:** Nonunion and pseudarthrosis of right hip.

absorption or removal of bone occurs near the ends of the fracture fragments within several days of a fracture. Because of this bone resorption, the fracture line may become more visible on subsequent radiographs. This explains why some subtle fractures are not be visible on radiographs obtained immediately following injury but are visible approximately 7 to 10 days following injury.

Self-explanatory terms used to describe problems in the fracture healing process include the following.

- **Nonunion** is a term used to describe permanent failure in normal healing of a fracture with formation of

a fibrous pseudarthrosis with adjacent sclerotic bone (Fig. 6.81). Nonunion has a variety of causes, including ischemia, infection, inadequate immobilization, and interposition of muscle or other structures between the fracture fragments.
- **Delayed union** is defined as continued, but temporary, lack of bony union at 6 months after the initial injury (Fig. 6.82).
- **Malunion** occurs when a fracture heals in less than anatomic alignment, producing a deficit or deformity (Fig. 6.83).

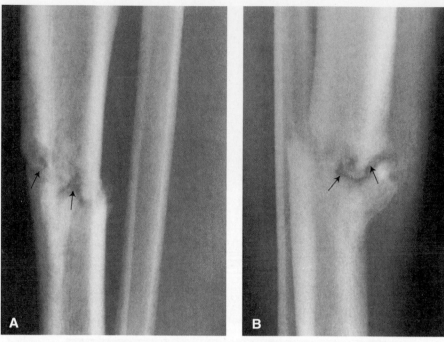

FIGURE 6.82. Osteomyelitis and nonunion of a tibia fracture. Left tibia and fibula AP **(A)** and lateral **(B)** radiographs showing a clearly visible fracture line (*arrows*) after 3 months indicating delayed union at the fracture site due to infection.

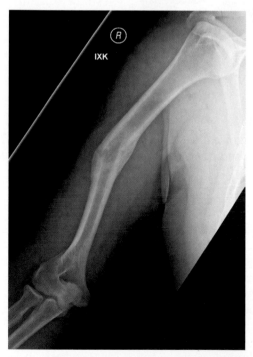

FIGURE 6.83. Malunion. Healing of angulated humeral shaft fracture.

STRESS, ATYPICAL, AND PATHOLOGIC FRACTURES

Atraumatic fractures including stress, atypical, and pathologic fractures[4] are commonly encountered. Misdiagnosis can result in delayed diagnosis of malignancy, failure to correct a metabolic derangement, or suboptimal surgical treatment and potential implant failure.

Stress fractures, in the broadest sense of the term, can be divided into **fatigue** fractures and **insufficiency** fractures: A fatigue fracture is a focal failure of *normal* bone caused by repetitive stress, for example, "march fractures" of the metatarsal bones, when the rate of accumulated microdamage outpaces the ability of the bone to regenerate through the normal remodeling process (Fig. 6.56). In comparison, an insufficiency fracture is a focal failure of abnormally *weakened* bone caused by repetitive stress such as a sacral insufficiency fracture. The term fragility fracture likewise signifies a fracture in abnormally weakened bone due to metabolic bone disease most commonly in a patient with osteoporosis.

Atypical femoral fractures in the lateral cortex of the femoral diaphysis can be seen in patients undergoing long-term therapy with bisphosphonate medications. When an atypical femoral fracture is identified, screening of the contralateral hip and entire femur is recommended with AP and lateral radiographs because up to one-half of patients will eventually develop a fracture in the contralateral femur.

The term **pathologic fracture** generally is reserved for fractures through tumor or osteomyelitis. The MRI appearance of many pathologic fractures with well-defined margins contrasts with the radiographic appearance of many aggressive-appearing lesions, which classically have a wide zone of transition. On MRI, the most important marrow signal intensity characteristic to differentiate benign from pathologic fractures is the margin and homogeneity of the T1-weighted signal intensity abnormality around the fracture. In benign fractures, the T1-hypointense signal abnormality represents acute edema and hemorrhage, which has indistinct margins, and a gradual bandlike transition to normal marrow signal intensity further from the fracture. In many pathologic fractures, however, the T1-weighted signal intensity abnormality is at least partially caused by the infiltrative tumor which causes a T1-hypointense signal abnormality with well-defined convex margins.

Soft-Tissue Injuries

Injuries to muscles and tendons are often diagnosed clinically. Some muscular injuries may require further evaluation—using ultrasound or MRI. Typical of these are muscle avulsions or tears of the hamstring (Fig. 6.84) or pectoralis muscles. A muscle may also tear in its body. The extent of the intramuscular tear and hematoma is particularly important to the elite athlete since length of rehabilitation and long-term prognosis are affected by the severity of the muscular injury. Muscle injury may be complicated by subsequent calcification and/or ossification at the injury site called *myositis ossificans*, now more commonly termed *heterotopic ossification*. Common locations for this complication include the quadriceps and brachialis muscles and near the hip following hip surgery (Fig. 6.85).

MRI is an excellent imaging tool for evaluating cartilage, menisci, tendons, and ligaments and usually radiographs are negative in such injuries (Figs. 6.86-6.90). In the wrist, MRI is used to evaluate the intrinsic wrist ligaments, triangular fibrocartilage complex, flexor and extensor tendons, and the nerves. The collateral ligaments and tendinous attachments of the elbow are commonly evaluated with MRI. In the shoulder, the tendons of the rotator cuff, the biceps tendon, and the glenoid labrum are evaluated with MRI.

Many foreign bodies in soft tissue and bone are radiopaque and readily identified on radiographs (Fig. 6.91A and B). Occasionally, a nonopaque foreign body in an extremity is suspected, and if not visible on a radiograph, an ultrasound, CT, or MR study can be requested to assist in its detection (Fig. 6.91C).

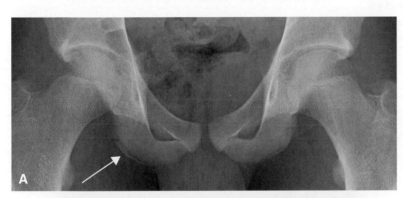

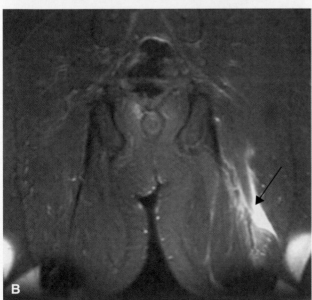

FIGURE 6.84. Hamstring muscle tears. A: AP radiograph of pelvis shows partial avulsion of the hamstring origin on the right ischium (*arrow*). **B:** Coronal T2-weighted MRI in a different patient shows increased signal in the left posterior thigh representing edema and blood around the biceps femoris of the hamstrings (*arrow*).

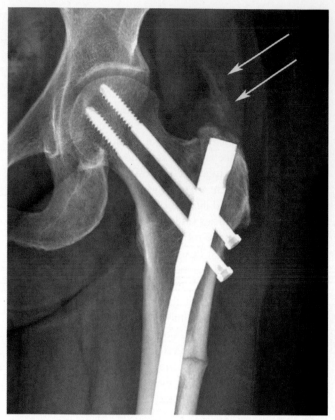

FIGURE 6.85. Heterotopic ossification. AP radiograph of left hip post placement of intramedullary nail. Heterotopic ossification is developed in the soft tissues of the surgical bed (*arrows*).

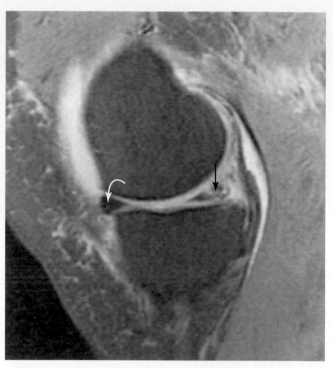

FIGURE 6.87. Posterior horn of medial meniscus tear. Sagittal proton-density MRI through the medial meniscus showing edema and synovial fluid within the tear (*straight arrow*). The anterior horn of the meniscus is normal (*curved arrow*).

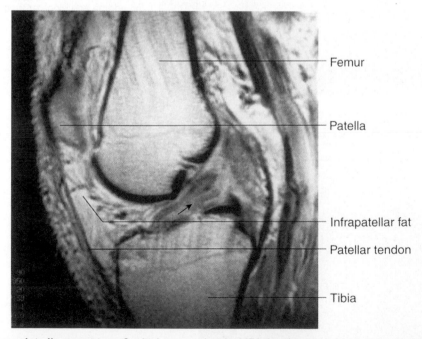

Femur

Patella

Infrapatellar fat

Patellar tendon

Tibia

FIGURE 6.86. Anterior cruciate ligament tear. Sagittal, proton-density MRI showing high signal at the site of the anterior cruciate ligament tear (*arrow*).

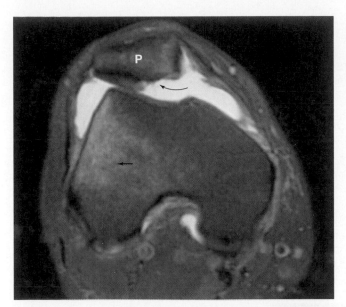

FIGURE 6.88. Recurrent patellar dislocation. Axial T2, MRI showing lateral subluxation of the patella, which normally articulates with the trochlea of the femur. Edema in the lateral femoral condyle (*straight arrow*) indicates where the patella impacted during dislocation. A cartilage defect (*curved arrow*) occurred in the posterior surface of the patella during the dislocation or relocation.

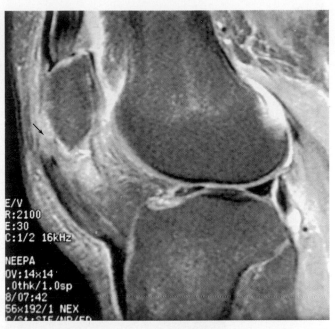

FIGURE 6.89. Patellar tendon tear. Sagittal proton-density MRI showing disruption patellar tendon and its attachment (*arrow*)

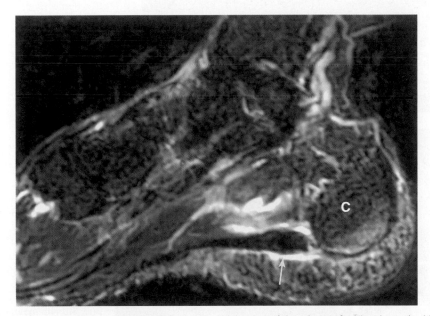

FIGURE 6.90. Plantar fasciitis. STIR MRI images of left foot show thickening of the plantar fashion (*arrow*) with surrounding edema.

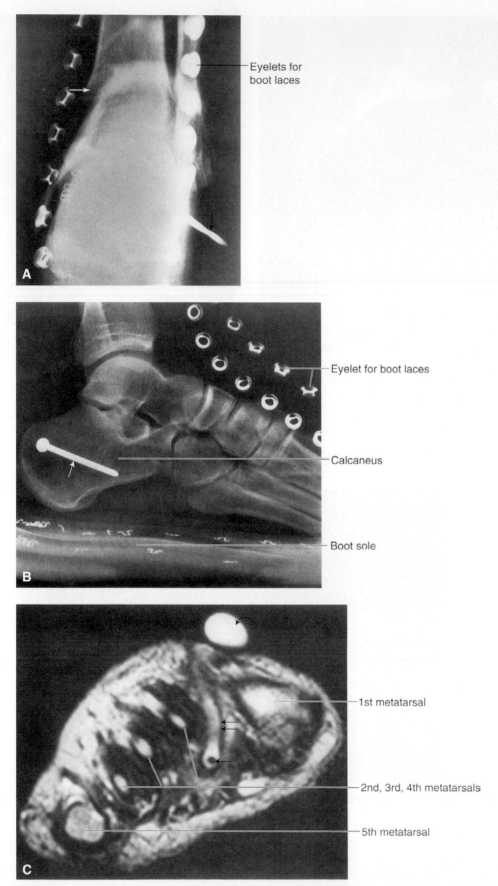

FIGURE 6.91. **Soft tissue foreign body. (A)** AP and **(B)** lateral foot radiographs showing metallic nail (*arrow*) lodged (driven by power tool) in the calcaneus. **C:** Left foot axial T2 image showing a foreign body wedged between the first and second metatarsals.

NONACCIDENTAL INJURY

In 2015, there were over 600,000 victims of child abuse and an average of 4 children per day died of abuse and neglect in the United States. Boys and girls are affected equally. Although 80% of nonaccidental injury (NAI) deaths are secondary to head injuries, NAI can occur in any part of the skeletal system with fractures occurring in up to 55% of cases. An appropriate workup for suspected NAI includes a radiographic survey of the long bones, pelvis, spine, ribs, and skull. Bone scintigraphy may also be useful if clinical suspicion remains high with normal radiographs. Metaphyseal fractures, probably due to a twisting mechanism, are typical findings in NAI (Fig. 6.92A) as are subperiosteal hemorrhage (Fig. 6.92B) and bucket-handle fractures (see Fig. 6.39).

Skeletal injuries and fractures that should make the observer highly suspicious for nonaccidental trauma are summarized in Table 6.8. Suspicious findings must be differentiated from normal periostitis found in infancy, osteogenesis imperfecta, congenital insensitivity to pain, and metabolic and vitamin deficiency disorders.

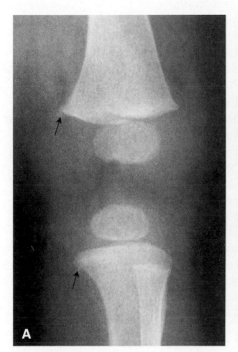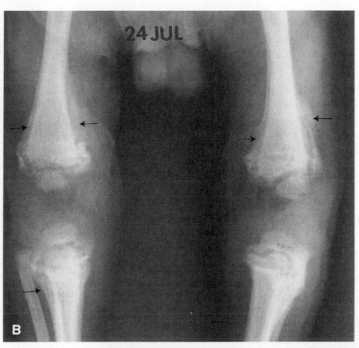

FIGURE 6.92. Nonaccidental injury. Metaphyseal corner fracture **(A)** following a twisting mechanism is a typical finding as is subperiosteal hemorrhage (*arrows*) **(B)** and a bucket-handle fracture (*arrows*) (Fig. 6.39).

TABLE 6.8	Fractures Associated With NAI (Child Abuse)
Type:	
Posterior rib fracture	
Metaphyseal corner	
Periosteal hemorrhage	
Bucket-handle fractures	
Multiple fractures of varying ages	
Common sites:	
Lower extremity: femur (most common), tibia	
Elbow	
Shoulder	
Ribs	

ARTHRITIDES

The radiograph is the initial imaging test for most arthritides. Features such as the joint distribution, the presence of periarticular osteoporosis, and erosions are helpful in making the diagnosis.

Osteoarthritis

Osteoarthritis (OA) is the most common form of arthritis and can be categorized into primary and secondary. **Secondary OA**, or degenerative joint disease (DJD), occurs with increasing age, is due to wear and tear, and may involve almost any joint of the extremities and spine but more commonly the PIP and DIP joints of the fingers and carpometacarpal joint in the thumb as well as the hips and knees (Fig. 6.95). In younger patients, OA may occur secondarily after trauma, osteonecrosis, or infection. **Primary OA** is more common in women and involves the DIP and PIP joints of the hands and the first carpometacarpal joint in a bilaterally symmetrical fashion (Fig. 6.93).

Clinical features and radiographic findings of OA are listed in Table 6.9 and include asymmetric, irregular joint space narrowing because of articular cartilage destruction, subchondral sclerosis, and osteophyte formation. Sclerosis may be less conspicuous in patients with osteoporosis. The presence of osteophytes in the absence of sclerosis or joint space narrowing favors diffuse idiopathic skeletal

TABLE 6.9	Typical Symptoms and Radiographic Findings in Osteoarthritis and Rheumatoid Arthritis

Osteoarthritis

Pain, deformity, and limitation of joint motion

Pain improves with rest

Involves virtually all joints of the extremities and spine

Typically involves the hand distal interphalangeal (DIP) joints and the first carpometacarpal (CMC) joint

Asymmetric joint narrowing

Sclerotic bone changes

Cysts or pseudocysts

Osteophyte formation

Usually absence of osteoporosis

Genu valgus and varus deformities (knees)

Cephalad and sometimes lateral migration of the femoral head

Rheumatoid Arthritis

Pain, stiffness, and limitation of motion, especially in the hands and feet, worse in the morning

Pain improves with activity

Involves all synovial joints of the extremities and spine

Typically involves the hand MCP and wrist joints

Symmetric joint narrowing (both within a joint and side-to-side)

Periarticular osteoporosis (prominent feature)

Periarticular soft-tissue thickening and swelling

Marginal osseous erosions

MCP joint subluxation and ulnar deviation

Medial migration of the femoral head and acetabular protrusio

Pencil tip appearance of the distal clavicle

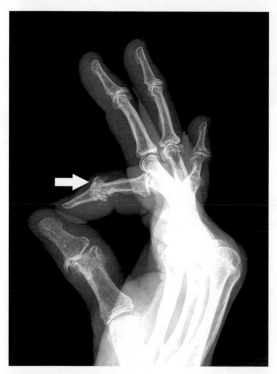

FIGURE 6.93. Osteoarthritis of the distal interphalangeal joints and the interphalangeal joint of the thumb. Note the loss of joint space, osteophyte formation (*arrow*), and preservation of bone density.

hyperostosis (DISH) rather than osteoarthritis. A common feature of osteoarthritis is a subchondral cyst or geode, which is always well defined and should not be mistaken for an aggressive lytic lesion (Fig. 6.94).

When advanced osteoarthritis involves the medial knee compartment, a genu varus deformity or bowed leg usually results (Fig. 6.95). Advanced OA in the **L**ateral knee compartment often results in a genu va**L**gus deformity or knock-knee appearance. When advanced OA involves the hip, the femoral head migrates cephalad because of asymmetric cartilage destruction primarily at the superolateral aspect of the acetabulum, whereas in rheumatoid arthritis the femoral head tends to drift centrally from uniform cartilage loss. Acetabular protrusion may result from softening of the bones due to osteoporosis (Fig. 6.96). Another frequent location of OA is the great toe (metatarsophalangeal [MTP]) joint where the apex at the joint is displaced medially to form a hallux valgus (Fig. 6.97). While OA technically only affects synovial joints, degenerative change of the

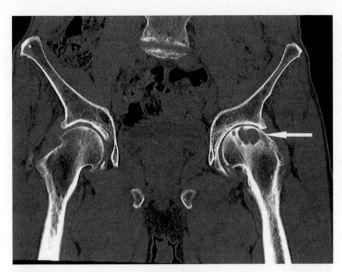

FIGURE 6.94. Geode. Coronal CT of pelvis showing a well-defined, subarticular lucency (*arrow*) associated with OA.

syndesmotic fibrocartilaginous joints (intervertebral disks) in the spine is referred to as **degenerative disk disease** (Fig. 9.51).

Rheumatoid Arthritis

Rheumatoid arthritis (RA) is an inflammatory arthritis of unknown etiology that involves synovial joints and is characterized by periarticular osteopenia, marginal erosions, and symmetric joint narrowing secondary to articular cartilage destruction by pannus, which is granulation tissue derived from the synovium. Clinical features and radiographic findings associated with RA are listed in Table 6.9. The most commonly affected joints, in decreasing frequency, are the MCP joints, carpal articulations, PIP joints, knees, MTP joints, shoulders, ankles, cervical spine, hips, elbows, and temporomandibular joints. The initial

symptoms of RA include morning stiffness and pain, limitation of movement, and swelling in the hands and/or feet. Usually, the first joints involved are the metacarpal and metatarsal phalangeal joints and this tends to be bilaterally symmetrical. Typical findings include periarticular osteoporosis due to hyperemia, symmetric joint narrowing, and marginal erosions (Figs. 6.98-6.101). As the disease progresses, characteristic joint deformity may develop because of subluxation and ulnar deviation of the fingers at the MCP joints. Despite widespread cartilage destruction, true bone ankylosis (fusion) is rare. Although radiographs are the standard modality in its evaluation and monitoring of progression, MRI can detect periarticular soft tissue thickening before any radiographic abnormality (Fig. 6.102).

The differential diagnosis of RA as shown in Table 6.10 includes gout and infection. In gout, osteoporosis is usually absent, and articular and juxta-articular erosions are more sharply defined, characteristically with overhanging margins. In osteomyelitis and infectious arthritis, the osteoporosis is maximal near the infection site. In OA, osteoporosis is usually absent and osteophytes and subchondral sclerosis are present. However, RA and OA can, and often do, occur simultaneously.

Psoriatic Arthritis

Psoriatic arthritis is found in 2% to 6% of patients with skin manifestations of psoriasis, although the vast majority of those with psoriatic arthritis have had a long history of psoriatic skin disease, particularly with psoriatic nail changes. The arthritis is characterized by involvement of small joints with asymmetric distribution. There are bone erosions with enthesiopathy—bony proliferation adjacent to joints and at muscle and tendon attachment sites (Fig. 6.103). Unlike RA, ankylosis is more frequent. There are five clinical spectra of the arthritis: (1) polyarthritis with DIP joint involvement;

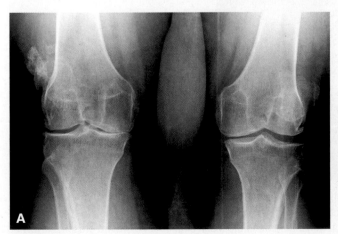

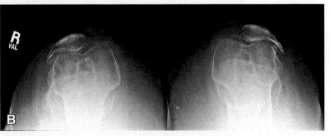

FIGURE 6.95. Osteoarthritis of the knees. A: Standing AP view of both knees shows bilateral osteoarthritis maximal in the right medial tibia femoral compartment. **B:** Sunrise view of both knees showing osteoarthritis in the patellofemoral compartments of the knees.

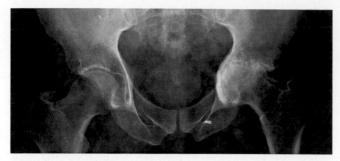

FIGURE 6.96. Osteoarthritis and protrusio acetabuli of the left hip. Note minimal loss of superior joint space in the right hip.

(2) a markedly deforming condition (arthritis mutilans) with widespread joint destruction and ankylosis (fusion across joints); (3) symmetric arthritis resembling RA; (4) single or asymmetric, few joint involvement (pauciarticular); and (5) asymmetric sacroiliitis and spondylitis, which may resemble ankylosing spondylitis.

Gout, Pseudogout, and Hemophilic Arthritis

Gout arthritis (Fig. 6.104) is secondary to hyperuricemia or elevated serum uric acid levels and involves the synovial spaces, with joint effusion and synovial hypertrophy. The (predominantly male) patients classically present with podagra, or pain and inflammatory changes near the

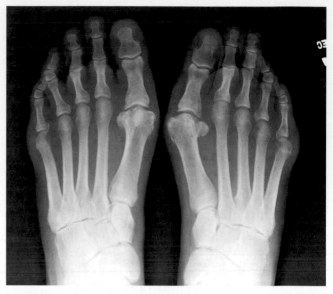

FIGURE 6.97. Bilateral hallux valgus. Bilateral loss of joint space at first MTP joint and valgus deformities.

medial aspect of the first MTP joint. Although the disease is characterized by exacerbations and remissions, gout is usually present for a number of years before it is detectable radiographically. Noncalcified soft-tissue tophi may appear

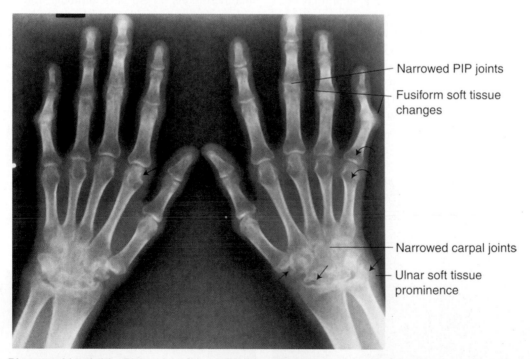

— Narrowed PIP joints
— Fusiform soft tissue changes
— Narrowed carpal joints
— Ulnar soft tissue prominence

FIGURE 6.98. Rheumatoid arthritis. Right- and left-hand PA radiographs showing periarticular osteoporosis (*curved arrows*), swan neck deformities of the little fingers, narrowing of the proximal interphalangeal (PIP) joints with associated fusiform soft tissue swelling, narrowing of the carpal and PIP joints, and soft tissue thickening or prominence around the distal ulna. Also, there are erosions involving the carpals, ulnar styloids, and metacarpal heads (*straight arrows*). The fusiform soft tissue swelling surrounding the joints represents edema and effusion. The soft tissue prominence around the distal ulna is secondary to edema and thickening around the external carpi ulnaris.

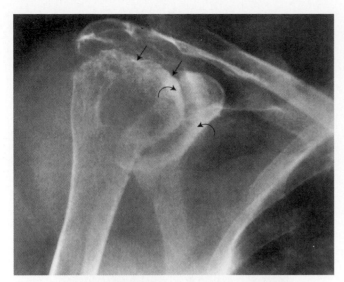

FIGURE 6.99. **Rheumatoid arthritis.** Right shoulder AP radiograph. There is characteristic osteoporosis, a pointed distal clavicle, and mild cephalad drift of the humeral head. The cephalad drift of the humeral head suggests rotator cuff damage that is common in this disease. There are articular bone erosions (*straight arrows*) and sclerosis (*curved arrows*). The sclerosis may be from some secondary osteoarthritis that may develop after cartilage loss when the inflammation from rheumatoid arthritis is quiescent.

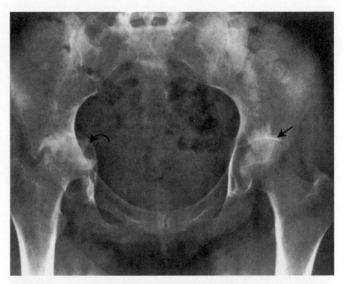

FIGURE 6.101. **Rheumatoid arthritis.** Pelvis AP radiograph showing generalized osteoporosis. The entire left hip joint space is symmetrically narrowed (*straight arrow*). There is characteristic medial drift of the right femoral head and acetabular protrusio (*curved arrow*). Note that the sacroiliac joints are not involved in this patient.

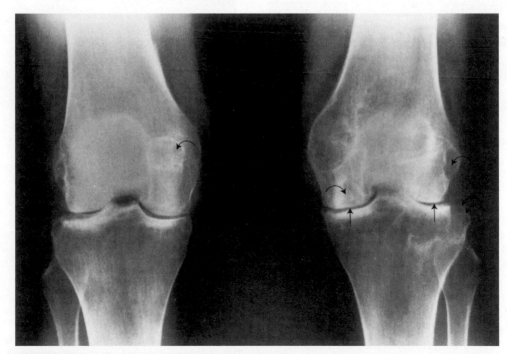

FIGURE 6.100. **Rheumatoid arthritis.** There are symmetric narrowing of the knee joints (*straight arrows*), periarticular cysts (*curved arrows*), erosions (*double arrows*), and osteoporosis.

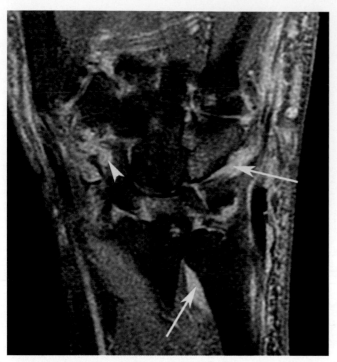

FIGURE 6.102. Rheumatoid arthritis. Coronal fat-suppressed T2-weighted MR of the wrist with synovial thickening/pannus formation (*arrows*) and erosions (*arrowhead*). Also compare the cartilage loss in this patient with the normal cartilage in the wrist in Figure 6.35D and E. The bones, particularly the hamate and the lunate have higher signal, likely owing to edema.

TABLE 6.10	Differential Diagnosis of Rheumatoid Arthritis

Gouty arthritis
Infectious arthritis
Sudeck atrophy
Psoriatic arthritis
Osteoarthritis
Ankylosing spondylitis
Scleroderma
Systemic lupus erythematosus

nonspecifically as focal increased opacity on plain films, but adjacent well-defined erosions and preservation of bone density are characteristic of the disease. The radiographic findings of gout arthritis are listed in Table 6.11.

The characteristic radiographic features of **pseudogout** are **chondrocalcinosis**, which describes the deposition of calcium pyrophosphate dihydrate crystals in the joint soft tissues including menisci, ligaments, articular cartilage, and the joint capsule, and the consequent arthritis, which resembles osteoarthritis (Fig. 6.105). The arthritis of calcium pyrophosphate deposition or the clinical

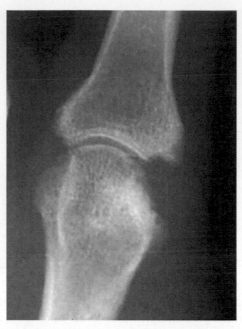

FIGURE 6.103. Psoriatic arthritis. Anterior radiograph of the left-hand second metacarpal–phalangeal joint showing joint space narrowing and small erosions with a fluffy proliferation of new bone at the joint margins.

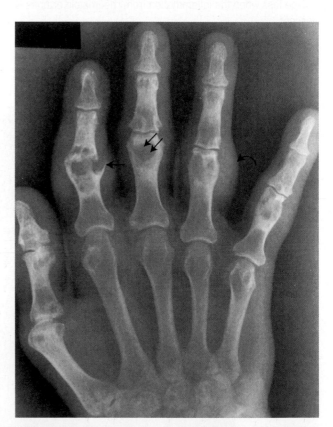

FIGURE 6.104. Gout arthritis. The proximal interphalangeal (PIP) joint spaces are at least partially preserved, and the lucent areas (*double arrows*) are typical of the sharply marginated peri-articular erosions. Erosions that extend into the joint often have an overhanging edge (*single straight arrow*). Note the classic appearance of a tophus (*curved arrow*). A tophus is an asymmetric swelling about the joint that may or may not be calcified.

TABLE 6.11 Radiographic Features of Gout

Sharply marginated and sometimes sclerotic-bordered erosions with overhanging edges near a joint

Tophus formation (paste-like calcium urate within the soft tissues) or soft tissue nodules

Normal bone mineralization

Occasionally joint deformity

exacerbation termed pseudogout has a predilection for the shoulder, elbow, patellofemoral and radiocarpal joints and joint aspiration of calcium pyrophosphate dihydrate crystals crystals, is diagnostic.

It can affect both fibro- and hyaline cartilage, with involvement of fibrocartilage more frequently related to aging and degeneration. There is a higher incidence of CPPD in patients with gout, primary hyperparathyroidism and hemochromatosis.

The joints in patients with **hemophilia** are gradually damaged by hemarthroses. Cystic change and osteoporosis are common features (Fig. 6.106). During childhood and adolescence, there may be periarticular overgrowth of bones possibly related to hyperemia.

Neuropathic Joints

Chronic trauma to a joint that lacks pain sensation may result in a neuropathic or Charcot joint (Fig. 6.107), the common causes of which are listed in Table 6.12. Diabetic neuropathic joints are more common in the

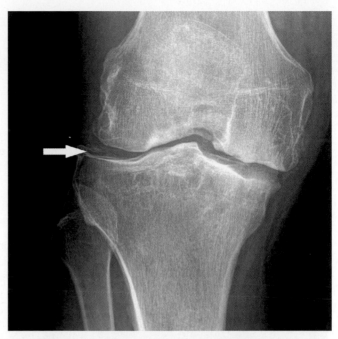

FIGURE 6.105. Calcium pyrophosphate deposition (CPPD) disease or pseudogout. Right knee AP radiograph. There are calcifications in the lateral meniscus (*single straight arrow*) and the medial meniscus.

lower extremity, whereas syringomyelia-related neuropathic joints usually occur in the shoulders and upper extremities. The radiographic findings include joint space narrowing, fragmentation of sclerotic subchondral

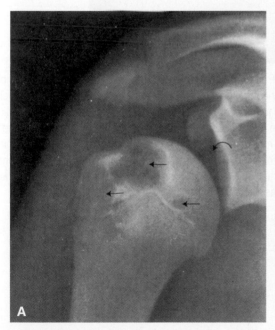
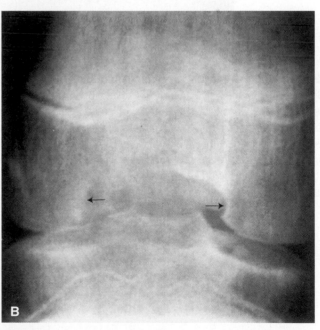

FIGURE 6.106. Hemophilia. A: Right shoulder AP radiograph with cystic changes (*straight arrows*) in the humeral head secondary to repeated bleeds and there is widening of the shoulder joint (*curved arrow*) due to hemarthrosis. **B:** Knee AP radiograph showing a widened intercondylar notch (*arrows*) secondary to repeated episodes of hemarthrosis. There is osteoporosis.

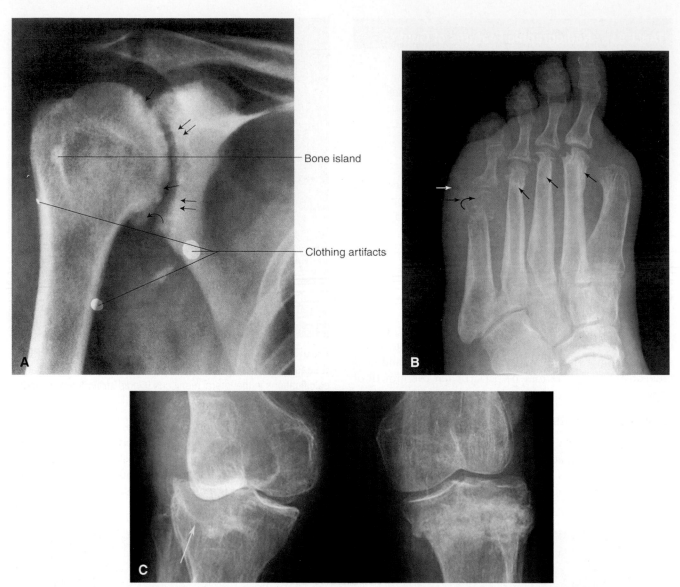

Bone island

Clothing artifacts

FIGURE 6.107. Neuropathic joint or Charcot joint. A: Right shoulder AP radiograph in a patient with **syringomyelia.** There is characteristic irregularity of the articular surfaces secondary to destruction of the bone and joint cartilage (*single arrows*). There are sclerotic changes or increased density (*double arrows*) of the bone surrounding the joint and an osteophyte (*curved arrow*). **B:** Oblique radiograph of neuropathic joints in the left foot of a **diabetic.** There are healed fracture deformities of the metatarsal heads (*arrows*). The great toe has been amputated because of infection. Note the destruction of the fifth metatarsal head (*curved arrow*) and adjacent ulcer (*white arrow*) from current osteomyelitis. **C:** Anterior views of the knees in a patient without specific trauma. There is a depressed fracture of the right tibial plateau (*arrow*). The left proximal tibial has a metaphyseal fracture with some sclerosis, which indicates there has been some healing and likely some persistent motion. The patient's mild pain was disproportionate to the appearance of the fractures.

TABLE 6.12 Causes of Neuropathic or Charcot Joints
Diabetes mellitus
Syringomyelia
Meningomyelocele
Peripheral nerve injury
Congenital indifference to pain

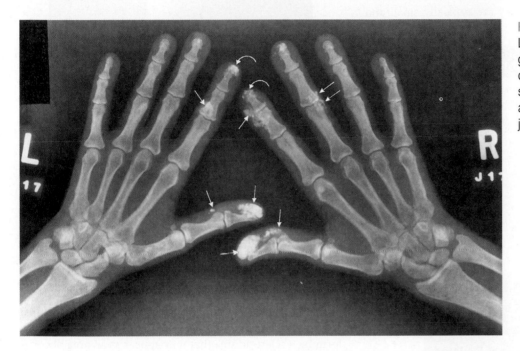

FIGURE 6.108. **Scleroderma.** Left- and right-hand PA radiograph showing soft tissue calcifications (*straight arrows*) and the soft tissues at the tip of the fingers are atrophic (*curved arrows*). The joints are normal.

bone, articular cortical destruction, joint loose bodies, and bone mass formation at the articular margins. Some of the neuropathic joint findings overlap those found in osteoarthritis. Arthralgia does not exclude a neuropathic joint; rather, the degree of pain is disproportionate to the amount of damage.

Other

Scleroderma is a connective tissue disorder characterized by multiple soft-tissue calcifications (Fig. 6.108), atrophy of the fingertips, and loss of bone at the tips of the distal phalanges (acro-osteolysis). Joint changes if present may resemble rheumatoid arthritis.

TUMORS

Key features in diagnosis of bone lesions include **skeletal maturity (have the epiphyses fused?), the number and location of lesions, the definition of lesion margins, and the presence of periosteal reaction.**

Radiography should be the initial test in a patient with a suspected bone lesion. If the lesion appears benign on radiography and is not an osteoid osteoma, no further imaging is usually required. One of the main challenges when evaluating bone tumors is to decide which ones do not require further workup such as biopsy. There are several **DO NOT TOUCH** benign lesions, all characterized by a well-defined or sclerotic margin, which is a key feature of benignity. If radiography is negative, or not consistent with the clinical findings, or indeterminate for malignancy with mineralized matrix or lytic or sclerotic features, then MRI should be performed. Other indications for MRI include lesions that are aggressive (poorly defined) in appearance and pathologic fractures. The aggressiveness of a lytic bony lesion is determined by the most aggressive part of the margin and is a sign that normal new bone formation cannot occur. CT is recommended if the radiographic or clinical pattern is suspicious for osteoid osteoma and CT is also preferred for evaluation of subtle cortical abnormalities and matrix mineralization. Tc-99m scanning may be helpful for assessing disease distribution but is typically negative in patients with myeloma.

Benign

Common benign bone lesions are listed in Table 6.13. A **bone island**, or enostosis, is the most common bone lesion. It is essentially cortical bone within the medullary cavity and appears as a small sclerotic focus. It blends with the surrounding trabeculae and has no aggressive features (Fig. 6.109). **Fibrous cortical defects (FCD) or nonossifying fibromas (NOFs)** may appear similar to an enostosis in adults but are more closely related to the cortex. These fibro-osseous lesions are lucent and may expand the cortex in children and adolescents. They are typically small and

TABLE 6.13 Common Benign Bone Lesions
Bone island
Nonossifying fibroma/fibrous cortical defect
Osteochondroma
Osteoid osteoma
Enchondroma
Bone cyst
Fibrous dysplasia
Chondroblastoma
Osteoblastoma
Hemangioma

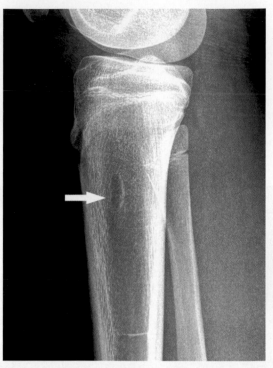

FIGURE 6.110. Fibrous cortical defect/nonossifying fibroma. The bony lesion has a sclerotic margin (*arrows*), is slightly lobulated, and arises from the cortex. This benign fibro-osseous lesion will eventually become sclerotic and appear as a focal area of cortical thickening when she is an adult.

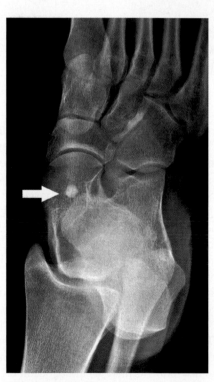

FIGURE 6.109. Bone island (*arrow*) (enostosis) in the calcaneus is a focus of mature compact (cortical) bone within the cancellous bone (spongiosa). Bone islands are usually ovoid or oblong with a spiculated contour that blends into the bone trabecula. They are benign and generally asymptomatic.

found incidentally, but may grow and cause a pathological fracture. FCDs and NOFs heal or involute with maturity, forming a sclerotic area that may appear as an area of cortical thickening (Fig. 6.110).

An **osteochondroma** or osteocartilaginous exostosis is bony projection of the cortex with a cartilage cap and is most commonly found in the metaphysis of long bones, especially around the knee and shoulder. These benign tumors can result in deformities and/or cause pressure on surrounding structures. The cartilaginous cap of osteochondromas may rarely (<1%) undergo malignant transformation to chondrosarcoma. Multiple osteochondromas are seen in multiple hereditary exostoses, a hereditary autosomal-dominant syndrome (Fig. 6.111). Growth abnormalities and malignant transformation (5%–15%) are more common in multiple osteochondromas than in a single osteochondroma. Features such as growth of an osteochondroma in a skeletally mature individual and the presence of pain may indicate malignant transformation.

A simple **bone cyst** (Fig. 6.112) is most commonly found in the metaphysis or metadiaphysis of the proximal humerus and femur in patients younger than 25 years and if large enough may cause a pathologic fracture.[5] A lucent bony lesion in an older adult is very unlikely to be a simple bone cyst. However, smaller subarticular lucencies in adults are likely degenerative cysts or, if large, termed geodes (Fig. 6.94).

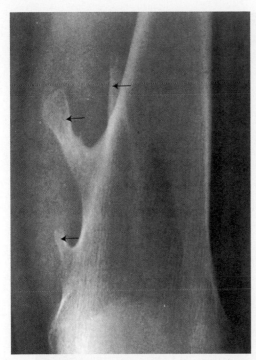

FIGURE 6.111. Multiple osteochondromas. Left femur AP radiograph. The osteochondromas (*arrows*) point away from the knee joint, simulating a coat hook.

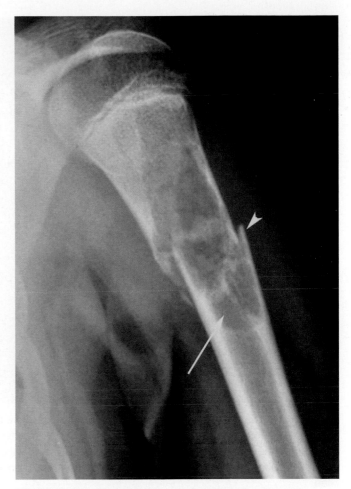

FIGURE 6.112. Benign cyst. Left shoulder AP radiograph with pathologic fracture through a benign bone cyst (*arrow*) in a 10-year-old child. There is mild lateral offset of the distal fracture fragment. Note the thinning of the bone cortex (*arrowhead*) caused by the expanding, benign cyst.

An **enchondroma** (Fig. 6.113) is a slow-growing cartilaginous tumor usually found in the hand phalanges and in the distal metacarpals. Small calcifications may be present within the lesions, and, occasionally, they may be difficult to differentiate from bone infarcts. **Bone infarcts** (osteonecrosis, AVN) (Fig. 6.114) are most frequent in long bones, may be asymptomatic, and typically have a well-defined and sclerotic border, whereas enchondromas are more likely to have central calcification.

Fibrous dysplasia is characterized by replacement of medullary bone by fibrous tissue in childhood. It can affect one bone (monostotic) or multiple bones (polyostotic). These lesions may be asymptomatic or present as a pathological fracture. The radiographic features include expansile radiolucency and cortical thinning.

Osteoid osteoma (Fig. 6.115) is a benign bone tumor typically presenting as pain worse a night, which is relieved by NSAIDs. They occur most commonly in the femoral neck and tibia. Most are cortical with sclerosis surrounding a small radiolucent center or nidus. In some instances, there may be calcifications within this lucent zone, mimicking a sequestrum of osteomyelitis.

Osteoid osteoma has intense activity on a radionuclide bone scan (Fig. 6.115B), whereas bone islands have none or very little activity. CT is usually diagnostic, demonstrating the classic nidus (Fig. 6.115C). MRI may also show the nidus but may be confusing because of the large amount of bone edema surrounding it (Fig. 6.115D). Treatment is either CT-guided radiofrequency ablation or surgical curettage of the nidus.

Chondroblastoma (Fig. 6.116) is an uncommon benign bone lesion found in the epiphysis, usually before skeletal maturity. These radiolucent lesions generally have sclerotic borders and sometimes contain scattered calcifications.

Giant cell tumors (GCTs) account for 5% of all primary bone tumors and occur in adults following skeletal maturity (Fig. 6.117). These lesions are eccentrically located in the end of long bones such as the tibia, femur, radius, and humerus where they are subarticular. The tumors usually have sharp, nonsclerotic, or ill-defined endosteal margins without periosteal reaction and may break through the cortex developing a soft tissue component. Approximately 15% of GCTs recur following simple curettage and packing and may require more aggressive surgery such as a wide margin of excision. Based on their radiographic appearance, it is difficult to determine whether they are benign or malignant. However, they are rarely (5%) malignant, and only

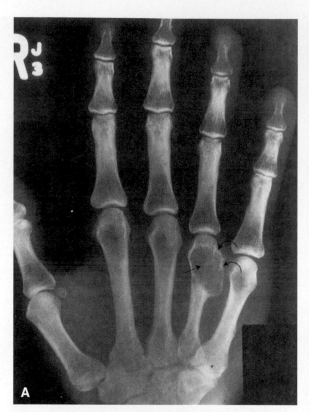

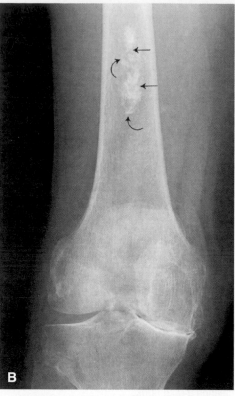

FIGURE 6.113. Enchondroma. A: Right-hand PA radiograph showing slow-growing tumor that typically causes thinning and scalloping (*curved arrows*) of the inner bone cortex of the distal fourth metacarpal (*straight arrow*). **B:** Right knee radiograph. In a large bone, scalloping of the cortex is less common. The calcification of cartilage often appears as small balls (*straight arrows*) or as arcs (*curved arrows*) and rings and occurs in the central part of the lesion. Note osteoarthritis affects predominantly the medial compartment of the knee.

FIGURE 6.114. Multiple bone infarcts. Bilateral knees AP radiographs. The multiple infarcts are manifested by thin zones of sclerosis surrounding lucencies (*straight arrows*) and marrow calcifications (*curved arrows*). The more peripheral calcification pattern helps distinguish infarcts from enchondromas. The etiology in this patient is unknown.

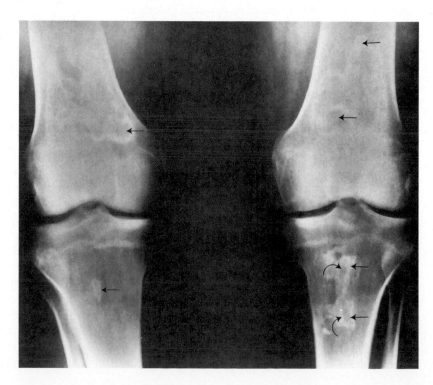

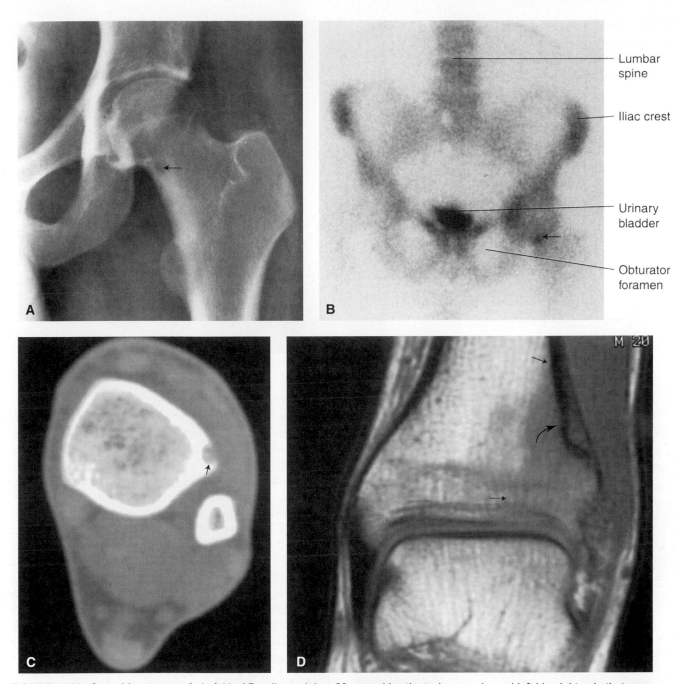

FIGURE 6.115. Osteoid osteoma. A: Left hip AP radiograph in a 20-year-old patient who experienced left hip night pain that was typically relieved by aspirin. The lucent zone (*arrow*) in the inferior aspect of the left femur subcapital region is the osteoid osteoma. **B:** Anterior pelvis radionuclide scan on the same patient. The single area of increased radionuclide uptake (*arrow*) in the left femoral neck corresponds to the radiolucent abnormality visualized in **(A)**. The bone scan is otherwise normal. Typically, the activity would be much greater, but is less in this patient since the lesion is within the joint. **C:** Axial CT distal tibia. Osteoid osteoma. The cortical lucent nidus (*arrow*) is nicely demonstrated by CT. Rarely, there is a central dot of calcification in the lucency. **D:** Coronal T1 MR in the same patient does not show the nidus as well as CT (*curved arrow*), but the large amount of edema (*gray*) is easy to see (*straight arrows*).

FIGURE 6.116. Benign chondroblastoma. Right shoulder AP radiograph showing the lesion in the proximal humerus epiphysis (*arrow*) of a 14-year-old patient. The typical sclerotic border is present (*curved arrows*).

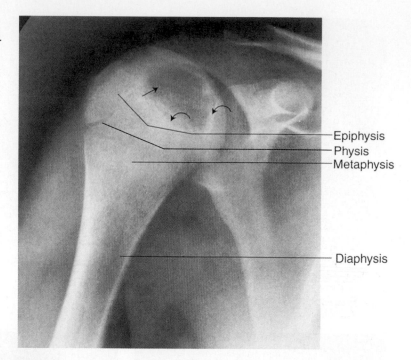

— Epiphysis
— Physis
— Metaphysis

— Diaphysis

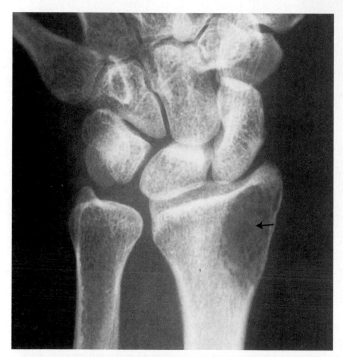

FIGURE 6.117. Giant cell tumor. Left wrist PA radiograph showing the classic appearance and common location of this tumor (*arrow*) in the distal radius.

distant metastases are considered a reliable radiographic finding to support malignancy.

Malignant

Bone metastases occur in up to 30% of patients with malignancy and are 20 times more common than primary bone tumors in adults. The most common primary tumors

with bone metastases are lung, breast, prostate, and kidney, which combined account for 80% of cases. Most bony metastases occur in red marrow (trunk, skull, and proximal humerus and femur) (Fig. 6.118). Radiographically, metastases have an ill-defined or wide zone of transition with little periosteal reaction. Moth-eaten and expansile lytic lesions also occur. The density of bone metastases varies widely, depending on the primary tumor (Table 6.14) and this density may change following chemotherapy or radiation. Bone scan and FDG PET are highly sensitive, compared with plain films with as many as one-third of metastases being demonstrated on either type of scan in the absence of any plain film abnormality. Although both bone scan and FDG PET are sensitive, they are relatively nonspecific and may show increased uptake in the presence of nonpathological fractures, arthritis, and infection. Bone biopsy is often required for confirmation of malignancy and tumor biomarker analysis.

Plasma Cell Tumors

Multiple myeloma originates from plasma cells in the bone marrow and is the most common primary malignant bone tumor in adults. This disease occurs in patients older than 40 years and the most common sites are the trunk and skull. The typical radiographic appearance of multiple myeloma (Fig. 6.119) consists of multiple osteolytic areas with a "punched-out" appearance, which may be indistinguishable from osteolytic metastatic disease. The lytic lesions of multiple myeloma tend to be more uniform in size than those of metastatic disease. Myeloma may also present as diffuse osteopenia. The solitary form of this tumor is a **plasmacytoma**, which is typically lytic and expansile (Fig. 6.120).

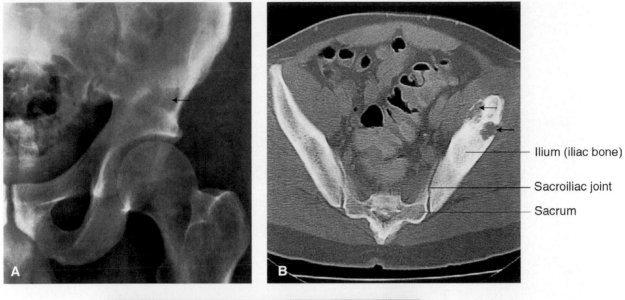

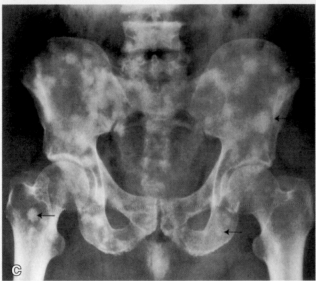

FIGURE 6.118. Bony metastases. A: Left hip AP radiograph. The radiolucent area in the left iliac bone (*arrow*) represents an osteolytic metastasis from carcinoma of the lung. **B:** CT image in the same patient. Two osteolytic metastases (*arrows*) in the left iliac bone. **C:** Pelvis AP radiograph. Osteoblastic metastases from carcinoma of the prostate. The *arrows* indicate multiple bilateral osteoblastic (*white*) metastatic lesions.

TABLE 6.14	Radiographic Appearance of Bone Metastases
Osteoblastic or Sclerotic	
Prostate	
Breast	
Carcinoid	
Neuroblastoma	
Mixed (lytic and blastic)	
Breast	
Cervix	
Bladder	
Osteolytic	
Nearly all neoplasms	

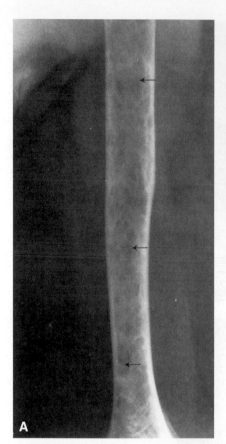

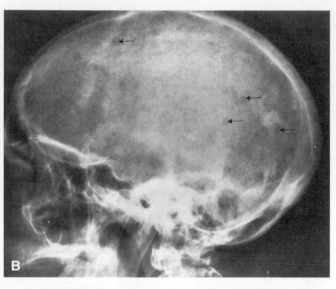

FIGURE 6.119. **Multiple myeloma.** Left humerus AP radiograph **(A)** and lateral skull radiograph **(B)**. The lucent or black areas indicated by the *arrows* represent the classic appearance of multiple myeloma in bone.

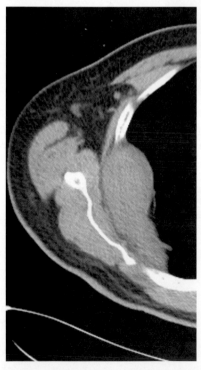

FIGURE 6.120. **Plasmacytoma.** CT shows a well-defined, grossly expansile rib lesion.

Ewing sarcoma is the most common primary malignant bone tumor in the first decade of life and in the second decade, it is second in frequency only to osteosarcoma (Fig. 6.121). The classic appearance is purely lytic with a permeative margin or a soft tissue mass with a periosteal reaction. It is usually diaphyseal or metadiaphyseal in location and occurs in the humerus, femur, and tibia in younger children and in the trunk in teens. Up to one-third of patients have systemic features which mimic infection, and up to 30% of patients have metastases to bone or lung at the time of diagnosis. Other causes of periosteal reaction in children include osteomyelitis, fracture, eosinophilic granuloma, neuroblastoma, and osteosarcoma. Because of its plasma cell origin, the soft tissue extension of Ewing sarcoma usually does not contain calcified tumor matrix, in contrast to the soft tissue extensions of osteosarcomas.

Osteogenic Tumors

Osteosarcoma is a primary malignant bone tumor occurring most commonly in the second decade of life but has a second peak in older adulthood. It is usually metaphyseal in location and most commonly occurs around the knee. These tumors are aggressive in appearance, having a wide zone of transition, and because it is a bone-forming tumor, it classically produces an abundance of

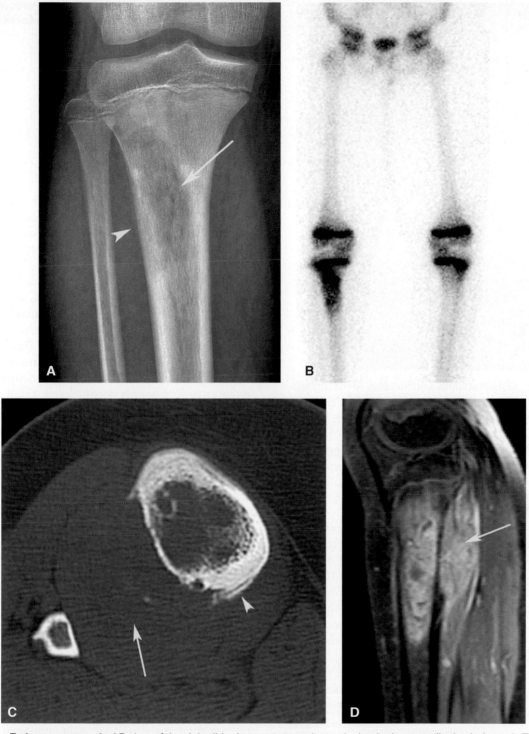

FIGURE 6.121. **Ewing sarcoma. A:** AP view of the right tibia demonstrates a lucent lesion in the metadiaphysis (*arrow*). There is subtle periosteal reaction laterally (*arrowhead*). Note the open physes. **B:** Anterior image from a radionuclide bone scan show normal increased activity of the growing physes and bladder (*black*), but abnormal increased activity in the right proximal tibia. **C:** Axial CT image through the lesion reveals that the normal marrow fat has been replaced by soft tissue density and some cortical thinning and destruction. There is periosteal reaction (*arrowhead*) and a large soft tissue mass (*arrow*). **D:** Sagittal fat-suppressed T1-weighted MRI was obtained after the injection of MR contrast. The tumor enhances both in the bone and soft tissue components (*arrow*).

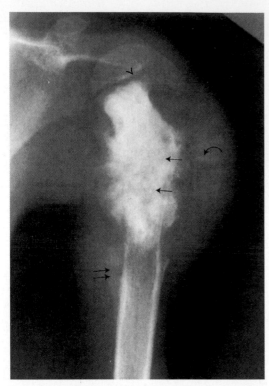

FIGURE 6.122. Osteosarcoma. Left humerus AP radiograph in a 6-year-old showing the lesion in metaphysis and diaphysis. The tumor (*single straight arrows*) has not crossed the physis (*arrowhead*). Codman triangle (*double straight arrows*) represents periosteal new bone formation reacting to the tumor growth, and the sunburst or ray appearance (*curved arrow*) represents tumor bone.

new, irregular bone with osteoid matrix (Fig. 6.122). An aggressive periosteal reaction (new bone formation in reaction to the growing tumor) in the form of a Codman triangle or sunburst pattern may also be seen. MRI allows superior imaging of the marrow and should be used to plan the biopsy as up to 10% of patients have skip lesions (metastases within the same bone). Distant metastases to the lung occur in up to 20% of patients and are the main source of relapse.

Differentiation of osteosarcomas from Ewing sarcoma may be difficult. In Ewing sarcoma, reactive bone formation is limited and does not extend into the soft tissue mass.

METABOLIC BONE DISEASES

Osteoporosis and Osteomalacia

Osteopenia is a generic term to describe reduced bone density due to reduced bone mineral density. **Osteoporosis** is defined as decreased bone mass with normal mineralization, whereas **osteomalacia** is a normal bone matrix (osteoid) with a reduced amount of mineralization. Osteoporosis

TABLE 6.15	Common Causes of Osteoporosis
Generalized	
Age-related	
Estrogen deficiency or postmenopausal	
Steroid or heparin therapy	
Hyperparathyroidism	
Malnutrition	
Local	
Disuse	

has become a major public health problem affecting over 10 million Americans (mostly women) and causing 2 million related fractures per year. Of those fractures, nearly 300,000 are hip fractures and roughly 700,000 are vertebral fractures. There are many causes of osteoporosis, the common ones of which are in Table 6.15. Multiple myeloma should be included in the differential diagnosis of diffuse osteopenia in adults. Radiographs are relatively insensitive for the evaluation of osteoporosis. Dual x-ray absorptiometry is currently the standard diagnostic method (Fig. 6.123) and is used to determine normal bone density versus osteopenia versus osteoporosis using the T-score, which compared the patient's values with those of a normal young adult.

Hyperparathyroidism is due to an excess of parathyroid hormone and may be primary (most commonly due to a parathyroid adenoma) or secondary, most commonly due to chronic renal disease. Subperiosteal resorption is the characteristic radiographic feature, most commonly found in the phalanges, distal clavicles, and SI joints (Fig. 6.124). Other radiographic features include a generalized increase in bone density and cystic lesions, which are sometimes expansile, termed brown tumors. Brown tumors occur in locations where bone loss is rapid and are a combination of hemosiderin and granulation tissue replacing the normal marrow. On MRI, they appear as cystic, solid, or combination of both.

Rickets

Rickets occurs in the growing portions of infant bones and is caused by poor calcification of the osteoid matrix that may result from vitamin D deficiency, renal disease, or intestinal malabsorption. The radiographic findings include widened and irregular physes, cupping of the metaphyses, bowing of the legs, and osteopenia (Fig. 6.125). Rickets only occurs in growing bone and is known as osteomalacia in adults.

Paget's Disease

Paget's disease is characterized by increased bone formation and occurs with increasing frequency from middle-age onward.

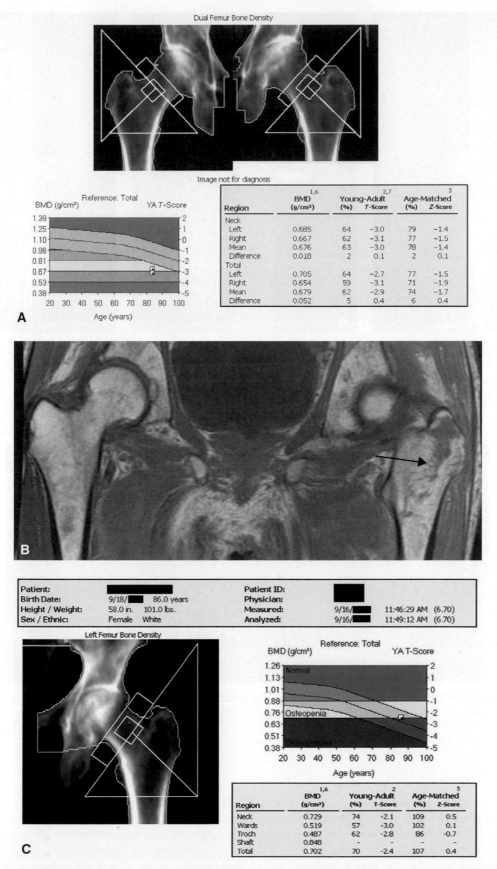

FIGURE 6.123. Osteoporosis. A: Dual X-ray absorptiometry (DEXA) scan of bone mineral density in the hips in an 83-year-old man. A T-score of −2.5 or less indicates osteoporosis. (The patient's score was −3 on the left and −3.1 of the right.) **B:** Coronal T1-weighted MRI of the hips obtained after a minor fall on the same patient demonstrates an incomplete intertrochanteric hip fracture (*arrow*). **C:** DEXA scan of the left hip in an 86-year-old woman. A T-score of −1.5 and −2.5 for the femoral neck indicates osteopenia. (This patient's score was −2.1.)

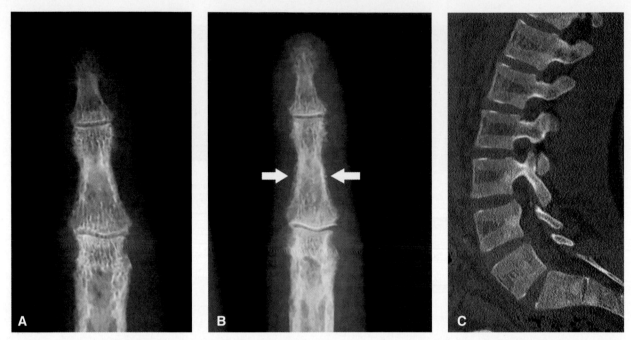

FIGURE 6.124. Hyperparathyroidism. A: Normal left index finger. **B:** Left index finger radiograph 1 year after a diagnosis of hyper-parathyroidism. Subperiosteal resorption is noted in the left index finger. **C:** Sagittal CT of lumbar spine showing transverse bands of vertebral body sclerosis, rugger jersey spine.

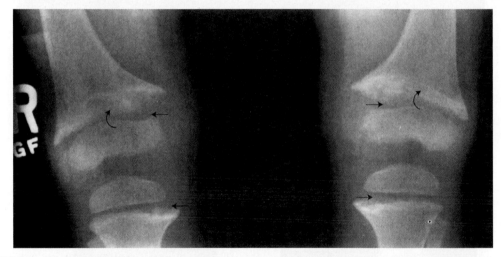

FIGURE 6.125. Rickets. Right and left knees AP radiographs. The physes are widened (*straight arrows*) and the metaphases are cupped (*curved arrows*).

The most commonly involved sites are the skull, trunk, and femur (Fig. 6.126). The radiographic features of Paget's disease are listed in Table 6.16. On radiographs, the bones are expanded, the cortices are thickened, and sclerotic and the trabecular pattern is thickened and prominent. Early in the disease, rarefaction, bone expansion, and bone destruction may occur. Deformities such as bowing of long bones and protrusio acetabuli develop as a result of bone softening. Complications include pathologic fractures and rarely sarcomatous degeneration. The differential diagnosis of Paget's disease includes osteoblastic metastatic disease, fibrous dysplasia, lymphoma, and osteosclerosis.

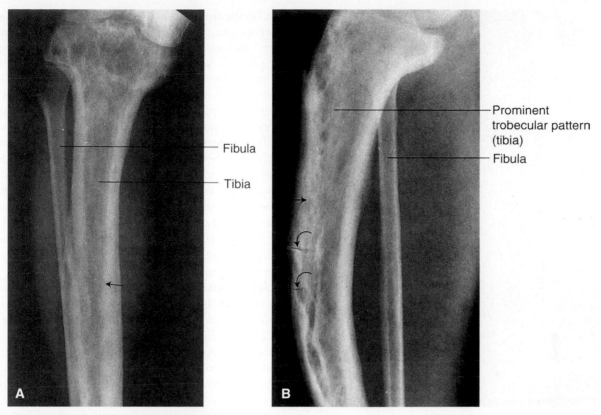

FIGURE 6.126. **Paget's disease.** Right tibia and fibula AP **(A)** and lateral **(B)** radiographs. The tibia cortices are sclerotic in appearance (*straight arrows*) because of widening and thickening of the cortices and a prominent trabecular pattern. The tibia is bowed anterolaterally. The fibula is spared. The typical transverse pathologic fractures are best visualized on the lateral radiograph (*curved arrows*), and they are the most common complication of this disease.

TABLE 6.16	Radiographic Features of Paget's Disease

Thick and sclerotic bone cortices with enlarged bone
Thick and prominent trabecular pattern
Long bone bowing
Acetabular protrusio
Pathologic fractures
Focal lucent area in the skull (osteoporosis circumscripta)

INFECTION

Osteomyelitis (infection of bone/bone marrow) can occur in all age groups and the classic clinical presentation is bone or joint pain and fever. Causes of osteomyelitis include local spread of infection from adjacent soft tissue, direct inoculation following trauma, and seeding during bacteremia (the predominant route in children). Unlike tumors, acute osteomyelitis is a more rapidly destructive process and may have gas in the soft tissues. The radiographic appearances are variable and may be normal. In adults, particularly diabetics, the risk of foot osteomyelitis is higher in the presence of a skin ulcer extending to the bone. However, barring an adjacent skin ulcer, the radiographic appearance of osteomyelitis can be identical to a bone tumor with a wide zone of transition marking it aggressive appearance with bone and joint destruction, periosteal reaction, and a soft tissue component (Fig. 6.127). Three-phase bone scanning will show increased uptake in all three phases compared with cellulitis.

Currently, MRI with contrast is the most sensitive and specific technique as it detects marrow edema, and enhancement with contrast is a very useful tool for the demonstration of bone and soft tissue involvement by infection. Typically, osteomyelitis appears as decreased signal on T1WI and increased signal on T2-weighted and short tau inversion recovery (STIR). MRI also allows evaluation of soft tissue involvement by infection. However, it can be a confusing picture in a diabetic foot, which may have additional abnormalities such as fractures and neuropathic changes (Fig. 6.128). Plain films and MRI are complementary, and both are indicated in diabetics with suspected osteomyelitis of the foot.

In **infants**, the metaphyseal vessels traverse the physis, and infections may involve the metaphysis, epiphysis, and joint resulting in a growth deformity. Osteomyelitis in **children** is usually confined to the metaphyseal regions of bones where the normal arterial supply does not traverse the fused physis (Figs. 6.129 and 6.130). However, in adults the metaphyseal and epiphyseal vessel anastomose across the physis remnant, increasing the risk of septic arthritis.

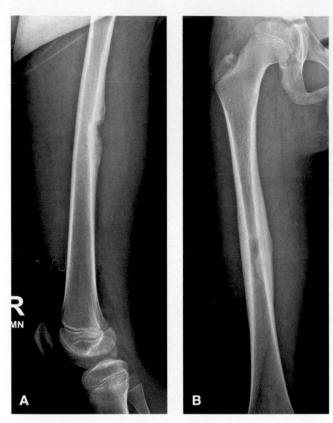

FIGURE 6.127. Osteomyelitis. A and B: AP and lateral views of femur showing sclerosis, lucency, and periosteal reaction in the mid shaft.

Chronic osteomyelitis is defined as infection longer than 6 weeks and results if infection is inadequately treated or refractory to therapy. There is a wide range of radiographic appearances including thickened cortex and a combination of lucency and sclerosis. Confirmatory imaging with MR depicting soft-tissue and marrow edema, as well as alterations in tissue perfusion or CT, is recommended as infection with aggressive features may be misdiagnosed as malignancy (Fig. 6.82). A **sequestrum** of necrotic bone, which appears relatively dense because of its lack of blood supply, may develop, followed by an **involucrum** (shell of bone surrounding a sequestrum) and a **cloaca**, which is a bony defect through which pus drains. Osteomyelitis can also occur at a prior fracture, where one may ascribe the changes to the fracture fragments. It is important to remember that when a fracture heals, the bone density should return to normal; persistent sclerosis is suggestive of chronic osteomyelitis.

Septic arthritis: Prompt diagnosis and treatment are essential in patients with septic arthritis as cartilage destruction can ensue rapidly, resulting in osseous erosions, osteomyelitis, and ankylosis. Synovial thickening and enhancement, joint effusion, and inflammatory change in the juxta-articular tissue are the typical imaging findings, although effusion can be absent in up to one-third of adult patients with septic arthritis. In children, a hip effusion may be more reliably detected on ultrasound than on plain films. Joint aspiration is recommended either under fluoroscopic or US guidance for needle placement.

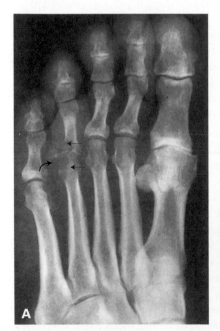

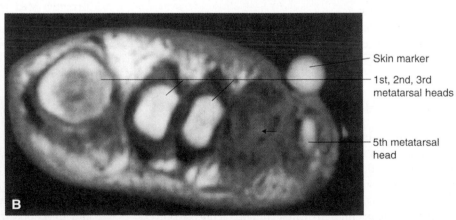

Skin marker

1st, 2nd, 3rd metatarsal heads

5th metatarsal head

FIGURE 6.128. Osteomyelitis. A: Left foot AP radiograph in a patient with diabetes mellitus. There are destructive changes (*straight arrows*) involving the base of the proximal phalanx of the fourth toe as well as the fourth metatarsal head. Also, there are destructive changes in the fourth metatarsophalangeal joint manifested by narrowing of the joint space. The infection has characteristically caused destructive joint changes as well as bone destruction on both sides of the joint. Loose bone fragments have resulted from the osteomyelitis (*curved arrow*). **B:** Left foot axial T1 MRI in the same patient. When compared with the other metatarsal heads, the fourth metatarsal head is not visible because the infection (*arrow*) has destroyed and replaced the bone marrow.

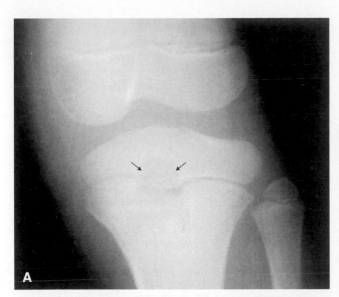
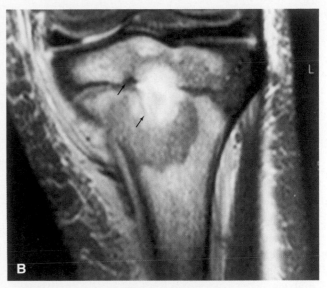

FIGURE 6.129. **Osteomyelitis. A:** AP radiograph of the left knee in a child. Focal lucency is noted in the epiphysis (*arrows*). **B:** Coronal fat-suppressed T2 MR in the same patient shows the abscess crosses the physis and involves the metaphysis as well (*arrows*).

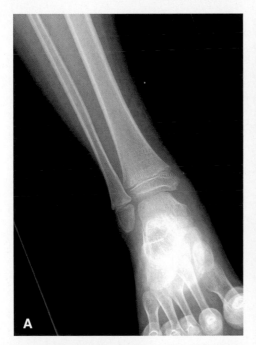
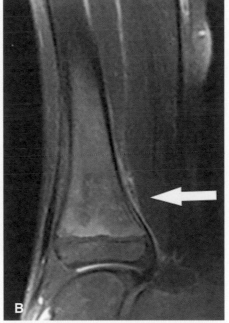

FIGURE 6.130. **Osteomyelitis. A:** AP radiograph of the right tibia was reported as normal. **B:** Increase in signal on T2 (*white arrow*) and cavity formation in the metaphysis consistent with acute osteomyelitis.

KEY POINTS

- Sesamoids are bones within a tendon or volar plate. Ossicles are extra or supernumerary bones next to the skeleton and usually named after the neighboring bone.
- Because fractures and other abnormalities may not be visualized on all radiographic views, always insist on at least two views of an injured or diseased area that are orthogonal to each other.

- Fractures may not be visible on the first radiographs but may become visible after time (7 days) because of bone resorption at the ends of the fracture fragments.
- MRI is useful for injuries to soft tissue structures such as the shoulder rotator cuff, knee ligaments and menisci, ankle ligaments, and Achilles tendon. CT imaging is good for bone detail, fracture diagnosis, locating fracture fragments, and evaluating matrix formation in bone tumors.

- The Salter–Harris classification describes fractures around the physis, which is considered the weakest point in a growing bone.
- Osteoarthritis is the most common form of arthritis and often results from asymmetric cartilage wear. The radiographic features of osteoarthritis include irregular joint narrowing, subchondral sclerosis and/or cyst formation, and osteophyte formation.
- The radiographic features of rheumatoid arthritis include periarticular soft tissue thickening, symmetric joint narrowing, marginal erosions, periarticular osteoporosis, and joint deformity.
- Metastatic cancer is the most common malignant bone tumor in adults. The most common cancers that have bone metastases are lung, breast, and prostate cancers.
- Multiple myeloma is the most common primary malignant bone tumor in adults, and it originates in the bone marrow.
- Ewing sarcoma usually occurs in children and young adults and typically has a permeative appearance and an onionskin-like periosteal reaction.

- Osteomyelitis and septic joints typically present with localized pain and fever. The radiographic features include bone and joint destruction, periosteal reaction, and occasionally, a soft tissue component.

Further Reading

1. Helms CA. *Fundamentals of Skeletal Radiology.* 5th ed. Saunders; 2019.

References

1. Jarraya M, Hayashi D, Roemer FW, et al. Radiographically occult and subtle fractures: a pictorial review. *Radiol Res Pract.* 2013;2013. doi:10.1155/2013/370169.
2. Stiell IG, McKnight RD, Greenberg GH, et al. Implementation of the Ottawa ankle rules. *JAMA.* 1994;271:827-832.
3. Stiell IG, Wells GA, Hoag RH, et al. Implementation of the Ottawa knee rule for the use of radiography in acute knee injuries. *JAMA.* 1997;278:2075-2079.
4. Marshall RA, Mandell JC, Weaver MJ, Ferrone M, Sodickson A, Khurana B. Imaging features and management of stress, atypical, and pathologic fractures. *Radiographics.* 2018;38:2173-2192.
5. Ha AS, Porrino JA, Chew FS. Radiographic pitfalls in lower extremity trauma. *Am J Roentgenol.* 2014;203:492-500.doi:10.2214/AJR.14.12626.

Questions

1. The second digit of the hand, when starting on the radial side is properly called
   a. Ring finger
   b. Index finger
   c. Long finger
   d. Second finger

2. Bones form by
   a. Endochondral bone formation
   b. Intramembranous bone formation
   c. Periossification bone formation
   d. a and b
   e. a and c

3. A small bone just lateral to the lateral epicondyle of the humerus in an 8-year-old is likely
   a. An apophysis
   b. An epiphysis
   c. A fracture
   d. A normal variant

4. In a child, a fracture line extending through the physis into the epiphysis is a Salter–Harris
   a. I
   b. II
   c. III
   d. IV
   e. V

5. Which finding is most common with a shoulder dislocation?
   a. Anterior location
   b. Greater tuberosity fracture
   c. Posterior location
   d. Glenoid fracture

6. The most appropriate imaging modality to better evaluate a calcaneal fracture is
   a. Ultrasound
   b. CT
   c. MR
   d. Bone scan

7. An elderly patient with a fall and hip pain has a fracture on radiograph. The next course of action is to
   a. Get an MR imaging study
   b. Obtain a CT scan to evaluate the fracture
   c. Call an orthopedic surgeon
   d. Order a bone scan

8. The best study to look at all the internal structures of the knee would be
   a. Radiograph
   b. Ultrasound
   c. Computed tomography
   d. Magnetic resonance imaging

9. Periarticular osteoporosis, marginal erosions, and morning stiffness best describe
   a. Osteoarthritis
   b. Gout
   c. Rheumatoid arthritis
   d. Septic arthritis

10. Which of the following is a malignant bone tumor?
    a. Osteoid osteoma
    b. Multiple myeloma
    c. Enostosis
    d. Osteochondroma

Brain Imaging

Bojan Petrovic, MD

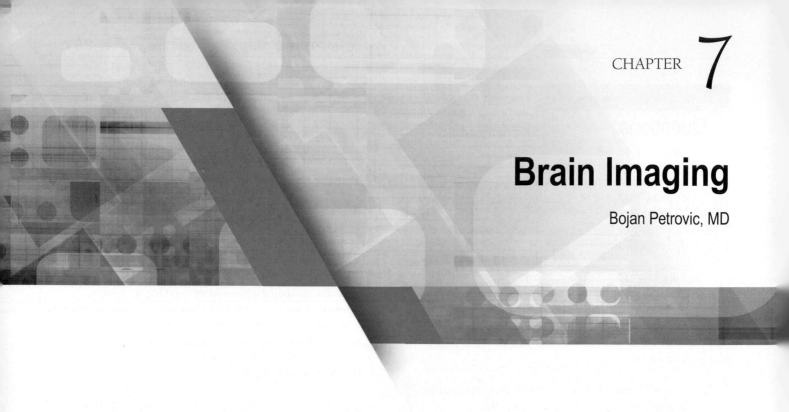

The use of computed tomography (CT) and magnetic resonance imaging (MRI) has revolutionized the subspecialty of neuroradiology, making these modalities central to the care of patients with neurologic conditions. The objectives of this chapter are to introduce the reader to common applications of brain imaging, to help the reader understand appropriate imaging modalities for various conditions, and to clarify when IV contrast is appropriate.

CT AND MRI

Multidetector **CT** data acquisition is usually performed in the axial (strictly helical) plane and allows near-isotropic voxel acquisition for generation of high-quality two-dimensional multiplanar and three-dimensional (3D) reformatted images.

The images can then be reviewed in the axial plane or the image data can be reconstructed for viewing in other planes (typically coronal and/or sagittal). Postprocessing with image reconstruction algorithms allow review of the images with a soft-tissue algorithm (optimal for evaluating the brain) or a bone algorithm (to optimize assessment of the calvarium and skull base). Additionally, the images can be windowed during review to adjust image contrast, which is helpful to diagnose pathology such as hemorrhage or stroke.

One of CT's major limitations is its lack of soft-tissue contrast resolution. If two different types of soft tissue adjacent to one another have a similar density, they will absorb roughly the same number of photons and appear almost identical on CT. In addition, artifact due to bone or other high-density items such as aneurysm clips can degrade the examination. For example, images through portions of the posterior fossa and inferior aspects of the middle cranial fossae are frequently degraded by bone artifact on CT, limiting the detection of subtle abnormalities in the posterior fossa, particularly within the brainstem.

Unlike CT of the brain, which is typically only a single image acquisition (unless pre- and postcontrast studies are obtained), **MRI** of the brain consists of multiple image acquisitions, each obtained with different parameters or "pulse sequences" designed to highlight different parts of

the brain or detect different diseases (Table 7.1). For example, normal brain anatomy is well depicted on T1-weighted images, while susceptibility-weighted images are used for detecting hemorrhage, and diffusion-weighted imaging (DWI) is invaluable for detection of acute infarcts. A head CT may be acquired in less than a minute, but each pulse sequence for an MR examination may take several minutes making the overall scan time relatively longer than CT.

MRI has superior soft-tissue contrast resolution to CT, which makes it more sensitive for imaging early infarcts, subtle tumors, or demyelinating lesions. By selecting appropriate pulse sequences the MRI scan can be customized to answer a clinical question. For example, a fat-suppressed T1-weighted sequence could be added in evaluation of a lesion that appears bright on a T1-weighted image because loss of signal on the fat-suppressed sequence would indicate that the lesion contains fat rather than proteinaceous or hemorrhagic contents. Limitations of MRI include susceptibility to artifacts of metal (e.g., aneurysm clips), cerebrospinal fluid (CSF) or vascular pulsation artifacts, motion artifact (especially in patients unable to tolerate lengthy examinations), as well as either contraindications or restrictions on imaging in patients with pacemakers/implanted defibrillator or metallic foreign bodies.

Because each modality has its advantages and disadvantages, the choice will depend on the clinical indication and question to be answered.

CONTRAST AGENTS

Intravenous contrast, iodinated contrast and gadolinium chelate, can greatly improve detection of disease on CT and MRI, respectively, most commonly when there is clinical concern for infection, tumor, or a vascular abnormality. Reviewing the American College of Radiology's Appropriateness Criteria can be quite helpful to aid in selection of the appropriate imaging examination for a clinical indication as well as whether contrast is indicated. However, if in doubt, radiologists are always available for consultation in individual cases. Administration of contrast material should only be performed after review of the patient's renal function and any contrast allergies.

The blood–brain barrier is a selectively permeable barrier separating blood from extracellular fluid of the brain and spinal cord. It is composed of endothelial cells of the capillaries and astrocytes, the combination of which allows passive diffusion of water- and lipid-soluble molecules as well as the active transport of molecules crucial to neural functions such as glucose and amino acids. The blood–brain barrier normally prevents movement of large molecules such as iodinated contrast and gadolinium chelates into the CNS. Disruption of the blood–brain barrier that occurs in tumor, infection, inflammation, infarction, etc. allows contrast into the CNS, resulting in contrast enhancement, which is abnormal.

TABLE 7.1	Summary of Use and Features of MRI Sequences	
Sequence	**Utility**	**Features**
T1	Good for normal anatomy	White matter is bright. Fat, subacute blood also bright.
T2	Fluid-sensitive sequence	Many types of CNS pathology are bright.
FLAIR	Fluid-sensitive sequence with suppression of CSF signal	Many types of CNS pathology are bright.
STIR or fat-suppressed T2	Fat-suppressed fluid-sensitive sequence	Useful when assessing for marrow signal abnormality. Many types of marrow pathology are bright.
Gradient echo sequence	Sensitive to calcium, iron, blood degradation products	Hemorrhage, calcifications appear dark.
SWI (susceptibility-weighted imaging)	Exceptionally sensitive to calcium, iron, blood degradation products	Hemorrhage, calcifications appear dark.
DWI (diffusion-weighted imaging)	Useful in evaluating pathology with restricted diffusion such as acute infarcts, pyogenic abscess, very cellular tumors	Restricted diffusion appears bright.

CNS, central nervous system; CSF, cerebrospinal fluid.

NORMAL ANATOMY

Normal anatomy is presented in Figures 7.1 and 7.2. Key features to note are size of the ventricles, position of the midline structures, gray matter–white matter differentiation, density, symmetry of the brain parenchyma, and abnormal density outside the brain. On CT, denser tissue (such as bone) is displayed in brighter shades, whereas low-density areas such as air in the sinuses or fat appear dark.

On MRI, CSF is dark on T1-WI, and on T2-WI it is bright. Figure 7.3 shows structures that are calcified and should not be mistaken for hemorrhage in a noncontrast CT scan.

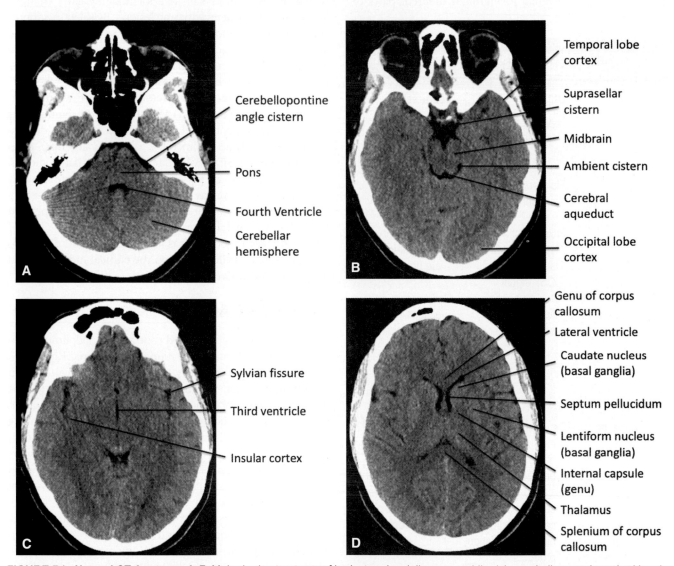

FIGURE 7.1. Normal CT Anatomy. A-F: Major brain structures of brainstem (medulla, pons, midbrain), cerebellum, and cerebral hemispheres (frontal, temporal, parietal, and occipital lobes). Note how the cerebrospinal fluid–filled spaces (suprasellar cistern, ventricles, sylvian fissure, sulcus) are low density (black). Also note that the gray matter structures (cortex, basal ganglia, thalamus) are relatively denser (appearing brighter on CT) than the lower-density white matter (e.g., subcortical white matter, centrum semiovale, internal capsule, corpus callosum).

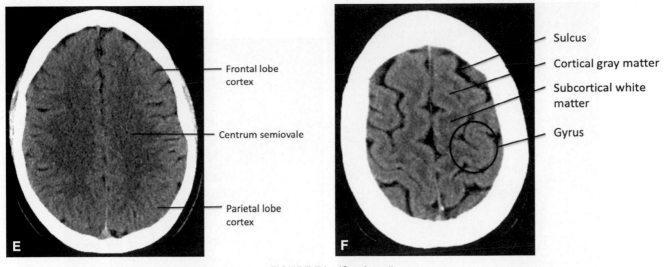

- Frontal lobe cortex
- Centrum semiovale
- Parietal lobe cortex

- Sulcus
- Cortical gray matter
- Subcortical white matter
- Gyrus

FIGURE 7.1. *(Continued)*

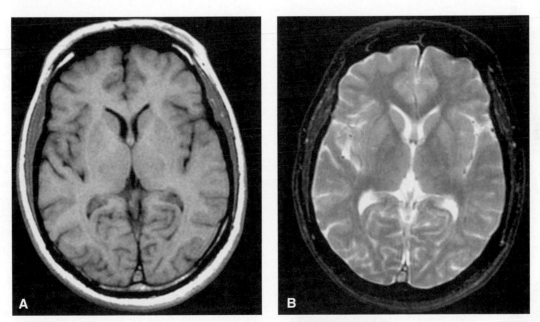

FIGURE 7.2. Normal MR Anatomy. Axial T1-weighted **(A)** and T2-weighted **(B)** MR images at the level of the foramen of Monro. On T1-weighted images, the cerebrospinal fluid in the ventricles is black and on T2-weighted images it is white. Notice the superb anatomic detail, much better than CT.

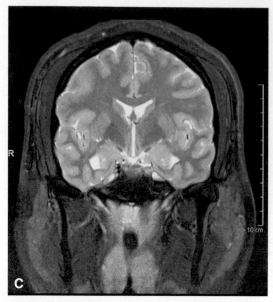

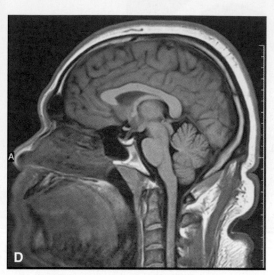

FIGURE 7.2. *(Continued)* **C:** Coronal T2-weighted image at the level of the Foramen of Monro in the same patient. The anatomical definition rivals that of a brain section in the neuroanatomy laboratory. **D:** Sagittal midline T1-weighted image of the same patient. The midline structures, face and foramen magnum, are seen in fine detail. Note how well you see the cerebellum and brainstem without the beam hardening artifacts of CT.

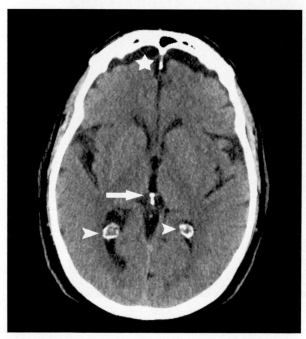

FIGURE 7.3. Normal variant. Intracranial calcification. Choroid plexus (*arrowheads*), pineal gland (*arrow*), and anteriorly the falx cerebri (*star*).

HEADACHE

The yield of CT and MR in patients referred with isolated, nontraumatic headache is low, with a 0.4% incidence of potentially treatable lesions, so imaging for chronic headache and normal neurological examination is rarely indicated.

Neuroimaging is more likely to be positive in populations at risk including pregnant patients, immunocompromised individuals, cancer patients, and patients with papilledema or systemic illnesses, including hypercoagulable disorders.

ALTERED MENTAL STATUS

Altered mental status (AMS) is not a diagnosis, rather a generic term for a wide range of symptoms of acute or chronic disordered mentation including confusion, drowsiness, disorientation, lethargy, somnolence, encephalopathy, unresponsiveness, and coma. The prompt diagnosis of acute intracranial pathology in patients with AMS is critical to guide appropriate management and ensure a positive outcome. An noncontrast CT (NCCT) of the head, which can be performed safely and rapidly, is the test of choice to exclude acute intracranial hemorrhage (ICH), infarct, brain mass, hydrocephalus, or mass effect. The use of IV contrast during head CT should be considered if infection, tumor, or inflammation is suspected, but more commonly NCCT of the head is followed by MRI of the brain with and without contrast because of its greater sensitivity for detecting ischemia, encephalitis, or subtle hemorrhage. MRI is also the test of choice in the evaluation of suspected multiple sclerosis, vasculitis, or neuropsychiatric systemic lupus erythematosus.

TRAUMA

Traumatic brain injury (TBI) is the leading cause of disability and death in children and young adults in the United States. The widespread availability and rapid examination time make CT an ideal modality for evaluating head trauma. Three major sets of criteria or guidelines have been independently developed to predict which patients with minor or mild acute closed head injury do not require a head CT. While the New Orleans Criteria (NOC), Canadian CT Head Rules (CCHR), and National Emergency X-Ray Utilization Study (NEXUS)-II each have a high sensitivity, there are trade-offs with a lower specificity for the detection of significant findings. Imaging may not be indicated in patients with a minor or mild acute closed head injury who score 13 or higher on the Glasgow Coma Scale (GCS). However, imaging, usually a NCCT, is indicated in patients with a moderate or severe acute closed head injury (GCS <13). NCCT or MRI is also indicated if there is neurologic deterioration, delayed recovery, or persistent unexplained deficits after acute TBI or new cognitive and/or neurologic deficit following subacute or chronic TBI. NCCT of the maxillofacial or temporal bone is recommended for suspected CSF rhinorrhea. **Penetrating head injury** should be investigated by NCCT followed by CT angiogram of the head and neck to include the aortic arch if there is an expanding neck hematoma.

Contusion is a cortical (gray matter) bruise frequently associated with small amounts of hemorrhage. Typically, it occurs at the point of contact of injury. Contusions may also occur at the diametrically opposite location of the brain and along the falx and tentorium. On CT, contusions appear as high density with adjacent low density representing edema (Fig. 7.4). On MRI, T2-WI of acute contusions show low signal in the hemorrhagic component of the contusion with surrounding high T2 signal edema. Contusions can show restricted diffusion in areas of hemorrhage or cell death (Fig. 7.5). Gradient echo or susceptibility-weighted images are more sensitive for detecting hemorrhage. **Diffuse axonal injury (DAI)** results from severe rotational acceleration/deceleration head movement that shears axons. Sites of maximum shear strain include

splenium and body of the corpus callosum, the gray matter/white matter junction, and the brainstem. DAI in most patients with significant closed head injury is associated with a poor prognosis. MR is more sensitive than CT in the diagnosis of DAI. On MRI, nonhemorrhagic DAI is seen as foci of T2/FLAIR hyperintensity. Hemorrhagic DAI is best detected as low signal foci on gradient echo or SWI sequences. DAI can also result in restricted diffusion (Fig. 7.6).

Head CT should be evaluated for contusion, intracranial mass effect, ventricular size and configuration, bone injuries, and acute hemorrhage in the parenchymal, subarachnoid, subdural, or epidural spaces. Additional coronal or sagittal multiplanar reformats are useful in diagnosing hemorrhage adjacent to bone. While CT is more sensitive than MRI in detecting bony injuries, MRI is more sensitive than CT in detecting all stages of hemorrhage, contusions, and DAI in the posterior fossa and brainstem. Skull radiography has limited use in head trauma such as the detection of radiopaque foreign bodies.

Acute intracranial hemorrhage is usually seen as increased density on CT but may be isodense if the patient is anemic (Fig. 7.7). Acute hemorrhage, less than 12 hours, is low intensity on T2-weighted images and isodense on T1. Subacute hematomas are usually high intensity on T1-weighted images. Once hemorrhage is identified, it is important to determine if it is **intra-axial** (within the substance of the brain itself), or **extra-axial** (outside the brain, but within the skull). The shape and distribution of extra-axial hematomas can be a clue to their location.

Epidural hematomas (interposed between the calvarium and the dura) usually appear as a lentiform mass or mass with convex margins on both sides (biconvex) (Fig. 7.8). Fractures of the temporal bone crossing the middle meningeal artery or less commonly middle meningeal vein are responsible for most epidural hematomas. In contrast, **subdural hematomas**, which are deep to the dura but

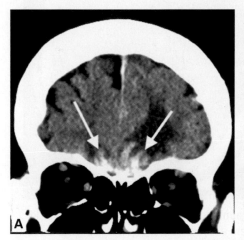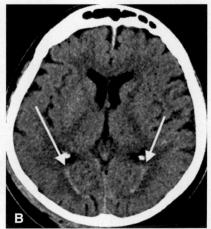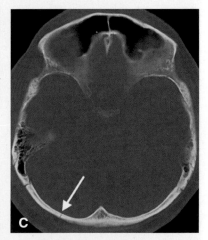

FIGURE 7.4. Skull fracture, intraventricular hemorrhage, and hemorrhagic contusions in the inferior frontal lobes. A: *Arrows* indicate small areas of parenchymal hemorrhage in the bilateral inferior frontal lobes. Note the presence of low-density edema in the frontal lobes adjacent to the areas of parenchymal hemorrhage. **B:** *Arrows* indicate small areas of high-density hemorrhage layering in the occipital horns of the lateral ventricles. **C:** *Arrow* indicates nondisplaced skull fracture opposite to the site of parenchymal hemorrhage in the inferior frontal lobes.

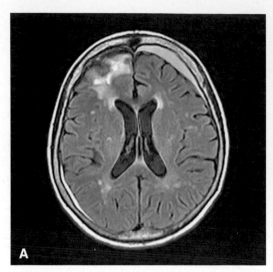
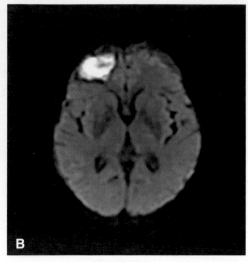

FIGURE 7.5. **Cerebral contusion.** Axial FLAIR **(A)** and DWI **(B)** images showing contusion in the right frontal lobe. A small subdural hematoma overlies the left frontal lobe as well as the right parieto-occipital region.

superficial to the arachnoid membranes, characteristically have a crescent shape and maintain a concave medial margin, which is somewhat parallel to the surface of the skull (Fig. 7.9). They are caused by shearing of the bridging veins between the pia-arachnoid and the dura. In the elderly, subdural hematomas may be larger at diagnosis because age-related parenchymal volume loss can permit accumulation of a larger volume of hemorrhage prior to development of mass effect. Subacute subdural hematomas are usually isodense to low density and may simulate the shape of an epidural hematoma. The presence of high density within a subacute subdural hematoma may indicate rebleeding. Chronic subdural hematomas are typically low density and may have only a minor history of head trauma in adults. In infants, chronic subdural hematomas are a feature of nonaccidental injury (Fig. 7.10).

Subarachnoid hemorrhage (SAH) occurs between the arachnoid membrane and the brain and diffuses into the

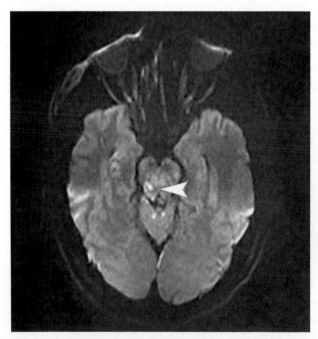

FIGURE 7.6. **Diffuse axonal injury (DAI).** DWI showing a hyperintensity in the right brainstem (*arrowhead*) consistent with DAI.

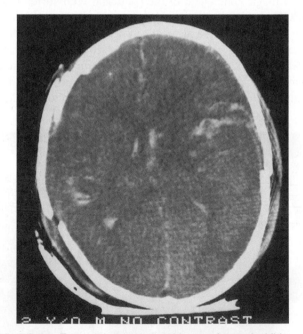

FIGURE 7.7. **Traumatic intracranial hemorrhage.** A child injured in a severe auto accident shows multiple white areas in the brain as well as disruption of the skull. The white areas are areas of intracranial hemorrhage in the parenchyma, ventricles, and extra-axial spaces. Also note the disruption of the normal brain architecture, reflecting the severe cerebral edema.

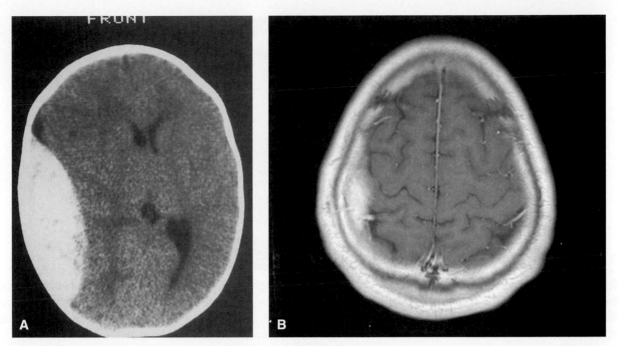

FIGURE 7.8. Epidural hematoma. A: CT shows a biconvex hyperdense mass characteristic of an epidural hematoma. Note shift of midline structures. **B:** MRI shows a small right parietal epidural hematoma.

sulci and filling the CSF cisterns surrounding the brain (Fig. 7.11). **Intra-axial** bleeding occurs within the brain parenchyma, may cause edema, and appear as a low density, often ring-like area, about the hematoma (Fig. 7.4).

Intraventricular hemorrhage appears as a high density within the normally low-density ventricles. If large enough, intraventricular hemorrhage may expand the ventricles. Typically, some component of intraventricular hemorrhage

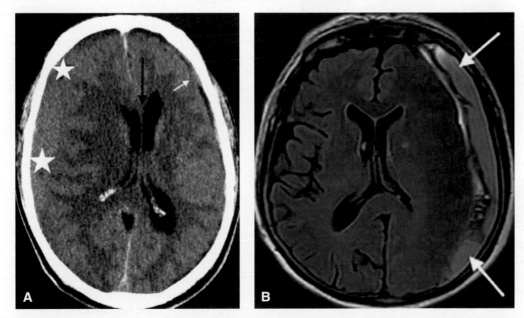

FIGURE 7.9. Subdural hematoma. A: Axial CT showing bilateral subdural hematomas. The right subdural hematoma is the same density as the cerebral cortex, a feature that can make a subdural difficult to identify if it is small. There is mass effect with effacement of cerebral hemispheric sulci and partial effacement of the right lateral ventricle. Note presence of right to left midline shift with the black *arrow* indicating the septum pellucidum, which has been displaced to the left of midline. *Arrow* indicates the high-density component of a mixed density subdural hematoma overlying the left frontal lobe. **B:** Different patient MRI FLAIR showing a left parietal subdural hematoma.

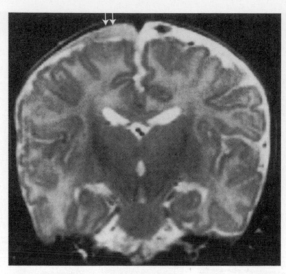

FIGURE 7.10. Subdural hematoma, nonaccidental injury. Coronal T2-weighted MRI of the brain shown to illustrate that MRI is also effective in showing trauma. This is an abused child who has a subdural space hematoma (*arrows*). Note that the surface is concave, reflecting the contour of the cerebral cortex, but not extending among the gyri. This configuration is typical for a subdural hematoma. Also note that the signal densities are different on MRI. Imaging of bleeding is more complex on MRI than by CT.

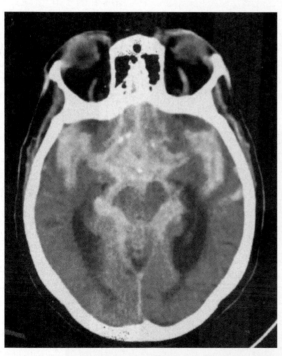

FIGURE 7.11. Subarachnoid hemorrhage. CT scan at the level of the suprasellar and ambient cisterns shows that the normally low density (black) basal cisterns have been filled with high density (white) material consistent with subarachnoid hemorrhage.

TABLE 7.2	**Characteristics of Intracranial Blood by Imaging**		
Time of Bleed	**CT**	**T1-weighted MRI**	**T2-weighted MRI**
Immediate	White (high density)	Gray (intermediate to slightly low signal)	White (high signal)
Acute	White (high density)	Gray (intermediate to slightly low signal)	Black (low signal)
Subacute	Gray (intermediate density)	White (high signal)	Black in early subacute White in late subacute
Chronic	Nearly black (low density)	Gray–black (intermediate to low signal)	Black (low signal)

will layer within the dependent portion of the ventricles (Fig. 7.4B). Note that while acute hemorrhage is denser (brighter) than adjacent brain, the density of hemorrhage decreases with time, and chronic hematomas may have a density similar to that of the CSF. Similarly, the signal characteristics of intracranial hemorrhage on MRI will evolve over time in a predictable pattern, providing an estimate of the age of the hematoma (Table 7.2).

Mass effect and midline shift are usually signs of raised intracranial pressure, indicating a neurosurgical emergency. Look for deviation of the midline structures such as the falx cerebri, septum pellucidum, and third ventricle. A large right subdural hematoma causes partial effacement of the right lateral ventricle as well as displacement of the ventricles and

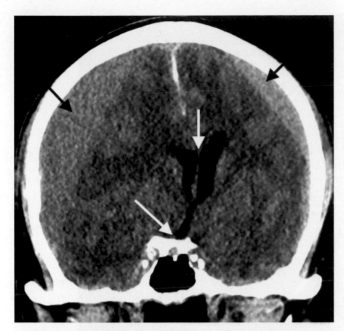

FIGURE 7.12. Bilateral subdural hematomas with mass effect and midline shift. Coronal CT showing bilateral subdural hematomas (*black arrows*). There is subfalcine herniation with *upper white arrow* showing right-to-left midline shift of the septum pellucidum. *Lower white arrow* indicates effacement of the suprasellar cistern with the floor of the third ventricle abutting the dorsum sellae.

right cingulate gyrus to the left of midline, beneath the falx cerebri (subfalcine herniation) (Fig. 7.12). This is an ominous finding because the midline shift may result in compression of the anterior cerebral arteries against the falx cerebri causing infarction. One caveat: midline shift is not always

a medical emergency. Although it is frequently the result of mass effect and displacement of brain away from a lesion, it may also occur following asymmetric volume loss in one cerebral hemisphere due to ipsilateral atrophy.

Effacement/decreased size of the cerebral sulci may be due to a focal abnormality such as hemorrhage or occur globally with cerebral edema. Assessment of the basal cisterns is also imperative as this signifies raised intracranial pressure and correlates with cerebral herniation syndromes, placing the patient at risk for infarcts as a consequence of impingement on cerebral arteries and/or veins. For example, herniation of the medial temporal lobe (uncal herniation) can result in compression of the posterior cerebral artery and infarction. Herniation syndromes can also result in obstructive hydrocephalus, which further increases intracranial pressure.

Gray matter/white matter differentiation. On CT, (counterintuitively) the gray matter (cerebral cortex, basal ganglia, thalami) appears denser (brighter) than the white matter (axons coated with myelin). A loss of gray–white differentiation occurs in cerebral edema or infarction. **Cerebral infarction** causes an influx of water into cells (**cytotoxic edema**), lowering the density of the brain parenchyma. A global anoxic injury such as that occurs following cardiac arrest may cause diffuse cerebral edema with effacement of the extra-axial spaces (the sulci and basal cisterns will be smaller or even obliterated) and partial effacement of the ventricles (Fig. 7.13). In severe anoxic injury, the cerebellum, brainstem, and deep gray matter (basal ganglia and thalami) can be of a higher density than the cerebral cortex. This is called the "reversal sign" or sometimes the "white cerebellum sign" and reflects preferential preservation of blood flow in the posterior circulation relative to that in the anterior circulation. Unfortunately, it usually indicates irreversible brain injury

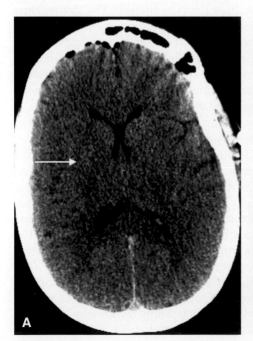

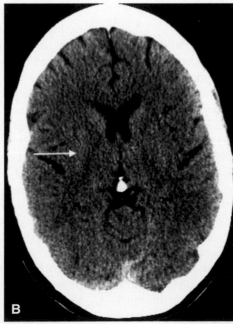

FIGURE 7.13. Global anoxic injury. A: Global anoxic injury with diffuse cerebral edema and diffuse loss of gray–white differentiation. *Arrow* illustrates poor definition of basal ganglia. Sulci are diffusely mildly effaced. **B:** Baseline head CT, prior to anoxic injury. *Arrow* shows how much better basal ganglia were seen on prior to anoxic event. Also note how much larger the sulci were on baseline CT, illustrating the degree of sulcal effacement in **(A)**.

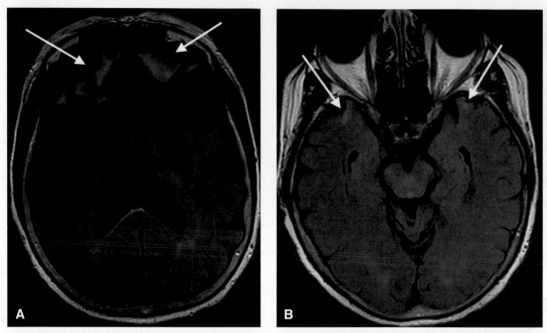

FIGURE 7.14. Posttraumatic encephalomalacia. A: Axial MRI FLAIR images with encephalomalacia (*arrows*) in the frontal lobes and **(B)** gliosis (*arrows*) in the temporal lobes bilaterally, a typical distribution for posttraumatic injury. The temporal lobe changes are quite subtle and could be difficult to identify on CT.

MRI is considered the modality of choice for patients with subacute and chronic TBI and is recommended for patients with acute head trauma when CT fails to explain the neurological findings. Susceptibility-weighted MR imaging is sensitive for minute hemorrhages, and FLAIR imaging can be helpful in the diagnosis of encephalomalacia resulting from prior brain contusions (Fig. 7.14).

VASCULAR DISEASE

Stroke

An ischemic stroke results from loss of blood flow to the brain. Typical scenarios are infarct as a result of vessel thrombosis, embolism, dissection, or a hypoperfusion event such as a cardiac arrest. Most commonly, ischemic brain infarcts are arterial, but venous infarcts (due to occlusion of a cerebral vein resulting in increased venous pressure and consequent loss of cerebral perfusion pressure) can also occur. Many infarcts are small and may be subclinical. However, when infarcts are large or involve critical areas of the brain, patients are symptomatic and neuroimaging is central to evaluation of these patients (Table 7.3).

Because of its wide availability and speed, NCCT is often the first examination. However, the sensitivity of CT for acute infarcts is limited in the first 24 hours after a stroke—particularly in the first 3 to 6 hours (hyperacute phase). The role of NCCT in the acute stroke setting is to exclude intracranial hemorrhage as this would preclude thrombolysis with tissue plasminogen activator (tPA) and to assess for

evidence of a large early infarct, which would also preclude administration of tPA. An infarct involving more than one-third of the middle cerebral artery territory on an early CT increases the risk of parenchymal hemorrhage after therapy with tPA.

Typically, CT findings seen with an acute infarct include loss of the normal gray–white differentiation (the gray and white matter become more similar in density making them difficult to differentiate from one another), a focal or regional area of low density in the brain parenchyma (brain appears darker than normal), which becomes more conspicuous over time, and mass effect related to swelling of acutely infarcted brain tissue. In some patients, acute intra-arterial thrombus can be seen on NCCT as an area hyperdensity (the blood vessel appears brighter than normal). This is most commonly seen in the middle cerebral artery and is referred to as the "hyperdense MCA sign" (Fig. 7.15A).

When considering endovascular intervention in stroke patients, it is important to know what portion of the brain is irreversibly infarcted, termed the infarct **core**, and what portion is ischemic but salvageable if promptly reperfused, termed the ischemic **penumbra**. The penumbra is dynamic and continues to shrink as ischemia time is prolonged. The goal of perfusion imaging is to determine which patients will benefit from intervention.

If the patient is not a candidate for administration of intravenous thrombolytic such as tPA, they may be still eligible for mechanical thrombectomy, which may be beneficial up to 24 hours from onset of stroke. CT angiography

TABLE 7.3 Algorithm for Investigation and Treatment of Stroke

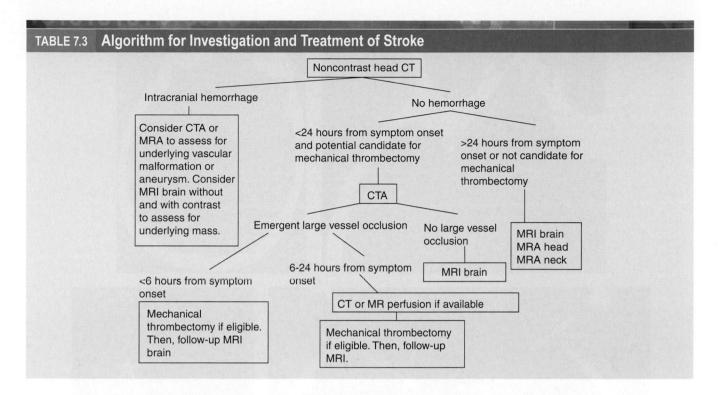

(CTA) is used to assess for a large vessel occlusion, which could be targeted for endovascular therapy (Fig. 7.15). With CT angiography, contrast is given IV and the brain imaged during the arterial phase of enhancement. In addition to being able to identify occlusions, CTA can diagnose significant stenoses or dissections, which may also cause stroke.

When the clinical diagnosis of stroke is in doubt, MRI may be helpful to more definitively determine whether an acute infarct has occurred. It can take 24 hours for an acute infarct to become apparent on CT, whereas MRI with DWI can detect an acute infarct in the hyperacute phase. As mentioned earlier in this chapter, infarcted cells undergo an influx of water producing cytotoxic edema. Compared with normal, healthy brain tissue where there is a random/ Brownian motion of water molecules, cytotoxic edema in acutely infarcted tissue results in a restricted motion of water molecules (i.e., restricted diffusion) that appears as high signal on the **diffusion-weighted** sequence of a brain MRI examination. Apparent diffusion coefficient (**ADC**) is a measure of the magnitude of diffusion (of water molecules) within tissue and is calculated from information acquired from the diffusion weighted sequence. Correlation with ADC map images should be performed to confirm that this represents true restricted diffusion (appearing dark on ADC map images) and is not artifactual in nature (7.15E). It should be noted that areas of restricted diffusion also occur in cerebral abscess, very dense tumors, or hematomas.

MR angiography (MRA) of the head is also a valuable tool in a patient with stroke and is typically performed without contrast. Flowing blood appears as bright signal on the images, whereas an occlusion will appear as an abrupt vessel cutoff (Fig. 7.16B). Sometimes, a high-grade stenosis causes reduction of blood flow to the point where it is not detected with MRA technique and can simulate an occlusion, appearing as a focal "flow gap." Neck MRA can also be helpful in assessing the status of the aortic arch, carotid, and vertebral systems. This is typically performed both without and with contrast as the noncontrast sequences are susceptible to artifact.

Chronic infarct result in focal or regional areas of atrophy or encephalomalacia (loss of brain tissue). Chronic cortical infarcts appear as thinning if small or as atrophic tissue if larger (Fig. 7.14). Chronic infarction is characterized by low density on CT and increased T2/FLAIR signal on MRI. With further brain volume loss, there will be corresponding increase in size of the sulci and ventricles (referred to as ex vacuo dilatation of the ventricles).

Small vessel ischemia occurs with aging, appearing as foci of hypodensity (dark) on CT or hyperintensity (increased signal) on T2 or FLAIR sequences on MRI in the white matter. Small vessel ischemia is frequently accompanied by subcentimeter "lacunar" infarcts of deep perforating arteries most commonly in the basal ganglia, thalami, and internal capsules.

Transient ischemic attack (TIA) is a sudden neurologic dysfunction limited to a vascular territory with complete resolution by 24 hours. This should not be regarded as a benign event because within 1 month of a TIA, 13% of patients will have a stroke. There is risk of infarction even when focal transient neurologic symptoms last less than 1 hour and about 50% of patients with TIA have corresponding ischemic lesions on brain on diffusion-weighted MRI.

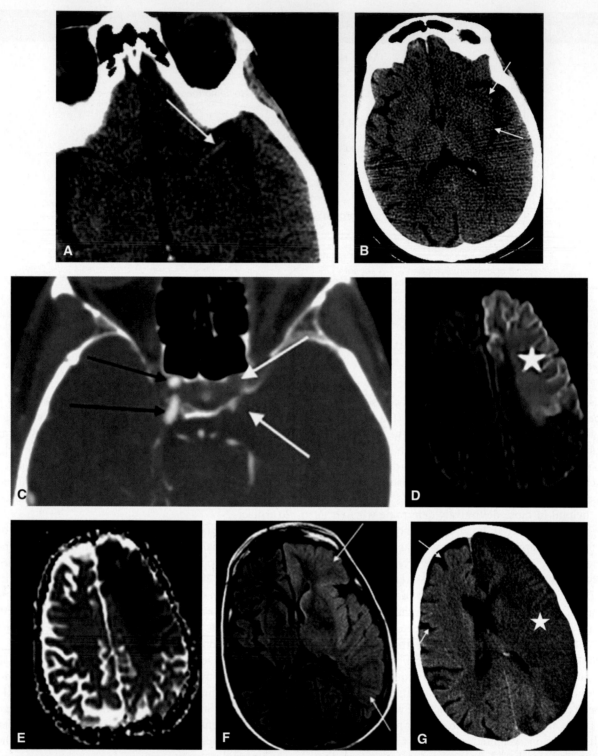

FIGURE 7.15. Stroke: Acute left middle cerebral artery (MCA) and anterior cerebral artery territory infarcts. A: Noncontrast head CT depicts the **hyperdense MCA sign**, indicating acute thrombus in the left middle cerebral artery (*arrow*). **B:** Noncontrast head CT shows loss of gray–white differentiation along the left insula (**insular ribbon sign**), consistent with acute infarction. **C:** CT angiogram shows occlusion of the left internal carotid artery (*white arrows*). *Black arrows* show normal contrast opacification in the patent right internal carotid artery. **D:** Diffusion-weighted image shows restricted diffusion in the left anterior cerebral artery and left middle cerebral artery territories (*star*). **E:** ADC map shows low signal in the left anterior cerebral artery and left middle cerebral artery territories, confirming true restricted diffusion. **F:** FLAIR images show diffuse increased signal in the area of the acute left anterior cerebral artery and left middle cerebral artery territories (*arrows*). **G:** Follow-up head CT shows expected evolution of the acute infarcts in the left anterior cerebral artery and middle cerebral artery territories (*star*) with greater hypodensity than on the initial head CT and development of mass effect with sulcal effacement. *Arrows* indicate preserved sulci along the right cerebral hemisphere, which contrast with the effaced sulci of the left cerebral hemisphere.

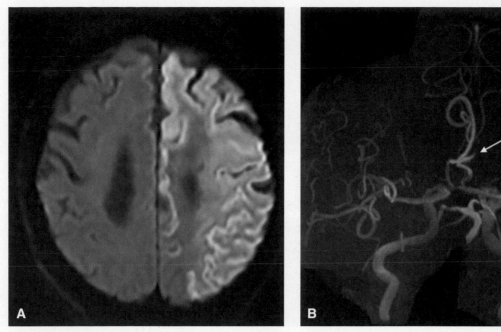

FIGURE 7.16. Acute left anterior cerebral artery (ACA) and left middle cerebral artery (MCA) infarcts. A: Diffusion-weighted imaging shows restricted diffusion in the acute left ACA and MCA territory infarct zones. **B:** MR angiogram shows occlusion in the left MCA (*black arrow*) and the left ACA (*white arrow*).

TABLE 7.4	Causes of Stroke in Young Adults

Arterial dissection
Cardiac defects: congenital heart disease, patent foramen
  ovale
Vasculitis
Recent pregnancy
Hypercoagulability
Illicit drug use

Diffusion-weighted MRI has a greater sensitivity than CT for detecting small acute infarcts in patients with TIA. Other useful tests in the workup following TIA include Duplex ultrasound and transcranial Doppler looking for a vascular stenosis in the carotid territory, a 12 lead ECG to exclude atrial fibrillation any echocariogram to exclude a cardiac source of embolus (Table 7.4).

Dissection

In an arterial dissection, there is a tear in the intimal layer, allowing blood to enter, forming an intramural hematoma. With further intramural accumulation of blood, the "false lumen" compresses the true lumen of the vessel, decreasing blood flow and may result in occlusion. When blood dissects to the outer layer of the blood vessel (subadventitial region), dilation of the outer wall of the vessel occurs (pseudoaneurysm—Fig. 7.17A). Dissection may occur intra- or extracranially with patients presenting with headache or neck pain.

Patients with internal carotid dissections can present with Horner syndrome, especially ptosis and miosis. Dissections can result in stroke because of hypoperfusion or thromboembolism. SAH can also occur in the setting of intracranial dissection with pseudoaneurysm. Hypertension and connective tissue or vascular disorders such as fibromuscular dysplasia or Ehlers-Danlos syndrome may predispose to dissection.

Dissections of the carotid or vertebral arteries may present as sudden, severe unilateral headache with radiation to the neck and may be diagnosed with CTA, MRA, or conventional (catheter) angiography. Although catheter angiography is considered the gold standard for diagnosis, it is an invasive procedure and therefore CTA or MRA are usually preferred for initial evaluation. CTA and MRA are nearly equivalent in their ability to detect dissection and both will show irregular, often eccentric narrowing of the dissected artery, with or without associated aneurysmal dilation. In some cases, a distinct curvilinear dissection flap may occur as a filling defect within the vessel on these studies (Fig. 7.17B). A fat-suppressed T1-weighted sequence can be helpful in confirming a subacute dissection on MRA because subacute intramural blood products (approximately 2–3 days to several weeks old) appear as a crescent of high signal surrounding the flow void in the vessel lumen on this sequence.

Aneurysm

The most common cause (70%) of nontraumatic SAH is a ruptured aneurysm. Aneurysmal SAH (Fig. 7.18) can be devastating as it may cause vasospasm and infarction. Saccular aneurysms (where the vessel outpouching is

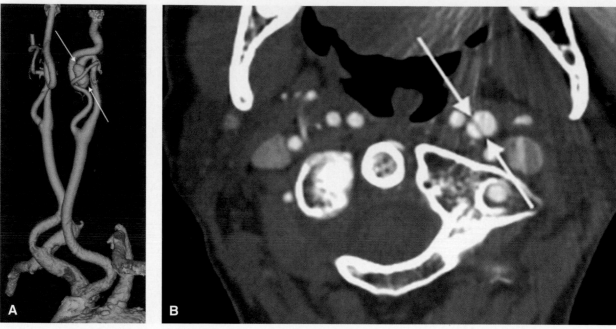

FIGURE 7.17. Left cervical internal carotid artery dissection with pseudoaneurysm. A: 3D MIP reconstructed image from a CT angiogram. *Arrows* indicate a left cervical internal carotid artery pseudoaneurysm. **B:** Axial source image from the CT angiogram shows a dissection flap (*arrows*).

eccentric, affecting only part of the artery's circumference) tend to occur at vessel branch points, most commonly in the anterior communicating artery region, posterior communicating artery region, middle cerebral artery bifurcation, or where the internal carotid artery bifurcates into the anterior cerebral and middle cerebral arteries. The risk of aneurysm rupture is related to its size.

In patients with sudden onset of severe headache, SAH is best diagnosed on NCCT. Lumbar puncture may be necessary if the CT scan is negative. In addition, patients with SAH will require vascular imaging (MRA, CTA, or catheter angiography) for identification of bleeding aneurysm or arteriovenous malformation (AVM). Both CTA and MRA have greater than 90% sensitivity for detecting aneurysms of 3 mm in size or larger. If an aneurysm is not identified on CTA or MRA, conventional (catheter) angiography should be done. There is increased incidence of intracranial aneurysms in patients with family history of first-degree relative with aneurysm and patients with fibromuscular dysplasia or polycystic kidney disease, all of whom may benefit from screening for aneurysm with MRA or CTA.

Arteriovenous Malformations

An AVM is the next most common cause of SAH after a ruptured aneurysm. AVM is characterized by a tangle of dysplastic vessels through which blood flows from arteries directly to veins without the normal intervening capillary bed. AVMs may also present as seizures. Modalities for evaluation include CTA, MRA, or conventional angiography with the last technique being the gold standard for diagnosis,

treatment planning, and follow-up. Angiographically, AVMs appear as a tangle of vessels with enlarged draining veins (Fig. 7.19). The feeding arteries are also typically enlarged and may contain aneurysms.

Cerebral Venous Thrombosis

Cerebral venous thrombosis is uncommon but may present as cerebral edema or infarction. Venous thrombosis leads to venous hypertension and decreases the arterial perfusion pressure. Risk factors for cerebral venous thrombosis include dehydration, hypercoagulable states, pregnancy, oral contraceptive use, and trauma. Acute dural sinus thrombosis or cortical vein thrombosis may be diagnosed on an NCCT as hyperdensity in the vessel (compared to the normal density of blood within the arterial structures, which serve as an internal reference). More commonly, dural sinus thrombosis is diagnosed on contrast-enhanced CT (CECT) or CT venography where it will appear as a filling defect in the enhancing vessel (Fig. 7.20). On MRI cerebral venous thrombosis appears as loss of the normal low-signal flow void or presence of abnormal high T1 signal in the vein or dural sinus if it is subacute. On MR venography, the thrombosis appears as focal flow gap (if the noncontrast time-of-flight MR venography technique is used) or a focal filling defect (if contrast-enhanced MR venography is performed). As the two techniques are complementary, it is often beneficial to perform MR venography both without and with contrast. Edema or infarction occurs in the territory drained by the thrombosed cerebral vein or dural sinus. Venous infarcts are hemorrhagic in about one-third of patients.

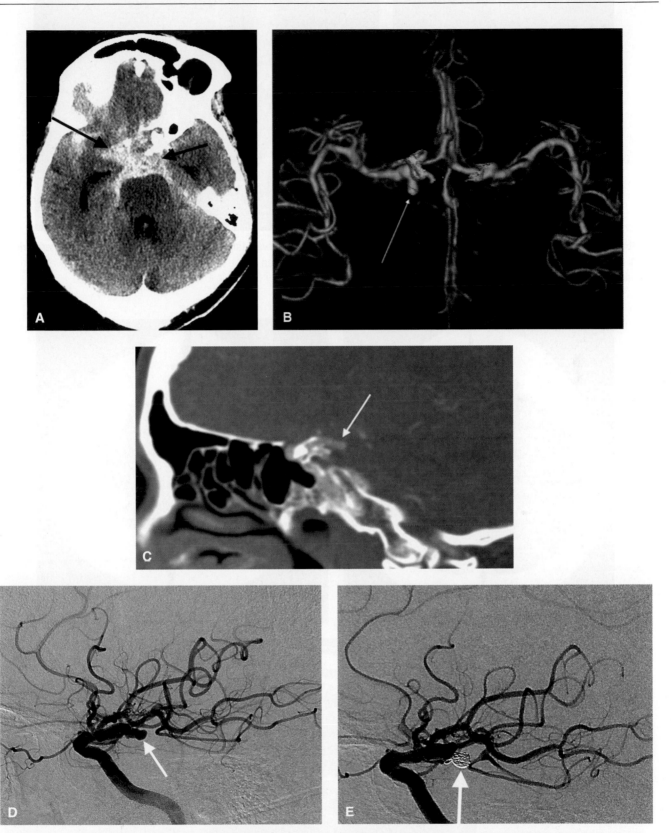

FIGURE 7.18. Aneurysmal subarachnoid hemorrhage. A: *Black arrows* indicate extensive subarachnoid hemorrhage in the basal cisterns. **B:** 3D-MIP reconstructed image from CT angiogram shows right posterior communicating artery aneurysm (*arrow*). **C:** Sagittal reformatted image from CT angiogram shows posterior communicating artery aneurysm (*arrow*). **D:** Lateral view from catheter angiogram again shows posterior communicating artery (aneurysm). **E:** Lateral view catheter angiogram after coil embolization of the aneurysm shows no residual flow in the aneurysm. *Arrow* indicates the coil embolization pack.

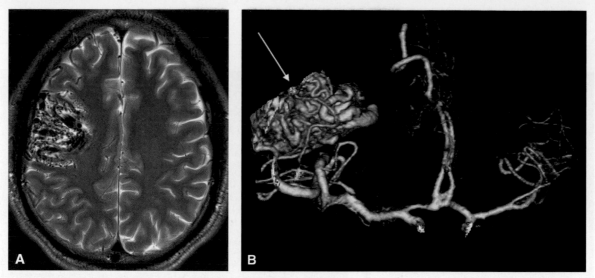

FIGURE 7.19. Arteriovenous malformation. A: Axial T2-weighted image shows a tangle of flow voids centered in the posterior right frontal lobe consistent with arteriovenous malformation. **B:** 3D MIP reconstructed image from CT angiogram shows arteriovenous malformation (*arrow*) with enlarged feeding right middle cerebral artery.

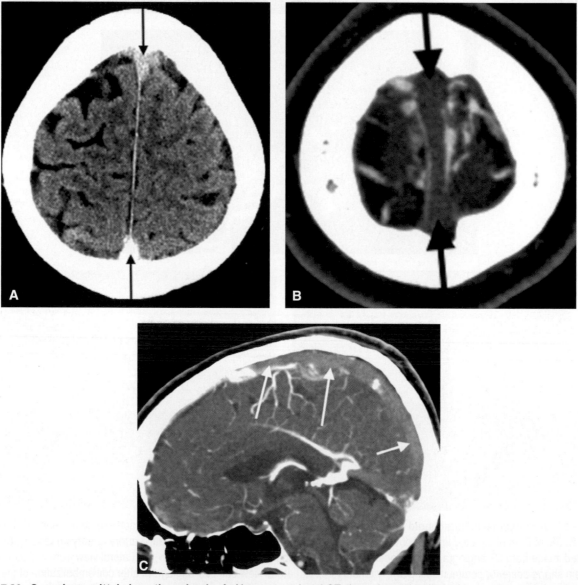

FIGURE 7.20. Superior sagittal sinus thrombosis. A: Noncontrast head CT shows hyperdensity in the superior sagittal sinus (*arrows*) due to acute superior sagittal sinus thrombosis. **B:** Axial CT venogram image shows filling defect in the superior sagittal sinus due to superior sagittal sinus thrombosis (*arrows*). **C:** Sagittal reformatted image from CT venogram shows filling defect in the superior sagittal sinus due to thrombosis.

TUMORS

Primary brain tumors are rare, and approximately half of them present with headache. MRI pre- and postcontrast is a study of choice in patients with suspected brain tumor. Metastases are the most common brain tumors in adults. In children, however, primary central nervous system tumors are more common than metastases. In adults, brain tumors are more commonly seen within the cerebral hemispheres. In contrast, in children posterior fossa tumors are more common than supratentorial tumors.

The use of IV contrast is recommended when a tumor is suspected as they enhance following contrast administration (especially higher-grade primary brain neoplasms or metastases) because of the breakdown of the blood–brain barrier. Extra-axial tumors such as meningiomas lack a blood–brain barrier and will also enhance. Although contrast-enhanced examinations aid in detection of brain tumors, this is typically done following a noncontrast examination as the presence of contrast can sometimes be difficult to distinguish from other substances such as acute hemorrhage or dense, cellular tumor.

Compared with CT, the superior soft-tissue resolution of MRI makes it preferable for diagnosing brain tumors, especially small tumors without surrounding edema and those located in parts of the brain prone to bone artifact on CT near the skull base.

Once a brain tumor has been identified, determination of its location, **intra-axial versus extra-axial**, is important. An extra-axial tumor, such as a meningioma, is located outside of the brain but within the calvarial vault. An intra-axial tumor, such as glioblastoma, arises within the brain. However, this determination based on location is not always possible. In general, an extra-axial tumor will display its widest base along the dura and will smoothly indent on the brain. As an extra-axial tumor indents the brain, it widens the CSF space between the brain and the mass (CSF cleft sign), which is in contrast to a claw sign, where a tumor is partially surrounded by normal brain tissue, indicating an intra-axial location. In cases where tumor is located at the level of the brain surface, review of imaging in multiple planes may be necessary.

Extra-axial brain tumors are the most common primary brain tumors in adults, with meningiomas being the most frequent. Meningiomas are dural-based masses and may be calcified (Fig. 7.21). Among **intra-axial** tumors in adults, metastases occur most commonly at the gray matter–white matter junction. They are usually circumscribed, have a round shape, and typically enhance. Primary brain tumors are most commonly of glial cell origin, with astrocytomas being most frequent. Astrocytomas can be circumscribed masses or they can be ill-defined or infiltrating, particularly if they are higher-grade tumors. The lower-grade astrocytomas tend to enhance less frequently than higher grade tumors (Fig. 7.22).

Once a tumor has been defined as intra-axial or extra-axial, the next task is to assess for **mass effect and midline shift**. It is important to determine whether the mass effect

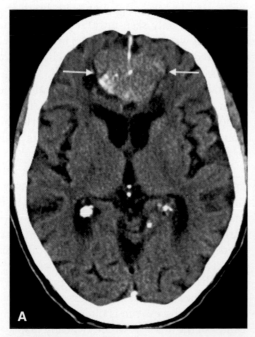 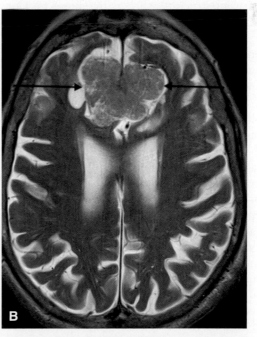

FIGURE 7.21. Anterior interhemispheric meningioma. A: Extra-axial hyperdense, partially calcified mass (*arrows*) in the anterior interhemispheric fissure is a meningioma. Note it mildly indents on the adjacent frontal lobes. **B:** Axial T2-weighted image shows that the meningioma is clearly extra-axial with CSF clefts seen between the mass (*arrows*) and the frontal lobes.

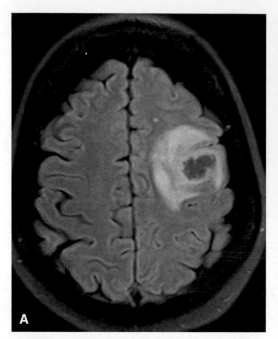 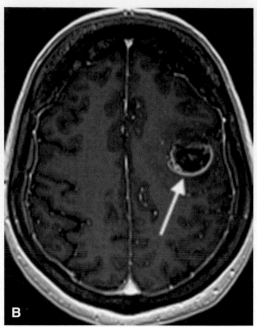

FIGURE 7.22. **Astrocytoma. A:** Axial MRI FLAIR image shows a focal mass in the posterior left frontal lobe with a small area of surrounding FLAIR signal due to a combination of edema and infiltrating tumor. **B:** Postcontrast axial T1-weighted image shows heterogeneously enhancing posterior left frontal mass.

or displacement will compromise function of critical brain structures (e.g. compression of the brainstem), compromise blood flow, or cause obstructive hydrocephalus (which would cause elevation of intracranial pressure).

If intervention such as biopsy or resection is planned, **mapping** of adjacent structures such as the motor tract or language centers (including Broca area or Wernicke area) using function MRI (fMRI) is important. With blood oxygen level dependent (BOLD) fMRI, patients are asked to perform certain tasks during imaging such as finger tapping, language or memory tasks, or reading tasks. The motor, language, and visual centers will be identified by detection of increased blood flow to these areas during these tasks as compared with the resting state. Another MRI technique that is increasingly being employed is diffusion tensor imaging (DTI), which allows for creation of visual representations of white matter tracts of interest.

Post tumor resection, imaging surveillance is done to detect recurrence of tumor. In patients treated with radiation therapy (as many brain tumors are), it can be difficult or impossible to differentiate the development of radiation necrosis from recurrent tumor as both appear as enhancing lesions with mass effect and edema on MR. MR perfusion imaging can differentiate between radiation necrosis and high-grade recurrent tumor by creating maps of relative cerebral blood volume (rCBV). Areas of radiation necrosis will classically display low rCBV, whereas high-grade tumors are associated with neovascularity, which results in higher rCBV.

INFECTION

Brain Abscess

Many of the typical features of infection may be absent in patients with brain abscesses. For example, fever may only be present in 50% of patients with brain abscess, and leukocytosis is only seen in 50% of these patients. Imaging, which allows earlier diagnosis of intracranial infections, has been credited with a significant decline in mortality of brain abscess with the use of CT and MRI.

Brain abscess can occur as a local spread of infection from adjacent structures (such as the sinuses or mastoids), or following head trauma or surgery. However, hematogenous spread is also possible in patients with lung abscess or endocarditis.

Typically, a brain abscess begins as a cerebritis, which appears as an ill-defined area of low-density edema on CT or a focal or regional area of T2 hyperintense signal abnormality on MRI. Contrast enhancement is variable in this early phase. As cerebritis evolves into an abscess, there will be development of a more conspicuous area of focal low density with adjacent edema, mass effect, and irregular rim enhancement. Similar findings are seen on MRI with a well-defined rim that is thinnest along its medial wall (Fig. 7.23). The abscess rim is often T2 hypointense (unlike the center of the abscess, which typically displays increased T2 signal). As ring enhancement is nonspecific for the diagnosis of abscess, DWI is helpful as it shows restricted diffusion within the center of a pyogenic abscess (central bright

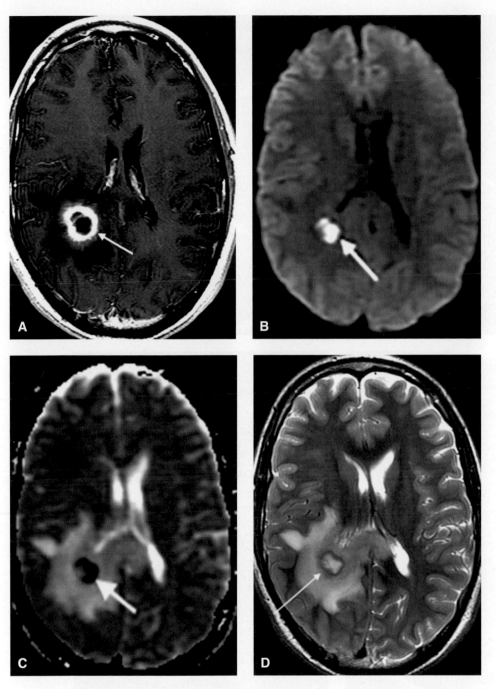

FIGURE 7.23. Cerebral abscess. A: Postcontrast axial T1-weighted image shows ring-enhancing lesion in the deep right parietal lobe (*arrow*). **B:** Diffusion-weighted image shows there is central restricted diffusion (*arrow*) within the ring-enhancing lesion, typical of pyogenic abscess. **C:** ADC map image shows low signal (*arrow*) within the center of the lesion, confirming true restricted diffusion. **D:** Axial T2-weighted image shows the wall of the ring-enhancing lesion is T2 hypointense, characteristic of pyogenic abscess. There is moderate confluent edema surrounding the ring-enhancing lesion.

signal on the DWI sequence and corresponding low signal in this location on the ADC map). This is in contrast to brain tumors, which will typically display restricted diffusion at the rim (where viable tumor is present), instead of the core of the lesion.

Encephalitis

Encephalitis is an inflammation of the brain most commonly caused by viral infection or autoimmune conditions. Up to 10% to 15% of cases encephalitis occur in patients with HIV. As with other CNS infections, clinical hallmarks include fever, headache, and mental status changes as well as seizures or focal neurological deficits. Many encephalitides have a predilection for the gray matter (cerebral cortex, basal ganglia, thalami) over white matter but involvement of cerebral white matter, brainstem, and cerebellum also occurs. MRI is the preferred diagnostic modality with increased T2/FLAIR signal in the gray matter, with or without associated white matter involvement. Diffusion restriction is common while enhancement can be variable.

Some encephalitides show characteristic locations of involvement. **Herpes encephalitis** caused by HSV1 has a strong predilection for the **limbic system** with T2 hyperintense signal abnormality and restricted diffusion in the

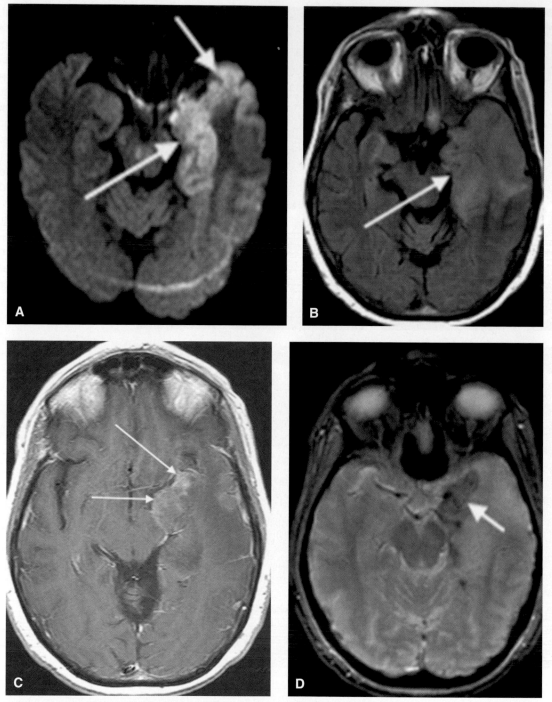

FIGURE 7.24. Herpes encephalitis. A: Diffusion-weighted MR image shows restricted diffusion in the medial and anterior left temporal lobe due to herpes encephalitis (*arrows*). **B:** Axial FLAIR image shows moderate confluent FLAIR hyperintense signal in the left temporal lobe (*arrow*). **C:** Postcontrast axial T1-weighted image shows mild patchy enhancement in the left temporal lobe (*arrows*). **D:** Axial gradient echo image shows mild patchy susceptibility artifact in the left temporal lobe due to petechial hemorrhage (*arrow*) associated with herpes encephalitis.

temporal lobes, inferior frontal lobes, cingulate gyri, and insula and associated brain swelling/mass effect (Fig. 7.24). The basal ganglia are typically spared in herpes encephalitis. As herpes encephalitis is frequently a hemorrhagic encephalitis, foci of low signal on gradient echo or

susceptibility-weighted sequences confirm hemorrhage. The differential diagnosis of herpes encephalitis (especially a unilateral herpes encephalitis) includes an acute infarct, infiltrating primary brain tumor, or an autoimmune or paraneoplastic "limbic" encephalitis. However, the clinical scenario and abrupt onset of symptoms that occurs with an acute herpes encephalitis (as opposed to a more subacute course seen with brain tumor or limbic encephalitis) should allow differentiation from these other entities.

Meningitis

Meningitis is an inflammation of the leptomeninges and is most commonly infectious—bacterial, viral, or granulomatous. The diagnosis is made on clinical grounds with analysis of CSF and only rarely on imaging. The primary role of imaging in meningitis is to diagnose its complications, which include cerebritis or brain abscess, empyema (an infected extra-axial collection, outside of the brain), ventriculitis (infection of the ependymal lining of the ventricles), hydrocephalus (dilated ventricles), and rarely infarcts. On MRI, meningitis appears as areas of enhancement filling in the sulci and basal cisterns or curvilinear enhancement on the surface of the brainstem. This appearance is referred to as leptomnenigeal enhancement and may also be seen with carcinomatous meningitis (spread of tumor to the meninges—Fig. 7.25) and neurosarcoid.

HIV-infected patients who present with altered mental status or abnormal neurologic examination may be a challenging diagnostic problem as they often have abnormalities on CT or MRI, the differential diagnosis of which depends on the degree of immunosuppression (Table 7.5).

TABLE 7.5	Differential Diagnosis of HIV-Related Brain Disease
CD4 Count/microL	**Differential Diagnosis**
>500	Benign, malignant tumors and metastases
>200 and <500	HIV-associated cognitive and motor disorders
<200	Opportunistic infections, primary CNS lymphoma

HYDROCEPHALUS

Ventriculomegaly (enlarged ventricles) is a common feature of aging and other causes of brain parenchymal volume loss (so-called ex vacuo ventriculomegaly). **Obstructive hydrocephalus** may present as ventricular enlargement due to an imbalance in the volume of CSF produced versus absorbed into the bloodstream. This imbalance is most commonly due to obstruction of the CSF circulatory pathway. The key to differentiating these two processes is that with ex vacuo ventriculomegaly the ventricular dilation will be in proportion to enlargement of the sulci, whereas with an obstructive hydrocephalus, dilation of the ventricles will be disproportionate with the size of the sulci (Fig. 7.26). There are two types of obstructive hydrocephalus: **noncommunicating hydrocephalus**, where the obstruction is within the ventricular system, preventing CSF from exiting the ventricles, and

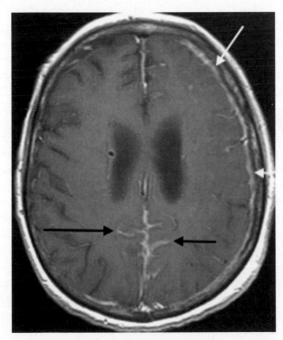

FIGURE 7.25. Leptomeningeal enhancement. White *arrows* show dural enhancement over the lateral aspect of the left cerebral hemisphere and (*black arrows*) show leptomeningeal enhancement within the medial parietal sulci due to lymphoma. The differential diagnosis includes infectious meningitis, leptomeningeal metastases, and neurosarcoid.

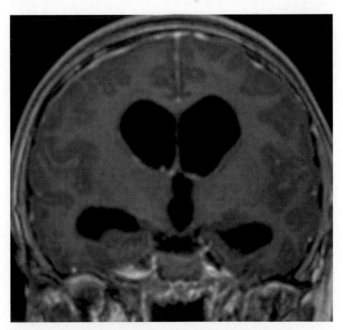

FIGURE 7.26. Hydrocephalus. Coronal postcontrast T1-weighted image shows marked hydrocephalus involving the lateral ventricles and third ventricle. Note how ventricular enlargement is out of proportion to the size of the sulci.

communicating hydrocephalus, where the obstruction is outside of the ventricular system and prevents the arachnoid villi from resorbing CSF. Causes of obstructive hydrocephalus include tumor and a congenital stenosis of the cerebral aqueduct, which connects the third ventricle to the fourth ventricle. Communicating hydrocephalus occurs most commonly as a complication of SAH although it can also result from meningitis or leptomeningeal carcinomatosis. Patients with obstructive hydrocephalus may present with headache, nausea, vomiting, or diplopia and may have papilledema on physical examination. Acute obstructive hydrocephalus may require placement of a ventriculostomy catheter to divert CSF and decrease intracranial pressure. Acute obstructive hydrocephalus is often accompanied by development of edema in the periventricular white matter referred to as transependymal flow of CSF. This is seen as low density on CT or high T2 signal on MRI in the periventricular white matter. In chronic hydrocephalus, compensatory pathways for CSF resorption have developed and the transependymal flow of CSF is minimal.

Normal pressure hydrocephalus is essentially a low-level chronic hydrocephalus, which occurs in the elderly with a classic clinical triad of dementia, gait abnormality, and urinary incontinence. The pathophysiology is poorly understood but is thought to be related to impaired resorption of CSF at the level of the arachnoid granulations. The ventricles are disproportionately enlarged compared with the sulci, but the patients have normal opening pressure on lumbar puncture. However, as mild normal pressure hydrocephalus can be difficult to differentiate from ex vacuo ventriculomegaly, this is not an imaging diagnosis. The diagnosis depends on imaging findings in conjunction with the clinical picture and requires confirmation with improvement of symptomatology following removal of large volume of CSF on lumbar puncture (high-volume LP). Treatment includes CSF shunting, which may cause symptomatic improvement.

DEMENTIA

Dementia is characterized by a significant loss of function in multiple cognitive domains without affecting the general level of arousal. Several types of dementia have been described, including Alzheimer disease (AD), Lewy body disease, frontotemporal dementia (FTD), and the vascular dementias. Traditionally, the primary role of imaging with CT and MR in patients with AD has been to exclude other significant intracranial abnormalities. In addition to structural imaging with CT and MRI, which may be nonspecific, single photon emission CT (SPECT) performed with hexamethylproyleneamine oxime (Tc-99m HMPAO) is used to assess regional cerebral blood flow (**rCBF**) and positron emission tomography (PET) using F-18 FDG for assessment of regional cerebral glucose metabolism (**rCGM**). Normally, there is significantly greater blood flow to gray matter compared with white matter seen on both SPECT and PET scans such that lesions in the white

matter often cannot be detected or even differentiated from CSF spaces, so MRI or CT correlation is necessary for identifying white matter changes and enlarged ventricles.

Although PET has higher sensitivity and higher resolution than SPECT, the overall patterns seen in dementia are similar for both rCGM and rCBF. The characteristic patterns of AD are well established for both PET and SPECT, with findings present before atrophy can be detected with MRI. Bilateral hypometabolism or hypoperfusion, initially asymmetrical, is seen in the early stages in the **posterior cingulate and the superior posterior parietal cortex**. As the disease progresses, **symmetric parietal and temporal lobe involvement predominates**. Reduced frontal lobe uptake, often asymmetric, is a late occurrence. The occipital visual cortex, primary somatosensory and motor cortices, basal ganglia, thalamus, and cerebellum are spared in AD. CT-based and MRI-based volumetric measurements confirm focal atrophy of the hippocampal formation in patients with mild AD compared with normal controls and those with other forms of dementia.

Dementia with Lewy bodies shows changes primarily in the **occipital lobes**. The involvement of the primary visual cortex accounts for visual hallucinations, which are a feature of the disease. In contrast to Alzheimer disease, hippocampal activity is preserved in patients with dementia with Lewy bodies.

In patients with FTD, hypometabolism occurs in the frontal, anterior cingulate and anterior temporal regions more frequently, whereas patients with AD demonstrate hypometabolism in the temporoparietal and posterior cingulate regions. **Vascular dementia** is diagnosed through a combination of clinical features and focal white matter lesions (subcortical encephalomalacia) on MRI.

MULTIPLE SCLEROSIS

Multiple sclerosis (MS) is a condition where immune system dysfunction leads to activated T-cells damaging myelinated axons and causing demyelination. The disease tends to affect younger adult patients, especially in the 20 to 40 year age range, and women are roughly twice as likely to develop as MS as men. Patients can present with virtually any neurologic deficit, depending on the location of the lesion, but weakness, paresthesias, and visual or urinary symptoms are among the most common. Demyelinating lesions may involve the white matter anywhere in the CNS. The diagnosis of MS is based on a combination of clinical symptoms, MRI findings, and laboratory evidence.

On MRI, patients with MS typically display T2 hyperintense lesions in the periventricular, subcortical, and juxtacortical white matter, the corpus callosum, brainstem, and the cerebellar peduncles. The characteristic periventricular lesions have an ovoid or flame shape and are oriented radially relative to the lateral ventricles (Fig. 7.27). Identification of periventricular lesions adjacent to the temporal horns of the lateral ventricles can also be helpful as a differentiating feature as this is not a typical location for involvement by small vessel ischemic change. Similarly, T2 hyperintense lesions in the cerebellar peduncles or medulla can be a helpful discriminating feature as these are areas that are not commonly affected by small vessel ischemic disease. Actively demyelinating multiple sclerosis plaques display contrast enhancement. Contrast enhancement patterns include nodular or ring enhancement; incomplete ring enhancement is a characteristic of demyelinating lesions.

Large (greater than 2 cm) and mass-like MS lesions are called **tumefactive MS** and may be mistaken for brain tumors or abscess. Incomplete ring enhancement and presence of other lesions typical of multiple sclerosis can be helpful in differentiating a tumefactive MS from a neoplastic process. In some cases, short interval follow-up imaging to assess for improvement of enhancement may be necessary for confirmation and to exclude tumor. MR perfusion imaging shows low relative cerebral blood volumes in tumefactive MS, whereas high-grade tumors typically show high relative cerebral blood volumes (hyperperfusion).

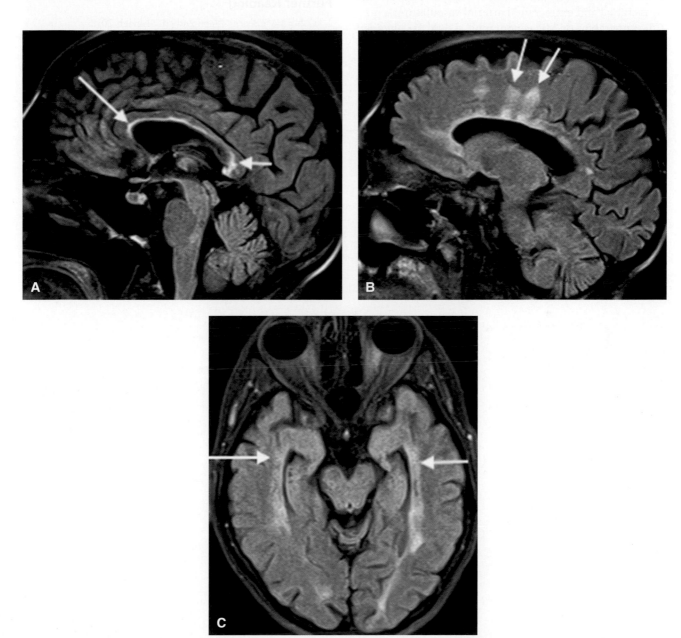

FIGURE 7.27. Multiple sclerosis. A: Sagittal FLAIR image shows increased signal in the corpus callosum at the callososeptal interface (*arrows*), typical of multiple sclerosis. **B:** Sagittal FLAIR image shows multiple finger-like flame-shaped lesions (*arrows*) oriented radially relative to the lateral ventricles, typical of demyelinating plaques in multiple sclerosis. **C:** Axial FLAIR image shows lesions in the periventricular white matter adjacent to the temporal horns of the lateral ventricles (*arrows*), typical of demyelination. This is not a common location for microvascular ischemic change.

KEY POINTS

- On NCCT performed for the acute head trauma patient, check for intracranial hemorrhage, mass effect, and midline shift.
- The role of NCCT in the acute stroke setting is to exclude intracranial hemorrhage as the cause of the stroke and to assess for evidence of a large early infarct.
- MRI with DWI imaging is very sensitive in detection of acute infarcts.
- CTA and MRA are noninvasive ways to evaluate the intracranial and extracranial arterial vasculature.
- CT venography or MR venography should be obtained when there is concern for cerebral venous thrombosis or dural sinus thrombosis.
- MRI of the brain without and with contrast is the optimal modality for evaluating most brain tumors. Advanced MR imaging applications such as MR perfusion, DTI, and fMRI can be helpful adjuncts in evaluation and management of patients with brain tumors.
- MRI without and with contrast is often the optimal modality in evaluation of patients with CNS infections although CT without and with contrast can be quite helpful when MRI is not an option.
- There are multiple causes of dilated ventricles including volume loss, communicating or noncommunicating hydrocephalus, or normal pressure hydrocephalus.
- MRI of the brain to evaluate for active demyelination in a patient with multiple sclerosis should be performed with and without contrast.

Further Reading

1. Osborn A. *Osborns' Brain*. 2nd ed. Elsevier; 2018.

Questions

1. True or False: Superior soft-tissue contrast with MRI makes this the ideal modality for initial screening in acute head trauma patients.

2. All of the following are typical locations for demyelinating plaques in multiple sclerosis EXCEPT:
   a. The corpus callosum
   b. Medulla
   c. Periventricular white matter adjacent to the temporal horns of the lateral ventricles
   d. Pineal gland
   e. Middle cerebellar peduncles

3. Typical areas involved with herpes encephalitis include all of the following EXCEPT:
   a. Medial temporal lobes
   b. Insula
   c. Cingulate gyrus
   d. Perirolandic cortex

4. Which of the following sequences is most helpful in identify hemorrhagic conversion of an infarct?
   a. Postcontrast T1
   b. FLAIR
   c. Gradient echo
   d. Proton density

5. A helpful feature in identifying brain abscess includes:
   a. Concentric ring enhancement
   b. Central restricted diffusion
   c. T1 bright rim
   d. Extensive susceptibility artifact

6. In the setting of acute stroke, identification of a hyperdense middle cerebral artery indicates:
   a. An underlying aneurysm
   b. Mild vessel narrowing
   c. Acute MCA thrombus
   d. An underlying dissection
   e. Associated AVM

7. True or False: When dissection is being considered, addition of fat-suppressed T1-weighted imaging to the typical MRA protocol can be helpful to assess for intramural thrombus.

8. True or False: Prominent transependymal flow of CSF is a sign of chronic, compensated hydrocephalus.

9. True or False: Meningitis is primarily a clinical and lab diagnosis and the role of imaging is to assess for complications of meningitis.

10. True or False: Primary CNS lymphoma may occur in HIV-infected patients.

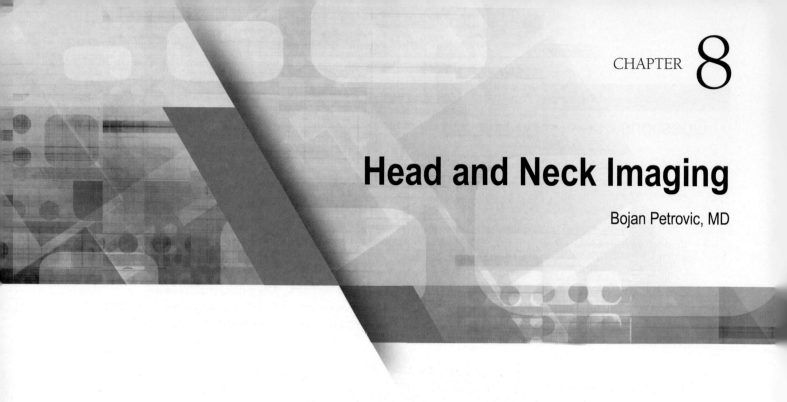

CHAPTER 8

Head and Neck Imaging

Bojan Petrovic, MD

CHAPTER OUTLINE

The term "head and neck" is used to refer to the portions of this region outside of the brain, including the sinuses, orbits, neck, skull base, and temporal bone.

Normal anatomy of the face, orbits, and neck is presented in Figures 8.1-8.3.

TRAUMA

CT is excellent at identifying facial bone fractures and alignment of fracture fragments (important in determining whether surgical fixation may be necessary). Contrast is usually not necessary unless vascular injury is suspected. Blood in a paranasal sinus can be a clue that there is a fracture, and air in the facial soft tissues suggests presence of either a sinus fracture or a skin laceration.

An orbital blowout fracture with displacement of a fracture fragment inferiorly into the maxillary sinus or medially into the ethmoid sinus can result in herniation of orbital contents through the fracture (Fig. 8.4). If the inferior rectus muscle is affected, this can result in diplopia. Hypoesthesias of the cheek and gums occurring after orbital blowout fracture can be explained by fractures traversing the canal for the infraorbital nerve. CT is useful to assess a retrobulbar hematoma or orbital emphysema which could compress the optic nerve causing blindness. Fractures involving the roof or lateral wall of the sphenoid sinus or cribriform plates or ethmoid roofs may be complicated by a cerebrospinal fluid leak, meningitis, or abscess.

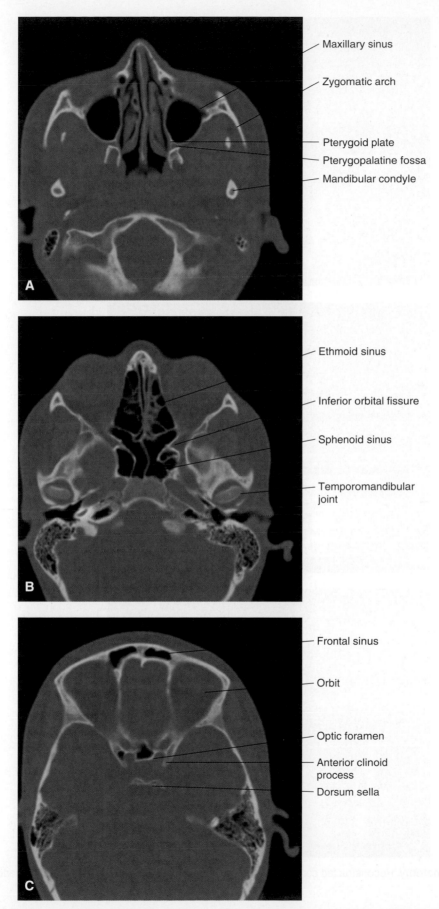

FIGURE 8.1. Normal anatomy. Axial CT images of the sinuses in bone windows: inferior plane **(A)**, middle plane **(B)**, and superior plane **(C)**.

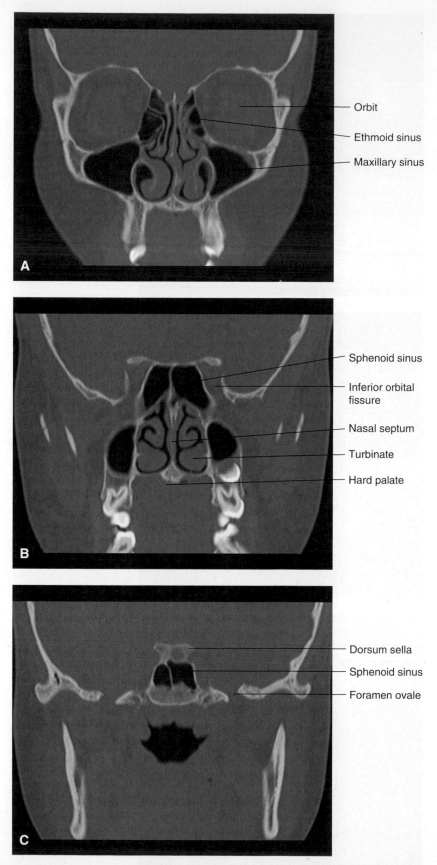

FIGURE 8.2. **Normal anatomy.** Reconstructed coronal CT images of the sinuses in bone windows: anterior plane **(A)**, middle plane **(B)**, and posterior plane **(C)**.

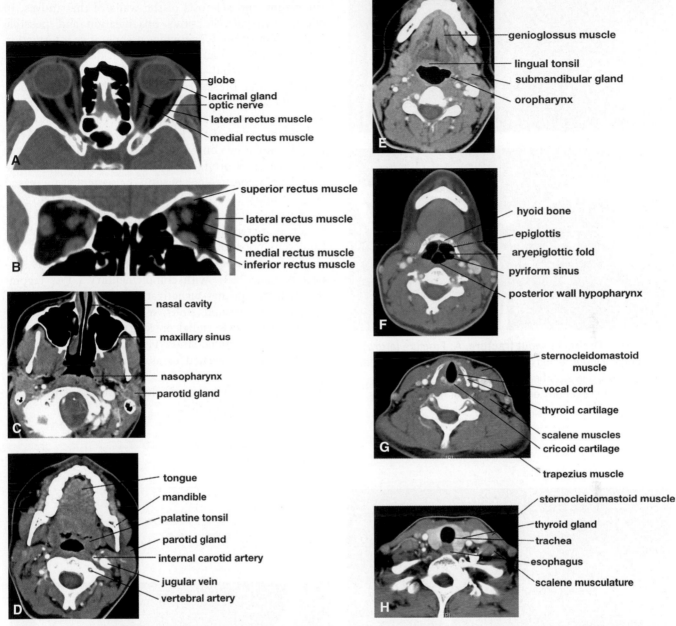

FIGURE 8.3. Normal anatomy of the orbits and neck. **A and B:** Axial and coronal images through the orbits. **C–H:** Axial images through the neck: **(C)** nasopharynx, **(D)** oropharynx, **(E)** floor of mouth, **(F)** epiglottis/hypopharynx, **(G)** vocal cords, and **(H)** thyroid gland.

SINUSITIS

Sinusitis is a clinical diagnosis based on facial pain or pressure, purulent nasal drainage, nasal obstruction, and fever. Imaging of patients with acute (<4 weeks) uncomplicated sinusitis is unnecessary unless a complication such as headache, facial swelling, orbital proptosis, and cranial nerve palsies or alternative diagnosis is suspected. Mucosal thickening is frequently seen in asymptomatic patients, and therefore sinusitis remains primarily a clinical diagnosis. In the absence of recent nasal lavage or presence of a nasogastric tube, however, layering of paranasal sinus fluid (so-called air–fluid levels) or presence of frothy/bubbly secretions in the sinuses are the most specific imaging signs for sinusitis (Fig. 8.5A). Radiography is relatively insensitive and rarely indicated in preference to noncontrast CT (NCCT).

In addition to identifying which sinuses are opacified, obstruction of paranasal sinus outflow tracts (frontal recesses, sphenoethmoidal recesses, ostiomeatal units)

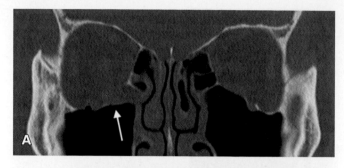

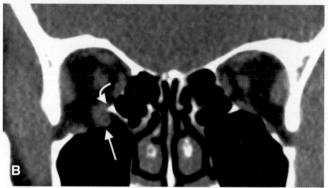

FIGURE 8.4. Orbital blowout fracture. A: Fracture (*arrow*). **B:** The right inferior rectus muscle herniates into the fracture defect (*arrow*), and a portion of the bony floor of the orbit impinges on the inferiorly displaced inferior rectus muscle (*curved arrow*).

should be sought. With chronic sinusitis, CT may show thickening and sclerosis of the walls of the sinuses, in addition to variable sinus opacification and possible sinus calcification. CT provides preoperative information for endoscopic surgery, with excellent delineation of the complex ethmoidal anatomy and anatomic variations, including the presence of **sphenoethmoidal (Onodi) air cells** which increase the risk of injury to the optic nerves or carotid arteries (Fig. 8.5B). Another abnormality is dehiscence of the lamina papyracea, whether due to old trauma or congenital dehiscence, that can result in herniation of orbital fat or even medial rectus muscle into the ethmoid region, placing the patient at increased risk of injury to orbital contents during sinus surgery. In-office use of cone beam CT (CBCT) for sinonasal evaluation is increasing in popularity but the technique is limited by poor soft tissue resolution.

If a sinus mass causing obstruction or fungus is suspected, then, MRI, with complementary CT is recommended for optimal visualization of brain and orbits. Chronic, inspissated sinus secretions can sometimes generate very little signal on MRI T2-weighted images, mimicking an aerated sinus. For this reason, the role of MRI is largely relegated to assessment for intracranial complications of sinusitis or when underlying obstructing neoplasm is suspected which can be identified on MRI as an enhancing mass.

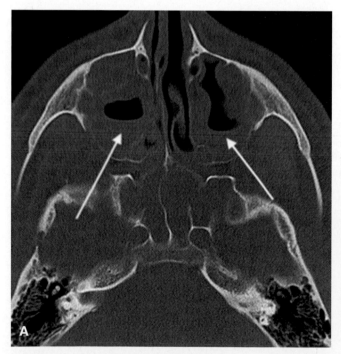

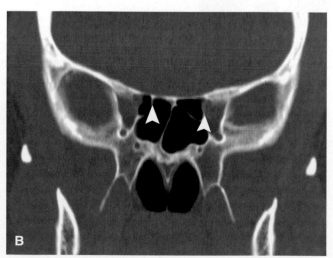

FIGURE 8.5. Maxillary sinusitis (A). Circumferential mucosal thickening in the maxillary sinuses with air–fluid levels (*arrows*) due to layering fluid. **B: Bilateral sphenoethmoidal air or Onodi cells** on coronal CT. Note proximity to the right optic canal (*arrowheads*).

NECK INFECTIONS

Tonsillar Abscess

CT can be helpful in evaluation of suspected tonsillar or peritonsillar abscess. Patients with tonsillitis typically present with sore throat, dysphagia, fever, and mild trismus. If the trismus is severe or antibiotics are unsuccessful, contrast CT allows differentiation of tonsillitis from a tonsillar or a peritonsillar abscess. Tonsillitis will appear as enlarged palatine tonsil(s) with either a solid enhancement pattern or a striated enhancement pattern (Fig. 8.6). In contrast, tonsillar abscess will appear as a discrete, low-density fluid collection with peripherally enhancing rim. When the tonsillar abscess extends beyond the tonsil into the adjacent soft tissue spaces, this is a peritonsillar abscess (Fig. 8.7), which may progress to airway compromise and will likely require incision and drainage in addition to IV antibiotic therapy.

Retropharyngeal Abscess

A retropharyngeal abscess may also present with fever, chills, dysphagia, and sore throat, which typically occurs as a complication of tonsillitis or pharyngitis, although it can also be seen as a complication of diskitis–osteomyelitis, a penetrating foreign body injury, or superior extension of a mediastinal infection. Retropharyngeal abscesses are most commonly seen in pediatric patients (especially in patients younger than 6 years) and in immunocompromised adults. A lateral radiograph of the neck soft tissues will typically display thickening

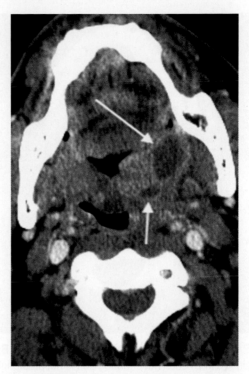

FIGURE 8.7. Tonsillar and peritonsillar abscesses. Discrete low-density, peripherally enhancing fluid collections (*arrows*) are compatible with abscesses. While the more medially located one is within the tonsil, the more laterally located collection is in the parapharyngeal region, and it is termed as a peritonsillar abscess.

of the prevertebral soft tissues. Normally, on a lateral radiograph, the prevertebral soft tissues will measure 7 mm or less in thickness at the C2 level. At the C6 level, the prevertebral soft tissues should measure 14 mm or less in a pediatric patient younger than 15 years or 22 mm or less in adults. One caveat is that pediatric patients should have the radiograph performed during inspiration with the neck extended because flexion of the neck can result in false thickening of the prevertebral soft tissues in younger patients. Ultimately, however, CT with contrast may be necessary to determine whether prevertebral soft tissue thickening is due to retropharyngeal abscess or another process. A retropharyngeal low-density fluid collection with a thick, peripherally enhancing wall indicates an abscess. In contrast, a retropharyngeal fluid collection without a recognizable wall or peripherally enhancing rim suggests a reactive effusion (Fig. 8.8). Complications of retropharyngeal abscess include airway compromise due to mass effect on the upper aerodigestive tract, mediastinitis, epidural abscess, and jugular vein thrombosis.

Epiglottitis

Inflammation of the epiglottis and surrounding soft tissues is most commonly due to a *Haemophilus influenzae*, the incidence of which has markedly decreased with vaccination. Swelling of the epiglottis places the patient's airway at risk and can be life-threatening. Patients will commonly display

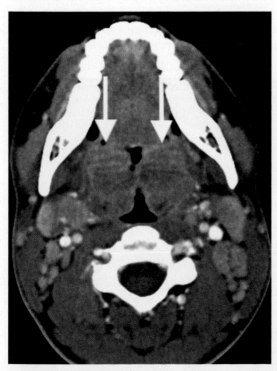

FIGURE 8.6. Enlarged bilateral palatine tonsils (*arrows*) have a "kissing" morphology and display a striated enhancement pattern typical of tonsillitis.

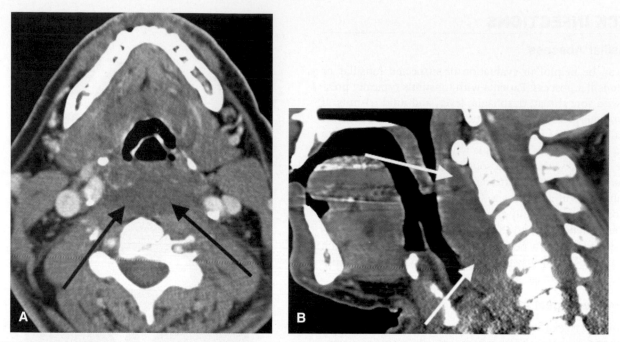

FIGURE 8.8. **Retropharyngeal effusion. A:** Axial and **B:** Sagittal CT with contrast shows a low-density retropharyngeal fluid collection (*arrows* in A and B) does not enhance and is not an organized, drainable retropharyngeal abscess.

difficulty breathing, drooling, and difficulty swallowing secretions, and they may require intubation to protect the airway in addition to therapy with steroids and antibiotics. On lateral radiographs obtained in the upright position, a thickened epiglottis is seen which has been described as having an appearance similar to a thumb. If the radiograph is not a true lateral and is obtained with obliquity, the epiglottis can take on an artificially widened shape (so-called omega epiglottis).

The presence of thickening of the aryepiglottic folds (soft tissues extending posteriorly and inferiorly from the epiglottis to the arytenoid cartilages) can be helpful in confirming epiglottitis in this scenario. When the aryepiglottic folds are abnormally thickened, they display a convex superior contour (as opposed to the typical concave orientation). CT should be reserved when the diagnosis is not clear or to exclude an abscess. Figure 8.9 illustrates epiglottitis on CT.

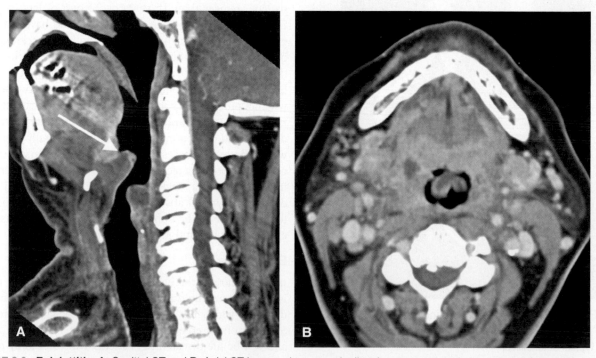

FIGURE 8.9. **Epiglottitis. A:** Sagittal CT and **B:** Axial CT images show a markedly edematous epiglottis (*arrow*) consistent with epiglottitis.

ORBITS

Infection

When patients present with a facial cellulitis about the orbit, it is essential to identify the extent of the infection and whether it is confined to the preseptal soft tissues (preseptal/periorbital cellulitis) or has spread posterior to the orbital septum (connective tissue that serves as the anterior boundary of the orbital compartment) into the orbit itself (i.e. postseptal/orbital cellulitis). Preseptal cellulitis (Fig. 8.10) is typically a mild condition that responds well to antibiotic therapy. In contrast, orbital cellulitis requires more aggressive treatment to avoid permanent loss of vision and intracranial extension of infection. In patients with proptosis, pain with eye movement, limitation of eye movements, double vision, or loss of vision, orbital cellulitis may be suspected on a clinical basis and

CT with contrast of the orbits can be helpful for confirmation. Preseptal cellulitis will be seen as soft tissue swelling and fat stranding in the periorbital region. Orbital cellulitis is diagnosed when there is fat stranding/edematous infiltration of the orbital fat (behind the orbital septum). If abscess has developed, it will appear as a well-organized, low-density, rim-enhancing fluid collection in the orbital compartment. Young children are more prone than adults to development of a subperiosteal abscess (collecting between the orbital wall and orbital periosteum). This is identified on CT as a rim-enhancing collection along the orbital wall. Most commonly, this is seen in the medial aspect of the orbit, occurring as a complication of ethmoid sinusitis (Fig. 8.11). Notably, infection can spread from the ethmoid sinus into the orbit without frank destruction of the medial orbital wall.

Optic Nerves

When clinical features suggest that vision loss is attributable to a process affecting the optic nerves, MRI without and with contrast is frequently the best imaging test. T2 hyperintense signal abnormality and/or enhancement within the optic nerves indicate an autoimmune, infectious, or granulomatous optic neuritis (Fig. 8.12) and can differentiate such a process from a tumor, such as optic glioma or an optic nerve sheath meningioma.

Thyroid Eye Disease

Thyroid ophthalmopathy, also referred to as Graves ophthalmopathy or thyroid eye disease, is an autoimmune inflammatory process involving the extraocular muscles, fat, and connective tissues. Most patients will have clinical or laboratory evidence of hyperthyroidism, although a minority will not. It results in a typically bilateral pattern of extraocular muscle enlargement with greatest predilection for the inferior rectus muscles followed by

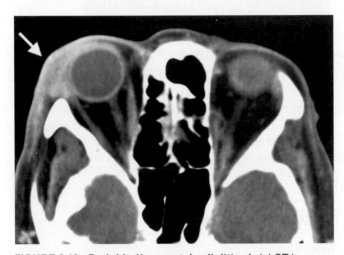

FIGURE 8.10. Periobital/preseptal cellulitis. Axial CT image shows soft tissue swelling and enhancement in the lateral right periorbital region (*arrow*) consistent with preseptal cellulitis.

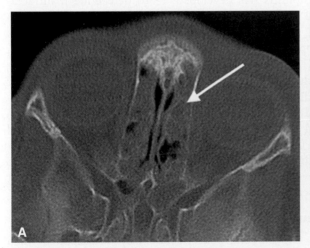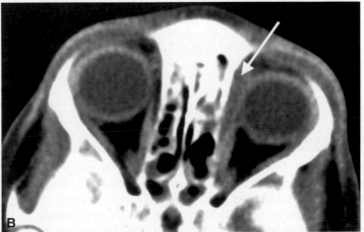

FIGURE 8.11. Orbital subperiosteal abscess. A: Axial CT shows ethmoid air cell opacification in a patient with ethmoid sinusitis (*arrow*). **B:** Subperiosteal abscess (*arrow*) which has developed between the lamina papyracea and the left medial rectus muscle.

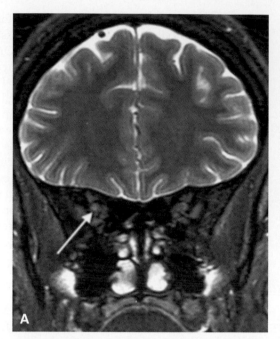
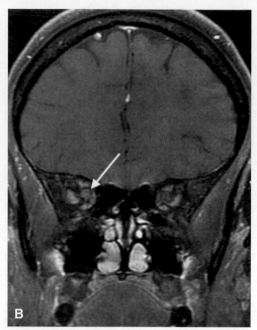

FIGURE 8.12. Optic neuritis. Coronal T2 weighted MRI **(A)** and postcontrast T1 weighted MRI **(B)** show T2 hyperintense signal and enhancement in the right optic nerve (*arrows* in A and B, respectively) in a patient with acute right optic neuritis.

the medial rectus muscles, superior rectus muscles, and lateral rectus muscles, in that order (Fig. 8.13). There is also proliferation of orbital fat in these patients which can contribute to proptosis. In severe cases, vision loss can occur due to compression of the optic nerve near the apex and surgical decompression may be necessary. Investigation can be performed with either CT or MRI of the orbits, but MRI is superior at identifying compression of the optic nerve.

TEMPORAL BONE

Infection

When characteristic clinical features are present, imaging is not necessary to make the diagnosis of mastoiditis. However, imaging can be helpful to confirm the diagnosis in atypical cases, to determine if an acute coalescent mastoiditis has developed, or to determine if intracranial complications (e.g. abscess, dural sinus thrombosis, meningitis) or extracranial complications (such as subperiosteal abscess or neck abscess) have developed. If CT shows clear mastoid air cells, mastoiditis can be excluded. Mastoid air cell opacification is a nonspecific finding that does not always correlate with acute mastoiditis. The destruction of the bony septae between mastoid air cells or of the cortex of the mastoid portion of the temporal bone is diagnostic of acute coalescent mastoiditis (Fig. 8.14), which may require mastoidectomy to prevent complications such as dural sinus thrombosis or abscess.

Trauma

On CT, temporal bone fracture may be suspected when mastoid or middle ear fluid is identified, if small foci of air

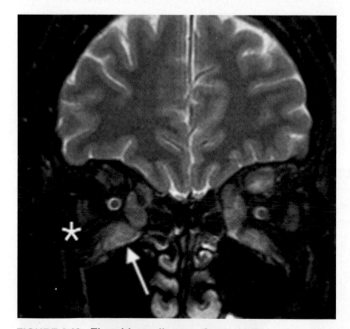

FIGURE 8.13. Thyroid eye disease. Coronal MRI is enlargement and T2 hyperintense signal abnormality involving the inferior and medial rectus muscles as the left superior rectus muscles. *Arrow* indicates the enlarged, T2 hyperintense right inferior rectus muscle compare with the much thinner right lateral rectus muscle (*asterisk*).

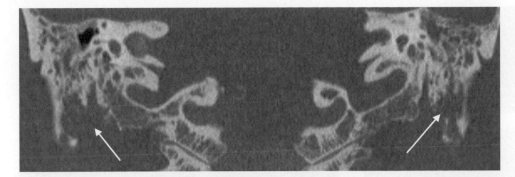

FIGURE 8.14. **Acute coalescent mastoiditis.** There is extensive opacification of mastoid air cells bilaterally. *Arrows* indicate areas of erosion of the bony cortex along the mastoid tips bilaterally.

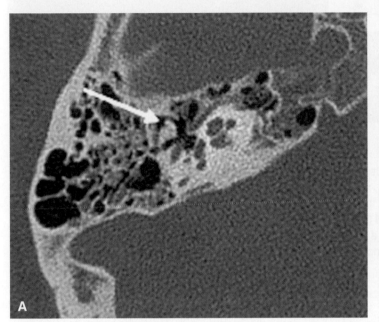

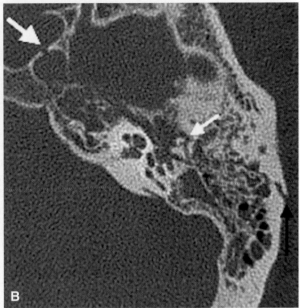

FIGURE 8.15. **Left temporal bone fracture. A:** Normal anatomy with "ice cream on cone" appearance of the right malleus and incus (*arrow*). **B:** The "ice cream" appears to have partially slid off the "cone" consistent with malleoincudal subluxation (*short white arrow*). *Black arrow* in (**B**) indicates the left temporal fracture bone line. *Large white arrow* shows the fracture line also traverses the left carotid canal. Correlation with CT angiography should be performed to exclude internal carotid artery injury.

(pneumocephalus) are seen within the cranial vault near the temporal bones, or if abnormal air is seen within the inner ear structures (cochlea, vestibular, or semicircular canals). When temporal bone fracture is suspected, dedicated CT of the temporal bones should be obtained to exclude complications such as fractures disrupting the ossicular chain (conductive hearing loss) (Fig. 8.15), fractures traversing the cochlea (sensorineural hearing loss), and fractures traversing the semicircular canals or vestibule (vertigo). Fractures traversing the canal for the facial nerve or internal auditory canal could cause facial weakness or paralysis. Fractures traversing the carotid canal or jugular foramen could result in injuries to the internal carotid artery or jugular vein which would be better evaluated with a contrast-enhanced examination (CT angiogram or CT venogram).

Cholesteatoma

Cholesteatoma is an epidermoid cyst composed of stratified squamous epithelium which enlarges over time. These are mostly acquired, occurring as a result of tympanic membrane retraction or perforation. Over time, a soft tissue mass develops within the middle ear cavity, which results in erosion of bony structures. While most cholesteatomas can be diagnosed on otoscopic examination, NCCT can assess size and extent of the lesion and diagnose bony erosion of middle ear ossicles (Fig. 8.16), the roof of the middle ear cavity (tegmen tympani), the bony covering of the facial nerve, and the bony covering of the lateral semicircular canal. MRI is useful to exclude intracranial complications such as intracranial infection or herniation of brain or meninges through a bony dehiscence in the roof of the middle ear cavity.

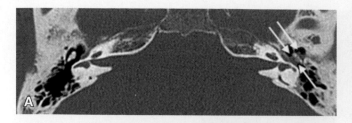

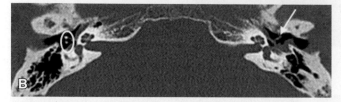

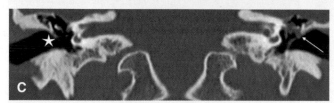

FIGURE 8.16. **Left middle ear cholesteatoma. A:** *Arrows* indicate abnormal soft tissue density surrounding the middle ear ossicles. **B:** Arrow indicates the manubrium of the malleus. Notice that the long head of the incus is absent, having been eroded by cholesteatoma. Note normal paired relationship of the encircled manubrium of the right malleus and long process of the right incus. **C:** Cholesteatoma has eroded scutum which has a blunted appearance (*arrow*). Note the normal sharp appearance of the right scutum (*star*).

Vestibular Schwannoma

The most common mass in the internal auditory canal and the second most common extra-axial intracranial mass is a vestibular schwannoma. This is a benign tumor that arises from the Schwann cells along the vestibular portion of the eighth cranial nerve. This may present as unilateral or asymmetric sensorineural hearing loss, tinnitus, or dizziness. Vestibular schwannomas may be found in the internal auditory canal and/or cerebellopontine angle cistern. When vestibular schwannoma is suspected, MRI is the modality of choice for imaging investigation. Thin section, heavily T2-weighted imaging through the internal auditory canals may display a low-signal "filling defect" within the normally very high signal internal auditory canals. Postcontrast imaging with show a nodular enhancing mass in the internal auditory canal and/ or cerebellopontine cistern (Fig. 8.17). It should be noted that not all enhancing masses in the internal auditory canals are a vestibular schwannoma. For example, facial nerve schwannomas can also occur; thin, curvilinear enhancement along the seventh and eighth cranial nerve complex can be seen with neuritis, and either curvilinear or nodular enhancement can be seen with leptomeningeal carcinomatosis.

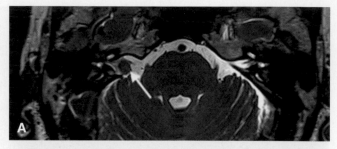

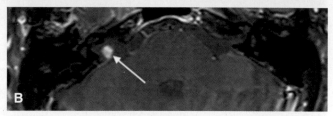

FIGURE 8.17. **Right vestibular schwannoma. A:** The *arrow* shows a mass-like "filling defect" outlined by fluid signal in the right internal auditory canal on this heavily T2-weighted image. **B:** This mass (*arrow*) demonstrates avid enhancement.

SIALADENITIS

Sialadenitis is a common indication for imaging the parotid or submandibular glands. This can be accomplished with either contrast-enhanced CT or MRI. However, in the acute care setting, CT is more commonly selected due to increased availability. Acute sialadenitis typically presents as an enlarged, prominently enhancing gland. Periglandular fat stranding is a common associated finding with acute sialadenitis (Fig. 8.18). In cases where sialadenitis is due to an obstructing stone, a dilated parotid or submandibular duct containing the calculus may be seen. When stone-associated sialadenitis is suspected, addition of a precontrast acquisition through the gland and its duct may be helpful as contrast can obscure very small calculi. Note that only a minority of sialoliths (approximately 20%) are radiopaque. These are best detected with conventional sialography, but this is a semi-invasive procedure where the parotid or submandibular duct is cannulated, iodinated contrast material is injected, and radiographs are obtained. MR sialography is an alternative technique for detection of nonradiopaque sialoliths as well as strictures involving the salivary ducts. Patients are typically given lemon juice before imaging to stimulate salivation. Heavily T2-weighted images of the glands and ducts are obtained to accentuate the fluid signal within the ductal structures. Sialoliths appear as low-signal defects within the ducts. The duct proximal to the level of obstruction may display intermitted dilatation and stricture formation (sequela of sialodochitis). In the setting of chronic sialadenitis, the gland will often be small and heterogeneous, with variable fatty infiltration.

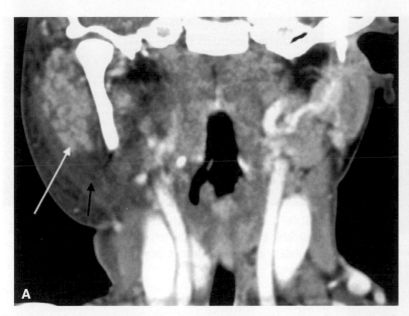
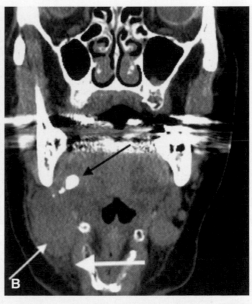

FIGURE 8.18. Acute sialadenitis. A: Acute right parotitis with enlargement and heterogeneous enhancement of the right parotid gland (*white arrow*) associated with periglandular edema and fat stranding (*black arrow*). **B:** Acute right submandibular sialadenitis with an enlarged right submandibular gland (*thin white arrow*), sialoliths along the course of the proximal right submandibular duct (*black arrow*), and periglandular edema/fat stranding (*thick white arrow*).

THYROID

The thyroid gland is best imaged initially with ultrasound (Fig. 8.19). True thyroid cysts are rare, as most thyroid cysts are nodules containing fluid. Ultrasound-guided aspiration is the treatment of choice with cytological analysis of the fluid (Fig. 8.20A, B).

Thyroid Nodules

Thyroid nodules occur in >50% of the population with thyroid cancer occurring in about 5% of thyroid nodules. While

ultrasonography is the most accurate and cost-effective method for evaluating and observing thyroid nodules, its widespread use has led to early detection of subclinical tumors and drastic increase in incidence of thyroid malignancy. Benign or malignant ultrasonographic features are listed in Table 8.1. The calcification may be either dystrophic or punctate (microcalcification); the latter is a finding suspicious for malignancy (Fig. 8.21). Additionally, extension of the nodule outside the thyroid or the presence of lobulation are findings suspicious for malignancy (Fig. 8.22). Fine-needle aspiration biopsy (FNAB) is the best way to determine whether a thyroid nodule is benign or malignant but not all thyroid nodules require biopsy.

The American College of Radiology Thyroid Imaging Reporting and Data System (ACR TI-RADS)[1] was developed to balance the benefit of identifying clinically important cancers against the risk and cost of subjecting patients with benign nodules or indolent cancers to biopsy and treatment.[1] The ultrasound features in the ACR TI-RADS are categorized as benign, minimally suspicious, moderately suspicious, or highly suspicious for malignancy. A scoring system based on all the ultrasound features in a nodule, with more suspicious features being awarded additional points to produce a TI-RADS level, which ranges from TR1 (benign) to TR5 (high suspicion of malignancy). For risk levels TR3 through TR5, a size threshold (in most cases over 1 cm) at or above which FNA is recommended. The American Thyroid Association has recommended biopsy of any 5 mm or greater nodule in high-risk patients (Table 12.5).

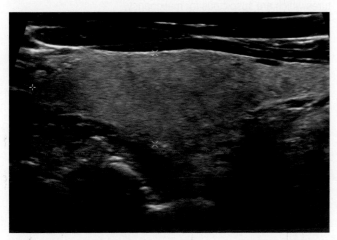

FIGURE 8.19. Normal thyroid. Sagittal view of thyroid ultrasound shows normal outline, echogenicity and consistency without any focal masses.

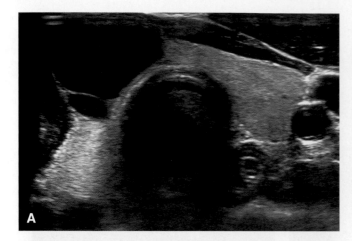

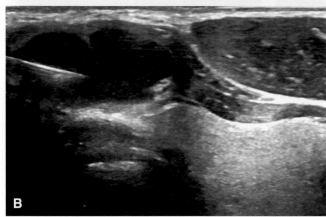

FIGURE 8.20. **Thyroid cyst. A:** Ultrasound shows a well-defined, hypoechoic lesion, with thorough transmission, consistent with a simple cyst. **B:** Ultrasound-guided needle aspiration of thyroid cyst.

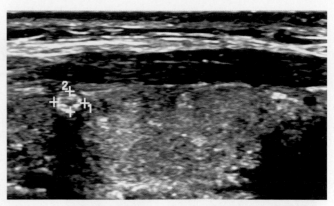

FIGURE 8.21. **Thyroid calcification.** Ultrasound showing dystrophic calcification on the left (cursors) and diffuse punctate or microcalcifications throughout the remainder of the gland.

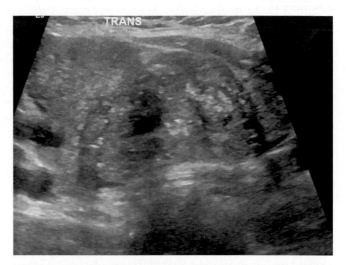

FIGURE 8.22. **Thyroid carcinoma.** Ultrasound showing diffuse punctate or microcalcifications with nodule lobulation, two features which are suspicious for malignancy.

TABLE 8.1	Ultrasonographic Features of Benign and Malignant Thyroid Nodules
Benign	**Malignancy**
Cystic or spongiform morphology	Hypoechogenicity
Smooth well-defined margin	Lobulated or irregular margins
Lack of calcifications	Microcalcifications
Large comet tail artifact	Taller than wide shape
	Solid composition with internal vascularity
	Extrathyroid extension

Thyroiditis

Thyroiditis (inflammation of the thyroid gland) can be caused by bacterial or viral infections or an autoimmune etiology (e.g. Hashimoto thyroiditis). On ultrasound, in the acute phase of thyroiditis, the thyroid gland appears enlarged and heterogeneous with increased vascularity (Fig. 8.23). In the chronic setting, the thyroid gland may become small and echogenic with decreased vascularity. Subacute thyroiditis is the most common cause of a reduced radioactive iodine uptake (RAIU) (see Chapter 10).

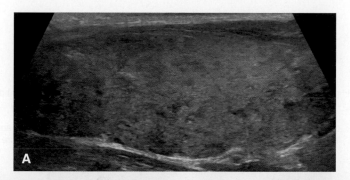

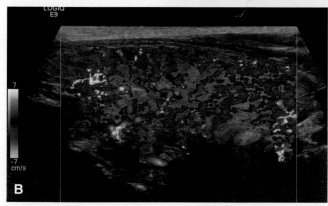

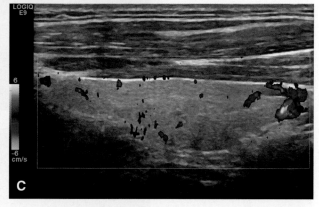

FIGURE 8.23. **Thyroiditis.** There is a diffusely heterogeneous appearance of the thyroid gland **(A)** which is also markedly hypervascular **(B)**, consistent with thyroiditis. **C:** Depicts a normal thyroid gland which is more homogeneous and shows much less color flow that the patient with thyroiditis.

CONGENITAL ANOMALIES

Craniosynostosis

There are multiple calvarial sutures which allow growth of the skull. They close in a predictable sequence (metopic, coronal, lambdoid, sagittal, in that order) once brain growth has slowed. Premature closure of a calvarial suture is referred to as craniosynostosis and results in restricted growth of the skull perpendicular to the long axis of the suture. This results in calvarial deformity as restricted growth in one suture will be compensated by increased growth along other sutures. Synostosis affecting the sagittal suture will result in a narrow, long head (scaphocephaly), whereas bilateral coronal or lambdoid synostosis results in a broad, short head (brachycephaly). Unilateral coronal or lambdoid suture synostosis will also result in an asymmetric contour of the head (plagiocephaly). Craniosynostosis may require surgical reconstruction. Craniosynostosis is readily identified by NCCT with 3-D reformats (Fig. 8.24).

Thyroglossal Duct Cyst

Thyroglossal duct cyst is a congenital abnormality that occurs in the anterior neck anywhere along the course of the thyroglossal duct from the foramen cecum at the base of the tongue to the level of the thyroid gland. Failure of involution of the duct can result in a thyroglossal duct cyst. Most are midline, but they can also occur slightly off midline, particularly when located more inferiorly, nearer to the thyroid gland. Ultrasound will typically show an anechoic or hypoechoic midline neck mass. On CT, this will appear as a low-density, nonenhancing, cystic lesion (Fig. 8.25) unless it is infected, in which case it may show a thin rim of peripheral enhancement. Presence of a solid nodular component within the mass should raise suspicion for development of papillary thyroid carcinoma within the cyst.

Fibromatosis Colli

Fibromatosis colli is a benign fibrous proliferation of the sternocleidomastoid muscle which is the most common cause of neonatal torticollis, usually identified by 6 months of age. The diagnosis is often clinically apparent, but in cases where the clinical presentation is atypical, ultrasound can be helpful in confirming the diagnosis. Ultrasound will show spindle-shaped enlargement of the sternocleidomastoid muscle, typically in the lower 1/3 of the muscle belly, which can be isoechoic, hyperechoic, or hypoechoic (Fig. 8.26).

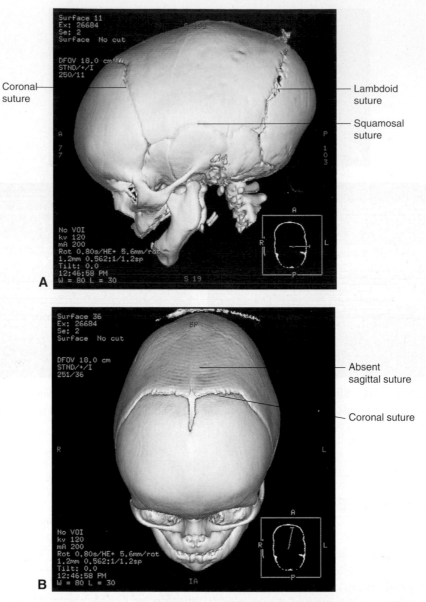

Coronal suture
Lambdoid suture
Squamosal suture
Absent sagittal suture
Coronal suture

FIGURE 8.24. Sagittal synostosis. A and B: Lateral/anterior view of the three-dimensional reconstructed CT images. The sagittal suture is fused, and the head is dolichocephalic.

FIGURE 8.25. Thyroglossal cyst. CT of the infra-hyoid neck shows a paramedian cystic mass anterior to the strap muscle.

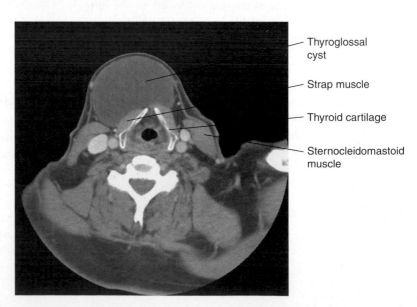

Thyroglossal cyst
Strap muscle
Thyroid cartilage
Sternocleidomastoid muscle

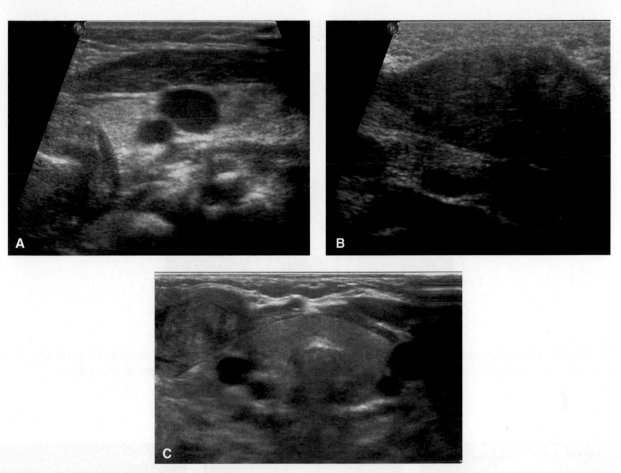

FIGURE 8.26. **Fibromatosis colli of the right sternocleidomastoid muscle (SCM) muscle. A:** Longitudinal ultrasound along the normal left SCM.Logitudinal **(B)** and transverse **(C)** images of the right SCM show a spindle-shaped enlargment of the lower one-third of the right SCM muscle.

NECK TUMORS

For patients older than 40 years with a palpable neck mass, the diagnosis overwhelmingly favors malignancy especially in those with a history of smoking. The most common malignant neck mass in an adult are nodes with metastases. Lymphadenopathy is identified by size criteria, abnormal morphology, or abnormal attenuation characteristics. Most neck lymph nodes are considered enlarged when they are over 1 cm in long axis dimension on axial imaging but submandibular and jugulodigastric lymph nodes may be up to 1.5 cm in size and lateral retropharyngeal lymph nodes should not be more than 0.8 cm in size. Normal lymph nodes typically have an elongated, ovoid morphology and a fatty hilum. Lymph nodes that become rounded or lose their fatty hilum should be viewed with suspicion. Nodes with a low-density center are suggestive of either central necrosis in a metastatic lymph node or an infected, suppurative lymph node (Fig. 8.27). Metastatic lymph nodes in patients with squamous cell carcinoma frequently display hypermetabolism on flurodeoxyglucose (FDG) PET scans (Fig. 8.28) which can be especially helpful when a metastatic lymph node does not show other morphologic or attenuation

characteristics to suggest a pathologic lymph node. In the setting of malignancy, presence of a lymph node with ill-defined margins and stranding/infiltration of the surrounding fat suggests spread of tumor beyond the lymph node capsule.

With the rise of human papillomavirus–related oral, pharyngeal, and laryngeal squamous carcinomas, awareness of malignancy is important for all adult age-groups. Contrast-enhanced neck CT or contrast-enhanced neck MRI is recommended for patients with a nonpulsatile neck mass followed by percutaneous needle biopsy. CTA or MRA are recommended for pulsatile masses to diagnose aneurysms or vascular tumors. For suspected thyroid or salivary masses ultrasound is an alternative.

Certain head and neck malignancies have a propensity to spread along nerve which can be detected on MRI as an enlarged, enhancing nerve replacing normal surrounding fat (Fig. 8.29). If the tumor surrounding the nerve has compromised the function of the nerve, denervation changes in muscles supplied by the nerve may be seen, typically showing up as high T2 signal and/or enhancement within the affected muscles in the acute denervation phase and atrophy of the muscle in the chronic phase.

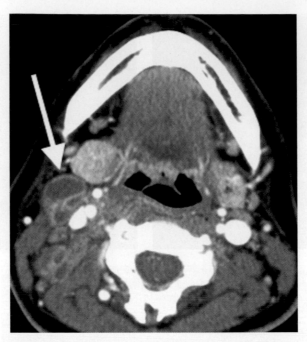

FIGURE 8.27. Tuberculous lymphadenitis. *Arrow* indicates one of several right neck lymph nodes demonstrating abnormal low density consistent with suppurative change. A centrally necrotic metastatic lymph node could have an identical appearance.

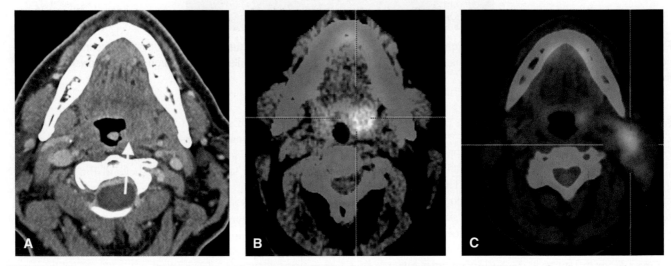

FIGURE 8.28. Squamous cell carcinoma. Left palatine tonsil with left neck metastatic lymphadenopathy. **A:** Small asymmetric mass of the left palatine tonsil (*arrow*) at the site of the primary tumor. **B and C:** 18F FDG PET-CT images demonstrating hypermetabolism at the site of the primary mass in the left palatine tonsil as well as in metastatic left neck lymph nodes.

The differential diagnosis of a neck mass in children is mostly benign, typically either congenital or inflammatory. Nevertheless, head and neck malignancies can occur in the pediatric patient, most frequently lymphoma or rhabdomyosarcoma. In a young adult, lymphoma is the most common malignancy.

While ultrasound allows differentiation of a cystic from a solid mass, it is rarely diagnostic and CT/MRI and biopsy are required. In patients with suspected thyroid cancer, CT of the neck should typically be performed *without* contrast, as this may impact imaging or treatment with radioactive iodine.

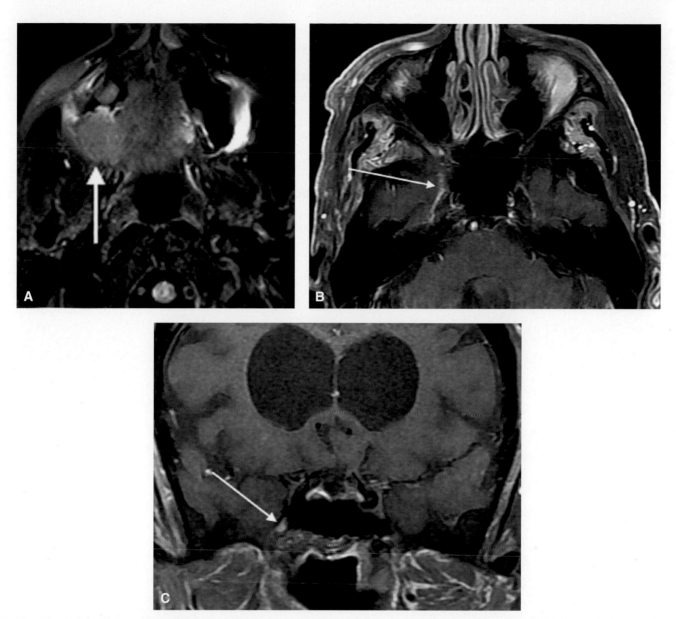

FIGURE 8.29. Maxillary carcinoma. There is perineural spread of cystic tumor along the V2 segment of the right trigeminal nerve. **A:** Arrow indicates the right maxillary sinus mass. **B and C:** *Arrows* demonstrate asymmetric enhancement in the right foramen rotundum consistent with perineural spread of tumor along the V2 segment of the right trigeminal nerve.

KEY POINTS

- CT is the imaging modality of choice in the evaluation of sinusitis. It helps identify extent of disease and important anatomic variants. MRI can be useful if intracranial extension of disease is suspected.
- Use of IV contrast material is helpful in evaluation of suspected neck infections like tonsillar abscess or retropharyngeal abscess.
- Epiglottitis is a life-threatening emergency. Look for a thumb-like appearance of the epiglottis on upright lateral radiograph and thickening of the aryepiglottic folds.

- Differentiation of preseptal/periorbital cellulitis from postseptal/orbital cellulitis has important management implications.
- MRI is the optimal modality for evaluation of the optic nerves.
- Acute coalescent mastoiditis is characterized by destruction of bony cortex and/or of the bony septae separating mastoid air cells.
- CT assessment of bony erosions is an important part of the workup/preoperative evaluation of middle ear cholesteatomas.

- Severe thyroid eye disease can lead to compression of the optic nerve at the orbital apex.
- CT is the modality of choice in evaluation of facial bone trauma.
- Either CT or MRI may be used in evaluation of sialadenitis, but MR sialography provides a noninvasive way to evaluate the submandibular or parotid ducts.
- CT is the optimal modality for assessment of craniosynostosis.
- Adult neck masses may be evaluated with either CT or MRI, but MRI is the best choice in evaluation for perineural spread of tumor.
- Although ultrasound can be used as an initial radiation sparing and relatively inexpensive assessment of a neck mass, it is rarely diagnostic. Unless the mass is suspected to be a benign lipoma or cyst, or an intrinsic thyroid lesion, CT or MRI should be considered as first-line imaging in an adult patient with a neck mass.

Further Reading

1. Harnsberger HR, Glastonbury CM, Michel MA, et al. *Diagnostic Imaging: Head and Neck.* 2nd ed. Salt Lake City: Amirsys; 2010.
2. Som PM, Curtin HD, eds. *Head and Neck Imaging.* 5th ed. St. Louis, MO: Mosby; 2011.
3. Brant WE, Helms CA, eds. *Fundamentals of Diagnostic Radiology.* 3rd ed. Philadelphia, PA: Lippincott Williams & Wilkins; 2007.

Specific Reference

1. Tessler FN, Middleton WD, Grant EG, et al. ACR thyroid imaging, reporting and data system (TI-RADS): white paper of the ACR TI-RADS Committee. *J Am Coll Radiol.* 2017;14:587-595. doi:10.1016/j.jacr.2017.01.046.

Questions

1. What is the most appropriate imaging modality to evaluate for facial bone fractures?
   a. Radiographs
   b. Ultrasound
   c. CT
   d. MRI

2. Abnormal low density within enlarged lymph nodes is suggestive of
   a. Suppurative change that can be seen with infection
   b. Central necrosis that can be seen with metastatic lymphadenopathy
   c. Both (a) and (b)

3. Administration of IV contrast for CT of the temporal bones in a patient with mastoiditis is helpful to assess for
   a. Epidural abscess
   b. Sigmoid sinus thrombosis
   c. Extracranial soft tissue abscess
   d. Concurrent middle ear infection
   e. (a), (b), and (c)
   f. None of the above

4. Branchial cleft cysts typically present in
   a. Adulthood
   b. Childhood

5. Differentiation between preseptal/periorbital cellulitis and postseptal cellulitis is important because
   a. It affects management/therapy.
   b. It determines risk of contagion.
   c. It determines the risk for developing other types of infections.

6. True or False: In patients with squamous cell carcinoma of the head and neck, regional lymph nodes under 1 cm in size are never pathologic.

7. The Onodi cell:
   A. Is the most anterior ethmoid air cell
   B. Is an important anatomical variant because of its relationship with the optic nerve, internal carotid artery, and sellar floor during sphenoid sinus surgery.
   C. Is rarely unilateral.
   D. Occurs in up to 60% of the population.

Options:
a. A and C
b. A, B, and C
c. B and D
d. All

8. True or False: Up to 20% of maxillary sinus infections may originate from underlying dental disease.

9. Acute fulminant invasive fungal sinusitis (AFIFS)
   A. Is rarely seen in immunocompetent patients.
   B. Is rapidly progressive over several weeks.
   C. Has a mortality rate of up 80%.
   D. Is best imaged using cone beam CT.

Options:
a. A and C
b. A, B, and C
c. B and D
d. All

10. Regarding vertigo and hearing loss:
    A. MRI is the modality of choice in patients with a suspected central cause for vertigo
    B. Causes of peripheral vertigo include posterior fossa neoplasms, Chiari malformation, posterior fossa infarcts, and demyelinating lesions.
    C. CT of the temporal bone provides excellent visualization of the bony labyrinth and is helpful in detecting possible causes of peripheral vertigo.
    D. CT of the temporal bone is the test of choice in patients with sensorineural deafness

Options:
a. A and C
b. A, B, and C
c. B and D
d. All

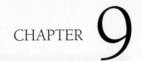

Spine Imaging

William J. Ankenbrandt, MD

Lower Back Pain and Radiculopathy

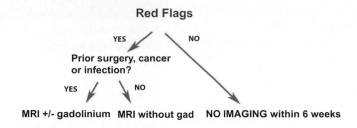

Lumbar Spine Trauma

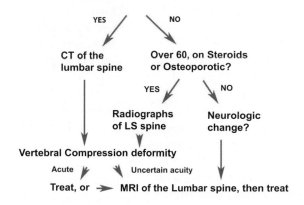

Neck and back pain are among the most common presenting symptoms in adult primary practice, the most common causes of which are included in Table 9.1. The decision to request imaging is based on the clinical scenario. This may be straightforward when dealing with a patient following high impact trauma, or it may be a challenge, as in the case of someone presenting with persistent or recurrent severe back pain without myelopathy, neurogenic claudication, or progressive motor weakness. The aim of this chapter is to describe commonly encountered conditions of the spine and their appropriate imaging.

IMAGING GUIDELINES

- Plain films have limited sensitivity and specificity for most causes of neck and back pain. They are most useful for follow-up after trauma or surgery to rule out osteoporotic compression fractures, in measuring angles in scoliosis, and to assess for fracture and joint instability.
- For high-impact trauma, CT, not plain film, is usually the first line of imaging.

TABLE 9.1 Back Pain Etiology
Congenital/Developmental
Meningocele and myelomeningocele
Syringomyelia
Transitional vertebra with pseudarthrosis
Sickle cell anemia
Scheuermann disease
Acquired
Disk herniation, annular tear
Arthritis—degenerative, rheumatoid, ankylosing spondylitis
Infection—staphylococcal, tuberculosis
Metabolic—osteoporosis, osteomalacia, Paget's disease
Neoplasm—benign and malignant primary bone tumors, metastatic
Trauma—fracture, muscle and ligament injury, spondylolysis, and spondylolisthesis
Extraspinal
Cardiovascular system—referred myocardial pain, aortic aneurysm
Gastrointestinal disease
Genitourinary system—renal and ureteral pain
Muscle strain
Psychosomatic or functional

- The spine is not just a stack of bones. Disks, cartilage, ligaments, joint capsules, and supporting muscles provide much of the stability of the spine, and these cannot be seen on plain films, only on CT or MRI.
- Contents of the spinal canal, supporting soft tissues and most bone lesions other than fractures, are best evaluated by MRI.
- In most cases where MRI is indicated, gadolinium is not needed. Gadolinium is helpful in diagnosing malignancy, infection, following diskectomy to exclude recurrent disk herniation and in the workup for myelopathy, cauda equina syndrome, and brachial or lumbar plexopathy.
- CT angiography (CTA) is used to exclude vertebral artery injury in cervical spine fractures and in patients with new stroke symptoms in the setting of significant cervical spine injury to rule out carotid or vertebral artery dissection.
- Myelography and diskography are rarely performed.

Imaging algorithms for three commonly encountered but different clinical scenarios are provided below:

1. Spine trauma in otherwise healthy adults:
   Imaging is not usually needed in patients who do not have palpable tenderness following minor trauma. However, CT is appropriate following high-impact trauma, or if there is significant pain and tenderness and in a patient who arrives in a cervical collar or is unable to be evaluated due to confusion or decreased level of consciousness:
   First line: CT
   Second line: MRI
- For patients with unstable fractures or new neurologic symptoms
- For patients with altered consciousness with severe mechanism of injury
- In children with suspected SCIWORA (see page 343) or craniocervical dissociation
   Third line: Plain films (X-rays), with flexion and extension views
- To assess for instability when
   – There is subluxation on CT but no obvious fracture
   – There is evidence of ligament injury on MRI
- To reevaluate alignment after immobilization or surgical fusion
2. Infection or tumor, suspected cord compression, myelopathy, or cauda equina syndrome:
   First line: Pre- and postgadolinium MRI
   Second line: CT—if pathologic fracture or instability, for surgical planning
   Plain films should be the initial test of choice in suspected thoracic or lumbar vertebral compression fractures after minor trauma in patients with osteoporosis. If a compression deformity is found, MRI is useful to detect vertebral edema on T1-weighted and STIR sagittal images, which confirm a recent fracture. MRI will also exclude cord

TABLE 9.2 "Red Flag" Conditions for Which Spine MRI is Indicated

History of malignancy
Unexplained weight loss
Immunosuppression
Urinary infection
IV drug use
Long-term corticosteroid use
Back pain not improved with conservative management (after 6 wk)
Significant trauma history (e.g., high-speed MVA, fall from a height)
Any back trauma or lifting injury in an osteoporotic or older individual
Urinary retention or overflow incontinence
Loss of anal sphincter tone or fecal incontinence
Saddle anesthesia
Global or progressive motor weakness or foot drop

compression or severe stenosis of the lumbar spinal canal due to significant retropulsion of bone into the spinal canal.

3. Low-back pain:

   Uncomplicated acute low-back pain (LBP) is usually a self-limited condition and does not require any imaging. Evidence suggests there is no difference in the primary outcome after 1 year for older adults who had imaging within 6 weeks after an initial visit for care for LBP compared with similar patients who did not have early imaging.

   Radiographs should be the initial study in patients with a history of low-impact trauma or osteoporosis. CT is preferred for structural bone disorders such as fracture, spondylolysis, pseudarthrosis, scoliosis, and lumbar stenosis and for the evaluation of fusion and bone graft integrity. Intradural and cord pathologies are better seen on MRI which is also recommended in those with a history of significant trauma or malignancy, infection, or cauda equina syndrome (bladder or bowel dysfunction and perianal or saddle numbness) or if symptoms are persistent or progress after 6 weeks of conservative treatment or the diagnosis is uncertain. Table 9.2 lists the **"red flag"** conditions for which MRI is indicated. MRI is also useful in evaluating post-op back surgery patients. Tc-99m-MDP bone scan has limited use as it is sensitive but relatively nonspecific for detecting infection or occult fractures. Not every patient fits into an algorithm, so exceptions can always be made depending on clinical circumstances.

PLAIN FILM INTERPRETATION

Radiographs help us understand the relationships of bones of the spinal column. Table 9.3 provides a checklist for evaluation of spine radiographs. Starting with vertebral

TABLE 9.3	Checklist for Spine Radiographs

Alignment
Must visualize seven cervical vertebrae
Vertebral body heights
Disk space heights
Bone density
Facet joints/pars interarticularis
Pedicles (lower cervical, T- and L-spine), on AP radiograph

alignment, there are 3 normal curves in the adult spine: cervical lordosis, thoracic kyphosis, and lumbar lordosis. Transient loss or reversal of these curves is most commonly due to muscle spasm following trauma.

Cervical Spine

Evaluate the craniocervical junction and to check the distance from the tip of the clivus (when visible) and the odontoid tip is less than 12 mm. The **atlantoaxial interval** is the space between the anterior arch of C1 and the odontoid process of C2, measured at the inferior aspect of the anterior atlantoaxial joint. It is normally 3 mm or less in an adult and up to 5 mm in a young child.

Evaluate the **anterior vertebral line**, **the posterior vertebral line**, and **the spinolaminar line** (Figure 9.1B). Make sure the spinolaminar line, the most posterior of the three lines, is a smooth arc without step-offs. Vertebral subluxation will offset all three lines and is better seen on oblique views. A unilateral perched or locked facet usually results in about 25% anterior subluxation and bilateral perched or locked facets cause about 50% subluxation. Articular pillar fractures can also cause subluxation. In adults, minor anterolisthesis of 2 mm or less is within normal limits. Check the anterior corners of the vertebral bodies for avulsion fractures.

On radiographs, the *open-mouth view* (Fig. 9.2B) allows visualization of the dens or odontoid process and alignment of the lateral masses of C1 with C2. Head tilt or turning can result in the lateral masses of C1 being offset *to the same degree in the same direction*, left or right. **A Jefferson fracture** (essentially a C1 burst fracture), caused by sudden axial loading from impact to the top of the head, results in lateral offset of the C1 lateral masses *in the opposite direction*.

Oblique views (Fig. 9.3) show the intervertebral foramina through which the spinal nerves pass. The cervical spine is unique in that there are synovial joints at the lateral aspect of the disks which can be affected by osteoarthritis with osteophyte formation which combined with facet joint osteophytes may result in foraminal stenosis.

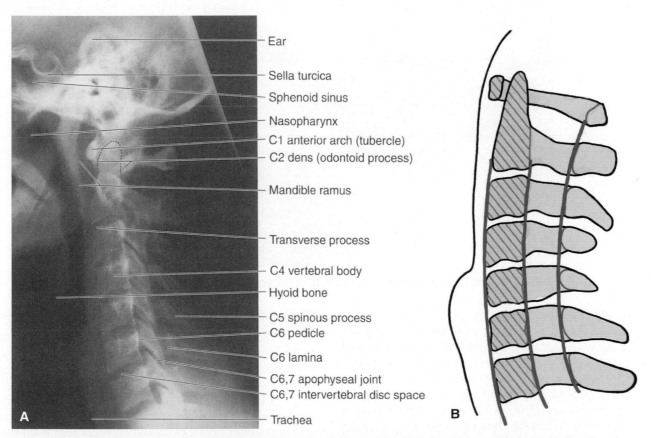

FIGURE 9.1. **Normal cervical spine. A:** Lateral view. **B:** Normal lines found on the normal lateral radiograph.

Labels for A and B:
- Ear
- Sella turcica
- Sphenoid sinus
- Nasopharynx
- C1 anterior arch (tubercle)
- C2 dens (odontoid process)
- Mandible ramus
- Transverse process
- C4 vertebral body
- Hyoid bone
- C5 spinous process
- C6 pedicle
- C6 lamina
- C6,7 apophyseal joint
- C6,7 intervertebral disc space
- Trachea

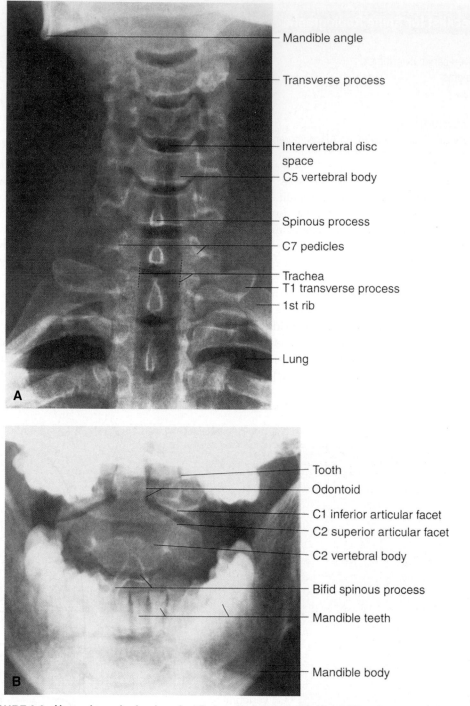

FIGURE 9.2. **Normal cervical spine. A:** AP view. **B:** Open-mouth view of the upper cervical spine.

Normally most motion occurs in the upper cervical spine. Lateral views of the neck in flexion and extension may be necessary to evaluate stability of the spine and assess for ligamentous injury following trauma. These views should only be done under supervision of a spine surgeon.

To "clear" a cervical spine in trauma patients, one must be able to clearly see all of the C7 vertebral body and the C7-T1 disk space. When the lower cervical vertebrae cannot be visualized on the lateral view, a swimmer's view is necessary (Fig. 9.4). Figure 9.5 shows normal anatomy on sagittal MRI images of the cervical spine.

Thoracic Spine

AP and lateral radiographs are standard views (Fig. 9.6), and sometimes a swimmer's view is necessary for better visualization of the upper vertebrae. Except for compression fractures and kyphoscoliosis, thoracic spine radiographs are generally low-yield studies because the rib cage adds stability and displaced fractures of the thoracic spine are not common. Pedicles should be easily seen at all thoracic levels on the AP view, unless there is severe kyphosis. Normal axial anatomy is seen pre and post myelogram in Figure 9.7.

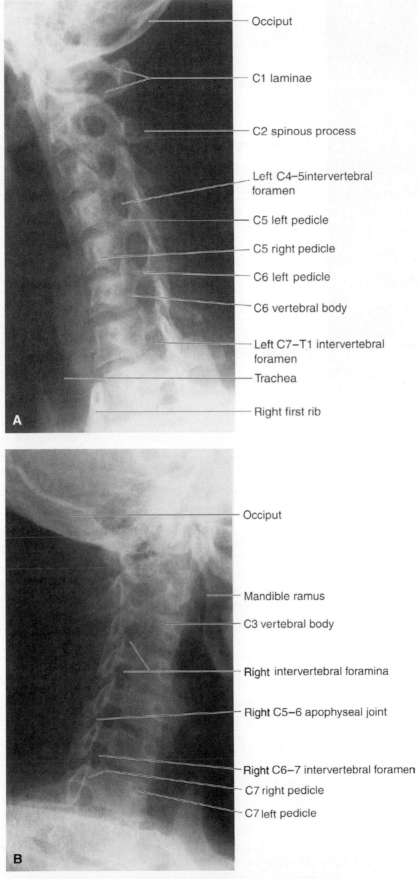

FIGURE 9.3. **Normal cervical spine.** Right **(A)** and left **(B)** oblique views.

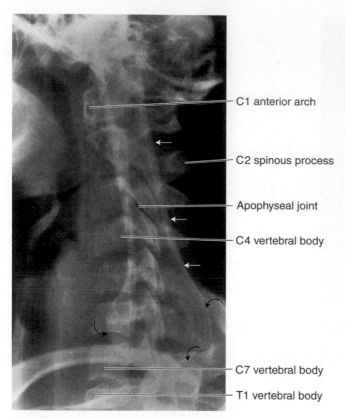

- C1 anterior arch
- C2 spinous process
- Apophyseal joint
- C4 vertebral body
- C7 vertebral body
- T1 vertebral body

FIGURE 9.4. **Normal cervical spine, swimmer's view.** The patient is usually radiographed supine with one arm, usually the left, abducted upward (*straight arrows*) alongside the head whereas the other arm is lowered. The *curved arrows* outline the humeral head.

Lumbar Spine

AP, lateral, and a coned, geometrically magnified lateral view of the lumbosacral junction are the standard views (Fig. 9.8). Approximately 15% of the population will have a **transitional lumbosacral segment**, and it may not be possible to ascertain, without thoracic spine imaging, whether there is sacralization of L5 or lumbarization of S1. To complicate the issue, the 12th ribs are frequently small, and some patients have hypoplastic L1 ribs making evaluation of the ribs an unreliable strategy for determining a vertebral level. Radiologists should explain their rationale for labeling the transitional segment L5 or S1. The standard convention is to count from the cervical spine caudally to the thoracic spine into the lumbar spine, so if thoracic spine imaging is available, there should be no ambiguity. One should not arbitrarily label a transitional lumbosacral segment as L5 or S1 before checking to see if thoracic spine imaging is available for comparison. Transitional vertebrae may become symptomatic especially after excessive back strain or when there is a **pseudarthrosis** (two bones articulating without a joint between them) as seen in Figure 9.17A. An angled anterior view may better evaluate L5 and the sacroiliac (SI)

joints (Fig. 9.9). Oblique views show the **pars interarticularis**, the narrow "isthmus" of bone connecting the superior and inferior articular processes (Fig. 9.10).

Evaluation of **bone density** is more easily done in the lumbar spine because of its greater size, and one must decide if the changes are generalized or focal. Metastases from prostate, breast, and other malignancies can result in an increased bone density or sclerotic appearance (Table 9.4).

The conus medullaris, the caudal tip of the spinal cord, normally lies between T12 and the bottom of L2, so cord compression does not occur below this level (Figs. 9.11 and 9.12). To rule out cord compression, in most cases MRI of the cervical and thoracic spine suffice, with a field of view large enough to include L2. If the cord terminates below L2, there may be cord tethering.

Figure 9.13 underscores the importance of understanding anatomic relationships of the spine. It is an oblique digital spot radiograph obtained during needle placement for **lumbar puncture**. When fluoroscopic guidance is used, the typical needle approach is **oblique interlaminar**, usually at the L2-3 level. The L2-3 level is usually chosen because it is caudal to the tip of the conus medullaris in a normal adult, and it is less likely to have spinal stenosis than the lower lumbar levels. The **interlaminar** approach is preferred over the **midline interspinous** space in people with degenerative disease.

Although largely superseded by MRI, **myelography** (intrathecal injection of water-soluble, iodinated contrast) allows visualization of spinal anatomy and was once the test of choice to evaluate for disk herniation and spinal stenosis, but it is invasive and has a 20% risk of CSF leakage through the needle track causing headache. Myelography shows the relationship of contrast-enhanced CSF in the thecal sac to adjacent bones and disks and outlines the spinal cord and cauda equina. Note how the nerve root sleeves containing the spinal nerves hug the *undersurface* of the pedicles in the lumbar spine. The L4 nerve root, for example, exits *below* the L4 pedicle (Fig. 9.14).

In addition to its multiplanar capability, MRI allows direct visualization of a wide variety of spinal structures including herniated and bulging disks, ligaments, synovial cysts, and nerve roots, which are not just inferred by mass effect on the contrast column or root sleeve cutoff with myelography. CT myelograms are still performed for the indications in Table 9.5.

Sacrum

The sacrum has an anterior concavity and is tilted posteriorly at the L5–S1 junction. The arcuate lines of the neural foramina should be smoothly curved and symmetric on the AP view (Fig. 9.15). Asymmetry may indicate fracture or tumor (Fig. 9.16). The sacroiliac (SI) joints are better imaged in a PA view as the orientation of the joint coincides with that of the divergent X-ray beam.

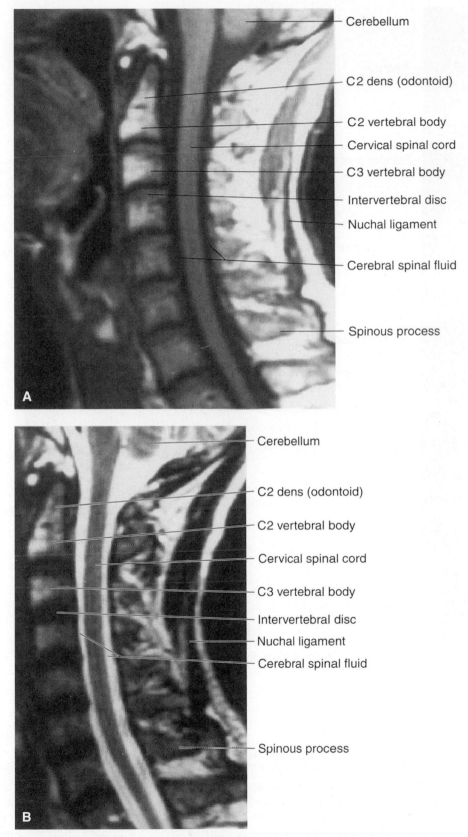

FIGURE 9.5. Normal cervical spine MRI. A: Midline sagittal T1WI. The CSF is nearly black on a T1-weighted image and white on a T2WI. The bone marrow fat appears whiter (high-intensity signal) on a T1 image than on the T2 image. **B:** Midline sagittal T2 MR image.

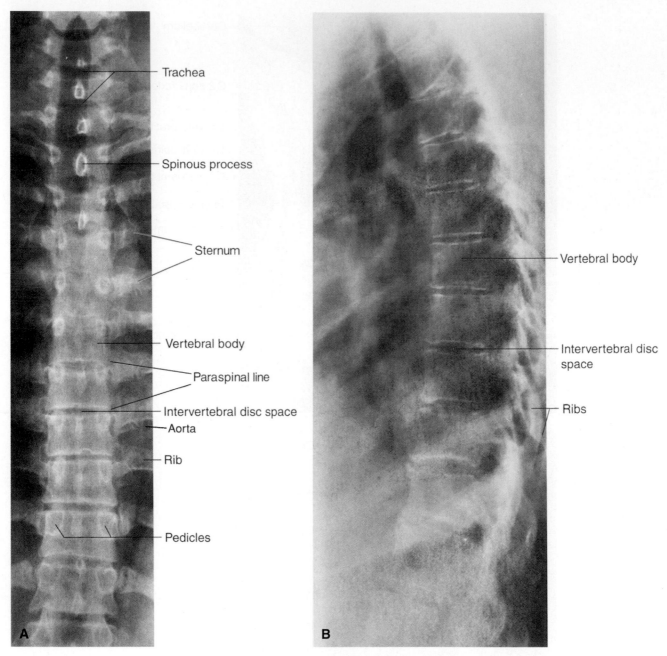

FIGURE 9.6. Normal thoracic spine. A: AP view. **B:** Lateral view.

Congenital Anomalies and Normal Variants

Accessory ossicles occurring in the cervical and lumbar spine are shown in Figure 9.17A and B. Ribs arising at C7 are called **cervical ribs** (Fig. 9.17C) and may cause symptoms due to extrinsic pressure on the brachial plexus and on the subclavian artery and vein. Less common anomalies are congenital atlantoaxial fusion and abnormal articulation between the C1 spinous process and the occiput (Fig. 9.18B).

Failure of neural tube closure in the fetus causes **neural tube defects** which can be divided into cranial anomalies (anencephaly, hydranencephaly, and encephalocele) and spinal dysraphism (spina bifida). Spina bifida occulta is common and usually asymptomatic (Fig. 9.19). Spina bifida aperta (those defects that can be seen externally) can be further divided into open and closed neural tube defects. Open tube defects are associated with neurological impairment and can be associated with Chiari II malformation,

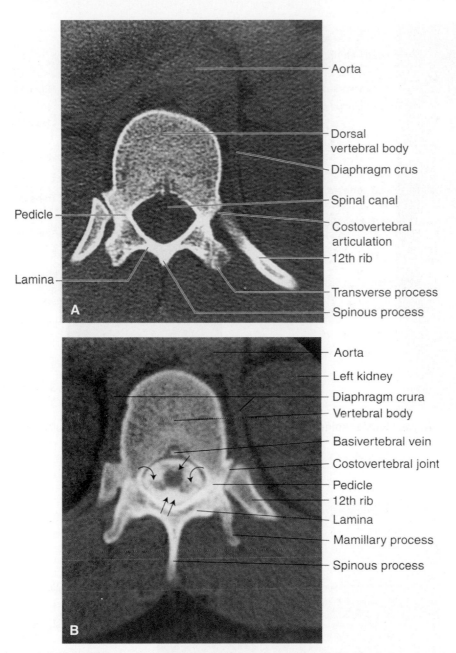

Aorta

Dorsal
vertebral body

Diaphragm crus

Spinal canal

Costovertebral
articulation

12th rib

Transverse process

Spinous process

Pedicle

Lamina

Aorta

Left kidney

Diaphragm crura
Vertebral body

Basivertebral vein

Costovertebral joint

Pedicle
12th rib

Lamina

Mamillary process

Spinous process

FIGURE 9.7. Normal thoracic spine, CT myelogram. A: Axial CT image at the T12 level. **B:** Thoracic spine axial CT image at the T12 level. Note the spinal cord (*single straight arrow*), nerve roots (*curved arrows*), and the contrast-filled subarachnoid space (*double straight arrows*).

with developmental hypoplasia of the posterior fossa with kinking of the cervicomedullary junction, tectal beaking, elongated low-lying cerebellar tonsils, and often a syrinx. A good way to remember which neural tube defects are open is that with the exception of terminal myelocystocele, if it has the prefix "myelo" it is an open defect (e.g., myelocele and myelomeningocele are open defects, whereas spina bifida occulta, meningocele, lipomeningocele and lipomyelomeningocele are closed defects).

A **meningocele** (Fig. 9.20) is a herniation of the meninges through a bone defect. In some sacral meningoceles, there is no external manifestation because they may project ventrally or expand the sacral spinal canal without protruding posteriorly. Symptoms are variable, and they are often discovered incidentally. Visceral innervation of the bladder and/or rectum may be affected, as well as sensory and motor nerves.

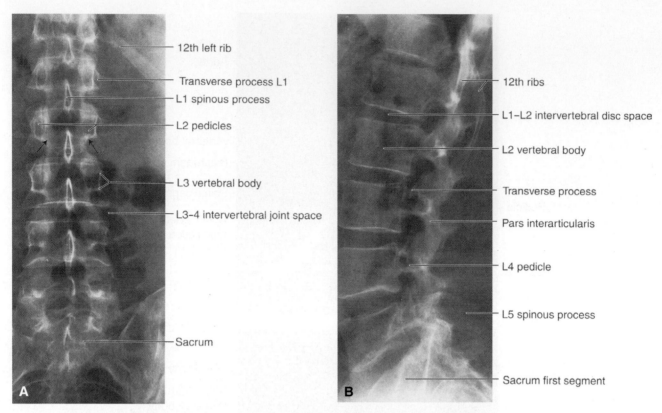

FIGURE 9.8. **Normal lumbar spine** AP **(A)** and lateral **(B)** views. Note the pars interarticularis region (*arrows*).

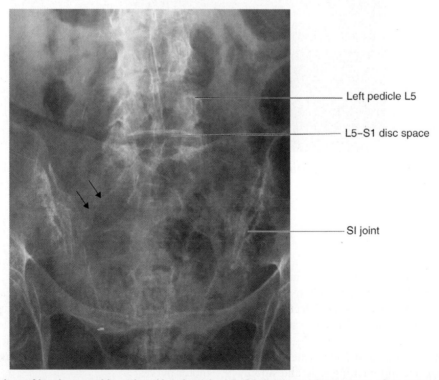

FIGURE 9.9. **Angled view of lumbosacral junction.** Note how the L5–S1 disk is now better seen when compared with Figure 9.8. The facets are prominent due to arthritis. Note the arcuate line of the right S1 anterior sacral foramen (*small straight arrows*).

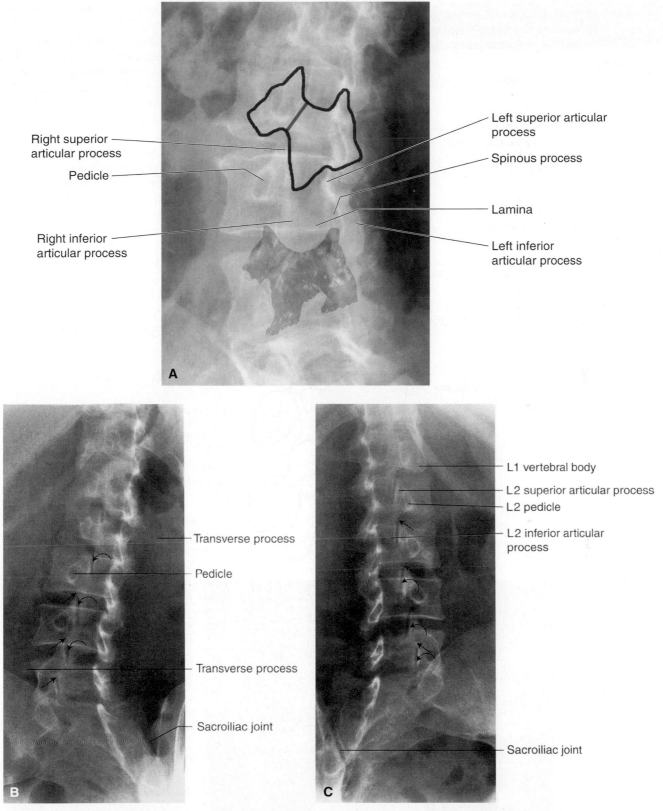

FIGURE 9.10. Normal pars interarticularis. A: Visible "Scotty dog" on oblique lumbar spine radiographs. **B and C:** Lumbar spine right **(B)** and left **(C)** oblique radiographs. Note the normal pars interarticularis or the neck of the Scotty dog (*straight arrows*) and the normal apophyseal (facet) joints between the superior and inferior articular processes (*curved arrows*).

TABLE 9.4	Common Causes of Increased and Decreased Bone Density

Decreased
Osteopenia, including osteoporosis
Osteomalacia
Osteomyelitis
Osteolytic metastases, multiple myeloma, and plasmacytoma
Rheumatoid arthritis, ankylosing spondylitis

Increased
Bone infarcts
Bone island
Callus formation–fractures
End plate sclerosis–disk degeneration
Fibrous dysplasia
Lymphoma
Osteoblastic metastases (prostate and breast)
Osteopetrosis
Paget's disease
Primary bone tumors (5% of multiple myeloma)

Scoliosis is defined as a lateral curvature of the spine in the coronal plane and is initially imaged with standing radiographs to measure the angle of curvature and pelvic tilt and to exclude vertebral segmentation anomalies, such as hemivertebra (Fig. 9.21). A **hemivertebra** is a vertebra with a body, pedicle, lamina, transverse process, and (if thoracic) a corresponding rib on only one side to absence of a contralateral ossification center. Most cases of scoliosis are idiopathic occurring in almost 5% of the population and are more common and severe in girls. Fig. 9.22 Approximately 10% of scoliosis cases are congenital with associated vertebral segmentation and rib abnormalities as shown in Fig. 9.23. A discrepancy in leg length caused by trauma, infection, or other injury to the physis may present as scoliosis. Painful scoliosis is most commonly due to a vertebral osteoid osteoma with the scoliosis typically concave toward the abnormality because of muscle spasm. Scoliosis due to neurofibromatosis may progress to severe angulation and subluxation with cord damage. Additional radiological features of neurofibromatosis include posterior vertebral body scalloping and enlarged neural foramina due to dural ectasia.

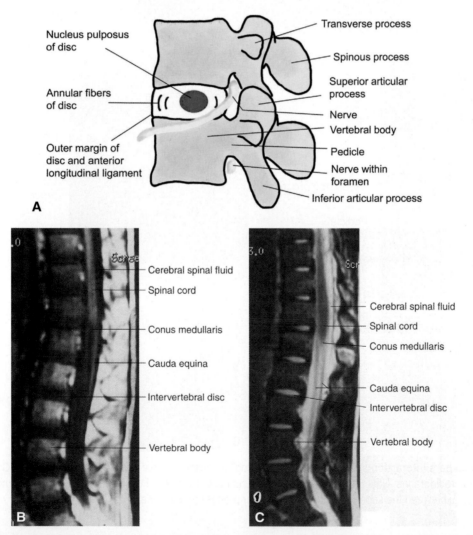

FIGURE 9.11. Normal lumbar spine MRI. A: Lateral diagram. **B:** Lumbar spine T1 **(B)** and T2 **(C)** sagittal MRI. The intervertebral disk is brighter on T2WI.

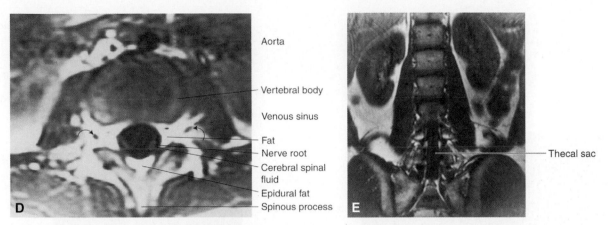

FIGURE 9.11. *(Continued)* **D:** Axial T1WI with nerve roots (*curved arrows*). **E:** T1 coronal plane passes through the upper lumbar vertebral bodies and the lower lumbar neural sac. (Illustration by CBoles Art.)

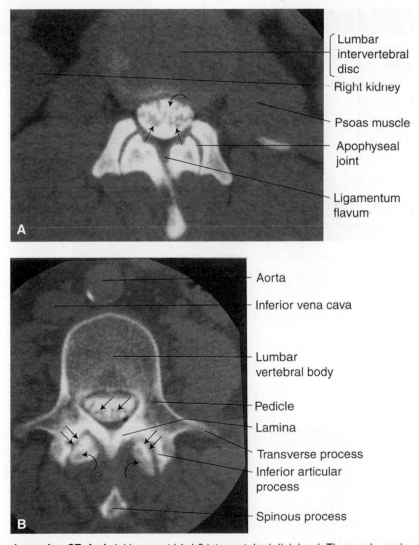

FIGURE 9.12. **Normal lumbar spine CT. A:** Axial image at L1–L2 intervertebral disk level. The cauda equina (*straight arrow*) is surrounded by iodinated contrast in the subarachnoid space CSF (*curved arrow*). **B:** Axial CT image through a lumbar vertebra. The *single straight arrows* indicate multiple nerve roots. The inferior articular processes of the vertebra articulate with the superior articular processes (*curved arrows*) from the vertebra below to form the apophyseal joints (*double straight arrows*).

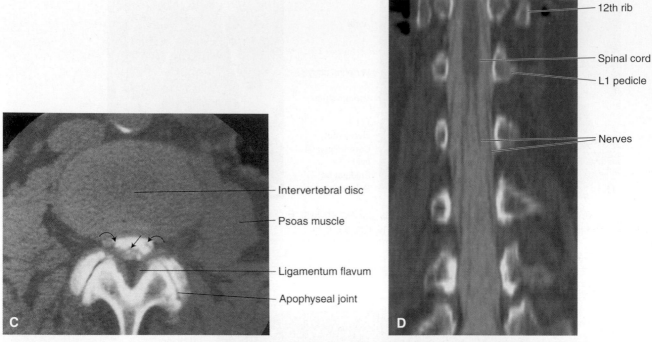

- 12th rib
- Spinal cord
- L1 pedicle
- Nerves
- Intervertebral disc
- Psoas muscle
- Ligamentum flavum
- Apophyseal joint

FIGURE 9.12. *(Continued)* **C:** Axial CT image through a lumbar intervertebral disk. The nerve roots (*straight arrow*) in the posterior aspect of the subarachnoid space whereas the *curved arrows* indicate nerve roots about to exit through the neural foramina. **D:** Coronal reformat of CT myelogram. This has a similar appearance to the conventional myelogram radiographs and shows the conus quite well.

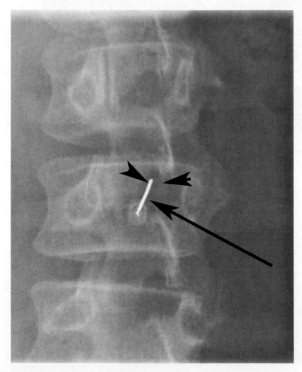

FIGURE 9.13. Fluoroscopically guided lumbar puncture. Oblique digital spot radiograph obtained during needle placement. Note spinal needle (*arrow*) is aligned with interlaminar space (*arrowheads*).

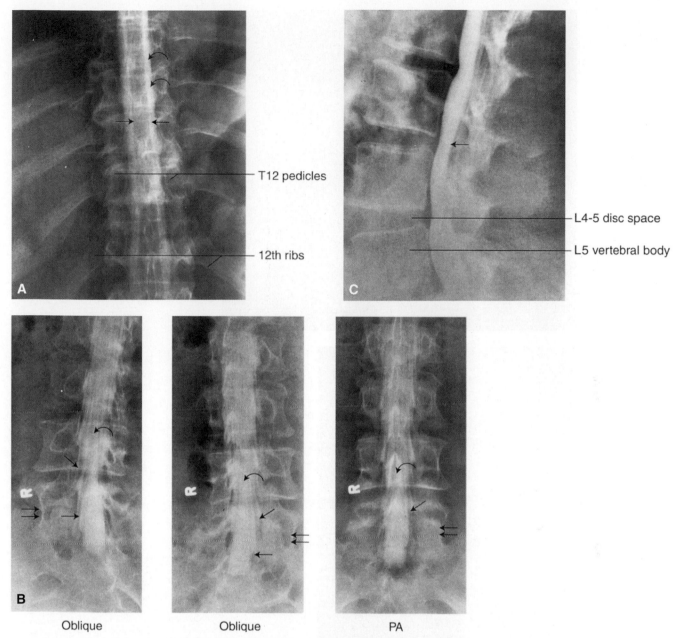

FIGURE 9.14. **Normal thoracic spine myelogram. A:** The spinal cord (between the *straight arrows*) is outlined by the injected subarachnoid contrast (*curved arrows*). **B:** Oblique and PA myelogram views. The *single straight arrows* show the nerve roots exiting the spinal canal surrounded by contrast. The *curved arrows* indicate nerve roots within the thecal sac. The *double straight arrows* indicate the L5 lumbar vertebra. **C:** Lateral view myelogram containing contrast (*arrow*).

TABLE 9.5	Indications for CT Myelography
Patients with pacemakers	
Post-op spine (ferromagnetic artifact)	
Metallic foreign bodies near vital structures	
Implantable devices	
Claustrophobia	
Suspected spinal dural leak	
Suspected spinal cord block	

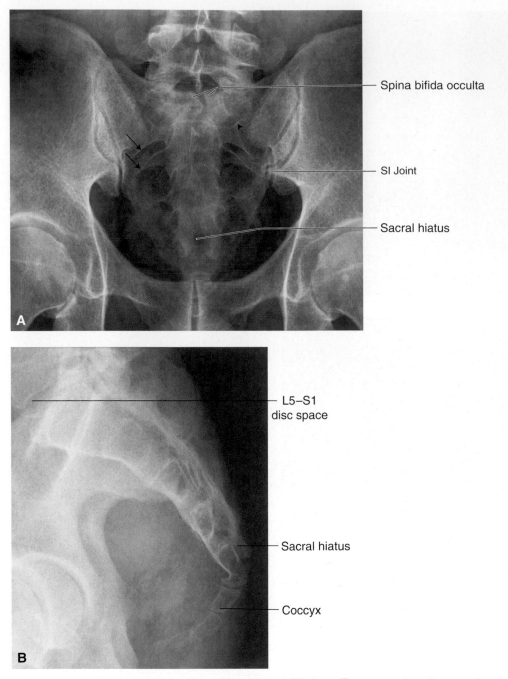

Spina bifida occulta

SI Joint

Sacral hiatus

L5–S1
disc space

Sacral hiatus

Coccyx

FIGURE 9.15. Normal sacrum AP with cephalad angulation **(A)** and lateral **(B)** views. The *arrows* show the normal arcuate lines of the anterior openings of the sacral neural foramina. The *arrowheads* demarcate the posterior margin of the left S1 foramen. There is a spina bifida occulta. The sacral hiatus represents the termination of the posterior elements at the midline.

When scoliosis is severe or rapidly progressive, it may be treated by fusion of a long segment of the spine (Fig. 9.24). Degenerative lumbar scoliosis (Fig. 9.25) may occur due to compression deformities, degenerative disk changes, leg length discrepancies, and lumbosacral anomalies including compression fractures.

As the sacroiliac joints are included in AP radiographs of the spine, it is important to be aware of an incidental finding of osteitis condensans ilii (Fig. 9.26).

FIGURE 9.16. **Symphysis pubis diastasis.** AP pelvis. Widening of the normal close relationship of the left and right pubic bones (*white arrow*) is due to trauma in this patient. Note the irregular margin from fracture of the right side of the symphysis. The disrupted arcuate line of the left sacral foramen (*black arrow*) should be identified as the pelvic "ring" typically breaks in at least two places.

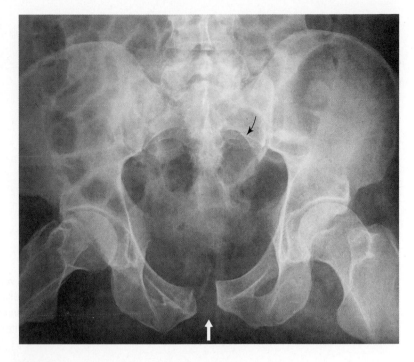

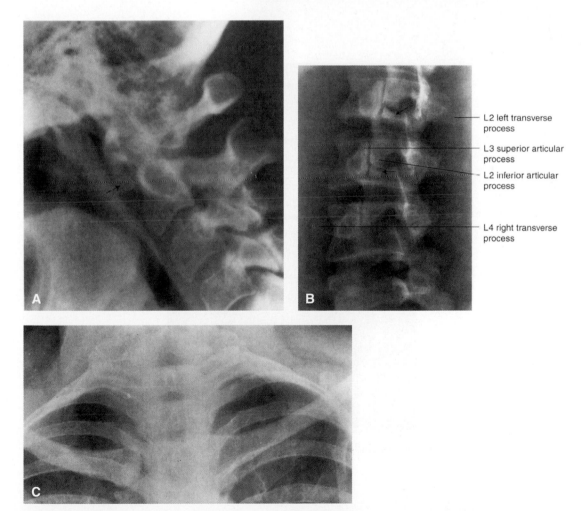

FIGURE 9.17. **Normal variants:** Accessory ossicles. **A:** Cervical spine, lateral view. An accessory ossicle (*arrow*) is located inferior to the anterior arch of the atlas or C1. **B:** Oblique view of lumbar spine with accessory ossicles (*arrows*). **C:** Bilateral cervical ribs. Lower cervical and upper thoracic spine AP view. The small bilateral ribs (*arrows*) arise from the C7 vertebra.

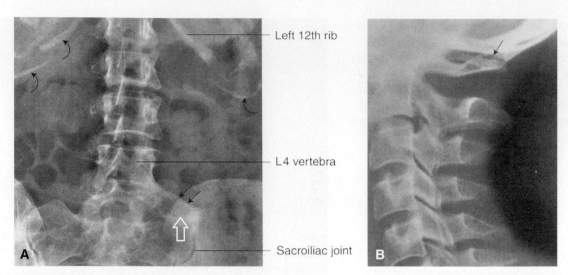

Left 12th rib

L4 vertebra

Sacroiliac joint

FIGURE 9.18. Normal variants. A: Partial sacralization of L5. L5 articulates with the left sacrum in an anomalous fashion (*straight arrows*). There is a pseudarthrosis (*white arrow*). Transitional vertebrae are described when L5 begins to look like a part of the sacrum or the sacrum begins to look like a part of the lumbar spine. The *curved arrows* indicate calcifications within the cartilaginous portion of the ribs. **B:** Partial occipitalization of C1. The spinous process of C1 articulates with the occiput (*arrow*).

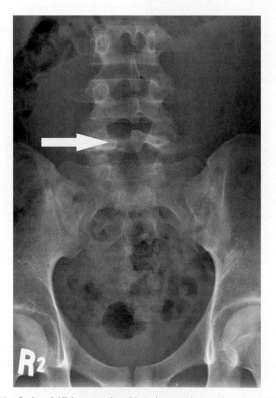

FIGURE 9.19. Spina bifida occulta. Note incomplete spinous process (*arrow*).

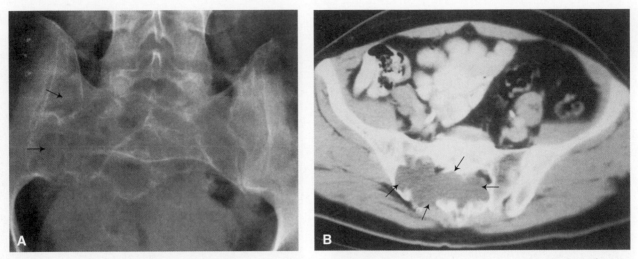

FIGURE 9.20. Sacral meningocele. A: Pelvis AP view. The lucent areas in the sacrum (*arrows*) indicate the bone defect secondary to the meningocele mass. **B:** Axial CT pelvis. The full extent of the meningocele mass within the sacrum is indicated by the *arrows*.

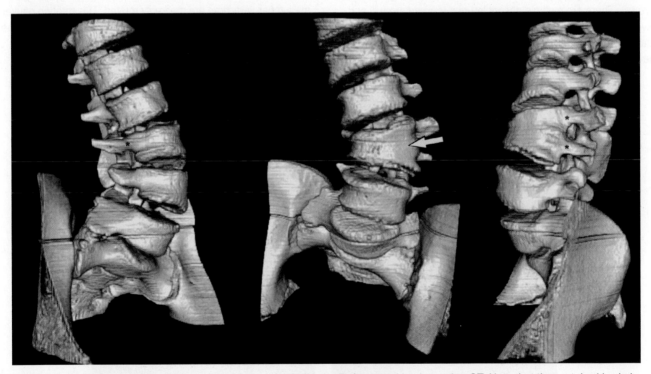

FIGURE 9.21. Midlumbar hemivertebra and fusion with scoliosis. Reformatted lumbar spine CT. Note that the vertebral body is shorter on the left side (patient's right) and has only one pedicle (*asterisk*) while the right side (patient's left) is taller due to fusion of a hemivertebra with the adjacent normal (*arrow*) and has two pedicles (*asterisk*). The line through L5 and the iliac bones is a movement artifact.

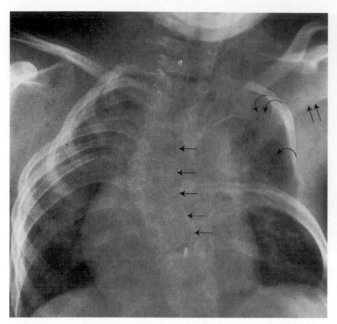

FIGURE 9.22. Congenital scoliosis. Thoracic spine AP view. The thoracic spine is convex to the right, and the thorax is markedly asymmetric. Underlying the scoliosis are multiple hemivertebrae or incompletely formed thoracic vertebrae (*single straight arrows*). There are multiple absent left ribs (*curved arrows*) and several left upper ribs are fused (*double curved arrows*). The left scapula is abnormally elevated (*double straight arrows*). Typically, the foramen magnum and sacrum usually form a vertical line.

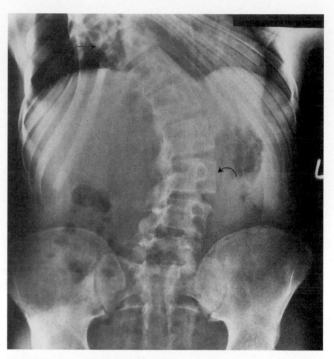

FIGURE 9.23. Idiopathic scoliosis. Thoracolumbar spine AP view. The lumbar spine is convex to the left (*curved arrow*), and the lumbar vertebrae are markedly rotated. This rotation causes the lumbar vertebra to appear oblique. The lower thoracic spine is convex to the right (*straight arrow*) resulting in asymmetry.

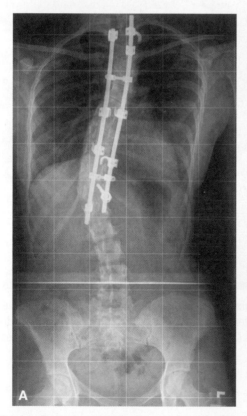

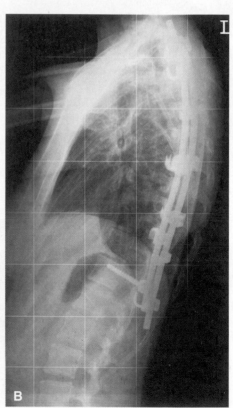

FIGURE 9.24. Posterior spinal fusion construct for idiopathic scoliosis AP **(A)** and lateral **(B)** thoracolumbar views.

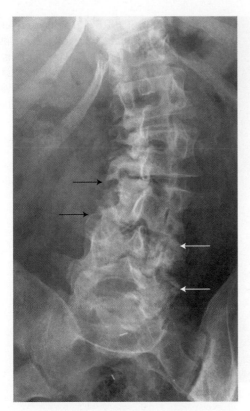

FIGURE 9.25. Scoliosis due to degenerative change. Lumbar spine AP view. The lumbar spine is convex to the left. The disks are asymmetrically narrowed, and there is prominent osteoarthritis of facets (*black and white arrows*), which is worse on the concave sides (*black arrows*).

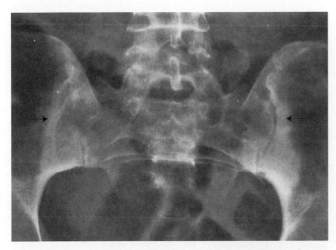

FIGURE 9.26. Osteitis condensans ilii. Pelvis AP radiograph. The bilateral, sharply marginated sclerotic areas (*arrows*) characteristically involve the iliac sides of the SI joints and spare the sacrum. This is a benign condition usually found in women in their childbearing years. This may be an incidental finding.

TRAUMA

Cervical Spine Injuries

Most cervical spine fractures occur between C5 and C7, followed by C1 and C2. Injuries can be caused by hyperflexion or hyperextension (Table 9.6). CT is the preferred method for initial evaluation. Radiographs are also helpful for evaluation of alignment.

The junction of C7 and T1 is an important site of potential injury between the mobile cervical vertebra and the fixed thoracic vertebral column (Fig. 9.27A and B). A swimmer's view should be obtained when the C7-T1 level is obscured by prominent shoulder and upper thoracic soft tissues. CT of the cervical spine must include the C7-T1 level.

Dens or odontoid process fractures are relatively common in the older patients, representing about 15% of all cervical spine fractures (C2 fractures of all types account for about 20%). They may result from hyperflexion or hyperextension injuries and are best diagnosed on CT. The lateral and open-mouth radiographic views can identify odontoid fractures, but detection can be challenging if there is no displacement, as overlapping structures can obscure the fracture line. **Type II** odontoid fractures are transverse fractures through the base of the odontoid and are unstable, often requiring surgical fusion, as up to 50% of type II fractures will have nonunion when treated with external immobilization in a hard collar or halo, increasing to more than 70% in patients older than 65 years (Fig. 9.28). **Type III** odontoid fractures extend into the body of C2 and are often asymmetrical and obliquely-oriented. They are treated with external stabilization in a hard collar, with around 85% rate of fusion. **Type I** fractures are the least common and involve the odontoid tip. They are typically stable, and they are treated with external immobilization in a hard collar with low rates of nonunion.

TABLE 9.6	Cervical Spine Injuries

Flexion
Anterior wedge fracture
Unilateral or bilateral locked or perched facet
Ligament disruption
Odontoid process fracture
Flexion teardrop fracture

Extension
Hangman fracture
Ligament disruption
Odontoid process fracture
Spinous process fracture
Extension avulsion fracture (aka "extension teardrop" fracture)

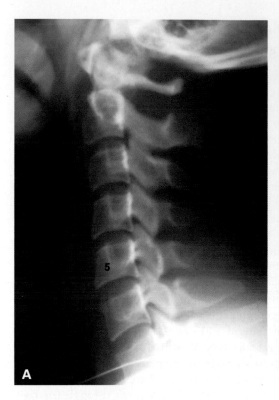

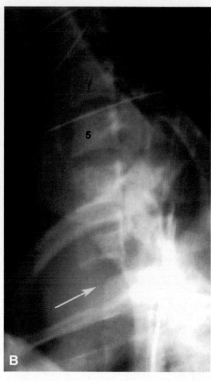

FIGURE 9.27. **Bilateral jumped facets at the C7–T1. A:** Lateral cervical spine radiograph is normal, but the inferior margin of C7 is not visualized. **B:** Swimmer's view in the same patient reveals the abnormality (*arrow*).

A **hangman's** or bipedicular C2 fracture (Fig. 9.29) occurs after forced extension with high-impact trauma to the anterior head or face and includes an oblique coronally oriented fracture through the C2 body. Surprisingly, except in the case of hanging, where there is the added abrupt distraction force, there is often no significant spinal cord injury. These fractures are unstable and require surgical fusion.

A **flexion teardrop fracture** (Fig. 9.30) is a severe injury that results following acute hyperflexion usually at C5 or C6. The teardrop shape describes the resulting compression at the anterior-inferior aspect of the vertebral body and retropulsion of the posterior cortex and is always associated with injury to the interspinous and supraspinous ligaments and often the ligamentum flavum. The fluid-sensitive MRI

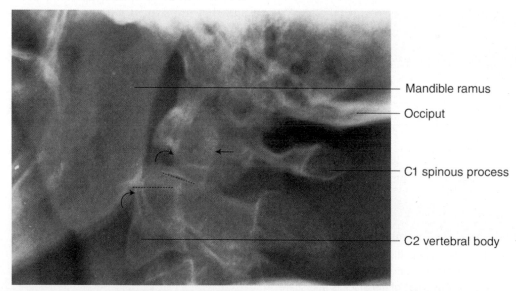

Mandible ramus
Occiput
C1 spinous process
C2 vertebral body

FIGURE 9.28. **Displaced fracture through the caudad or inferior aspect of the dens or odontoid process of C2.** Cervical spine lateral view. The fracture edges are indicated by the *dotted lines*, and the dens (*arrow*) is displaced posteriorly approximately 8 mm. The *curved arrows* indicate the amount of displacement of the dens.

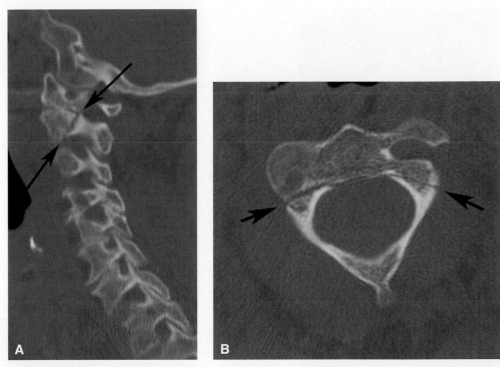

FIGURE 9.29. Hangman's fracture. A: Extension of fracture through the base of the pedicle (*arrows*). **B:** Axial view of the fracture (*arrows*).

sequences, the T2-weighted, inversion recovery fat suppression sequence (STIR) is used to exclude spinal cord contusion and edema while gradient echo images are the most sensitive for detecting spinal cord hemorrhage. A hemorrhagic cord contusion predicts poor outcome and is associated with permanent neurologic deficit.

Locked and perched facet joints also occur following neck hyperflexion, often with a twisting component. A locked facet occurs when the inferior articular process of the upper vertebra moves forward over the superior articular process of the lower vertebra, with anterior subluxation of the upper vertebra (25% subluxation if unilateral, 50% if bilateral). If the inferior articular process gets stuck on top of, rather than in front of, the superior articular process, it is called a **perched facet**. Articular pillar fractures are similar and unstable as there is usually posterior and sometimes anterior ligament disruption with cord injury (Figs. 9.27 and 9.31A). Oblique plain films or reconstructed CT images best demonstrate facet joint disruptions (Fig. 9.31B and C). **Unilateral locked facet** (Fig. 9.31C) has a rotational component and may not have as extensive ligament disruption. A **unilateral facet fracture–dislocation** may be difficult to diagnose as there is less displacement as a result of the fracture of the superior articular process (Fig. 9.32A-C). The distance between the spinolaminar line and the articular pillars, **the laminar distance**, will abruptly change at the level of unilateral perched or locked facet and may have a classic "bow tie" appearance.

Extension avulsion fractures result from acute hyperextension of the neck, usually from high-velocity impact to the face, resulting in anterior longitudinal ligament injury and bone avulsion. Radiographs and CT show an anterior-inferior corner fracture separated from a cervical vertebral body. MRI will confirm disruption of the anterior longitudinal ligament, with the avulsed fragment of bone still attached to the ligament.

Occasionally hyperflexion injury results in ligamentous injury without fracture (Fig. 9.33A-D). As with other hyperflexion injuries, this has the potential to cause spinal instability and cord injury and is best demonstrated on MRI which show edema in the injured ligaments and adjacent tissues. Flexion/extension radiographs can assess stability in patients with suspected ligament injury without demonstrable fracture but should only be done under the supervision of a spine surgeon.

Injury to the **brachial plexus** most commonly occurs when the head is forced away from the shoulder, resulting in stretching of the nerves. This mechanism occurs in football injuries and motorcycle accidents, where the helmet protects the head, but it and the shoulder pads increase the length of the lever arm. The spectrum of nerve injury ranges from mild neuropraxia and axonotmesis (minor and major stretch injuries) to neurotmesis (complete disruption of the nerve) as nerve rootlets are avulsed from the spinal cord. MRI is the optimal modality and the most sensitive ancillary finding in **nerve root avulsion** is posterior paraspinal muscle which most often

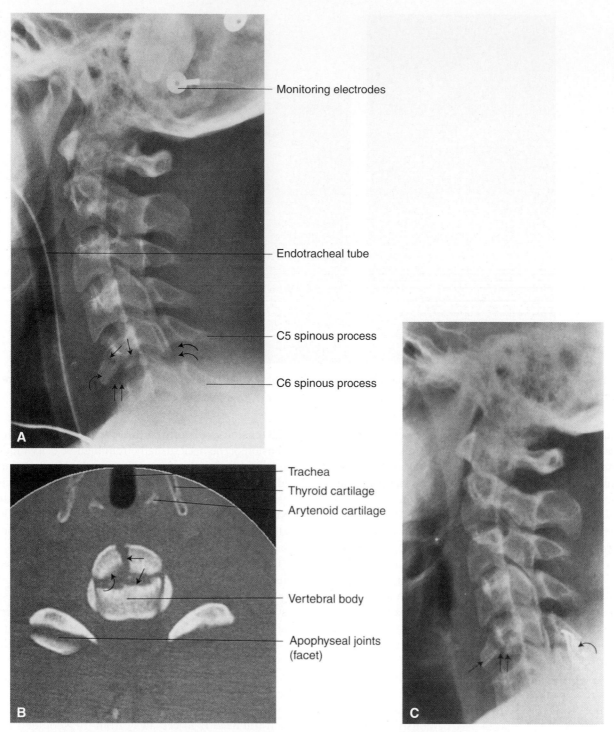

FIGURE 9.30. C5 flexion teardrop fracture. A: Lateral cervical spine view. There is mild compression anteriorly of the C5 vertebral body secondary to the comminuted fracture (*single straight arrows*), and there is mild separation of the fracture fragments. The major fracture fragment has a teardrop shape (*single curved arrow*) due to avulsion at the site of the anterior longitudinal ligament. The hyperflexion injury has resulted in a mild separation or fanning of the space between the C5 and C6 spinous processes secondary to ligamentous disruption (*double curved arrows*). The disrupted ligaments are the interspinal and supraspinal ligaments and possibly the ligamentum flavum. Also, the hyperflexion injury created minimal widening of the C5–C6 disk space (*double straight arrows*) and mild angulation of the spine at this level with minimal retrolisthesis of C5 on C6. This type of cervical fracture usually is associated with severe cord injury as the vertebral body is often displaced posteriorly into the spinal canal. **B:** Cervical spine axial CT image of the C5 vertebra. The comminuted fracture lines in the vertebral body are separated or distracted (*straight arrows*), and the anterior fracture fragments are displaced anteriorly approximately 3 mm (*curved arrow*). **C:** Lateral cervical spine radiograph. Posterior wire stabilization of the cervical spine between the spinous processes of C5 and C6 vertebrae (*curved arrow*). The major fracture fragment (*single straight arrow*) is in good alignment with mild offset of the fragments (*double straight arrows*), but no attempt is made to reduce this fragment.

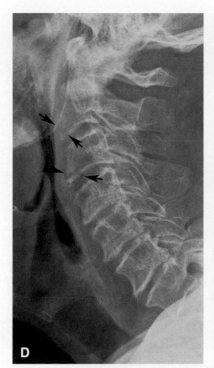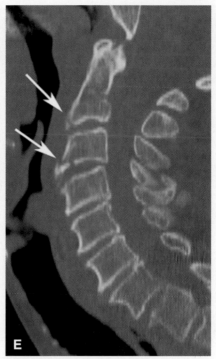

FIGURE 9.30. *(Continued)* **D and E:** Lateral view **(D)** and sagittal CT **(E)** of a fracture with less severe consequences, the extension avulsion fracture. Note that the anterior-inferior corners of C2 and C3 have been avulsed, a finding more conspicuous on CT than on the radiographs (*black arrows* on the radiograph; *white arrows* on the CT).

involves the multifidus muscle, a segmentally innervated obliquely oriented muscle immediately adjacent to the lamina.

Craniocervical Dissociation and SCIWORA in Children

In infants and young children, injury to the neuroaxis can occur in the absence of an obvious cervical spine fracture. In craniocervical dissociation, the ligament disruption allows the head to become dislocated from the cervical spine and the only clue on radiographs may be an increased distance from the tip of the clivus to the odontoid tip.

In patients with **spinal cord injury without radiographic abnormality** (SCIWORA), there can be significant spinal cord injury with little or no abnormality on imaging because the distensible ligaments and joint capsules have essentially snapped back in place immediately following trauma. Because the supporting structures of the vertebral column are much more distensible than the spinal cord, the cord can be injured without radiographic or CT evidence and MRI is necessary cord hemorrhage or edema.

Thoracic Spine Fractures

Most fractures of the thoracic spine occur in the lower thoracic region and are usually wedge-shaped compression fractures, involving the anterior column (anterior

two-thirds of the vertebral body), often with no canal compromise (Fig. 9.34). MRI is also useful in patients with multiple compression fractures of different or uncertain durations. The STIR sequence on MRI, detects bone marrow edema, indicating an acute or subacute nature of the fracture.

Lumbar Spine Fractures

Fractures of the lumbar spine are diagnosed on radiography, but CT should be the first imaging modality in patients with a high-impact mechanism of injury (Fig. 9.35A-E). MRI is useful for assessing the effect of the fracture fragments on the thecal sac and to exclude other abnormalities such as traumatic disk herniation or spinal epidural hematoma.

Epidural hematomas can occur anywhere in the spine either spontaneously or following a fracture. It is a neurosurgical emergency in terms of priority of neurological examination. Treatment of the hematoma depends on the presence of cord compression or cauda equina compression. Most hematomas will have markedly decreased signal on gradient echo sequences, but the caveat is that in the hyperacute phase (within about 6 hours of onset), there is still intracellular deoxyhemoglobin, which is diamagnetic rather than paramagnetic making it indistinguishable for less "urgent" epidural masses (Fig. 9.36A and B).

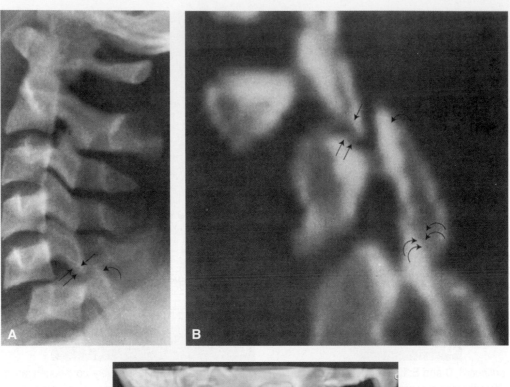

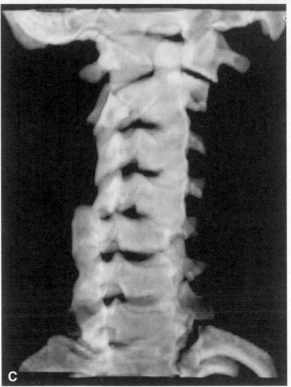

FIGURE 9.31. Bilateral locked facets at C5–C6. A: Cervical spine lateral view. The inferior articular process of C5 (*straight arrow*) is anterior to the superior articular process of C6 (*curved arrow*). The *double straight arrows* indicate the expected normal position for the superior articular process of the C6 vertebra. There is obvious anterior dislocation of the C5 vertebral body referable to the C6 vertebral body. No fractures are apparent. **B:** Cervical spine sagittal reconstructed CT image on a different patient. Bilateral facet lock. The inferior articular processes of the upper vertebra (*straight arrow*) are in an abnormal relationship with the superior articular process of the lower vertebra (*single curved arrow*). The *double straight arrows* indicate the expected normal location of the displaced superior articular process. A normal apophyseal articulation is visible at the level below (*double curved arrows*). **C:** Reformatted CT image in another patient with unilateral locked facets at C4–C5 on the right. Note how the upper cervical spine appears rotated while the lower cervical spine is straight. The left facets are not shown on this 3D reformat but were normal.

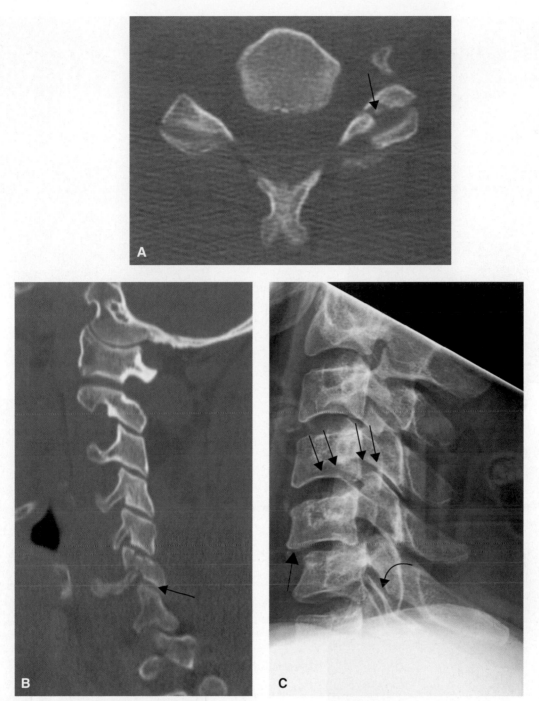

FIGURE 9.32. **Unilateral facet fracture–dislocation. A:** Axial CT image through C6. The left inferior articular process of C5 is broken, but not displaced (*arrow*). **B:** Sagittal reformatted image from the CT scan through the facet joints. There is a normal relationship between the fractured C5 inferior articular process and the superior articular process of C6 (*arrow*). **C:** Lateral view of the cervical spine obtained 1 month later demonstrated mild anterolisthesis of C5 on C6 (*single straight arrow*) and rotation of the articular pillar above this level. Note the overlap of bilateral facets below (*curved arrow*) compared with the "bow tie" appearance above with this (*double straight arrows*).

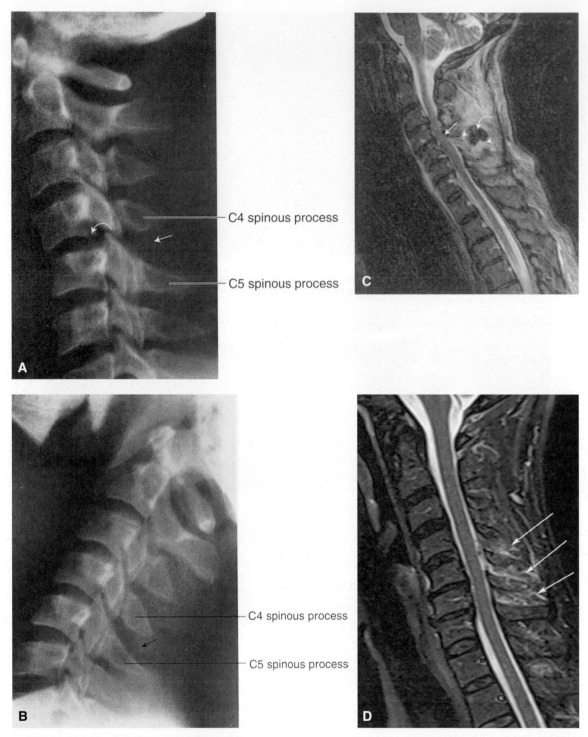

FIGURE 9.33. Posterior ligament disruption at C4–C5. A: Cervical spine cross-table lateral view with the patient supine. There is an increase in the height of the interspinous space between the C4–C5 spinous processes (*straight arrow*) secondary to disruption of the C4–C5 interspinal ligament, supraspinal ligament, and possibly the ligamentum flavum. Compare the height of the C4–C5 interspinous space with those above and below. The mild anterior spondylolisthesis of C4 referable to C5 (*curved arrow*) has resulted in mild kyphotic angulation and reverse of the normal cervical curvature at the C4 level. **B:** Cervical spine extension lateral view in the same patient. When the cervical spine is in full extension, the C4–C5 interspinous space (*straight arrow*) is now normal in height and the anterolisthesis of C4 on C5 has been reduced. **C:** Sagittal T2-weighted MRI cervical spine in a different patient. Ligament disruption without fracture. There is widening between the spinous processes at C5–C6 and increased signal (white) (*arrowheads*). Disruption of the ligamentum flavum (*straight arrow*) is also seen. A hematoma (*curved arrow*) can be seen, which would explain persistent widening of spinous processes on radiographs. There is a small amount of high signal within the posterior aspect of the C5–C6 disk which may suggest a disk injury as well. **D:** Sagittal STIR image in another patient with less severe injury involving spinous process fracture. Note the interspinous ligament edema (*arrows*).

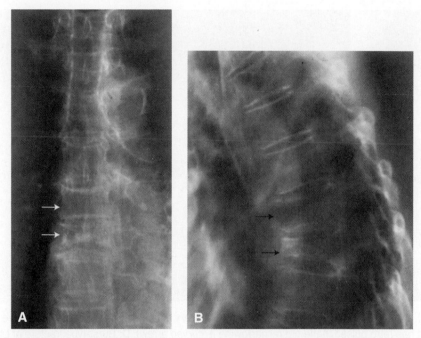

FIGURE 9.34. **Osteoporotic compression fractures.** Thoracic spine AP **(A)** and lateral **(B)** views show compression fractures of the T7 and T8 vertebral bodies (*white arrows* on the AP and *black arrows* on the lateral radiograph). Notice the overall decreased density (osteopenia) of all the osseous structures due to osteoporosis. Patients with multiple myeloma have a similar appearance. Figure 9.60.

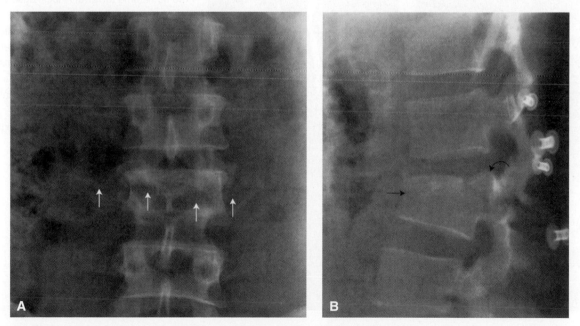

FIGURE 9.35. **Chance (seat belt) fracture of the L3 vertebrae lumbar spine** AP **(A)** and lateral **(B)** radiographs. There is a transverse fracture through the L3 vertebra involving the vertebral body and the transverse processes (*straight arrows*). A large fracture fragment arising posteriorly from the vertebral body is displaced into the neural canal (*curved arrow*) **(B)**). The L3 vertebral body height is less than normal secondary to compression or collapse caused by the fracture. There is mild dorsal angulation of the spine at the level of the L3 fracture.

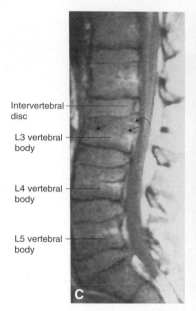

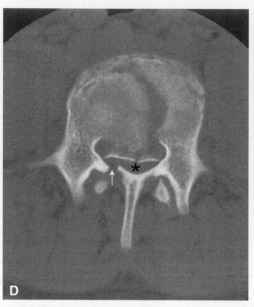

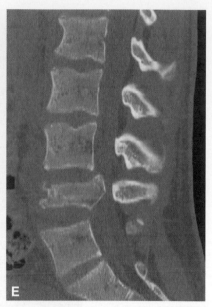

Intervertebral disc
L3 vertebral body
L4 vertebral body
L5 vertebral body

FIGURE 9.35. *(Continued)* **C:** MRI sagittal. The L3 vertebral body is mildly compressed secondary to a fracture (*straight arrows*), and a posterior fracture fragment has retro pulsed in the neural narrowing it (*curved arrow*). **D:** Burst-type fracture of L5. Axial CT image. There is severe compromise of the neural canal (*asterisk*) with resultant neurologic injury. The *straight arrow* demonstrates a fracture of the right lamina in this unstable fracture. **E:** Sagittal reformatted CT image on the same patient shows the severity of the canal compromise compared to the other levels.

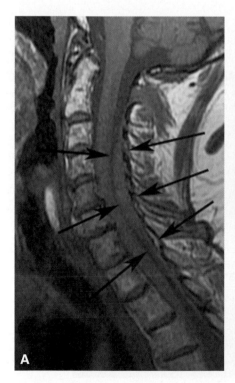

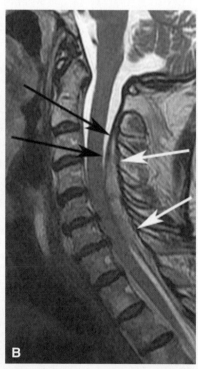

FIGURE 9.36. Hyperacute spontaneous spinal epidural hematoma. A: Sagittal T1. The hematoma (*arrows*) is isointense to the spinal cord, which is compressed and displaced anteriorly. B: Sagittal T2. The hematoma (*white arrows*) elevates the posterior dura (*black arrows*). Note that the hematoma is predominantly hyperintense on T2, indicating presence of intracellular oxyhemoglobin. Deoxyhemoglobin, which would be very dark on T2, takes several hours to form, so this hematoma is hyperacute.

Sacral Fractures

Sacral fractures may occur following major pelvic trauma but may occur as **insufficiency** fractures after minor trauma in osteoporotic patients. When the fracture extends into the sacral foramina, the arcuate lines are disrupted (Fig. 9.37A-E) but the fracture may be missed on plain films due to osteoporosis. On a Tc 99 MDP bone scan, a sacral insufficiency fracture appears as a classic "Honda sign" for the car-maker's trademark letter H since the fractures typically involve both sacral ala symmetrically and extend through the midline at approximately S2 or S3. On MRI, the fracture is most conspicuous on STIR images.

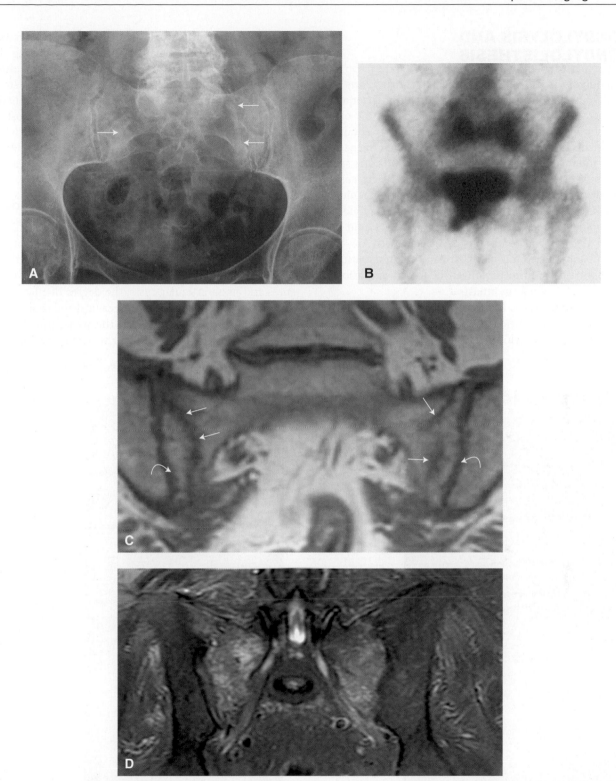

FIGURE 9.37. **Insufficiency fractures of the sacrum. A:** Sacrum AP view. There is vertically oriented subtle sclerosis involving each sacral ala (*arrows*). Compare this to the normal sacrum in Figure 9.14A and B: A bone scan shows increased activity to confirm the presence of fractures. The vertical orientation of each side with a horizontal connecting fracture line has been termed the "Honda sign." **C:** Coronal T1WI MR pelvis shows characteristic sacral insufficiency fracture lines that are easily seen (*straight arrows*), but should not be confused with the normal SI joints (*curved arrows*). **D:** Coronal T2-weighted MRI in another patient. Increased signal (bright) due to edema and blood is present in both sacral ala. A discrete fracture line is not always seen depending on the acuity of fracture or degree of healing.

SPONDYLOLYSIS AND SPONDYLOLISTHESIS

Spondylolysis is a defect in the pars interarticularis, the isthmus of bone connecting the superior and inferior articular processes of a vertebra and occurs in about 5% of the population. On oblique views, the posterior vertebral elements form a radiographic "Scotty dog" of which the neck is the pars interarticularis, which if disrupted, indicates spondylolysis or a pars defect (Fig. 9.10A). This defect can be acquired or congenital. If acquired, rather than congenital, it is thought to be the result of a stress fracture. Spondylolysis is readily identifiable on oblique radiographs, CT, and MRI (Fig. 9.38A-E) and is commonly associated with low-back pain, probably due to muscle spasm and occurs in athletes whose activities require prolonged or forced extension of the lower back, such as gymnasts.

Spondylolisthesis is the forward movement of a vertebra relative to the one below. Forward movement is possible due to bilateral spondylolysis defects (see above) or severe facet joint arthropathy. When associated with bilateral spondylolysis, there is usually no central stenosis (Fig. 9.39A and B). When the pars interarticularis are intact, there is often significant central spinal stenosis. Foraminal stenosis occurs in both types of spondylolisthesis. Spondylolisthesis with spondylolysis occurs in the lumbar spine, most commonly at L5-S1. Spondylolisthesis without spondylolysis occurs most commonly at L4-L5 (Fig. 9.40). If additional disk herniation is present, it is more commonly at an adjacent level than at the level of spondylolisthesis.

Degenerative Disk Disease and Spinal Stenosis

MRI is the imaging test of choice for degenerative disk disease and spinal stenosis because it not only demonstrates the contour abnormalities of bulging and herniated disks, it also shows osteophytes, thickened ligaments, annular fissures and juxta-articular cysts, the degree of effacement of CSF in the thecal sac, and in the cervical and thoracic spine shows the degree of flattening of the spinal cord. MRI also allows diagnosis of cord edema or scarring (myelomalacia).

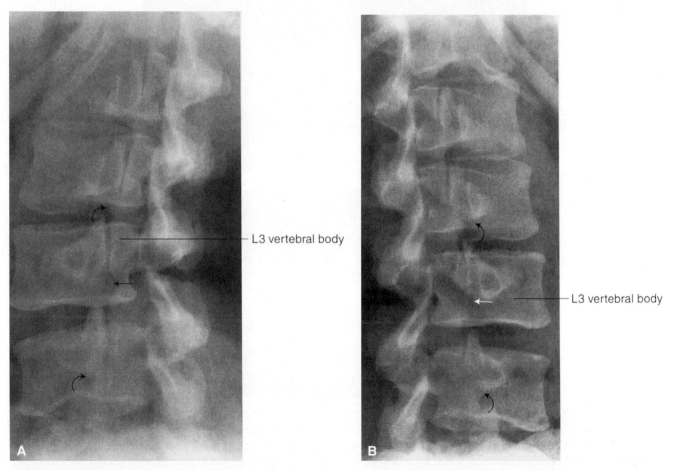

L3 vertebral body

L3 vertebral body

FIGURE 9.38. Bilateral spondylolysis of L3. A and B: Lumbar spine right **(A)** and left oblique **(B)** view (*straight arrows*). The pars interarticularis or the Scotty dog neck is disrupted bilaterally in the L3 vertebra (*black and white straight arrows*) compared with the normal appearing L2 and L4 vertebrae bilaterally (*curved arrows*).

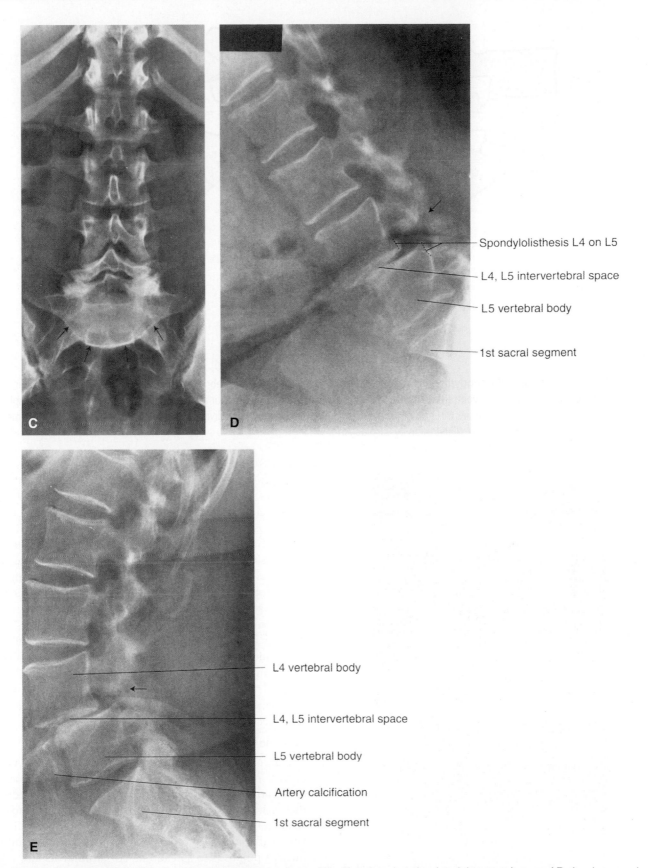

FIGURE 9.38. *(Continued)* **C:** AP view. The classical appearance of the Napoleon hat sign *(straight arrows)* on an AP view is secondary to severe (grade 4) spondylolisthesis of L5 referable to S1. The Napoleon hat is inverted or upside down. **D and E:** Lumbar spine lateral flexion **(D)** and extension **(E)** views. This patient has L4 spondylolysis and grade 2 anterior spondylolisthesis of the L4 vertebral body referable to the L5 vertebral body. The spondylolysis defect in the pars interarticularis *(straight arrows)* can be visualized on both views but the flexion radiograph opens the defect for easier visibility.

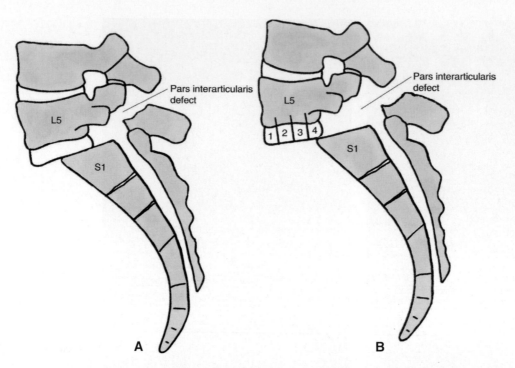

FIGURE 9.39. Comparison of spondylolysis and spondylolisthesis. A: The L5 vertebral body, pedicles, and superior articular processes have moved forward (or ventral) relative to the sacrum. However, the L5 inferior articular processes, laminae, and the spinous process remain in their normal position. **B:** Grading of spondylolisthesis. The sacrum is divided into fourths and the forward movement of L5 is simply given a grade of 1 to 4. (Illustration by CBoles Art.)

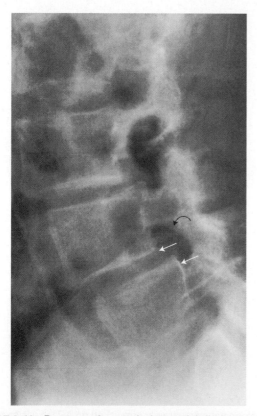

FIGURE 9.40. Degenerative grade 1 spondylolisthesis of L4 on L5. Lumbar spine lateral view. The pars interarticularis is intact (*curved arrow*). The spondylolisthesis (*straight arrows*) is secondary to the degenerative changes in the intervertebral space and the apophyseal joints that allow L4 to move forward relative to L5.

With the widespread use of MRI, it is evident that patients frequently have asymptomatic vertebral disk bulges and protrusions but not extrusions which are rarely asymptomatic. Spinal stenosis in general, not accounting for grade of stenosis, is not more prevalent in patients with back pain compared to asymptomatic controls. Severe lumbar spinal stenosis can cause neurogenic claudication, but until it becomes severe, stenosis may not cause back pain.

A common pitfall to avoid is "treating the image." MRI predicts favorable surgical outcome only when the imaging and clinical presentations are concordant (e.g., a disk extrusion compressing the L5 nerve root in a patient with foot drop). There is a lot of extraneous information on an MRI scan which needs to be filtered when approaching management decisions.

Terminology

The normal disk structures are shown in Figure 9.11A. The current nomenclature is as follows: Normal drying out or **desiccation** of disks occurs with aging, resulting in reduced disk space height. The term disk **degeneration** refers to desiccation, loss of disk height, and/or diffuse loss of integrity of the annulus fibrosis in all directions, allowing the nucleus pulposus to spread out. An **annular fissure** refers to disruption in the fibers of the disk (Fig. 9.41A). A **bulging disk** means that 50% or more of the circumference of the disk is mildly displaced outward relative to the margin of the vertebral body (Fig. 9.41). Lumbar disk herniation occurs most commonly at the L4–L5 and L5–S1 levels.

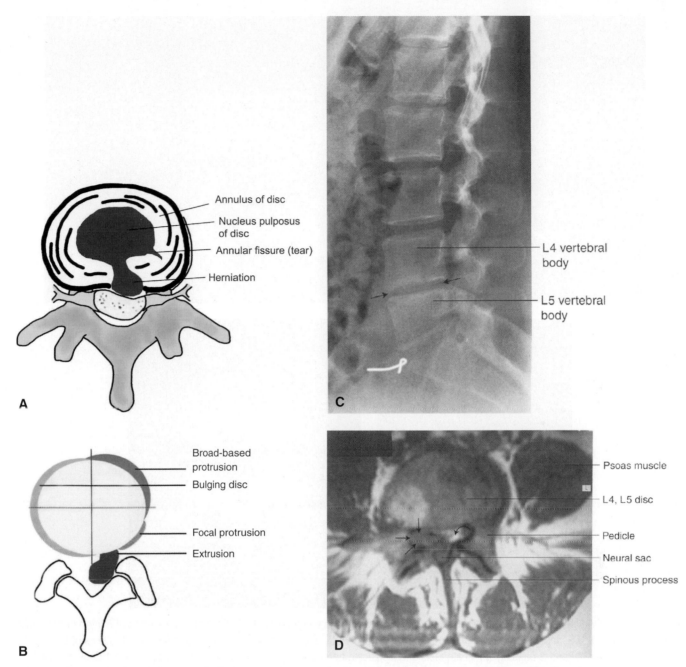

FIGURE 9.41. A and B: Lumbar intervertebral disk anatomy illustration. **A:** Disk herniation is a tear extending from the nucleus pulposus through all the layers of the annulus fibrosis. There may be compression of the thecal sac and nerve roots. Smaller annular fissures tears may cause pain. **B:** Lumbar intervertebral disk illustration. The disk has been divided into quadrants (blue lines) based on percentage of disk involved. **C:** Lumbar spine lateral radiographs. Herniated L4–L5 intervertebral disk. The patient is a 30-year-old woman with bilateral leg weakness greater on the right than the left. There is significant narrowing of the L4–L5 intervertebral disk space (*arrows*) suggesting disk disease at this level. Again, the disk is not visible on the radiograph. The disk space narrowing is more apparent when you compare the L4–L5 disk space to the other lumbar disk spaces. Normally the L4–L5 disk space height is greater than the other lumbar spine disk spaces. **D:** Lumbar spine axial T1 MRI in the same patient showing a large disk is extruded posterolaterally to the right (*straight arrows*), creating extrinsic pressure on the neural sac and obliterating the epidural fat on the right side. Normal epidural fat is present on the left (*curved arrow*).

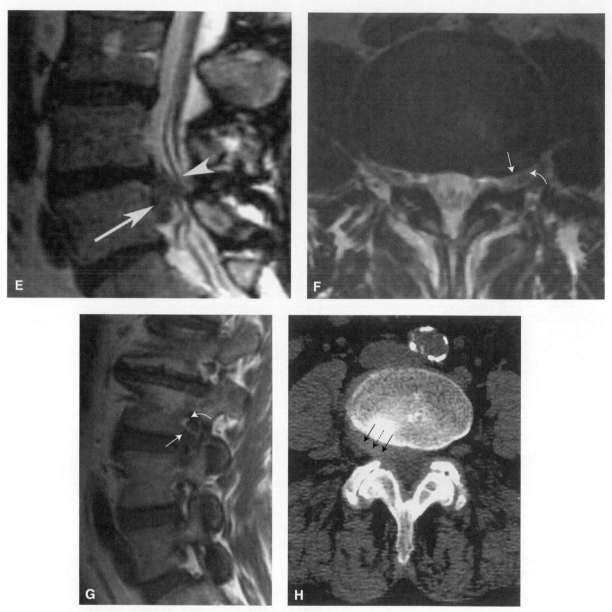

FIGURE 9.41. *(Continued)* **E:** Lumbar spine sagittal T2-weighted MRI in a different patient. Caudally extruded L4–L5 intervertebral disk and a protruding L5–S1 intervertebral disk. Notice that the extruded L4–L5 disk (*arrow*) has migrated inferiorly to the level of the L5–S1 disk space posteriorly and is causing spinal stenosis and displacing nerve roots (*arrowhead*). A bulging disk at L5–S1 does not touch the thecal sac at this level. Note a small vertebral hemangioma in L3 (*rounded bright signal*). **F:** Axial T2 MRI at L3–L4 in a 43-year-old man. Foraminal disk protrusion. The disk protrusion (*straight arrow*) narrows the left foramen and displaces the L3 nerve (*curved arrow*). **G:** Sagittal PD (proton density) MR on the same patient. This view shows the disk extension into the neural foramen (*straight arrow*) and relationship to the nerve (*curved arrow*). There are degenerative disk changes at L2–L3 as well with some foraminal narrowing seen at that level. **H:** Lumbar spine axial CT image. Protruded L4–L5 intervertebral disk. The *arrows* mark the protruded disk with narrowing of the right foramen by the disk and facet arthritis.

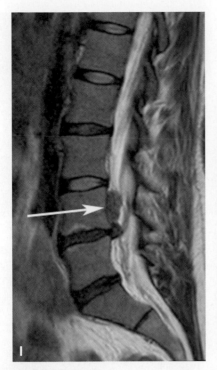

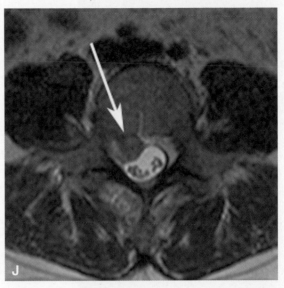

FIGURE 9.41. *(Continued)* **I and J** Sagittal and axial T2-weighted images of the sequestered disk or free fragment disk herniation (*white arrows*). (Illustration by CBoles Art.)

TABLE 9.7	Intervertebral Disk Herniation Nomenclature

Bulge— > or = 50% width of disk displaced beyond vertebral body margin

Protrusion—depth of extent of disk and/or dome width < width of base at disk margin

Extrusion—depth of extent of disk and/or dome width > width of base at disk margin

Sequestration—detached disk fragment

Schmorl node—herniation of disk axially through the end plate

Disk herniation can be categorized by form: **protruded, extruded, and sequestered** (Table 9.7; Fig. 9.41B-J). A **protrusion** implies the depth of disk extension (or dome of the herniated disk) is less than the width of its base at the disk margin. A **broad-based protrusion** involves over 25% of the circumference of the disk while a **focal protrusion** involves less than 25% of the disk margin. If the extension of disk material is greater than the width of its base or extends superior or inferior to the end plate, it is termed an **extrusion**. If the fragment becomes detached, it is termed a **sequestered fragment** (previously "free fragment"), or simply a *sequestration*.

Disk herniation can also be categorized by location: **central, paracentral, subarticular, foraminal, far-lateral foraminal, or extraforaminal**. The subarticular zone of the disk is adjacent to the facet joint. At the L4-5 disk level, the L5 nerve root is in the subarticular zone. Just caudal to this, the L5 root sits in the true lateral recess, at the level of the L5 pedicle. It then exits the L5-S1 foramen just under the L5 pedicle. Hence, a paracentral or subarticular disk extrusion originating from a radial annular fissure of the **L4-5** disk may impinge on the **L5** nerve root, whereas a foraminal or far-lateral foraminal disk extrusion at **L4-5** may impinge on **the L4** nerve root. A paracentral disk extrusion with cephalad migration into the L4 lateral recess may impinge on the L4 nerve root whereas extrusion with caudal migration into the L5 lateral recess may impinge on the L5 root. One important normal variant to be aware of is a conjoint nerve root which should not to be confused with a sequestered fragment or a synovial cyst, all of which can be distinguished on MRI. The epidural space surrounding a nerve root is targeted under fluoroscopic guidance for injection of a combination of steroid and local anesthetic for an epidural steroid injection (Fig. 9.42).

When a disk herniates anteriorly into the vertebral body, this results in a vertebral defect with a classical appearance called a **limbus vertebra**. When a disk herniates superiorly or inferiorly into a vertebral end plate, the resulting defect is called a **Schmorl node** which can

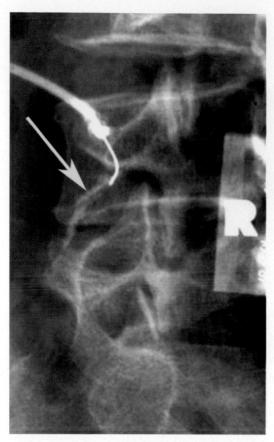

FIGURE 9.42. Epidural steroid injection. Oblique radiograph showing a needle is placed adjacent to the nerve in the foramen. Contrast is then injected which outlines the perineural sheath adjacent to the nerve (*arrow*). Contrast will also track proximally into the epidural space. After needle tip and location is confirmed, a combination of steroid and anesthetic are typically injected.

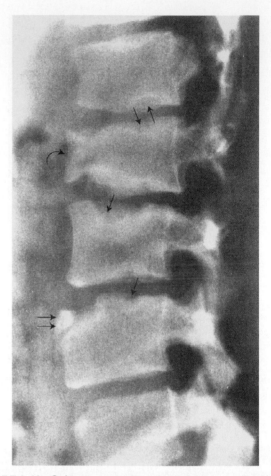

FIGURE 9.43. Scheuermann disease. Lumbar spine lateral view. The involvement of three or more vertebrae by Schmorl nodes (*single straight arrows*) is called Scheuermann disease. Anterior wedging and increased AP diameter of the vertebral bodies (*curved arrow*) may result from this process. There is a limbus vertebra (*double straight arrows*). Note the wavy appearance of the end plates.

be seen in up to 20% of MRI studies in patients without back pain. Although they are associated with degenerative changes in the lower back, they are not an independent risk factor for back pain. **Scheuermann disease** is osteonecrosis of the vertebral epiphyseal plates in teenagers and appears as fragmented and sclerotic epiphyseal plates of the vertebrae, wedge-shaped vertebral bodies with increased AP diameter, and narrowed disk spaces. Limbus vertebrae and Schmorl nodes may coexist (Fig. 9.43).

Modic type end plate changes represent a classification of vertebral body end plate MRI signal. They occur in up to 10% of asymptomatic adults and are common in patients with back pain. The prevalence of Modic changes increases with age and are associated with degenerative disk changes. The changes themselves are of unclear clinical significance and of unclear benefit in guiding the selection of treatment options. The type of Modic change in a single patient may progress or regress

over time. In Modic type 1, there is end plate inflammation and edema, but no trabecular damage or marrow changes. In Modic type 2, there is fatty replacement of red, marrow of the subchondral bone. In Modic type 3, there are fractures of the trabecular bone, resulting in subchondral sclerosis.

Disk herniations in the cervical and thoracic spine are easier to describe as the nerve root extends straight laterally through the foramina, in contrast to the lumbar spine where the roots extend caudally within the cauda equina before exiting the foramina. As there are seven cervical vertebrae and eight cervical nerve roots, the nerve roots are essentially shifted up a level, such that at C4-5, it is the C5 nerve root that exits the foramen, whereas at T4-5 and L4-5 it is T4 and L4, respectively.

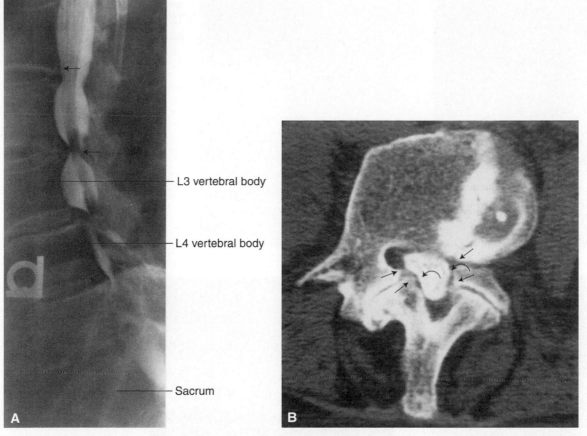

FIGURE 9.44. Spinal stenosis. A: Lumbar myelogram, lateral view. The *straight arrows* indicate multiple levels of neural sac compression secondary to thecal sac narrowing that is in turn secondary to degenerative changes in and around the neural canal. The L3–L4 and L4–L5 intervertebral disk spaces are also markedly narrowed (*curved arrow*). **B:** Axial CT image with contrast. Spinal stenosis at the L3–L4 level secondary to hypertrophic facet changes. The *straight arrows* outline the marked narrowing of the spinal canal, and the *curved arrows* indicate the deformity of the thecal sac secondary to the spinal stenosis.

Spinal stenosis describes a narrow vertebral canal or intervertebral foramen. In the lumbar spine stenosis is due to a combination of **bulging disk, facet arthritis with osteophytes, and thickened ligamentum flavum** (Fig. 9.44A and B). Clinically significant spinal stenosis in the thoracic spine is not as common as stenosis in the cervical and lumbar spine because of the relative immobility of the thoracic spine due to the supportive rib cage. Cervical spinal stenosis and thoracic spinal stenosis, when it occurs, can cause spinal cord flattening and myelopathy which is diagnosed on MRI. Lumbar spinal stenosis rarely causes cord symptoms because the cord terminates at or above the L2 level, and most lumbar spinal stenosis occurs at the lowest three disk levels. However lumbar spinal stenosis may cause neurogenic claudication with pain and lower extremity weakness with prolonged standing or walking.

DISKITIS AND OSTEOMYELITIS

Diskitis and osteomyelitis are most commonly due to staphylococcal infections. As with osteomyelitis elsewhere, patients with vertebral osteomyelitis usually have fever and localized pain. The lumbar spine is the most frequent spine site, followed by the cervical and then the thoracic spine (Fig. 9.45). The most common source is hematogenous spread, with a nidus of infection initially involving the interface between disk and end plate. MRI is the most appropriate diagnostic modality as the initial radiographic findings are subtle with poor definition of a vertebral end plate as the only early finding (Fig. 9.46A) The usual imaging pattern forms the "I" of infection, as the organism initially infects the disk and adjacent end plates, resulting in a narrow vertically oriented region of bone marrow and disk edema and

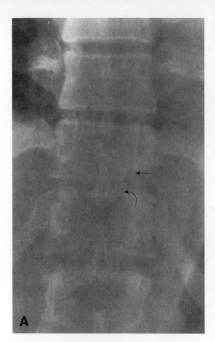

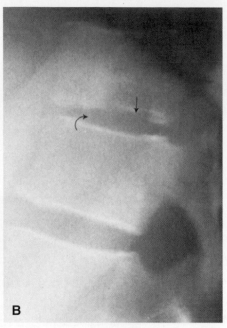

FIGURE 9.45. **Osteomyelitis.** Lower thoracic and upper lumbar spine AP **(A)** and lateral **(B)** radiographs showing destruction of the posterior T11 inferior end plate (*straight arrows*) and the marked narrowing of the T11–T12 intervertebral disk space (*curved arrows*) suggesting disk and joint destruction.

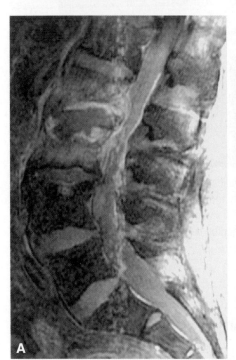

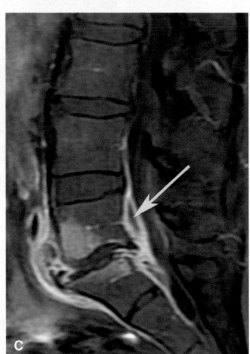

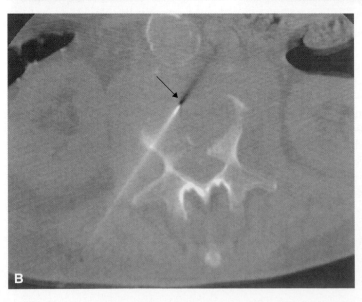

FIGURE 9.46. **Diskitis. A:** Sagittal T1 MRI with contrast. The L2–L3 disk appears enlarged because the adjacent end plates have been destroyed by infection. There is contrast enhancement (bright) surrounding the infected disk and of the vertebral bodies. **B:** Sagittal fat-suppressed MR images with contrast showing diskitis at L5–S1 with extension of infection to an epidural abscess (*arrow*). **C:** Axial CT during biopsy shows the tip of the needle (*arrow*) is in the infected disk.

pathologic enhancement, which then progresses to erode the end plates, often extending posteriorly into the epidural space (Fig. 9.46B). Epidural extension can take the form of a phlegmon or can progress to epidural abscess causing cord compression and septic thrombophlebitis resulting in cord edema, infarction, and paralysis. This is a surgical emergency. Disk biopsy (Fig. 9.46C) is necessary to determine the causative organism although an organism will only be identified in approximately 50% of disk biopsies.

POSTOPERATIVE IMAGING

When evaluating the **postoperative spine**, fractured hardware is best shown on radiographs and CT (Fig. 9.47A; Table 9.8). Loosening of hardware on CT is suspected when there is more than 2 mm lucency adjacent to the screw threads (Fig. 9.47B). Junctional degeneration (adjacent level degeneration) occurs at the level or levels immediately adjacent to a fusion construct. Disk degeneration and facet arthropathy at the level adjacent to a fused segment can lead to recurrent symptoms due to disk herniation, spinal stenosis, or sometimes synovial cyst.

Recurrent herniated disk occurs after 5% of micro-diskectomies. MRI should be avoided within 6 weeks of surgery except to rule out compression of the thecal sac, cauda equina, or spinal cord due to post-op fluid or hematoma because it can be difficult to determine what sort of soft tissue, fluid, and/or blood is present at the site of surgery in the early post-op period. After 6 weeks, enhancing granulation tissue will be mature enough to distinguish it, which has a solid enhancement pattern, from recurrent disk herniation, which enhances peripherally (Figs. 9.48 and 9.49).

Most post-op **infections** are superficial, but when they extend deeply, they can result in phlegmon and/or abscess in the paraspinal or epidural compartments. Unlike the pattern of hematogenous diskitis, which often starts at the interface between end plate and disk toward the center of the disk, post-op diskitis usually spreads directly from the surgical site to the edges of the disk (Fig. 9.50). As with hematogenous diskitis/osteomyelitis, improvement in imaging often lags that of clinical improvement, and the improvement in the thickness of inflammatory soft tissue may be a better imaging metric for treatment response.

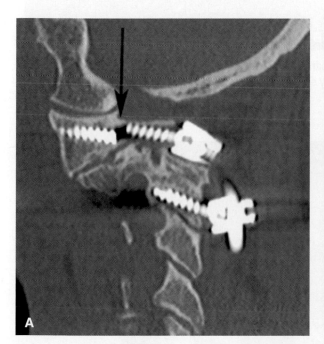
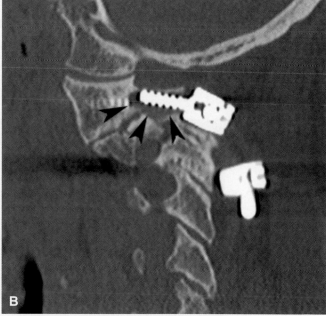

FIGURE 9.47. Hardware failure. A and B: Reformatted images showing fractured screw (*arrow*) with band of abnormal lucency (*arrowheads*) adjacent to the screw indicating loosening secondary to abnormal motion and bone reabsorption.

TABLE 9.8	Checklist for the Postoperative Spine

Evaluate integrity of hardware, positioning, and evidence of loosening
Check for stability of the fused segments and adjacent segments
Rule out postoperative hematoma or infection
Rule out recurrent herniated disk
Look for junctional (adjacent level) degeneration

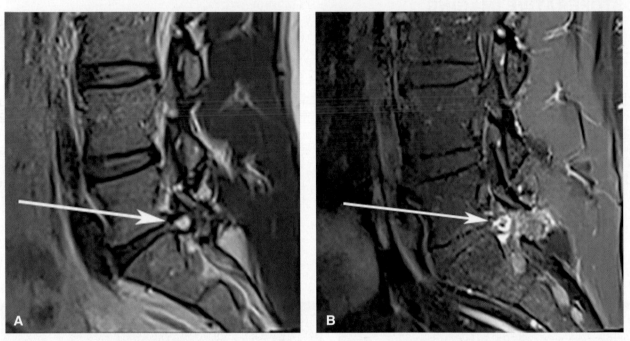

FIGURE 9.48. Recurrent disk herniation. A: The T2 hyperintense extradural mass (*arrow*) could be granulation tissue or recurrent disk herniation, but on **(B)** the postgadolinium sequence, the mass only enhances peripherally (*arrow*), confirming a recurrent disk herniation.

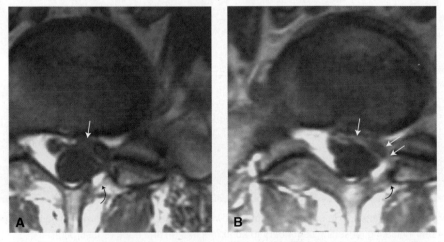

FIGURE 9.49. Post-op scar tissue. Axial T1 MRI at L5–S1 without **(A)** and with **(B)** intravenous contrast. The *curved arrow* demonstrates a surgically absent lamina. The *arrow* in **(A)** shows abnormal signal which could be a new disk herniation or scar tissue. **B:** Enhancement (*arrow*) indicates that it is scar tissue as disk does not enhance. The left S1 nerve root (*double arrow*) is displaced and enhances suggesting that it is affected by the scar tissue.

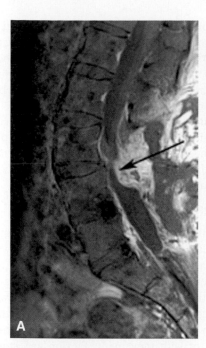
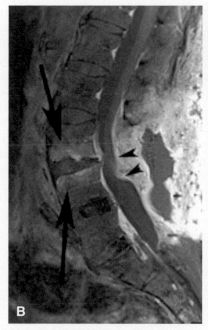
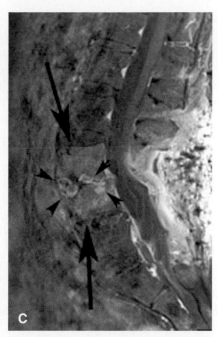

FIGURE 9.50. Post-op wound infection. **A:** *Arrow* depicts dorsal epidural enhancing tissue compressing the thecal sac. **B:** A subsequent scan shows development of enhancement at the edge of the disk and in the adjacent endplates (*arrows*). There is persistent dorsal epidural enhancing tissue (*arrowheads*). **C:** Follow-up imaging several weeks later shows improvement in posterior enhancing tissue but progression of enhancement of the disk with loss of height of the disk and endplate irregularity (*arrowheads*). There has also been progression of enhancement of the vertebral bodies (*arrows*). Imaging findings in the disk and bone can lag behind clinical signs of improvement on antibiotic therapy.

ARTHRITIDES

Because the spine has multiple joints, including 139 synovial joints such as the uncovertebral joints in the cervical spine, costovertebral joints in the thoracic spine and facet joints throughout, it is not surprising that arthritis may affect the spine.

Osteoarthritis

Osteoarthritis (Fig. 9.51) most commonly involves the facet joints of the spine. As elsewhere, the typical radiologic features of osteoarthritis include joint space narrowing, sclerosis, and osteophyte formation in addition to subchondral cysts. Complications of OA include spinal stenosis and spondylolisthesis.

FIGURE 9.51. Osteoarthritis. Thoracic spine AP (**A**) and lateral (**B**) views. Multiple osteophytes (*curved arrows*) are present and several disk spaces are narrowed (*straight arrows*) secondary to degenerative disk disease.

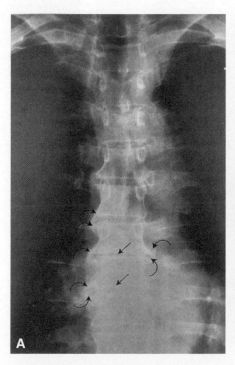
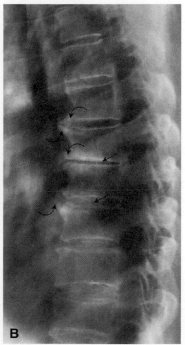

Axial Spondyloarthropathies

The axial spondyloarthropathies are a group of inflammatory arthritides that include ankylosing spondylitis, psoriatic arthritis, reactive arthritis, and inflammatory bowel disease–related spondyloarthropathies. These disorders involve the sacroiliac (SI) joints or the spine and usually begin in early adulthood. Their diagnosis is based on a combination of physical examination, laboratory tests (rheumatoid factor negative, HLA-B27, C-reactive protein), and imaging findings which include erosions, enthesitis, and bone proliferation.

The main limitation of conventional radiography in axial spondyloarthropathies is a low sensitivity for detecting abnormalities in the early stages of the disease as the radiographic findings of inflammatory change often lag the onset of clinical symptoms by several years. MRI (T2WI or STIR) best shows the characteristic bone marrow lesions and soft tissue inflammatory change. The SI joints become symmetrically narrowed with erosive change which then progresses to ankylosis. Following SI joint fusion, ankylosing spondylitis causes squaring of the vertebral bodies with syndesmophyte formation and ossification between the outer margin of the vertebral bodies and the disk annulus producing a "bamboo spine" appearance and because of the rigidity of the spine and relatively weak fusion across disks, even mild trauma may lead to fractures at the disk levels (Fig. 9.52).

Psoriatic sacroiliitis occurs in up to one quarter of patients with psoriasis but may coincide or even predate the skin changes in 20% of patients. The arthritis features both erosions and bony proliferation and SI joints involvement is usually asymmetrical (Fig. 9.53). Sporadic paravertebral ossification will connect adjacent vertebral bodies.

Reactive arthritis formerly called Reiter Syndrome consists of conjunctivitis, urethritis, and arthritis. The spine and SI joint findings are indistinguishable from psoriatic spondyloarthropathy, but the arthritis is more likely to involve the foot than the hand.

Rheumatoid Arthritis

Rheumatoid arthritis may involve any of the synovial joints in the spine. The disease severity varies from mild narrowing of cervical disk spaces to involvement of the odontoid and the atlantoaxial joint and the transverse ligament holding the odontoid close to the anterior arch of C1. When the transverse ligament becomes inflamed, subluxation, impaction, or even dislocation of the atlantoaxial joint may cause neck pain either at rest or with movement. Flexion and extension lateral cervical spine radiographs are indicated in rheumatoid arthritis patients when they experience pain with head movement and before undergoing general anesthesia or any other procedure which requires neck hyperflexion

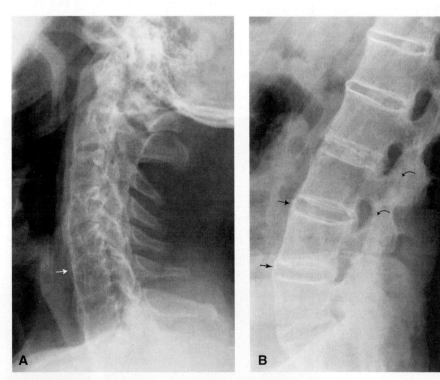

FIGURE 9.52. Ankylosing spondylitis. Lateral cervical **(A and B)** and AP lumbar **(C)** views. *Straight arrows* demonstrate syndesmophytes which bridge across disk levels forming a solid "bamboo" spine.

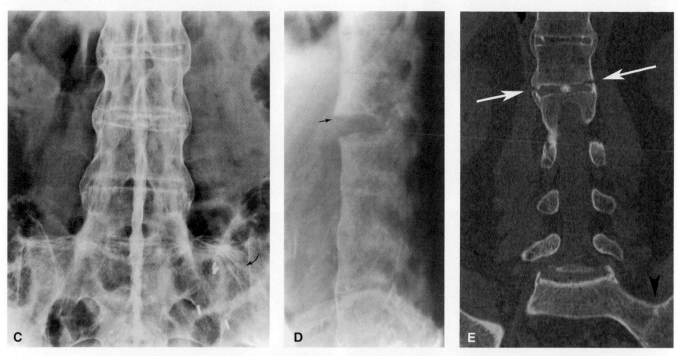

FIGURE 9.52. *(Continued)* The *curved arrows* in **(B)** mark the fused apophyseal joints, while the *curved arrow* in **(C)** is in the expected location of the SI joint, which has fused. **D:** Lateral lumbar view shows anterolisthesis of L1 on L2 and a widened L1–L2 disk (*arrow*) due to a fracture through this disk level. **E:** Coronal CT image of a fractured and potentially unstable "bamboo spine" (*white arrows*). Note that the fracture plane extends through the fused, calcified disk. The fused left sacroiliac joint is also visible (*black arrowhead*).

FIGURE 9.53. **Psoriatic sacroiliitis.** Pelvis AP view showing sclerosis and irregularity of the right SI joint (*straight arrow*) due to sacroiliitis associated with psoriatic arthritis. Compare the appearance to the sharply defined margins of the left SI joint (*curved arrows*).

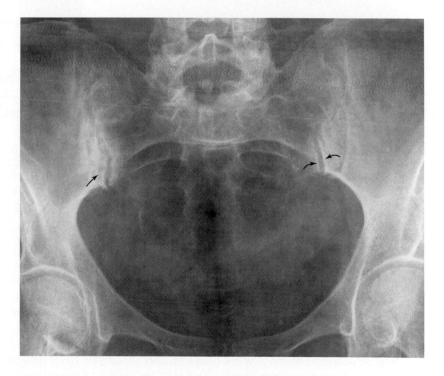

or hyperextension. On a lateral radiograph, the normal distance between the anterior border of the odontoid and posterior aspect of the C1 anterior arch is usually less than 3 mm in adults. With **subluxation or dislocation of the atlantoaxial joint**, this distance exceeds 3 mm, especially when the cervical spine is flexed (Fig. 9.54A-I).

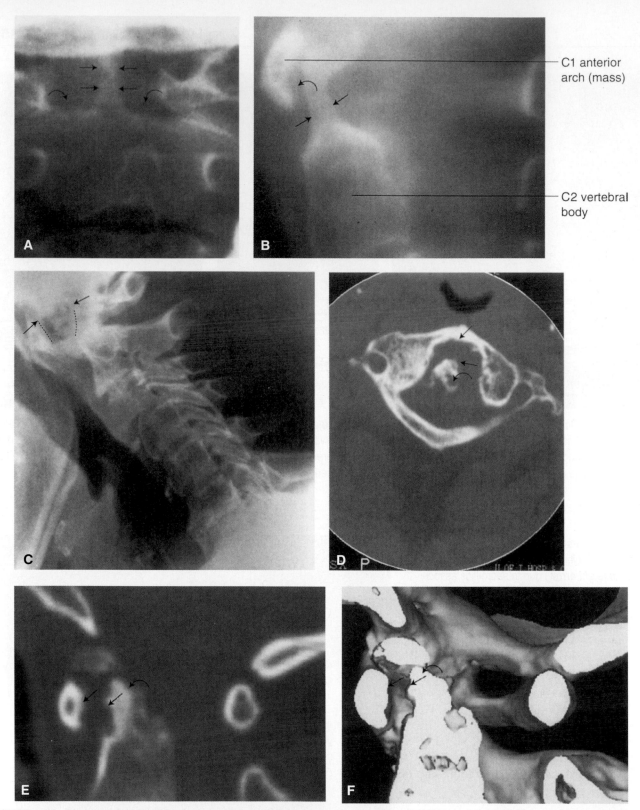

FIGURE 9.54. Rheumatoid arthritis. A: Cervical spine AP open-mouth view. The odontoid process (*straight arrows*) is narrowed, osteopenic, and poorly marginated. Note the increased distances between the odontoid process of C2 and the inferior articular processes of C1 (*curved arrows*) due to partial loss of odontoid bone. **B:** Lateral tomograph confirming the odontoid (*straight arrows*) is markedly narrowed. The space between the anterior odontoid and the anterior arch of C1 (*curved arrow*) is greater than the 2.5 mm. **C:** Lateral cervical spine flexion view in a different patient showing the space (*straight arrows*) between the anterior surface of the odontoid and the posterior aspect of the anterior arch of C1 (*dotted lines*) is dramatically widened indicating an unstable dislocation of C1 relative to C2. There is also grade 1 anterior spondylolisthesis of C2 relative to C3. Note the narrowing of all the cervical disk spaces and the generalized osteopenia. **D:** Cervical spine axial CT image. Rheumatoid arthritis with spinal stenosis in a 55-year-old man. The C1–C2 joint is abnormal with a distance of 8 mm between the anterior arch of C1 and the odontoid (between the *straight arrows*). There are advanced erosive changes in the odontoid (*curved arrow*). Cervical spine CT sagittal reconstruction **(E)** and sagittal CT 3D reconstruction **(F)** in the same patient as **(D)**. The odontoid has erosive changes and a distal penciled appearance (*curved arrows*). There is redemonstration of the abnormal C1–C2 joint (between the *straight arrows*).

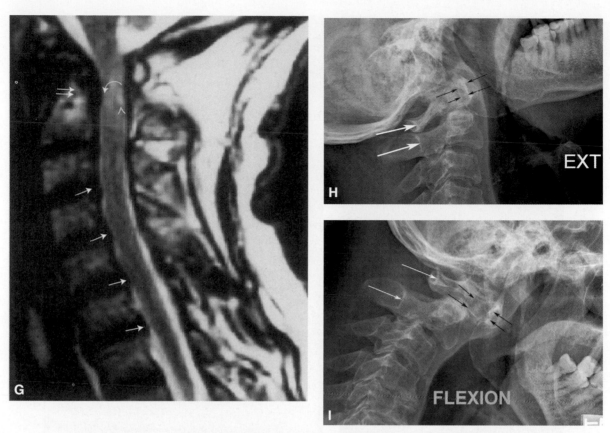

FIGURE 9.54. *(Continued)* **G:** Cervical spine sagittal T2 MRI in the same patient as shown in **(D)** and **(F)**. The odontoid (*double arrows*) is displaced posteriorly resulting in spinal stenosis and cervical cord compression (*curved arrow*). The increased signal in the compressed cord (*arrowhead*) probably represents edema. The *single straight arrows* indicate multiple levels of mild spinal stenosis. **H and I:** Ligament laxity: Note the increase in the atlantoaxial interval in flexion compared with extension (*small black arrows*). The spinolaminar line is more disrupted in flexion (*large white arrows*).

TUMORS OF BONE AND BONE MARROW

The most common benign vertebral tumor is a **hemangioma** which is usually asymptomatic and an incidental finding. The classic appearance of a hemangioma is of thickened vertical trabeculae that simulate corduroy fabric (Fig. 9.55). Hemangiomas do not require treatment unless symptomatic, such as a pathological fracture or when the lesion extends outside the vertebra and compresses the spinal cord or nerve roots. Table 9.9 lists common vertebral tumors.

Metastases are the most common cause of vertebral malignancy. The process may be osteolytic, most commonly breast carcinoma and lung carcinoma (Fig. 9.56), or

osteoblastic (sclerotic) (Fig. 9.57) or a combination of both. Table 9.10 lists the causes of osteoblastic metastases. In contrast to the spread by infection described above, metastases and lymphoma may involve contiguous vertebral segments, but the most typical pattern is the "C" of cancer, with the tumor growing around the edge of the disk to infiltrate the corner of the adjacent vertebral bodies. In contrast to benign diseases, malignancy may also involve the posterior vertebral elements (pedicles, laminae, spinous process).

The importance of visualizing the vertebral pedicles is emphasized in Figure 9.58. When one or both pedicles are missing in patients with known or suspected cancer, metastatic disease should be suspected. MRI is very useful to confirm the presence and extent of metastatic disease (Fig. 9.59).

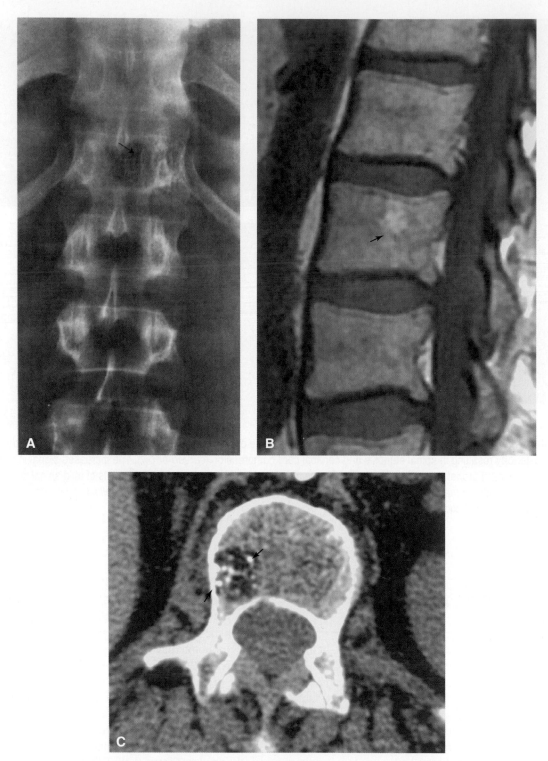

FIGURE 9.55. Vertebral hemangioma. A: Thoracolumbar spine AP view. The prominent vertical trabecular pattern of T12 is characteristic of bone hemangioma (*arrow*). **B:** Sagittal T1 MRI of the lumbar spine. The round, focal area of higher signal (*arrow*) represents fat and is characteristic of vertebral hemangioma. **C:** Axial CT of a thoracic vertebral body demonstrates the punctate appearance of the cross section of coarse trabeculae (*arrows*).

TABLE 9.9	Common Primary Vertebral Tumors

Benign
Hemangioma
Osteoid osteoma
Osteoblastoma
Aneurysmal bone cyst
Osteochondroma

Malignant
Multiple myeloma (most common)/plasmacytoma
Chordoma
Chondrosarcoma
Osteosarcoma
Ewing sarcoma

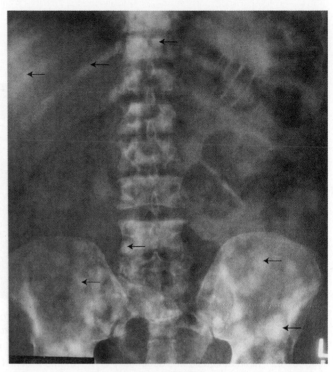

FIGURE 9.57. **Osteoblastic metastases.** Abdominal radiograph shows multiple areas of increased density (*arrows*) involving the pelvis, lumbar spine, dorsal spine, and ribs due to metastases from carcinoma of the prostate.

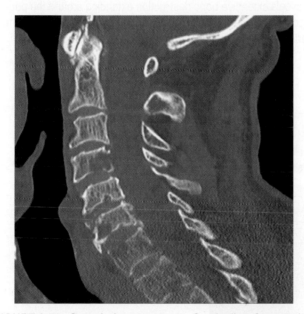

FIGURE 9.56. **Osteolytic metastases.** Sagtittally reformatted CT of the cervical spine showing several lytic metastases (areas of low attenuation).

TABLE 9.10	Source of Osteoblastic (Sclerotic) Metastases

Prostate Cancer
Breast Cancer
Lymphoma
Carcinoid
Neuroblastoma (occasional)

Multiple Myeloma

Multiple myeloma should be considered in the differential diagnosis of osteopenia and lytic lesions on radiographs and CT. Plasmacytoma, which may develop into multiple myeloma, appears similar to an osteolytic metastasis. Several patterns of marrow involvement are described on MRI, which can be used for staging of multiple myeloma (Fig. 9.60). Following treatment, the normalization of marrow appearance on MRI is associated with a better prognosis. Over half of all patients with multiple myeloma develop painful vertebral compression fractures which respond to vertebroplasty.

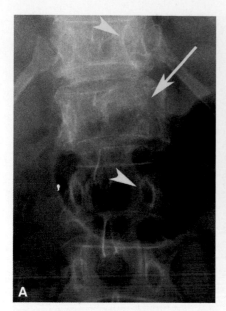
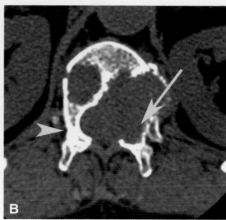
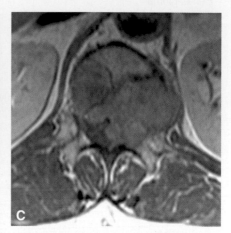

FIGURE 9.58. **Absent pedicle. A:** Thoracolumbar spine AP view. The left T12 pedicle is not visualized (*arrow*). Note the normal appearance of the pedicles at adjacent levels (*arrowheads*). **B:** Axial CT reveals extensive bone destruction extending around the pedicle on the left (*arrow*). The *arrowhead* shows points to the normal right pedicle. **C:** Axial T1-weighted MRI confirms the mass and bone destruction. This metastasis was secondary to melanoma which characteristically is not as dark on T1 as some other tumor types.

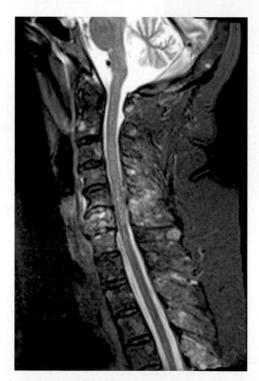

FIGURE 9.59. **Bony metastases:** Cervical spine sagittal T1 MRI shows several metastatic lesions of carcinoma of the breast. The metastatic lesions appear bright or gray on T2 images and involve both anterior and posterior elements of the vertebra.

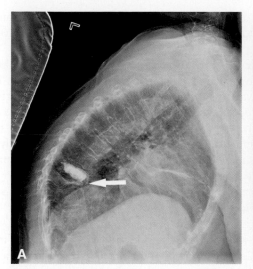
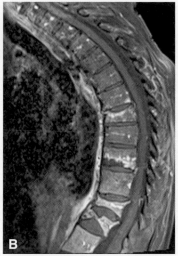
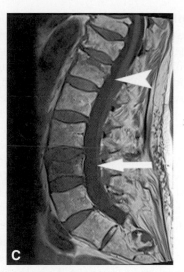

FIGURE 9.60. Multiple myeloma with osteoporotic compression fractures. Even in the absence of typical stippled marrow or obvious focal lesions, patients with multiple myeloma often become osteoporotic. **A:** Lateral thoracic radiograph showing kyphosis and severe compression deformity, or "vertebra plana" (*arrow*) just inferior to the vertebroplasty level. Note the methyl methacrylate in the vertebral body, which contains added radiopaque material, often barium sulfate, making it white on the radiograph. **B:** Fat-suppressed T1-weighted sagittal image of the thoracic spine showing compression fractures in a patient with multiple myeloma, with enhancement of the compressed part of the vertebral bodies. Note that benign compression fractures also enhance. **C:** T1-weighted sagittal image of the lumbar spine without gadolinium showing low signal indicating bone marrow edema in partially healed (*arrowhead*) and acute (*arrow*) compression fractures.

MISCELLANEOUS DISEASES

Osteopenia, osteoporosis, and osteomalacia have been discussed in the Metabolic Disease section of Chapter 6. The typical patient with osteoporotic vertebral compression fractures is elderly (Fig. 9.61). Vertebral fractures not only cause back pain but will also often result in loss of height and kyphosis. Severe thoracic kyphosis may decrease lung volume causing a restrictive defect. See Chapter 13 IR for vertebroplasty.

FIGURE 9.61. Osteoporosis. Lumbar spine lateral view shows multiple compression fractures secondary to osteoporosis (*straight arrows*). The fractures of L1, L3, L4, and L5 are manifest by a loss of the vertical body heights compared with the normal vertical heights of the T12 and L2 vertebral bodies. Note the multiple fish-mouth deformities (*curved arrows*) and the overall decreased density or osteopenia of the spine.

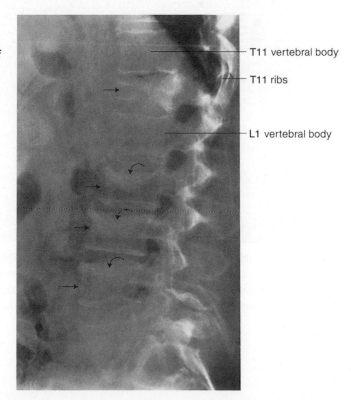

Diffuse idiopathic skeletal hyperostosis (DISH) or Forestier disease is characterized by flowing ossification of the anterior longitudinal ligament and exuberant para-articular osteophyte formation causing the spine to become a rigid tube which fractures like a long bone, obliquely and transversely. Intervertebral disk space is preserved, and the facet joints are not typically involved. The overall appearance is similar to the bamboo spine of ankylosing spondylitis and is best seen on a lateral spine radiograph (Fig. 9.62A). Because of reduced range of motion, mid-vertebral transverse fractures occur (Fig. 9.62B). The lower portion of the SI joints is typically spared. Spinal stenosis is a significant risk of DISH.

Paget's disease is characterized by expansion of bone and a predominantly sclerotic pattern, with coarsened trabeculae. When Paget's disease involves the spine, the finding of vertebral body expansion helps distinguish Paget's disease from other causes of bone sclerosis, such as sclerotic metastases (Fig. 9.63). The disease may present as back pain due to facet arthropathy or spinal stenosis. Malignant transformation to osteogenic sarcoma occurs in less than 10% of patients.

Sickle cell anemia involvement of the spine is characterized by microvascular thrombosis and infarction leading to avascular necrosis. The central portion of vertebral bodies collapses superiorly and inferiorly and presents an H shape when viewed laterally (Fig. 9.64). Patients with sickle cell anemia are susceptible to osteomyelitis especially due to *Salmonella*, but *Staphylococcus* is still the most common causative organism.

The cauda equina normally floats in a pool of CSF. In **arachnoiditis**, the nerve roots clump to each other or to the thecal sac which may become distorted (Fig. 9.65). Patients with arachnoiditis present with leg pain or motor deficit. Causes of arachnoiditis include previous spine surgery and use of Pantopaque (oil-based contrast) for myelography. The differential diagnosis includes leptomeningeal carcinomatosis.

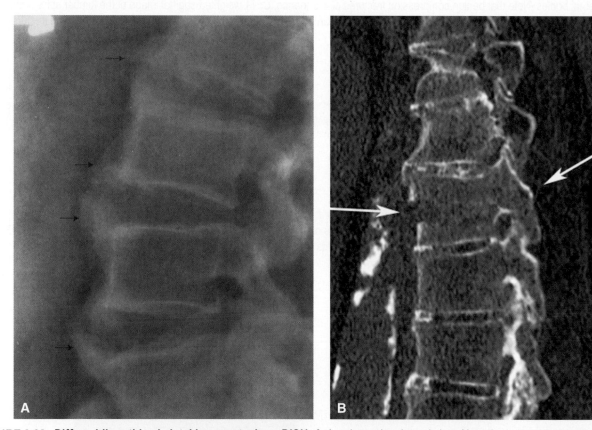

FIGURE 9.62. Diffuse idiopathic skeletal hyperostosis or DISH. A: Lumbar spine, lateral view. Note the large osteophytes (*arrows*) along the anterior vertebral bodies that extend anteriorly across the disk spaces and ossification of the anterior longitudinal ligament. The intervertebral disk spaces are normal in height. **B:** Sagittal image of a CT scan in a different patient showing a fracture extending transversely through the vertebral body (*left arrow*) into the posterior elements (*right arrow*) in this patient with "broken DISH".

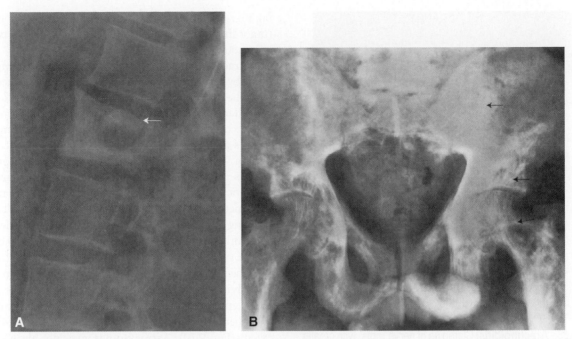

FIGURE 9.63. **Paget's disease. A:** Lumbar spine lateral view shows the classic picture frame appearance secondary to the increased trabecular density in the cortex (*arrow*) of the L2 vertebral body. There is mild loss of the L2 vertebral body height compared with the vertical heights of L1 and L3, due to a mild compression fracture. **B:** Pelvis AP view. The bone trabeculae are coarse (*arrows*) with an overall increased density.

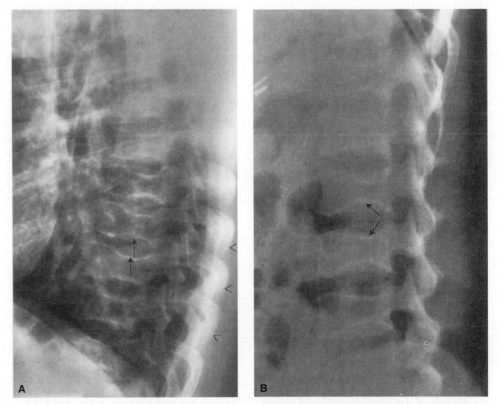

FIGURE 9.64. **Sickle cell anemia.** Thoracic spine **(A)** and lumbar **(B)** spine lateral views. There is overall osteopenia with the fish-mouth deformities of the vertebral bodies (*arrows*) like those in senile osteoporosis (see Fig. 9.63). Note the ribs in A (*arrowheads*).

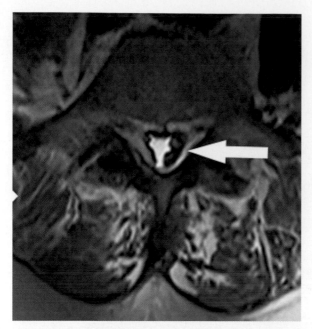

FIGURE 9.65. Arachnoiditis. Clumping of nerve roots, with greater than normal peripheral distribution of the nerve roots (*arrow*). Axial MRI. Compare with normal nerve root arrangement in Figure 9.12B.

DISORDERS OF THE SPINAL CORD

Spinal Cord Tumors

Traditionally the spinal canal and its contents have been divided into three compartments: the **extradural compartment, the intradural extramedullary compartment, and the intramedullary compartment**. Table 9.11 lists the common masses in each of these compartments.

Extradural masses are almost always benign and include disk herniation, osteophyte, or if it is posterior a juxta-articular (synovial) cyst (Fig. 9.66). Extradural tumors, when they do occur, most commonly develop secondary to epidural extension of bone marrow metastases, most commonly from breast or prostate carcinoma or from bone marrow involvement with lymphoma or multiple myeloma (Fig. 9.67A and B). Extension into the epidural compartment may cause radiculopathy due to extrinsic nerve root compression or, if large enough, spinal cord compression or diffuse cauda equina compression. A tip in the evaluation of these lesions is to evaluate the dorsal epidural fat on T1-weighted sagittal images. Normally the dorsal epidural fat is uniformly bright

on T1-weighted images. Have a high suspicion for epidural tumor in a patient with known bone marrow metastases or lymphoma when the fat turns from white to gray.

Intradural masses are those within the compartment lined by the dura mater. The lesions in this space that do not arise from the spinal cord are termed intradural *extra*medullary lesions, and those predominantly involving the spinal cord are *intra*medullary. **Intradural extramedullary** tumors and cysts (Fig. 9.68A and B) are most commonly benign, either schwannomas, neurofibromas, or meningiomas. However, metastatic disease particularly breast carcinoma and lymphoma can also present as intradural extramedullary nodules as they have a predilection for growing along the surface of the spinal cord or nerve roots and infiltrating the epidural compartment (Fig. 9.69).

The most common **intramedullary** tumors are cellular ependymoma, astrocytoma, and hemangioblastoma. **Ependymomas** are lesions with variable enhancement that are often associated with syrinx and can sometimes have dark hemosiderin "caps" at their cephalad and/or caudal extent (Fig. 9.70). **Astrocytomas** may not always enhance with gadolinium, but typically present as a persistent expansile T2-hyperintense spinal cord lesion that does not evolve or change over short interval scans (Fig. 9.71). **Hemangioblastoma** can be sporadic or occur as part of Von Hippel Lindau syndrome. These tumors have an enhancing nodule, are markedly hypervascular, and can occur on the surface of the cord. Intradural **metastases** are rare, usually only occurring in long-term survivors of systemic metastases.

Always review the extraspinal tissues including the retroperitoneum and the pelvis for possible causes of back or radicular pain (Figs. 9.72 and 9.73).

Demyelination and Myelitis

Multiple sclerosis involvement of the spinal cord is manifested as multiple short-segment lesions with increased T2 signal, the most active of which may enhance with gadolinium. The lesions are usually in the posterior or lateral columns (Fig. 9.74). As many as 20% of patients with spinal involvement do not have intracranial disease, but this is not predictive of poor outcome unlike spinal cord atrophy which is associated with progressive physical disability.

Neuromyelitis optica (NMO), previously called Devic syndrome, is characterized by optic neuritis and spinal cord demyelination and is no longer considered a variant of multiple sclerosis. Unlike MS, it tends to cause longer lesions in the spinal cord, often spanning three or more vertebral segments (Fig. 9.75).

Acute disseminated encephalomyelitis (ADEM) is an acute form of demyelination usually occurring a short time after a viral illness or following vaccination and can occur in children and young adults. It is a monophasic illness with multiple brain lesions which often enhance with gadolinium and, like other demyelinating diseases, can involve subcortical U-fibers. When it involves the spinal cord, lesions may extend contiguously for the length of two or more vertebral segments and often enhance with gadolinium.

TABLE 9.11	Spinal Masses by Location	
Extradural	**Intradural Extramedullary**	**Intradural Intramedullary**
Disk	Schwannoma	Ependymoma
Osteophyte	Neurofibroma	Astrocytoma
Synovial cyst	Meningioma	Hemangioblastoma
Metastases	Metastases	Metastases (rare)

Viral myelitis (Fig. 9.76) also extends over multiple segments and is characterized by central gray matter enhancement.

Subacute combined degeneration is usually caused by vitamin B12 deficiency and presents as sensory and sometimes also motor symptoms. It manifests on MRI as extensive longitudinal lesions with atrophy of the posterior and often also the lateral columns of the spinal cord (Fig. 9.77A and B).

Transverse myelitis is a rapidly developed myelopathy (spinal cord disease) with rapidly progressive paraplegia,

FIGURE 9.66. **Synovial cysts. A and B:** Sagittal and axial T2-weighted images show a typical T2-hypointense rim (*arrows*). There may be loss of the usual central bright T2 signal due to hemorrhage into the cyst or proteinaceous material. Note facet arthropathy (*arrowheads*).

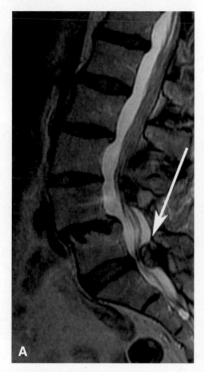

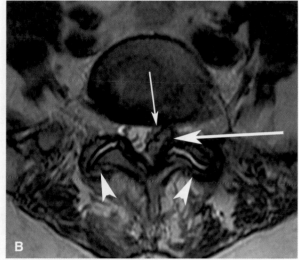

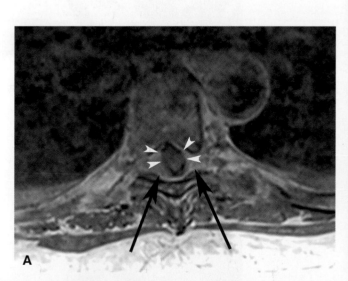

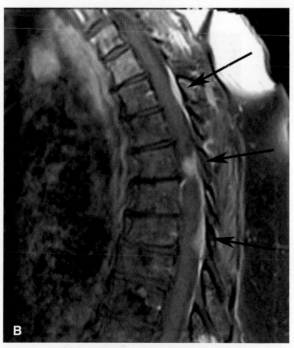

FIGURE 9.67. **Multiple myeloma. A:** Axial image shows epidural enhancing tumor (*arrows*) compressing the spinal cord (*arrowheads*) in the transverse dimension. B: Midline sagittal image in the same patient shows the dorsal epidural tumor (*arrows*)

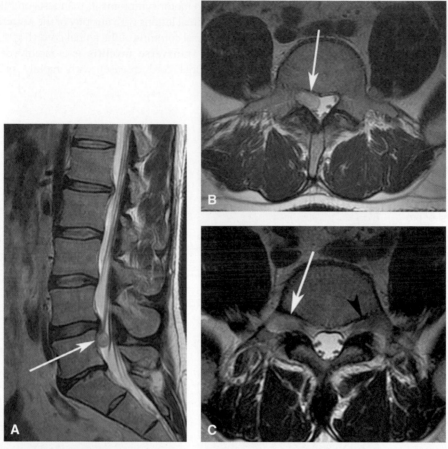

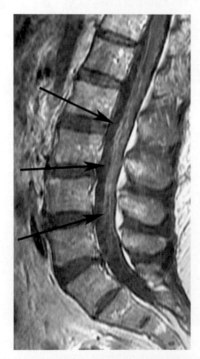

FIGURE 9.68. Schwannoma. A: This extradural tumor (*arrow*) has an appearance similar to an extruded disk but has higher signal than the adjacent disk. **B:** Axial T2-weighted image at L5 shows the schwannoma (*arrow*) expanding the right L5 nerve root in the lateral recess. **C:** Schwannomas are called dumbbell lesions because they have a narrow waist as they squeeze through the foramen. Note the foraminal component of the schwannoma (*white arrow*) compared to the contralateral normal L5 dorsal root ganglion (*black arrowhead*).

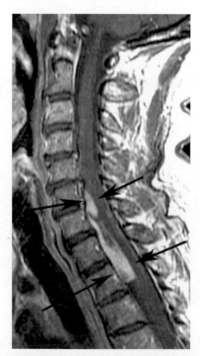

FIGURE 9.69. Lymphoma. Lymphoma is usually extradural and often grows along the surface of structures. In this case it is intra-dural extramedullary, coating the cauda equina with enhancing tumor (*arrows*).

FIGURE 9.70. Ependymoma. Atypical appearance of a spinal cord ependymoma, in that it is partially extramedullary. *Arrows* depict the main enhancing component of the tumor, which extends into the extramedullary space ventral to the spinal cord.

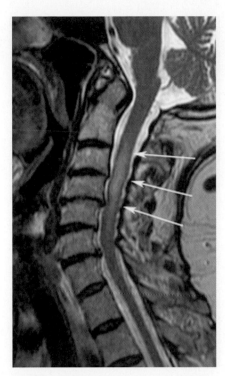

FIGURE 9.71. **Astrocytoma.** This tumor did not enhance but was mildly expansile. This T2-hyperintense tumor (*arrows*) did not enhance but was mildly expansile, the only hint of neoplasm. Note that benign lesions can also cause spinal cord expansion, but the persistence of spinal cord expansion without enhancement and slowly progressive myelopathy led to biopsy in this case.

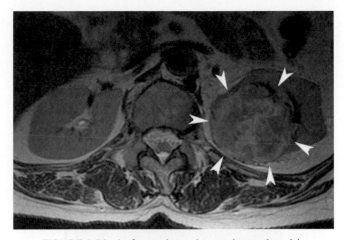

FIGURE 9.72. **Left renal carcinoma (*arrowheads*).**

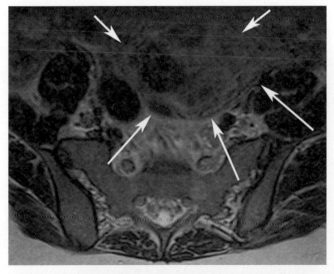

FIGURE 9.73. **Large uterine fibroids** *(arrows)* **impinging on the left lumbosacral plexus.**

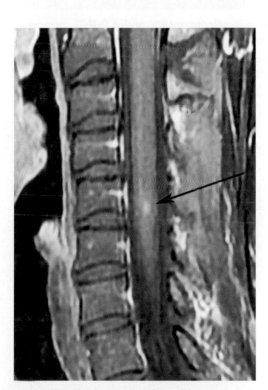

FIGURE 9.74. **Multiple sclerosis (MS).** Enhancing plaque (*arrow*) in the lateral column of the spinal cord, indicating active demyelination.

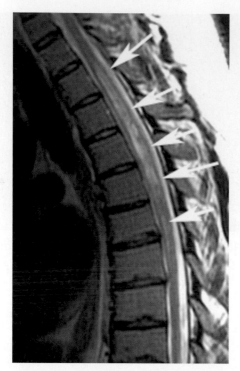

FIGURE 9.75. Neuromyelitis optica (NMO). Increased T2 signal (*arrows*) in the spinal cord extends over multiple contiguous spinal segments. Note that the spinal cord is expanded, and there was patchy enhancement following gadolinium (not shown).

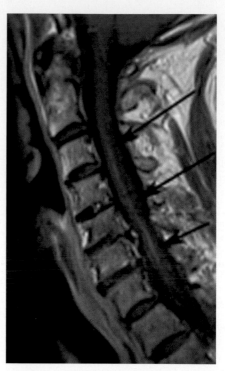

FIGURE 9.76. Viral myelitis. Linear longitudinal enhancement (*arrows*) involving the central gray matter.

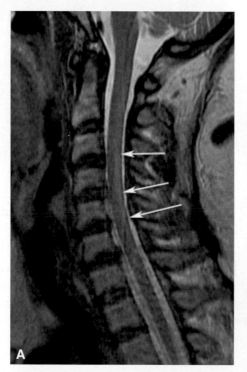

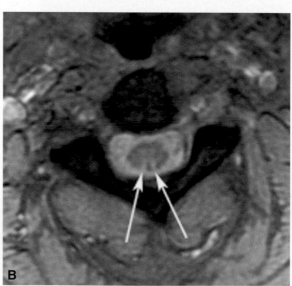

FIGURE 9.77. Subacute combined degeneration, due to vitamin B12 deficiency. A: Sagittal T2 shows contiguous increased T2 signal in the posterior columns (*arrows*) without cord expansion. **B:** *Arrows* on the axial T2-weighted GRE image shows symmetrical involvement of the posterior columns (the lateral columns may also be involved).

sensory loss, and bladder dysfunction typically following an upper respiratory tract infection. In all patients presenting with an acute/subacute myelopathy, exclusion of cord compression by abscess, tumor, or disk is essential by MRI. A disorder known for its imaging mimicry that should be considered in cases of transverse myelitis is **neurosarcoidosis**, which can look tumor-like, with an intramedullary-enhancing lesion, surrounding edema and spinal cord expansion.

Spinal Cord Infarction

The anterior spinal artery is supplied by the vertebral arteries, variably by other neck arteries and by the radiculomedullary arteries, so-named because they travel along and supply the nerve roots and spinal cord. The anterior spinal artery supplies anterior sulcal arteries which branch laterally in the central gray matter. Both the anterior spinal artery and the smaller and shorter posterior spinal arteries, located along the posterolateral surface of the cord, supply circumferential and surface penetrating arteries.

Infarction of the anterior spinal artery causes increased T2 signal within the anterior two-thirds of the spinal cord and involves gray and white matter (Fig. 9.78A). Spinal cord infarction may be a difficult diagnosis to make in the absence of diffusion-weighted imaging (DWI) on MRI. Like brain infarction and unlike many causes of transverse myelitis, a spinal cord infarct may take up to a week to enhance (Fig. 9.78B and D). A border-zone pattern of infarction produces the classic "owl's eyes" appearance on axial

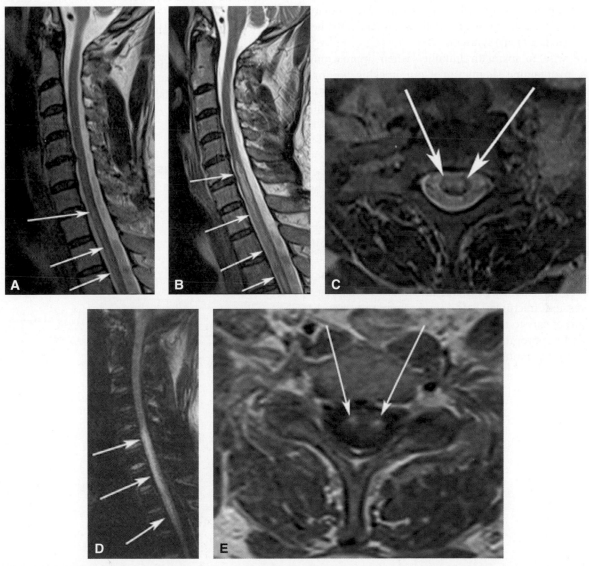

FIGURE 9.78. Spinal cord infarct, anterior spinal artery territory. A: On day 1, there is relatively subtle increased T2 signal in the lower cervical and upper thoracic spinal cord (*arrows*). **B:** By day 5, the spinal cord is expanded (*arrows*), with greater conspicuity of the signal abnormality. **C:** On axial images, the infarct involves central gray and adjacent white matter of approximately the anterior two-thirds of the spinal cord (*arrows*). **D:** Diffusion-weighted imaging (DWI), on day 6, shows subtle restricted diffusion (*arrows*). **E:** Note the early enhancement on day 6. The "owl's eyes" appearance of enhancement on the axial image (*arrows*) represents the vascular "watershed", as this was the most vulnerable part of the cord to ischemia and the first to infarct.

T2-weighted images because of bilateral symmetrical infarcts at the watershed between deep penetrating branches of the sulcal artery and surface-penetrating arteries (Fig. 9.78C and E). The infarcts are centered near the interface between central gray matter and the lateral columns.

CONCLUSIONS

The causes of neck and back pain and radiculopathy can be categorized as *soft, inflamed, edematous*, or *potentially unstable*. While not inclusive, the causes include herniated and bulging disk, synovial cyst, diskitis/osteomyelitis, fracture, spondylolysis, and tumor. These four categories notably do not include spinal stenosis, which is not more common in patients with back pain compared with asymptomatic people, and they also do not include spondylolisthesis, which is not more common in people with pain. However, spondylolisthesis with spondylolysis is included, as is spondylolisthesis with severe facet joint synovitis.

We are wise to maintain humility when approaching diagnosis, maintaining skepticism if our imaging findings are not concordant with the clinical presentation. Consult the medical record when available, rather than relying only on a few (sometimes misleading) words provided on the imaging requisition. Have empathy for the patient and for the clinical team. Try to integrate the findings with clinical data and comparison studies to create a narrative that is useful to all members of the health care team that are working diligently to help the patient.

KEY POINTS

- Radiographs are most helpful in postoperative follow-up, to assess for stability and in patients with suspected compression fractures. Standing radiographs are the standard of care to measure scoliosis.
- CT is the appropriate initial study (instead of radiographs) in the trauma patient.

- MRI is the principal imaging study for most diseases of the spine, including disk disease, myelopathy, spondylosis, stenosis, infection, and tumor.
- Odontoid fractures, flexion teardrop fractures, and perched or locked facets have a high association with spinal cord injury.
- Disk extrusion is more commonly associated with radiculopathy than disk bulge or protrusion.
- Structures causing neck and back pain and radiculopathy tend to be soft, inflamed, or associated with abnormal motion.
- Spinal stenosis and spondylolisthesis are not more common in patients with back pain compared with asymptomatic people.
- Diskitis and osteomyelitis cause contiguous signal abnormality and enhancement involving disk and adjacent end plates.
- CT myelography should be reserved for cases where MRI is nondiagnostic due to ferromagnetic artifact from hardware, in patients with implanted devices that are not MRI compatible, and in the evaluation of spontaneous intracranial hypotension to find the source of CSF leak.

References

General References

1. Naidich TP, Castillo M, Cha S, et al. *Imaging of the Spine*: Saunders; 2011.
2. Ross JR, Moore KR. *Diagnostic Imaging: Spine*. 3rd ed. Elsevier; 2013.

Questions

1. A patient presents to the emergency department with suspected neck trauma. The appropriate initial imaging study is
   a. lateral radiograph of the cervical spine
   b. four-view series of the cervical spine
   c. CT of the cervical spine
   d. MR of the cervical spine

2. A defect in the pars interarticularis is called
   a. spondylolisthesis
   b. spondylolysis
   c. limbus vertebra
   d. retroisthmic cleft

3. Which term best fits a disk abnormality in which a disk extends beyond expected margin of the annulus by less than 25% circumference and the depth of extension is less than the base of the abnormality?
   a. Sequestration
   b. Extrusion
   c. Protrusion
   d. Bulge

4. The most common cause of scoliosis is
   a. hemivertebra
   b. pedicle bars
   c. radiation in childhood
   d. idiopathic

5. The most common organism causing diskitis is
   a. *Streptococcus*
   b. *Staphylococcus*
   c. *Mycobacterium*
   d. *Enterococcus*

6. In a patient with a cervical spine injury and neurologic symptoms, the primary reason an MRI may be obtained is to
   a. determine the extent of fracture
   b. evaluate the spinal cord for edema or hemorrhage
   c. search for additional fractures
   d. assess for ligamentous injury

7. The following cervical spine injury is due to hyperextension
   a. locked facet
   b. C5 teardrop fracture
   c. burst fracture
   d. hangman fracture

8. An osteoblastic tumor in the spine is most likely due to which of the following?
   a. Multiple myeloma
   b. Prostate cancer
   c. Hemangioma
   d. Lung cancer

9. True or False: Multiple myeloma may present as osteopenia and a vertebral compression fracture.

10. A spinal cord infarct
    a. is often misdiagnosed on initial MRI
    b. enhances within a few hours of the onset of symptoms
    c. will have restricted diffusion in the acute phase
    d. requires emergency spinal angiogram
    e. a and c

CHAPTER 10

Nuclear Medicine

Thomas A. Farrell, MB, BCh

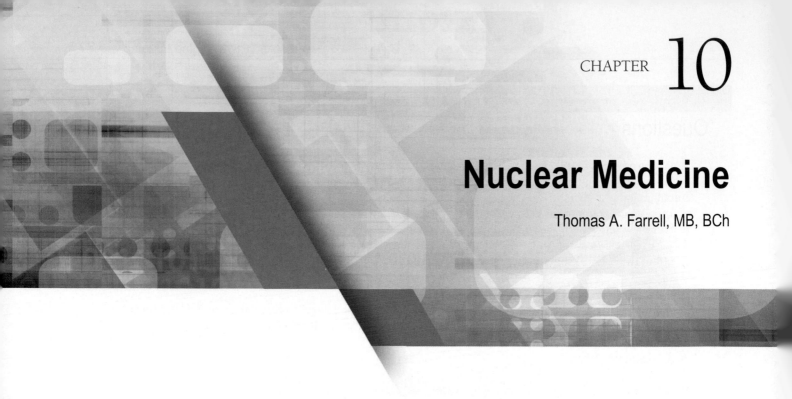

CHAPTER OUTLINE

Nuclear medicine uses small amounts of radioactive materials to diagnose and treat disease. The subspecialty is unique because it provides information about both organ structure and function in patients, and the techniques used often identify abnormalities early in the progress of a disease—often before other diagnostic tests. Nuclear imaging represents a physiologic map with minimal anatomic detail usually require correlation with other imaging modalities.

RADIOTRACERS AND RADIOPHARMACEUTICALS

When molecules with radionuclide components are prepared for administration, they are called radiopharmaceuticals (or technically, radiotracers if they are subpharmacologic doses because they participate in, but do not alter, various physiologic processes). The term radiopharmaceutical will be used generically in this chapter, but the distinction is important when diagnosing and treating disorders of the thyroid gland. Specific radiopharmaceuticals with physiochemical properties are used to study an organ or organ system. The radionuclide portion of the radiopharmaceutical typically emits gamma rays and/or x-rays that can be detected and create a scintigraphic image (often referred to as scan). There are several possible routes of patient administration of radiopharmaceuticals including intravenous, oral, and inhaled.

Over 30 radiopharmaceuticals use **technetium-99m (Tc-99m)**, which has many useful properties as a gamma-emitting tracer nuclide. It is eluted from a Tc-99m generator as a soluble pertechnetate and then either used directly as a soluble salt or combined with one of several Tc-99m–based radiotracers, which determine its uptake by various organs. Other agents incorporate a radioactive tracer atom into a larger active molecule, which is localized in the body, after which the radionuclide tracer atom allows it to be detected with a gamma camera. An example is F-18 **fluorodeoxyglucose (FDG)** in which fluorine-18 is incorporated into deoxyglucose to give 18-FDG, which is commonly used in positron emission tomography (PET) scanning. Some radioisotopes such as gallium-67 and radioiodine (I-123, I-131) are used directly as soluble ionic salts, without further modification.

The most commonly used nuclear medicine imaging system is a **gamma camera**, which is composed of an array of photomultiplier tubes. Each photomultiplier tube contains a sodium iodide crystal, that produces light when struck by gamma or x-rays. The light scintillations are digitized and processed into an image for interpretation. The image is essentially a physiologic map of the radiotracer distribution within the body. Table 10.1 lists commonly used radiotracers and radiopharmaceuticals and their applications.

Tomography is a basic imaging technique, which improves the visualization of an organ in a certain plane by blurring the adjacent tissue. This technique is widely used in nuclear medicine to improve image quality, for example, **single photon emission computed tomography (SPECT)**, involves an array of gamma cameras mounted on a gantry rotating around the patient. Spatial resolution of the organ of interest is improved by obtaining images in multiple projections to produce a 3D image. In **PET**, positrons undergo annihilation by combining with negatively charged electrons with the emission of two 511-keV photons in opposite directions. A PET scanner uses two detector elements or crystals on opposite sides of the patient to detect paired annihilation photons. If these photons are detected synchronously, the "annihilation" is assumed to have originated from a line between the two detectors. PET uses annihilation coincidence detection by several thousand crystals to acquire data over 360 degrees.

BONE SCINTIGRAPHY

Bone scintigraphy, more commonly referred to as a bone scan, is a valuable tool for the investigation of disorders such as tumor, infection, and fractures of the skeletal system. A Tc-99m–labeled diphosphonate derivative is used because this radiolabeled agent is adsorbed onto the surface of newly forming hydroxyapatite crystal during **osteogenic activity** (bone growth and repair), which occurs in response to almost all skeletal disorders. Scintigraphic images will demonstrate increased gamma-ray activity at the site of increased bone turnover. A typical protocol includes a whole-body scan with high count spot views reserved for specific areas of interest. Normal whole-body bone scans in an adult and child are shown in Figure 10.1. Note the multiple areas of increased activity in the child's epiphyses.

A bone scan is a sensitive but relatively nonspecific test and usually requires correlation with clinical features and other imaging modalities. The skeletal system is a common site for metastatic spread of many malignancies such as breast, lung, prostate, and renal carcinomas. Because **bony metastases** are a result of hematogenous seeding of tumor cells in the red marrow, they commonly occur in the axial skeleton and appear as numerous foci of increased radionuclide uptake (Fig. 10.2). Metastases that are osteoclastic or lytic (myeloma, renal cell carcinoma) are more difficult to detect because they appear cold or isointense on scintigraphy.

Like metastases, **osteomyelitis** can be detected earlier with a bone scan than with a plain film (Fig. 10.3). A **triple-phase bone scan** is used in the differential diagnosis of cellulitis and osteomyelitis. In osteomyelitis the scan appears positive on all three phases of the study: (1) early (arterial) hyperemia with (2) increased radiotracer uptake on blood pool images and (3) progressive local accumulation at the site on delayed images. By contrast, cellulitis appears as (1) delayed or venous phase hyperemia and (2) increased blood pool activity but (3) no local bone uptake on delayed images.

Stress fractures (Fig. 10.4) and shin splints (Fig. 10.5) are readily detected on a bone scan but may not be seen on a radiograph. Although MRI is more commonly being used for this indication, a bone scan may also be useful to detect **fractures**, which may not be easily seen on plain films. Some full-thickness cortical fractures, such as those in the sacrum, scapula, femoral neck, and small bones of the wrist and ankle, may be difficult to visualize on a radiograph but are detectable by a bone scan (Fig. 10.6).

TABLE 10.1	Commonly Used Radiopharmaceuticals and Their Applications
Radiopharmaceutical	**Application**
Tc-99m diphosphonate	Bone
Tc-99m iminodiacetic acid (HIDA)	Hepatobiliary
I-123, I-131	Thyroid
Tc-99m sestamibi	Parathyroid
Tc-99m MAG3	Renal ERPF split
Tc-99m DTPA	Renal GFR
Tc-99m macroaggregated albumin (MAA)	Lung perfusion
Xenon-133, Tc-99m DTPA aerosol	Lung ventilation
F-18 fluorodeoxyglucose (FDG)	Oncology
Indium DTPA octreotide	Neuroendocrine tumors
Prostate-specific membrane antigen (PMSA)	Prostate Ca
Thallium-201, Tc-99m sestamibi, rubidium-82	Cardiac
F-18 fluorodeoxyglucose (FDG), Tc-HMPAO	Brain

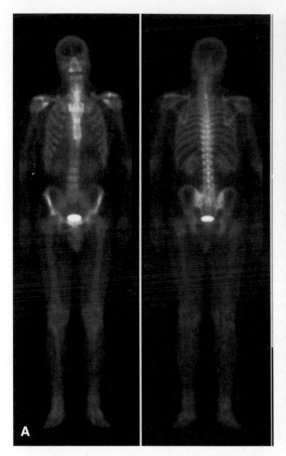
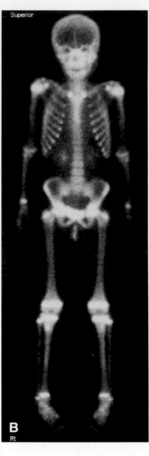

FIGURE 10.1. **Normal bone scans.** Whole-body images of a normal bone scan in an adult **(A)** and child **(B)**. Note the increased epiphyseal activity on the child's scan.

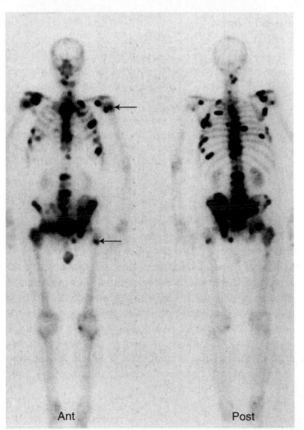

FIGURE 10.2. **Bony metastases.** Whole-body bone scan in anterior and posterior projections of a 65-year-old man with diffuse skeletal metastases from prostate carcinoma. There are numerous foci of increased uptake, primarily in the axial skeleton and in the proximal femurs and humeri (arrows).

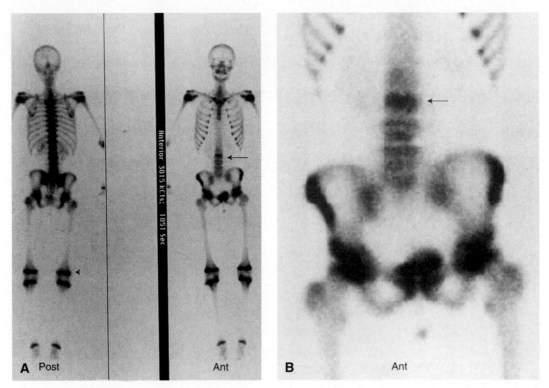

FIGURE 10.3. **Acute osteomyelitis.** Skeletal scintigraphic images (whole body **(A)**; regional view **(B)**) from an 18-year-old girl with diabetes who presented with 3 to 4 wk of low back pain. Radiographs of the vertebra were unremarkable. The images show increased Tc-99 MDP activity in the L3 vertebral body (arrows). Biopsy of the site confirmed osteomyelitis. The increased uptake of Tc-99m MDP at the growth plates in the lower extremities (arrowhead) on the whole-body images is a normal feature. Ant, anterior; Post, posterior.

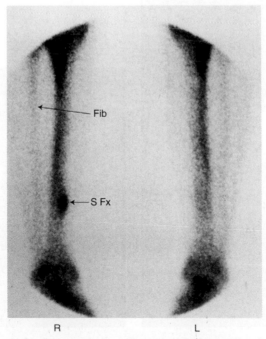

FIGURE 10.4. **Stress fracture.** A 20-year-old runner with pain in the right calf. Radiographs were normal. Scintigraphic images of the distal lower extremities show focal increase in uptake in the right distal tibia consistent with a stress fracture (arrow S Fx). The stress fracture does not involve the full thickness of the tibia. Fibula indicated by arrow Fib.

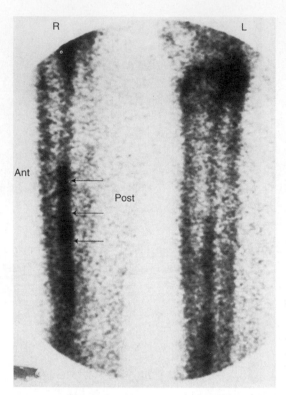

FIGURE 10.5. **Shin splint.** Bone scan of a patient with calf pain, showing a linear pattern of increased uptake (arrows) along the posterior aspect of the tibia (enthesopathy). Ant, anterior; Post, posterior.

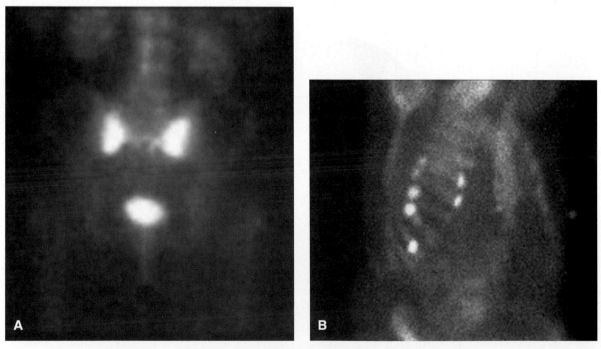

FIGURE 10.6. **Fractures. A:** Sacral insufficiency fracture. **B:** Multiple rib fractures.

TABLE 10.2	Causes of Nonosseous (False-Positive) Uptake on a Bone Scan
Location	**Cause**
Brain	Stroke
Chest	Myocardial infarct
	Hyperparathyroidism
	Lung metastases
Abdomen	Spleen (sickle cell disease)
Soft tissues	Trauma (IM injection)
	Myositis

TABLE 10.3	Causes of Photopenic Bone Lesions (False-Negative Bone Scan)
Multiple myeloma
Osteonecrosis
Post radiation therapy
Rarely metastatic bone disease (renal cell carcinoma, anaplastic)
Paravertebral soft tissue lesion invading bone

Although regarded as a sensitive test, bone scintigraphy may have false-positive and false-negative results (Tables 10.2 and 10.3). Evaluation of the kidneys is an important component of interpreting a bone scan because most of the administered dose undergoes renal excretion. Increased renal uptake is seen in urinary obstruction and acute tubular necrosis. Reduced or no renal uptake occurs in renal failure and on "superscan" because of metastases and metabolic bone disease.

HEPATOBILIARY IMAGING

Patients with **acute cholecystitis** classically present with right upper quadrant pain/tenderness, fever, and leukocytosis. However, the signs and symptoms of acute cholecystitis often vary and there are several conditions that may present in a similar fashion. The provisional diagnosis of acute cholecystitis typically requires confirmatory testing with ultrasound and/or hepatobiliary scintigraphy. Hepatobiliary scintigraphic imaging is performed using a Tc-99m–labeled iminodiacetic acid **(HIDA)** derivative that is an analogue of bilirubin. This radiopharmaceutical is actively transported into hepatocytes like bilirubin and excreted unchanged into the biliary tract. Normally HIDA accumulates within the gallbladder within 1 hour of intravenous injection (Fig. 10.7). However, in acute cholecystitis, the gallbladder fails to fill with the radiotracer

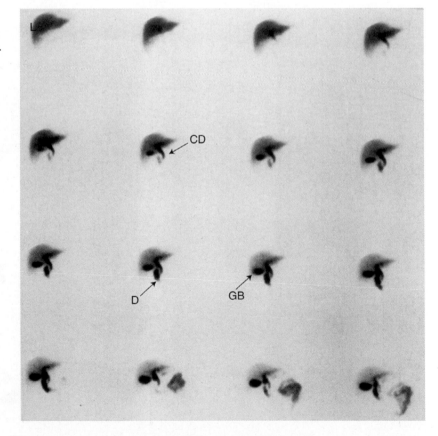

FIGURE 10.7. Normal hepatobiliary (HIDA) study. Anterior view images obtained every 2 min (moving from left to right and top to bottom) following injection of the hepatobiliary radiotracer show good extraction of the agent by the liver (L). The common bile duct (arrow CD) is seen as are the duodenum (arrow D) and gallbladder (arrow GB).

TABLE 10.4	Causes of False-Positive Results With Hepatobiliary Imaging in the Evaluation of Acute Cholecystitis

Prolonged fasting
Ingestion of food within 2 h of the study
Chronic cholecystitis
Chronic alcohol abuse
Pancreatitis

because of cystic duct obstruction. This test is extremely sensitive, and a normal result (i.e., visualization of the gallbladder) virtually excludes acute cholecystitis. False-positive scans are caused by prolonged fasting or recent ingestion of food (Table 10.4). The use of IV morphine has been found helpful in reducing the number of false-positive HIDA scans, thereby improving the specificity of the test. Morphine causes constriction of the sphincter of Oddi, which augments bile flow through the cystic duct, improving gallbladder visualization (Figs. 10.8 and 10.9). HIDA scanning is also useful in the diagnosis of postoperative **bile leaks** (Fig. 10.10).

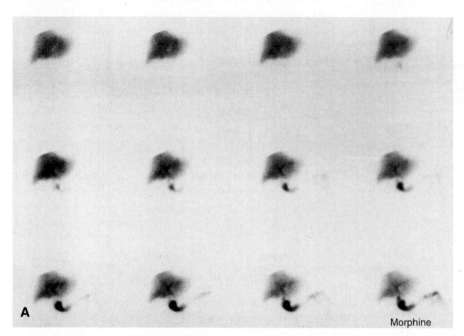

FIGURE 10.8. Normal HIDA study with IV morphine. A: Initial images show normal uptake and excretion by the liver, but nonvisualization of the gallbladder. **B:** Images obtained immediately following administration of morphine show the gallbladder visualization (arrow GB), which excludes acute cholecystitis. Note activity in the small bowel (arrow SB).

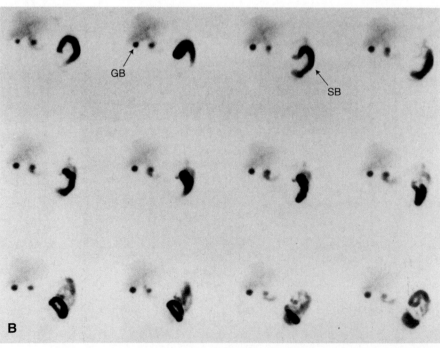

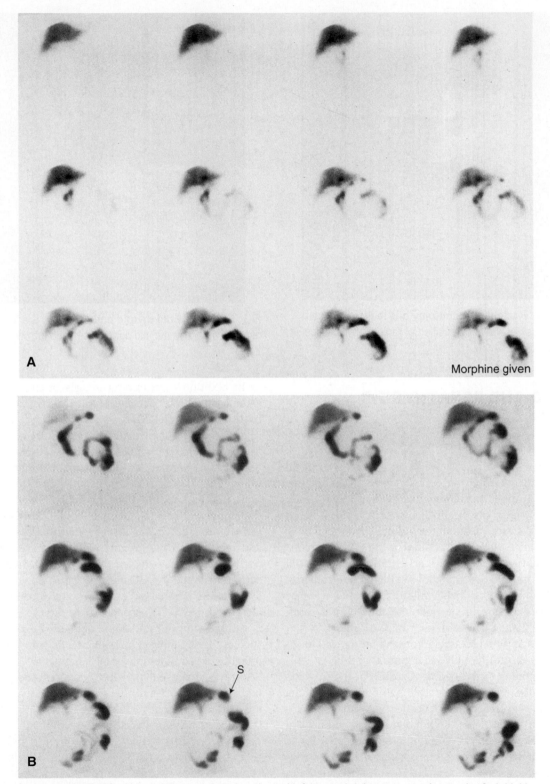

FIGURE 10.9. Acute cholecystitis. Hepatobiliary study in a patient with fever and right upper quadrant pain. **A:** Initial images show normal uptake and excretion by the liver, but the gallbladder is not visualized and consequently morphine is given at approximately the time of the image at bottom right. **B:** Images obtained immediately following injection of morphine continue to show absence of gallbladder activity, indicating cystic duct obstruction and acute cholecystitis. Note the reflux of radioactive bile into the stomach (arrow S).

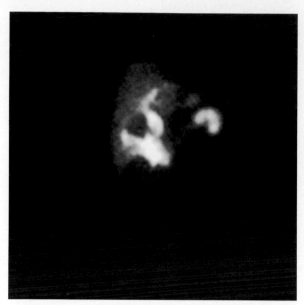

FIGURE 10.10. Postcholecystectomy bile leak. HIDA scan shows extravasation and accumulation of radiopharmaceutical in the gallbladder bed.

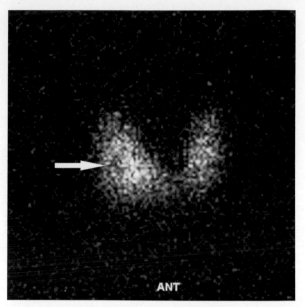

FIGURE 10.11. Cold thyroid nodule. There is a focus of reduced uptake in the mid right thyroid lobe (arrow).

THYROID AND PARATHYROID IMAGING

Thyroid

Radioiodine in the forms of I-123 and I-131 is an ideal radiotracer and radiopharmaceutical, respectively, as they are selectively trapped, and organified by the thyroid gland. Although Tc-99-m is also trapped by the thyroid, it is not organified and is rarely used in thyroid imaging.

I-131 has an 8-day half-life and its 364-keV photons result in a high radiation dose, particularly to the thyroid and are not optimal for imaging with gamma cameras. However, the high-energy beta emissions are effective therapy for Graves disease, toxic nodules, and thyroid carcinoma making them a true radiopharmaceutical.

The advantages of **I-123** as a radiotracer for thyroid imaging include its shorter half-life (13.2 hours) and better suitability for gamma camera imaging. Because of the thyroid's relatively small size, a pinhole collimator on the gamma camera provides geometric magnification with image resolution superior to parallel-hole collimators. The gland's lateral lobes extend along each side of the thyroid cartilage. While visualization of the thyroid isthmus is variable, the thin pyramidal lobe, which ascends anteriorly and superiorly from the isthmus, is normally not seen except in Graves' disease. Up to 90% of all thyroid nodules are cold (hypofunctional) on thyroid scans, 20% of which are malignant (Fig. 10.11). A hot or warm nodule is an autonomous follicular adenoma with a very low incidence of malignancy. Scintigraphy has largely been replaced by ultrasound and ultrasound-guided biopsy in the diagnostic workup of thyroid nodules.

In addition to obtaining images of the thyroid gland, estimation of the percent of **radioactive iodine uptake by the thyroid (%RAIU)** is useful in the diagnosis of thyroid disorders. Whereas imaging scans are acquired with a gamma camera, an uptake study is usually acquired with a nonimaging gamma scintillation probe detector and is useful in the differential diagnosis of thyrotoxicosis. The normal range for the %RAIU is approximately 4% to 15% at 4 to 6 hours and 10% to 30% at 24 hours. Causes of increased %RAIU include Graves disease, multinodular toxic goiter, and metastatic thyroid carcinoma. Increased uptake may occur in patients who are hyperthyroid, hypothyroid or euthyroid so the %RAIU must be evaluated with the clinical features and laboratory results. The most common cause of a reduced %RAIU is subacute thyroiditis.

Suppression of radioiodine uptake by exogenous iodine such as radiographic contrast media may prevent successful imaging or accurate uptake measurements.

Graves disease is the most common cause of thyrotoxicosis. Patients have a diffuse goiter, infiltrative ophthalmopathy, and occasionally infiltrative dermopathy. The thyroid scan shows a symmetrically enlarged gland with homogeneous tracer distribution and a prominent pyramidal lobe (Fig. 10.12). The %RAIU is increased. While there is no cure for Graves disease, the goal of treatment is to reduce the thyroid's ability to produce hormones. Three treatment options are available: medical therapy, I-131 therapy, and less commonly surgery.

Typical doses for diagnosis (radiotracer) are measured in **microcuries** and for therapy (radiopharmaceutical) in **millicuries** underscoring the dual nature of this agent. The radiopharmaceutical dose of I-131is dependent on

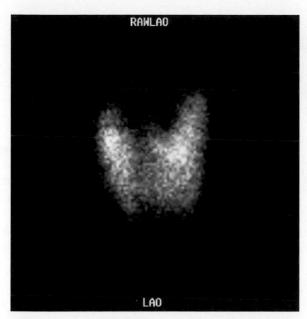

FIGURE 10.12. **Graves disease.** Tc-99m pertechnetate scan shows a diffusely increased uptake with visualization of a pyramidal lobe (superiorly from the midline). The diagnosis was confirmed by an elevated radioactive iodine uptake.

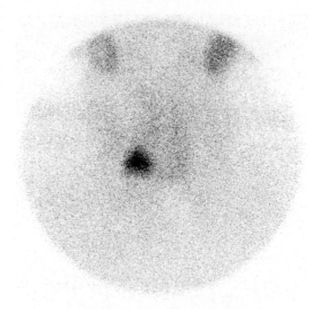

FIGURE 10.13. **Parathyroid adenoma** in a patient with hypercalcemia. Delayed imaging after Tc-99m sestamibi injection shows increased uptake in the right neck consistent with a parathyroid adenoma.

the gland weight and %RAIU. Other indications for I-131 therapy include multinodular toxic goiter and metastatic thyroid cancer. Radioiodine I-131 is a suitable option for toxic nodules because the radiation is delivered selectively to the hyperfunctioning nodules while sparing suppressed nonnodular thyroid tissue, which results in a low incidence of posttherapy hypothyroidism. Medullary and anaplastic thyroid carcinomas do not concentrate radioiodine and consequently are not detected with radioiodine scintigraphy or are suitable for I-131 therapy.

Parathyroid

An elevated parathyroid hormone (PTH) level in a patient with hypercalcemia is diagnostic of hyperparathyroidism. Surgical resection is the initial treatment and is usually curative with scanning reserved for localization of a residual hyperfunctioning parathyroid gland, which may be ectopic (e.g., mediastinal). Fewer than 1% of patients with hyperparathyroidism have parathyroid carcinoma. Typically, **Tc-99m sestamibi** is injected followed by rapid uptake in both the parathyroid and thyroid glands. However, thyroid gland washout occurs more rapidly, so at 2-hour a hyperfunctioning parathyroid gland is a seen as a focus of residual activity (Fig. 10.13). The use of **single photon emission computed tomography (SPECT)** results in improved target-to-background ratio compared with planar imaging improving 3D localization of the hyperfunctioning gland(s). Normally functioning parathyroid glands are not visualized. The most common cause for a false-positive parathyroid scan is a thyroid adenoma.

RENAL IMAGING

Cross-sectional imaging (US, CT, and MRI) has largely replaced Tc-99m DMSA imaging, which was used to demonstrate renal anatomy (Fig. 10.14). Because of its more efficient extraction in the proximal renal tubules, **Tc-99m MAG3** is preferred over Tc-99m DTPA in cases of impaired renal function and suspected obstruction. The MAG3 clearance is a measure of the effective renal plasma flow (ERPF) and can be used to estimate split renal function. In contrast, **Tc-99m DTPA** is filtered by the renal glomerulus and is a more reliable measure of

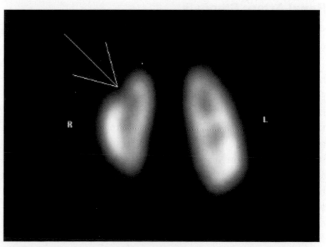

FIGURE 10.14. **Renal DMSA scan.** Upper pole cortical loss in the right kidney (arrow).

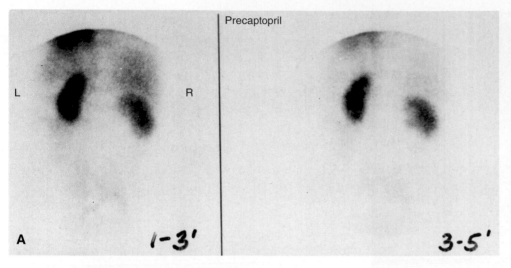

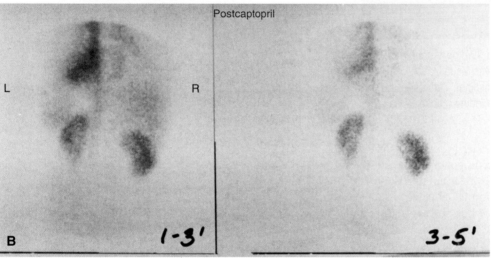

FIGURE 10.15. Captopril renogram positive for renal artery stenosis. A: Scintigraphic images of the kidneys in the posterior projection, 1 to 3 min and 3 to 5 min following injection of Tc-DTPA. **B:** Repeat images following administration of captopril show a significant decrease in the concentration of this agent (and, therefore, decrease in GFR) in the left kidney compared with the precaptopril images indicating the presence of renal artery stenosis.

glomerular filtration rate **(GFR)**. Its normal mean renal transit time is 3 minutes and at 2 hours there is less than 10% renal retention.

Renal Artery Stenosis

Scintigraphic imaging of glomerular filtration combined with administration of an angiotensin-converting enzyme (ACE) inhibitor, such as captopril, is used to diagnose hypertension caused by **renal artery stenosis**. In these patients, renin secretion is increased secondary to the hemodynamic effects of a functionally significant stenosis in the renal artery. Decreased perfusion pressure as a result of the arterial stenosis causes the juxtaglomerular cells to increase secretion of renin. Renin acts on angiotensinogen to form angiotensin I, which is converted to angiotensin II by ACE. Angiotensin II stimulates release of aldosterone, which acts as a potent vasoconstrictor of the peripheral vasculature, including vasoconstriction of the efferent renal arterioles distal to the glomerulus in the underperfused kidney with the renal artery stenosis. The efferent vasoconstriction acts to preserve the transglomerular pressure

gradient and maintain the GFR in the affected kidney. If an ACE inhibitor such as captopril is administered to a patient with renal artery stenosis, angiotensin II levels will drop and the efferent arterioles will dilate, leading to a fall in GFR (Fig. 10.15).

VENTILATION/PERFUSION LUNG IMAGING FOR THE DIAGNOSIS OF PULMONARY EMBOLISM

Pulmonary embolism (PE) is the third most common cause of cardiovascular mortality in the United States. The clinical diagnosis of PE is often difficult as symptoms and signs such as dyspnea, chest pain, tachypnea, and tachycardia are nonspecific. A chest radiograph should be obtained in all patients suspected of having PE to exclude other causes of the patient's symptoms such as pneumonia, pneumothorax, and heart failure. However, a normal chest radiograph does not exclude PE and even if the chest radiograph is abnormal and consistent with PE, this alone is rarely enough to make an accurate diagnosis necessitating further testing.

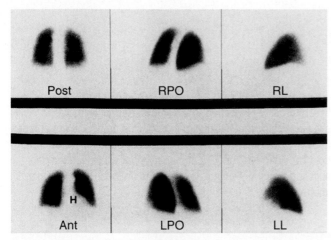

FIGURE 10.16. Normal lung perfusion in six projections. Ant, anterior; LL, left lateral; LPO, left posterior oblique; Post, posterior; RL, right lateral; RPO, right posterior oblique. H designates area of absent activity due to the heart.

Ventilation–perfusion (V/Q, Q is the physiologic symbol for flow rate) imaging is accurate for diagnosing PE. Images of regional pulmonary **perfusion** are obtained by intravenously injecting several hundred thousand tiny particles of macroaggregated human albumin that are radiolabeled with Tc-99m. These albumin particles measure between 10 and 40 μm and lodge on their first pass in pulmonary capillaries and precapillary arterioles in concentrations directly proportional to the regional pulmonary blood flow, which is normally greater in the lung bases (Fig. 10.16). Because less than 0.1% of the total cross section area of the pulmonary vasculature is occluded by the injected radiolabeled particles, complications are rare. Pulmonary emboli are often large enough to occlude the segmental pulmonary arteries, and hence the perfusion defects on the images will often appear segmental in configuration (Fig. 10.17A). Segmental defects are wedge shaped and pleural based. Perfusion defects are also seen in pneumonia, chronic obstructive pulmonary disease (COPD), and atelectasis because of localized reflex vasoconstriction. So a perfusion defect alone is not diagnostic of PE, and for this reason ventilation scintigraphy of the lungs is correlated with the perfusion study. Images of regional pulmonary **ventilation** are obtained by having the patient inhale either radioactive xenon gas or an aerosolized form of Tc-99m DTPA. The

FIGURE 10.17. Pulmonary embolism. A: Six-view perfusion scan showing numerous mismatched bilateral segmental defects. **B:** Single-breath ventilation images showing normal ventilation indicating a mismatch pattern consistent with PE. Ant, anterior; LL, left lateral; LPO, left posterior oblique; Post, posterior; RL, right lateral; RPO, right posterior oblique.

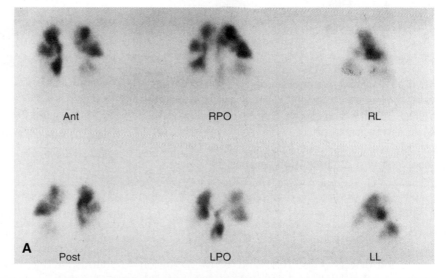

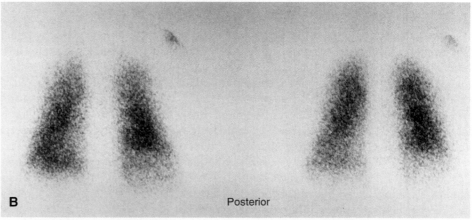

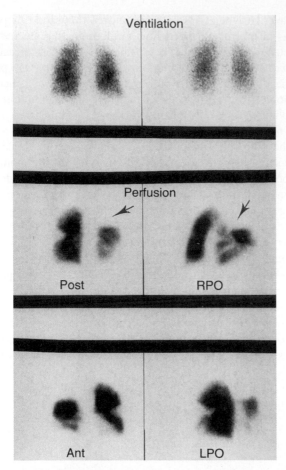

Ventilation

Perfusion

Post   RPO

Ant   LPO

FIGURE 10.18. Pulmonary embolism. Top two images are posterior ventilation images with xenon-133 showing uniform ventilation to both lungs. Bottom four images are from the perfusion study showing multiple segmental defects. Arrow points to mismatched perfusion defects in the right upper lobe. Ant, anterior; LPO, left posterior oblique; Post, posterior; RPO, right posterior oblique.

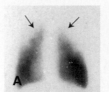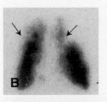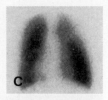

FIGURE 10.19. Matched V/Q defects. Patient with COPD showing matched ventilation and perfusion defects in upper lobes (arrows). **A:** Posterior perfusion image. **B:** Posterior initial breath-hold ventilation image. **C:** Later equilibrium ventilation image showing eventual filling of defects seen on the initial ventilation image.

TABLE 10.5	Causes of Matched Ventilation/Perfusion Defects With an Abnormal Chest Film
Pneumonia	
Chronic obstructive lung disease	
Atelectasis	
Asthma	

TABLE 10.6	Interpretation of Ventilation/Perfusion Scans	
Result	**Probability of PE**
Normal	0%
Low probability	<20%
Intermediate probability	20%–80%
High probability	>80%

combination of ventilation and perfusion scans improves the accuracy for the diagnosis of PE. A **mismatched defect** is described if ventilation is normal in regions of the lung that show perfusion defects (Figs. 10.17 and 10.18). Perfusion defects that are larger than the ventilation abnormality are also categorized as mismatched. In contrast, matched defects characterized by abnormal regional perfusion and corresponding abnormal regional ventilation are found in other lung diseases (Fig. 10.19 and Table 10.5). A **triple matched defect** describes the matching abnormalities on ventilation, perfusion, and chest radiograph.

The **Modified PIOPED** criteria are the most widely used for reporting V/Q scans and are used to estimate the **probability** that acute PE has occurred. A normal perfusion scan indicates virtually no chance that the patient has a PE, while multiple perfusion defects with a normal ventilation scan indicate a high probability that the patient has PE (Table 10.6). The current examination of choice in patients with suspected PE is CTA chest with a modified protocol so the patient is scanned when the contrast bolus maximally opacifies the pulmonary arteries. V/Q scans are still performed in patients who are allergic to intravenous contrast, in the presence of renal failure, during pregnancy, and in women of childbearing age. In pregnancy, a reduced dose perfusion only scan to reduce fetal exposure is recommended. In women of childbearing age, the absorbed radiation dose to the breast is 100 times greater in women undergoing CTA for PE than those having a V/Q scan. However, compared with V/Q scans, CTA has fewer non-diagnostic studies and can also estimate right ventricular strain, which has prognostic implications (see Table 2.8).

Neuroendocrine tumors (NET) originate from neuroendocrine cells most commonly in the GI tract or the bronchopulmonary system. Up to 50% of patients with NET have synchronous regional or distant metastasis at the time of diagnosis. Whole-body scanning with 68Ga DOTATOC PET/CT has proven useful and reliable in the diagnosis and staging of NET.

Prostate Carcinoma

Indium-111 ProstaScint is a murine monoclonal antibody that targets **prostate-specific membrane antigen (PSMA)** (not PSA), a transmembrane protein expressed on the cell surface of prostate carcinoma. PSMA has shown high selective expression in prostate carcinoma, metastatic lymph nodes, and bone metastases, allowing accurate diagnosis and staging of primary prostate carcinoma and restaging after biochemical recurrence, even in case of low prostate-specific antigen values.

Positron Emission Tomography and PET/CT

Positron emission tomography (PET) differs from the nuclear medicine techniques described so far because the radioisotopes that are used emit positrons rather than gamma or x-rays. Positrons have a higher energy (0.5 MeV vs. 140 keV for Tc-99m) and are imaged using a different type of scanner. After a positron is emitted, it travels a very short distance (a few millimeters) in body tissue and combines with an electron. The combined mass of the positron and electron is converted into energy in the form of two gamma rays that travel in opposite directions. These "simultaneous" gamma rays are detected by the PET scanner, which then creates a three-dimensional image of the distribution of the radioisotope in the body.

Positron-emitting radioisotopes include C-11, N-13, O-15, and F-18. They have a short half-life and in theory can be labeled to virtually any organic molecule such as glucose (or glucose analogues), water, or ammonia, or into molecules that bind to receptors. Currently, the main PET radiopharmaceutical used clinically is fluorine-18 fluorodeoxyglucose (F-18-FDG), which is a glucose analogue, imaging of which depicts the distribution of glucose metabolism in the body.

ONCOLOGIC IMAGING

Because many malignant tumors demonstrate enhanced metabolism of glucose relative to normal organs, whole-body PET imaging with F-18-FDG can be used to detect and stage malignancy (Fig. 10.20). Although PET can be used to measure the absolute level of tumor glucose metabolism, in practice this is time-consuming and requires arterial blood sampling of F-18-FDG levels. An alternative semiquantitative measurement is used and referred to as the **standardized uptake value (SUV)**, which is directly related to glucose metabolism and much simpler to determine from PET images. The SUV serves as a normalized target-to-background measure, and in general, lesions with

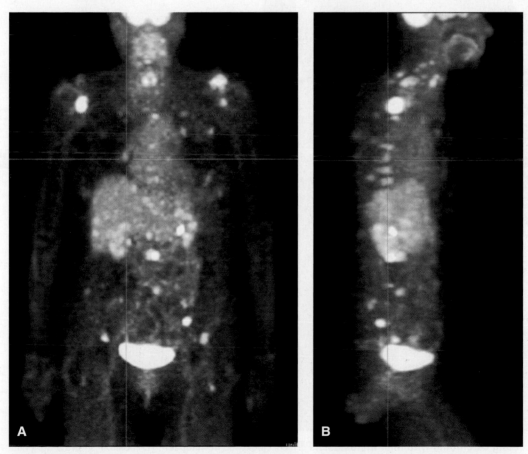

FIGURE 10.20. Lung carcinoma with widespread metastases. Frontal **(A)** and lateral **(B)** projections of a whole-body F-18-FDG PET scan showing numerous foci of increased uptake (including the spine) consistent with metastatic disease.

an SUV of 2.5 or greater are likely to be malignant, whereas values below 2.5 are more likely to be physiologic in origin or caused by benign lesions. One hour after intravenous administration, high F-18-FDG activity is normally present in the brain, heart, and urinary tract (excretory route). Sites of variable physiologic tracer uptake include the digestive tract, thyroid, and skeletal muscle. Elsewhere in the body, tracer activity is typically low.

To further improve localization of lesions detected on PET, patients are usually scanned on combined **PET/CT** scanners. These superimposed scans improve both the sensitivity and the specificity for malignant tumor detection. Tumor types commonly referred for PET/CT evaluation in clinical practice include lung, head and neck cancers, lymphomas, colon cancer, breast cancer, and melanoma. There are many clinical applications including initial staging, detection of recurrent tumor, and evaluation of response to chemotherapy (Figs. 10.21 and 10.22).

Limitations of PET

Some malignancies are known to be "not PET avid" for reasons including low glucose metabolism as seen in well-differentiated tumors, low proliferation rates, high mucin content, and tumor necrosis (Table 10.7). PET is not useful within 2 months of surgical resection because of a high false-positive rate, which may be the result of inflammation or granulation tissue. Furthermore, when performed within 4 weeks of chemotherapy, PET has a false-negative rate of over 80%, and surgical decisions should not be based on the results of PET without further investigation. Future developments include the use of a PET/MR combination, which may produce as good anatomic images with less radiation exposure.

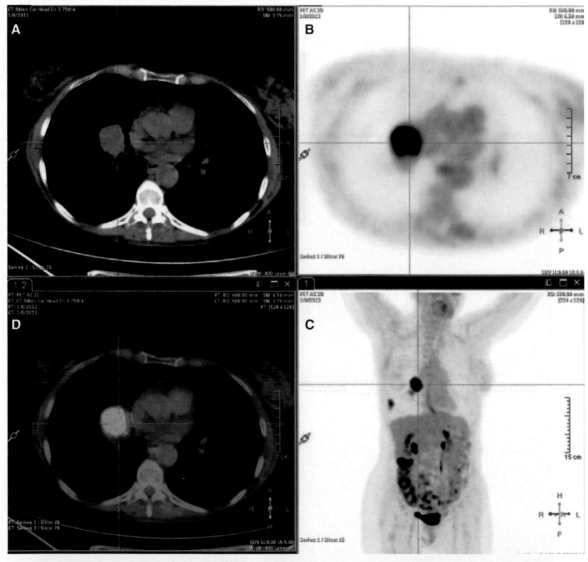

FIGURE 10.21. Lung carcinoma with hilar metastasis. PET/CT clockwise from top left. **A:** Axial CT shows a right hilar mass. **B:** Axial PET showing increased uptake in the mass. **C:** Coronal PET showing increased uptake in a smaller peripheral right lower lobe mass. **D:** Fusion of PET/CT images.

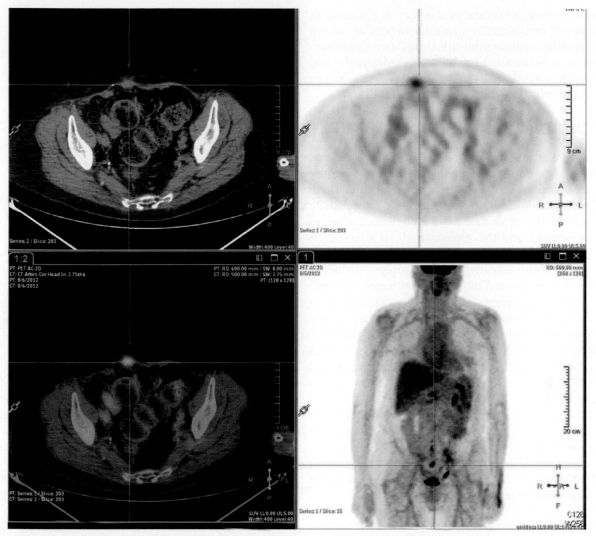

FIGURE 10.22. Postoperative carcinoma recurrence. PET/CT (clockwise from top left image is an axial CT of the pelvis, axial PET image at the same level, coronal PET and a combined axial PET/CT image) showing a focus of increased uptake in a soft tissue nodule in the anterior abdominal wall of a patient who had a hemicolectomy for colonic carcinoma. Biopsy confirmed recurrence.

TABLE 10.7	Causes of a False-Negative PET Scan/Low PET Avid Tumors

Lesion size <1 cm
Prostate carcinoma
Mucinous adenocarcinoma
Carcinoid

CARDIAC IMAGING

Cardiac imaging accounts for nearly 50% of all nuclear medicine tests. The two main areas of interest are cardiac function, specifically left ventricular function and myocardial perfusion imaging (MPI) in patients with known or suspected coronary artery disease (CAD).

VENTRICULAR FUNCTION IMAGING

Radionuclide ventriculogram (or multigated acquisition scan—MUGA) may be used to assess ventricular function and can be performed in two ways. A first pass technique involves scanning a rapid bolus of a Tc-99m radiotracer as it passes through the heart chambers—this is more accurate for right ventricular evaluation as there is no chamber overlap. The second and more commonly used technique is called **equilibrium scanning** as it requires Tc-99m RBC imaging, gated to the ECG over several hundred cardiac cycles. Ventricular function is evaluated by calculating the ejection fraction (EF), which is the volumetric fraction of blood pumped out of the ventricle during the cardiac cycle. The normal EF range is 55% to 70%. Common causes of poor ventricular function are ischemia, aortic and mitral valve disease and chemotherapy drugs such as **doxorubicin** and **trastuzumab (Herceptin)**, viral infections, and alcohol.

In patients receiving doxorubicin, a decline of 10% or more in absolute left ventricular EF to a value of 50% or less is a recommendation to discontinue the drug. Ventricular function may also be measured using echocardiography and MRI. Cardiac arrhythmias during image acquisition can limit reproducible assessment of ventricular function.

MYOCARDIAL PERFUSION IMAGING

There is consensus across national and international guidelines in favor of **myocardial perfusion imaging (MPI)** as a noninvasive diagnostic tool for the detection of obstructive CAD in patients with intermediate pretest probability of disease. The American College of Cardiology (ACC) and the American Heart Association (AHA) support the exercise ECG as the initial test but recommend stress imaging in subgroups including women with diabetes and those in whom a poor exercise performance is anticipated. ACC/AHA guidelines rely on the size and magnitude of stress-induced nuclear perfusion defects in order to determine "appropriateness" of revascularization therapy. As a secondary test, MPI is indicated in patients with nondiagnostic or unexpected exercise ECG results, that is, patients with a low or high pretest likelihood of CAD and an abnormal or normal exercise ECG, respectively. Stress MPI is not indicated for cardiovascular risk assessment in low- or intermediate-risk asymptomatic adults.

MPI is usually done using intravenously injected **thallium-201 chloride (Tl-201)** and/or **Tc-99m–labeled agents** such as **sestamibi** or **tetrofosmin**. Thallium is a potassium analogue (indicator of cell membrane integrity) and is the only SPECT radionuclide that assesses myocardial redistribution and viability. It cannot be extracted by infarction or scar. SPECT is used to obtain myocardial perfusion images using one of these agents by rotating in a 180-degree arc during which data are acquired and formatted to give a 3D image. Short-axis (Fig. 10.23) and coronal (horizontal long axis) and sagittal (vertical long-axis) views are used for interpretation. On short-axis views, the normal left ventricle has a doughnut appearance. The normal lateral left ventricular wall usually has slightly more uptake than the anterior or inferior wall. Reduced uptake is normally seen near the base of the heart corresponding to the membranous septum.

Stress testing improves the sensitivity of MPI for the detection of CAD and can be performed during either exercise or IV injection of adenosine, dipyridamole, or regadenoson, which increases coronary blood flow by as much as five times. Distal arterioles in a normal coronary artery will dilate substantially in response to either exercise or pharmacologic stimulation. As a result, perfusion (and radiotracer concentration) will increase considerably in the myocardium supplied by a normal artery, whereas myocardial perfusion will change little if at all distal to a significant stenosis. Therefore, significant

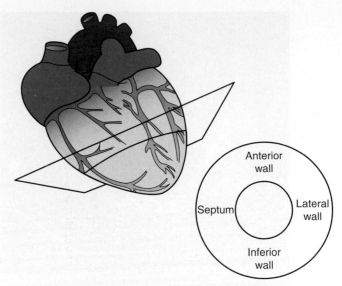

FIGURE 10.23. Normal myocardial SPECT views. The short-axis cross-sectional view is obtained by slicing the three-dimensional image of the heart muscle in planes perpendicular to the long dimension of the heart.

CAD will cause a perfusion defect immediately following stress. Perfusion defects seen on stress imaging that become less severe or normalize on delayed images are referred to as **reversible** and almost always contain viable myocardium (Fig. 10.24). Reversible defects typically also have wall motion at rest. Defects that do not change from stress to the delayed images are called **fixed** and usually contain scar tissue (Fig. 10.25). However, in some instances fixed defects may still contain viable tissue. Stress-induced thallium-201 uptake by the lung is evidence of ventricular dysfunction and a poor prognostic sign. In addition, poststress ventricular dilatation suggests multivessel disease.

One major limitation of using **Tl-201** scintigraphy alone is the high false-positive rate that is attributed predominantly to attenuation artifacts, which may be misinterpreted as perfusion defects. Although quantification of Tl-201 improves specificity, the false-positive rate remains problematic, particularly in women where breast attenuation may be mistaken for perfusion abnormalities owing to anterolateral ischemia or in obesity where inferior perfusion defects may be seen. The presence of a left bundle branch block can also lead to a false-positive stress test anteriorly during exercise, in which case pharmacologic agents listed above can be used.

The **Tc-99m**–labeled perfusion agents (sestamibi, tetrofosmin) enhance the specificity of SPECT and provide information on regional and global left ventricular systolic function via ECG gating of images. Because of the more optimal imaging characteristics of Tc-99m, there is less gamma-ray scatter and attenuation than with Tl-201, which results in fewer false-positive artifacts and a lower radiation dose. These agents also allow better gated acquisition,

FIGURE 10.24. Abnormal thallium scan. SPECT in a patient with a stenosis of the left anterior descending coronary artery; short-axis stress images column **(A)** showing a severe perfusion defect in the septum, which is reversible on rest/redistribution images column **(B)**.

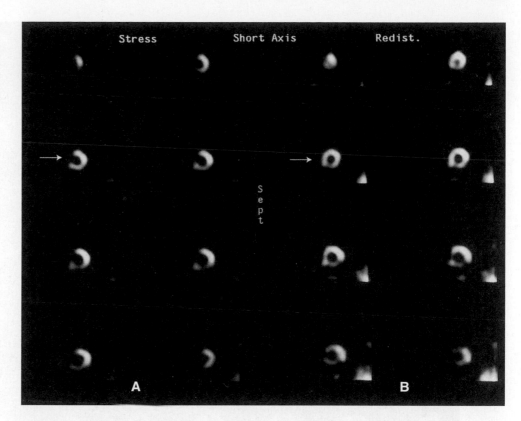

FIGURE 10.25. Abnormal thallium scan. SPECT in a patient with previous anterior myocardial infarction. Short-axis images show defects in the anterior (arrows) and lateral walls, both of which are fixed (unchanged from stress to rest/redistribution images). These findings are consistent with scarring.

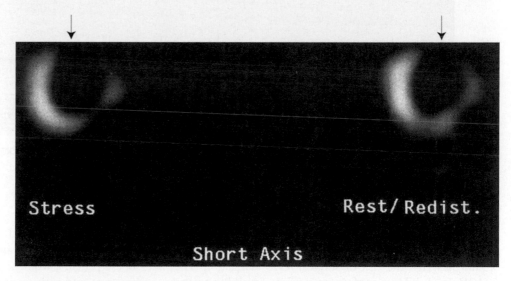

permitting the simultaneous evaluation of regional systolic thickening, global left ventricular function, and myocardial perfusion.

Several 1- and 2-day protocols using one or both agents have been described depending on workflow and equipment availability. Performing the stress phase of the examination first followed by a resting phase allows identification and characterization of myocardial perfusion defects due to ischemia. Typically, a combination of Tl-201 and Tc-99m perfusion agents are used at rest and stress, for example, same day Tl-201 at rest and Tc-99m agent

at stress (Fig. 10.26). Alternatively, low and high doses of a Tc-99m agent can be given at rest and during stress, respectively (Fig. 10.27).

Historically, it was believed that ischemic LV dysfunction was due to a combination of repetitive ischemia myocardial stunning and hibernation and was therefore potentially reversible in patients undergoing revascularization. This generated the concept of a **viable myocardium**, that is, the distinction between reversible and irreversible dysfunction due to myocardial necrosis. Several imaging techniques evaluating myocardial viability including those already described

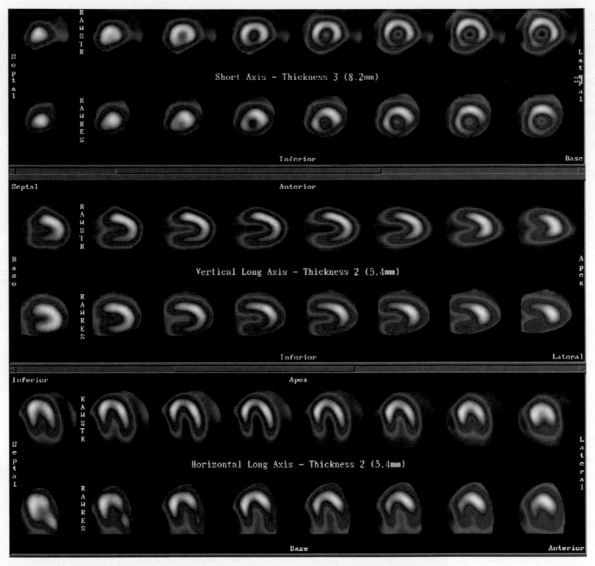

FIGURE 10.26. Normal stress rest thallium–Tc scan. Rest myocardial perfusion images were obtained after thallium (second, fourth, and sixth rows). Stress images were obtained after Tc-tetrofosmin (first, third, and fifth rows).

were developed with the aim of identifying patients in whom recovery of LV function and improvement of prognosis would outweigh the risk of surgical revascularization. The **STICH Trial** did not confirm an impact of viability on the outcome of patients undergoing revascularization or medical therapy and cautioned against relying on the concept of viability alone in the management of patients with LV dysfunction. The study concluded that one should not use viability studies such as SPECT Tl-201 or dobutamine echo to exclude patients from surgical revascularization.

Cardiac PET

As PET/CT scanners become more prevalent, myocardial PET perfusion imaging is being increasingly used in place of SPECT. Certain patient categories that are difficult to image with conventional SPECT are likely to benefit from PET, such as obese patients, women, patients with previous nondiagnostic tests, and patients with poor left ventricular function. The radioisotope **rubidium-82 (Rb-82)** acts physiologically like thallium in the heart yet unlike thallium or technetium it emits a positron giving superior spatial resolution and superior attenuation correction compared with SPECT (Fig. 10.28). The use of Rb-82 reduces the radiation dose to the patient by a factor of 10 compared with Tc-99m. In addition to viability imaging, cardiac PET imaging allows quantification of resting and stress blood flow, coronary flow reserve, and subclinical microvascular abnormalities in response to pharmacologic stress.

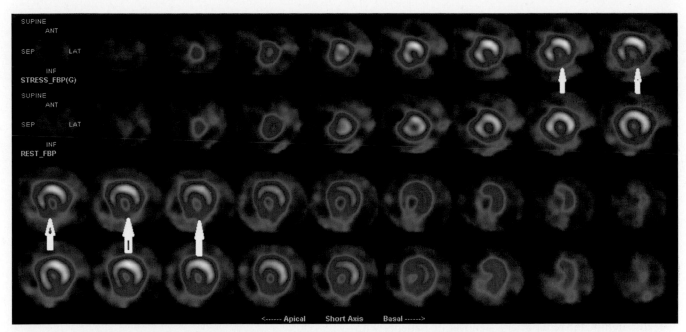

FIGURE 10.27. Abnormal stress nuclear imaging (Tc-99m tetrofosmin). The first and third rows are stress images showing an inferolateral defect (white arrows). The second and fourth rows are rest images showing normal inferolateral perfusion at rest. The "reversible" stress-induced defect is consistent with viable myocardium in the inferolateral wall.

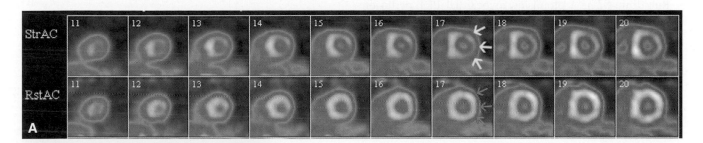

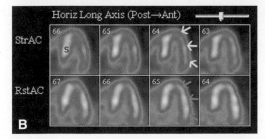

FIGURE 10.28. Myocardial rubidium imaging. Rb-82 cardiac PET images from a patient with chest pain ultimately found to have a high-grade stenosis of the circumflex artery, which supplies the lateral wall of the left ventricle. **A:** The short-axis stress images reveal decreased perfusion (white arrows on one of the slices) to the lateral wall of the left ventricle (LV) in the top row, which then appears "reversible" (the signal improves) on rest images in the bottom row (light gray arrows). **B:** The horizontal long-axis images demonstrate the same defect in perfusion by revealing much diminished rubidium signal in the lateral wall (white arrows on one of the images) in the stress images, which again shows significant improvement on the rest images (reversibility) as depicted by light gray arrows. RstAC, rest attenuation corrected; S, septum; StrAC, stress attenuation corrected.

- Nuclear imaging involves the use of subtherapeutic dose radiotracers, which are injected or inhaled creating a physiologic or functional map. Although used interchangeably with radiotracers, the term radiopharmaceutical applies to similar molecules used for treatment purposes.
- Technetium-99m is a widely used radionuclide and is imaged using a gamma camera.
- Ventilation–perfusion lung still has a role in the workup of certain patients with suspected PE.
- Visualization of the gallbladder with hepatobiliary scintigraphy almost always rules out the diagnosis of acute cholecystitis.
- Bone scintigraphy is a sensitive test for detecting skeletal metastases, osteomyelitis, and fractures.
- Patients with multiple myeloma may have a negative bone scan.
- Captopril renal imaging accurately detects hemodynamically significant renal artery stenosis in patients with renovascular hypertension.
- PET/CT imaging is widely used to detect and stage many malignant tumors.
- Myocardial stress perfusion imaging is an accurate technique for detecting CAD and can be performed with either SPECT (Tl-201, Tc-99m) or PET.
- Rubidium-82 is a promising myocardial PET perfusion agent.

Further Readings

1. Mettler FA, Gilberteau M, eds. *Essentials of Nuclear Medicine Imaging.* 7th ed. Philadelphia, PA: Saunders Elsevier; 2018
2. Ziessman HA, O'Malley JP, *Thrall JH Nuclear Medicine: The Requisites.* 4th ed. Elsevier Mosby; 2013

Cardiac Imaging

1. Expert Panel on Cardiac and Thoracic Imaging. ACR appropriateness criteria acute chest pain – suspected pulmonary embolism. *J Am Coll Radiol.* 2017;14:S2-S12.
2. Bonow RO, Maurer G, Lee KL, et al; STICH Trial Investigators. Myocardial viability and survival in ischemic left ventricular dysfunction. *N Engl J Med.* 2011;364(17):1617-1625.
3. Hendel RC, Berman DS, Di Carli MF, et al. Appropriate use criteria for cardiac radionuclide imaging: a report of the American College of Cardiology Foundation Appropriate Use Criteria Task Force, the American Society of Nuclear Cardiology, the American College of Radiology, the American Heart Association, the American Society of Echocardiography, the Society of Cardiovascular Computed Tomography, the Society for Cardiovascular Magnetic Resonance, and the Society of Nuclear Medicine. *J Am Coll Cardiol.* 2009;53(23):2201-2229.
4. Husain S. Myocardial perfusion imaging protocols: is there an ideal protocol? *J Nucl Med Technol.* 2007;35:3-9.
5. McArdle BA, Dowsley TF, deKemp RA, et al. Does rubidium-82 PET have superior accuracy to SPECT perfusion imaging for the diagnosis of obstructive coronary disease? A systematic reviewandmeta-analysis. *J Am Coll Cardiol.* 2012;60(18): 1828-1837.

Questions

1. Regarding thyroid scintigraphy, which is true?
   a. Most cold spots are malignant
   b. It is a good screening test for thyroid disease
   c. Uptake in the pyramidal lobe is seen in thyroiditis
   d. I-123 is the preferred agent for suspected retrosternal goiter

2. Regarding ventilation perfusion scanning for pulmonary embolism, the following are true except:
   a. Most PEs do not cause pulmonary infarcts
   b. The perfusion abnormality should be smaller than the corresponding chest film abnormality
   c. Most matched perfusion defects are due to vasoconstriction associated with an airway abnormality
   d. Up to 80% of patients with an intermediate probability V/Q scan have pulmonary embolism

3. The following tumors are usually not F-18-FDG avid on PET scan except:
   a. Mucinous colon carcinoma
   b. Bronchoalveolar carcinoma
   c. Neuroendocrine
   d. Small cell lung carcinoma

4. When performing a V/Q scan for suspected pulmonary embolism, radionuclide dose modification is recommended for patients who have/are except:
   a. Contrast allergy
   b. Pulmonary hypertension
   c. Pulmonary AV shunt
   d. Pregnancy

5. Patient instructions prior to a PET/CT for malignancy include all except:
   a. Nothing by mouth within 6 hours
   b. High-carbohydrate diet within 24 hours
   c. May take artificial sweeteners
   d. Diabetics avoid short-acting insulin

6. The following features are regarded as advantages of Tc-99m sestamibi over thallium for cardiac imaging except:
   a. Shorter half-life means a higher dose can be given
   b. Higher myocardial extraction fraction
   c. Higher count rate
   d. Optimal energy for use with standard gamma camera

7. In FDG PET scanning of the head and neck, physiological FDG uptake is often seen in
   A. Waldeyer's ring
   B. Salivary glands
   C. Brown adipose tissue
   D. Tongue

   Options:
   a. A and C
   b. B and D
   c. A, B, and C
   d. All

8. True or False: Synthroid should be discontinued for 4 weeks before a thyroid uptake or scan and iodinated contrast for CT should not have been received within 6 to 8 weeks.

9. True or False: The sensitivity of HIDA scanning for acute acalculous cholecystitis is higher than for acute calculous cholecystitis.

10. True or False: FDG PET is a sensitive test for the detection of intracranial tumors.

CHAPTER 11

Breast Imaging

Limin Yang, MD, PhD • Laurie L. Fajardo, MD, MBA

Approximately one in eight women in the United States will develop cancer of the breast during her lifetime, and this incidence appears to be increasing. Unfortunately, there is no known cause of most breast cancers, and therefore the best way to prevent mortality is early detection of the nonpalpable and potentially curable disease using mammography. It is generally believed that the earlier breast cancer is diagnosed, the smaller the chance of metastases and the better the long-term prognosis. Consequently, mammography is widely used as a screening test for breast cancer in the general asymptomatic female population. Clinical breast examinations and breast self-examination were formerly also recommended; however, the latest American Cancer Society (ACS) Breast Cancer Screening Guideline (Table 11.1) no longer includes these because research has not shown a clear benefit of regular clinical or self-breast examinations. However, it is recommended that women be familiar with how their breasts normally look and feel and report any changes to a health care provider right away.

Diagnostic mammography is also a key tool in the evaluation of patients with known or suspected breast disease. There is little doubt that mammograms are best interpreted by qualified radiologists. In addition, a radiologist may perform image-guided breast biopsy, allowing an accurate and cost-effective diagnosis of nonpalpable breast lesions. Given the prevalence of breast disease, all physicians should be aware of the clinical applications and limitations of breast imaging. The purpose of this chapter is to review the importance of screening mammography for early cancer detection and the use of diagnostic mammography, ultrasound (US), and magnetic resonance imaging (MRI) in the management of breast disease.

TABLE 11.1	General Screening Mammography Guidelines

1. **Women between 40 and 44 y of age** have the option to start screening with a mammogram every year.
2. **Women aged 45–54 y** should get mammograms every year.
3. **Women 55 and older** can switch to a mammogram every other year, or they can choose to continue yearly mammograms. Screening should continue as long as a woman is in good health and is expected to live 10 more years or longer.
4. The ACS does not recommend clinical breast examination for breast cancer screening among average-risk women at any age.
5. **All women** should understand what to expect when getting a mammogram for breast cancer screening—what the test can and cannot do.

Based on guidelines from American Cancer Society.

TABLE 11.2	ACR/SBI Recommendations for Age at Which Annual Screening Mammography Should Start

Age 40
- Women at average risk

Younger than Age 40
- Women with genetics-based increased risk (and their untested first-degree relatives) or with a calculated lifetime risk of 20% or more, beginning at age 30. Women with history of chest radiation therapy before age 30, beginning at age 25 or 8 y after radiation therapy, whichever is later. Women diagnosed with breast cancer, ADH, or lobular neoplasia before age 40, beginning at time of diagnosis.

From Monticciolo DL, Newell MS, Moy L, et al. Breast cancer screening in women at higher-than-average risk: recommendations from the ACR. *J Am Coll Radiol.* 2018;15 (3 pt A):408-414; copyright © 2018 Elsevier.
ADH, atypical ductal hyperplasia.

SCREENING MAMMOGRAPHY

The mortality rate for breast carcinoma has fallen by almost 30% over the past 20 years. Several large reputable studies have linked this reduction in mortality to both earlier detection of breast carcinoma due to screening mammography and improvements in breast cancer treatment. Critics of routine screening argue that women may go through unnecessary treatment such as surgery, radiotherapy, and chemotherapy for cancers that would not have posed a risk as some cancers will be diagnosed and treated that would never have caused any harm. In the United Kingdom, it is estimated that screening prevents about 1,300 deaths per year, but it also may result in about 4,000 women receiving treatment for a condition that would not have been threatening.

In 2013 the U.S. Preventive Services Task Force (USPSTF) revised their recommendations for screening mammography for women younger than 50 years because there was moderate certainty that the net benefits for this age group were small. For this age group, there is not a routine screening recommendation, but the recommendations allow for individualized decisions for biennial screening. For women aged 50 to 74 years, the USPSTF current recommendation is biennial rather than annual screening. No recommendation was made by the USPSTF for women older than 74 years, citing insufficient evidence. The Society of Breast Imaging (SBI) and the American College of Radiology (ACR) strongly criticized the USPSTF recommendations, and they have jointly published their own recommendations for screening mammography (Table 11.2). These recommendations are based upon evidence-based medicine where available. Where evidence is lacking, the recommendations are based on consensus opinions. The ACR and SBI firmly stand behind their recommendation that screening mammography should be performed annually beginning at age 40 for women at average risk for breast cancer.

For women with known risk factors for breast cancer, there are additional recommendations for when to initiate screening and type of screening. One of these risk factors is a *BRCA* gene mutation, which is associated with a rare hereditary breast–ovarian carcinoma syndrome. As many as two-thirds of women born with a deleterious mutation in *BRCA1* will develop breast cancer by age 70, and one-third will develop ovarian cancer by age 70. Approximately one-half of women with a deleterious mutation in *BRCA2* will develop breast cancer by age 70, and up to one-quarter will develop ovarian cancer by age 70. The ACR/SBI recommendations include annual screening mammograms and screening breast MRI of women with BRCA mutations.

Technique for Screening and Diagnostic Mammography

The importance of a well-performed mammogram cannot be overemphasized. A standard screening mammogram consists of two views: a *mediolateral oblique* (MLO) view with the central x-ray beam traversing the breast obliquely in a medial to lateral direction (Fig. 11.1A) and a *craniocaudal* (CC) view (Fig. 11.1B) with the central x-ray beam traversing the breast in a head to foot direction. It is necessary to compress the breast during the examination to visualize

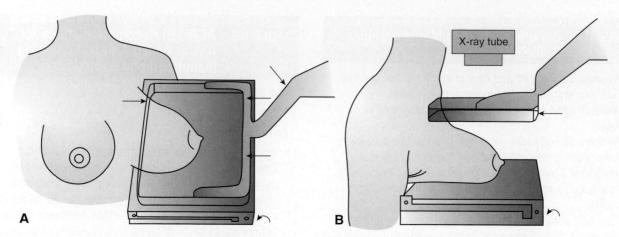

FIGURE 11.1. Mammographic technique. A: Illustration of patient positioning for a mediolateral oblique (MLO) mammogram. The x-ray beam passes obliquely through the breast in a medial to lateral direction. The breast is routinely compressed between the compression device (*straight arrows*) and the radiographic cassette (*curved arrow*). The cassette contains a radiographic film on which the image will be recorded. Compression improves the diagnostic quality of the images by reducing the breast to a more uniform thickness. **B:** Illustration of patient positioning for a craniocaudal (CC) mammogram. The x-ray beam passes through the breast in a head to foot or cephalad to caudad direction. The compression device (*straight arrow*) is more easily visualized in this illustration. Again, the image will be recorded on the film in the radiographic cassette (*curved arrow*).

all the breast tissue and to minimize radiation dose, and patients should be warned that compression may be uncomfortable. As with other forms of imaging, mammography has limitations, and adjunct screening using ultrasound (US) or breast MRI is becoming more widely accepted. If a potential abnormality is detected on a screening mammogram, a diagnostic workup is recommended. A diagnostic workup may require specific mammographic views including microfocus magnification compression views for microcalcifications and focal (spot) compression views for mass or focal asymmetry and possibly the need for US and/or MRI. For women younger than 30 years who present with a breast mass, US is the best initial examination to perform.

Diagnostic mammography is also performed when a breast mass is palpated. The vast majority of screening and diagnostic mammograms performed in the United States use digital technology, which has replaced film-screen mammography. The advantages of digital mammography include the ability to use image-processing techniques to enhance the images, the use of computer-assisted diagnostic (CAD) techniques in lesion detection and characterization, and the ease of electronic transmission and storage of images. Compared with film-screen mammography, digital mammography has been shown to be superior in detecting breast cancer in women younger than 50 years, pre- or perimenopausal women, and those with dense breasts.

It is important that the mammographer (technologist) be properly trained and qualified and that the federally mandated mammography quality controls (MQSA, Mammography Quality Standards Act) are met.

WHAT WE SHOULD SEE ON A MAMMOGRAM

In general, breast tissue is composed predominately of fibroglandular tissue in younger women and gradually replaced with adipose tissue in older women. Correspondingly, normal mammograms show a mixture of fat and fibroglandular tissue. Normal MLO and CC views of the breast are shown in Figure 11.2. Notice that breast images are a combination of fat (black) and parenchymal soft tissue (gray to white). This background of black and gray, especially the black, enhances visualization of masses and calcifications.

Approximately 85% of breast carcinomas are of ductal origin (ductal carcinoma in situ and invasive ductal carcinoma) and a lesser percentage arise from the breast lobules (lobular carcinoma).

The two most important and most frequent mammographic findings suspicious for malignancy are masses and microcalcifications. Other suspicious abnormalities include focal asymmetry, architectural distortion, and skin or nipple deformity. Any structural changes over time on mammograms require attention and further workup, unless otherwise explained (such as surgical scar).

The Breast Imaging Reporting and Data System (BI-RADS) initiative was instituted by the ACR in the late 1980s to address a lack of standardization and uniformity in mammography practice and reporting. An important component of this system is the lexicon, a dictionary of descriptors of specific imaging features which historically have been shown to be predictive of benign and malignant disease.

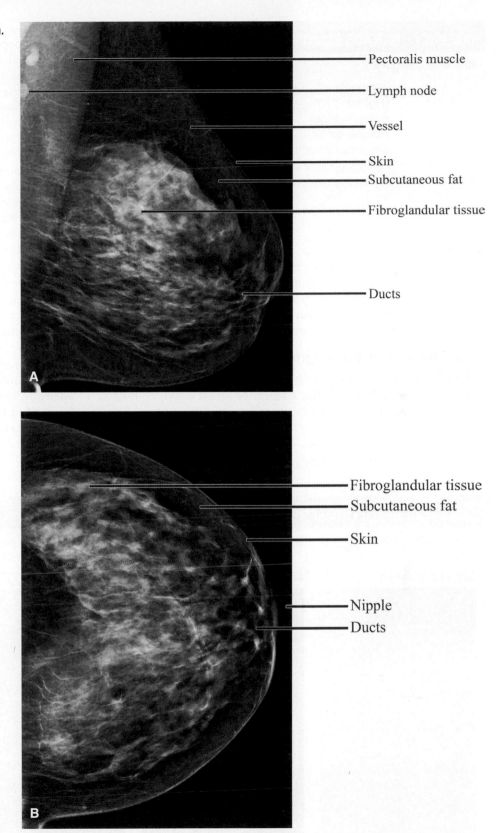

FIGURE 11.2. Normal mammogram.
A: Left breast mediolateral oblique (MLO) digital mammogram. Normal.
B: Left breast craniocaudal digital mammogram. Normal.

Pectoralis muscle

Lymph node

Vessel

Skin
Subcutaneous fat
Fibroglandular tissue

Ducts

Fibroglandular tissue
Subcutaneous fat

Skin

Nipple
Ducts

TABLE 11.3	BI-RADS Classification
BI-RADS Category	
0	Incomplete
1	Negative
2	Benign finding(s)
3	Probably benign
4	Suspicious abnormality
5	Highly suggestive of malignancy
6	Known biopsy-proven malignancy

BI-RADS Category 4 or 5 warrants biopsy.

Use of the BI-RADS lexicon promotes communication, quality assurance, standardization, and improved patient care. Initially, BI-RADS was developed for mammographic findings, but it now includes US and MRI findings (Table 11.3). This system is continuously revised on the basis of experts' opinions and evidence-based research.

Breast Density on Mammography

The BI-RADS lexicon describes breast density according to four categories, based on the amount of breast tissue (dense on a mammogram) and fatty tissue (not dense on a mammogram). Breast density is classified using the denser of a woman's two breasts. The breast composition categories are: (1) the breasts are almost entirely fatty (about 10% of the population); (2) there are scattered areas of fibroglandular density (about 40% of the population); (3) the breasts are heterogeneously dense, which may obscure small masses (about 40% of the population); and (4) the breasts are extremely dense, which lowers the sensitivity of mammography (about 10% of the population) (Table 11.4). High breast density is relatively common; 40% to 50% of women aged 40 to 74 have dense breasts. Mammograms of dense breasts are harder to read than mammograms of fatty breasts. In addition, women with moderately dense and extremely dense breast tissue have a higher risk for breast cancer than women with average breast density (Table 11.4). Women with the most extreme density have a 2.1 times increased risk, which is approximately equal to the risk of having one first-degree relative with unilateral postmenopausal breast cancer. Currently, 33 states require some level of breast density notification in the report given to a woman after having a screening mammogram. A concern is that while the significance of breast tissue density is uncertain, reporting it may alarm women and lead to an avalanche of needless screening tests and biopsies. Thus, to be able to answer questions a woman may have about her breast density and breast cancer risk, it is important that physicians who care for women to understand breast density and its associated risks.

TABLE 11.4	Breast Cancer Risk Associated With Varying Breast Density

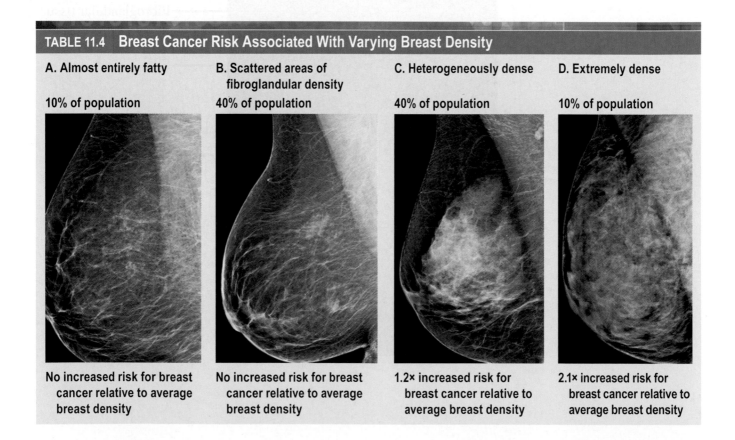

A. Almost entirely fatty	B. Scattered areas of fibroglandular density	C. Heterogeneously dense	D. Extremely dense
10% of population	40% of population	40% of population	10% of population
No increased risk for breast cancer relative to average breast density	No increased risk for breast cancer relative to average breast density	1.2× increased risk for breast cancer relative to average breast density	2.1× increased risk for breast cancer relative to average breast density

TABLE 11.5	Common Causes of Benign Breast Disease

- Cystic disease
- Mastitis, abscess
- Fibroadenoma, benign phyllodes tumor
- Lipoma, hamartoma
- Sclerosing adenosis, fibrocystic changes
- Fat necrosis

Masses

Using BI-RADS terminology, a mass is a space-occupying lesion seen on two different mammographic projections. Masses are described in terms of their shape, border (margin), density, location, size, and associated findings such as microcalcifications and architectural distortion.

Benign Masses

Benign breast disease (Table 11.5) may or may not be symptomatic or have associated masses. A fibroadenoma (Fig. 11.3) is a common benign mass that generally occurs in young

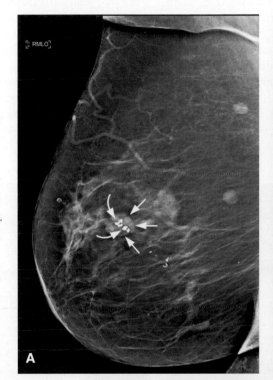
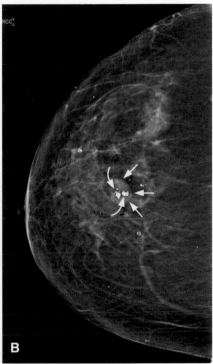
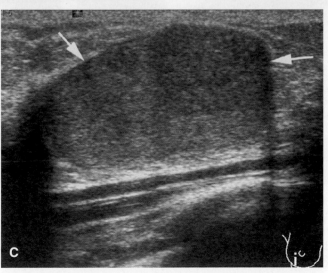

FIGURE 11.3. **Fibroadenoma.** Right breast MLO **(A)** and CC **(B)** mammograms. Calcified benign fibroadenoma. The fibroadenoma is oval and isodense with circumscribed borders (*straight arrows*). The benign calcifications within the fibroadenoma are typically globular, coarse, and variable in size (*curved arrows*). **C:** Ultrasound of the right breast shows a well-circumscribed homogeneous isoechoic solid mass, which is corresponding to a palpable mass (*arrows*).

women and may be single or multiple. On physical examination, fibroadenomas are often movable. The mammographic appearance is an oval circumscribed mass sometimes associated with coarse "popcorn" calcifications. On sonography, fibroadenomas will usually appear isoechoic, or similar in echotexture to normal breast parenchyma.

Benign cystic disease is another common clinical entity, which may present as a tender or nontender palpable mass or as an incidental nonpalpable mammographic finding. The mammographic appearance of a cyst is usually an isodense mass with well-defined borders (Fig. 11.4A). Although a cyst is usually rounder and more circumscribed than a solid mass on a mammogram, mammography cannot differentiate a solid mass from a cyst and US is needed to make this distinction. US of a breast cyst (Fig. 11.4B) usually shows a well-defined anechoic mass with characteristic posterior acoustic enhancement. Cysts may be treated with US-guided needle aspiration. Some benign lesions, such as breast hamartoma, are easily diagnosed on mammography without any additional imaging or intervention needed (Fig. 11.5).

When breast implants are placed for augmentation, implant displaced mammography views are required to visualize the breast tissue surrounding the implant. When implants are placed following mastectomy, routine screening mammography is not required for the postmastectomy breast. Implants may vary in appearance from less dense (saline) to dense (silicone) and in their location—either posterior (retropectoral or subpectoral) (Fig. 11.6) or anterior (prepectoral) to the pectoralis muscle. MR is useful in evaluating implant integrity.

Malignant Masses

Common mammographic and ultrasonographic findings of malignancy are listed in Table 11.6. Malignant masses are usually irregularly shaped and of high density with ill-defined or spiculated borders (Fig. 11.7). Microcalcifications are frequently associated within and/or outside of the mass. When suspicious findings are present, it is important to evaluate the extent of the disease such as multifocality/multicentricity on the imaging studies. Multifocality means that there are other disease foci in the same breast quadrant. Multicentricity means that there are other disease foci in a different breast quadrant. Asymmetric densities and architectural distortions are also suspicious for malignancy, especially if they are new.

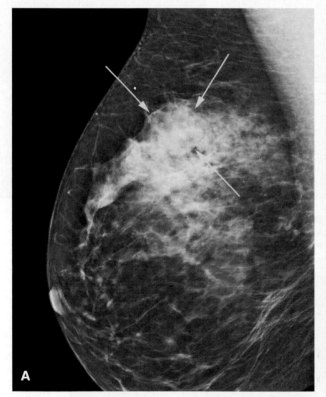
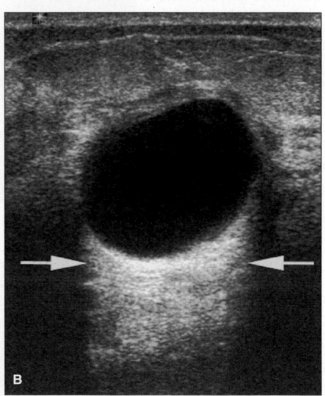

FIGURE 11.4. A simple cyst. A: Right breast MLO digital mammogram. The isodense cyst (*arrows*) has sharp borders and no calcifications. Note the difference between the smooth sharp borders of this benign cyst compared with the irregular and poorly defined borders of the carcinoma in Figure 11.7. **B:** Right breast ultrasound of the lesion **(A)**. This is the classic appearance of a benign simple cyst. The cyst is a round well-circumscribed anechoic mass with very thin cyst–parenchymal transition. Posterior acoustic enhancement (*arrows*) is commonly found immediately posterior to a cyst.

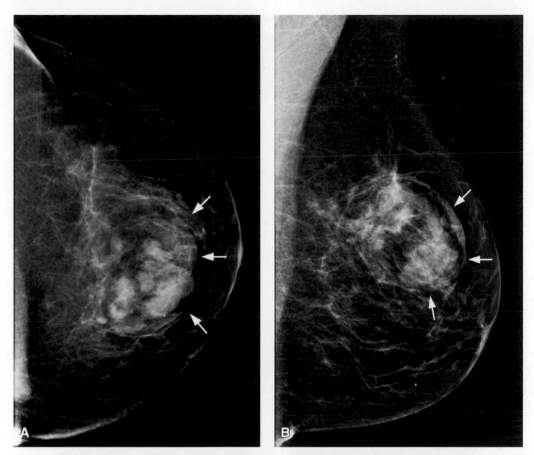

FIGURE 11.5. **Hamartoma (fibroadenolipoma).** The CC **(A)** and MLO **(B)** views of the left breast show a well-defined mass with heterogeneous internal density, which is not different from the surrounding normal breast tissue except it is confined within a thin wall in the upper inner left breast (*arrows*). This benign mass is usually impalpable due to its soft nature. This mammographic appearance is diagnostic.

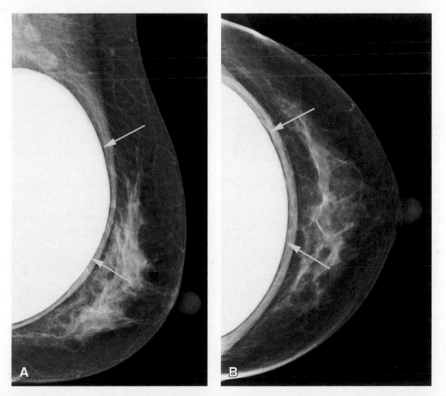

FIGURE 11.6. **Breast augmentations.** Left breast MLO **(A)** and CC **(B)** digital mammograms. The well-defined radiopaque areas represent the silicone augmentation implants (*arrows*).

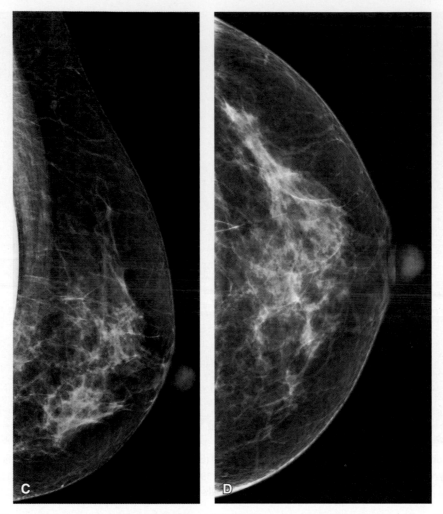

FIGURE 11.6. *(Continued)* Implant displaced MLO **(C)** and CC **(D)** views show breast parenchyma better than routine views.

TABLE 11.6	Mammographic/Ultrasonographic Findings Suspicious for Malignancy

1. A mass on a mammogram with
   a. ill-defined or spiculated borders
   b. Malignant calcifications
   c. High radiopaque density
   d. skin retraction or thickening
2. Microcalcifications that are (with or without a mass)
   a. pleomorphic
   b. fine linear branching or segmental
   c. clusters
3. Architectural distortion or focal asymmetry
4. Irregular hypoechoic solid mass on ultrasound with ill-defined/spiculated border, thick boundary echogenicity, and/or surrounding architectural distortion

Microcalcifications

Microcalcifications may be the first indicator of malignancy, especially if they are new, pleomorphic, or branching (Fig. 11.8A). However, it should be emphasized that most breast calcifications are benign. Benign microcalcifications are homogeneous in size and shape (usually punctate, round, or coarse) and more diffusely scattered (Fig. 11.8B). Malignant microcalcifications are more heterogeneous in shape and size (pleomorphic), more clustered in a small area, and linearly or segmentally distributed (see Fig. 11.8A). Some calcifications are so small (100–200 microns) that magnification mammography is needed to best evaluate their morphology and distribution. The description of microcalcifications using BI-RADS terminology includes the shape, distribution, location, and associated findings such as a mass.

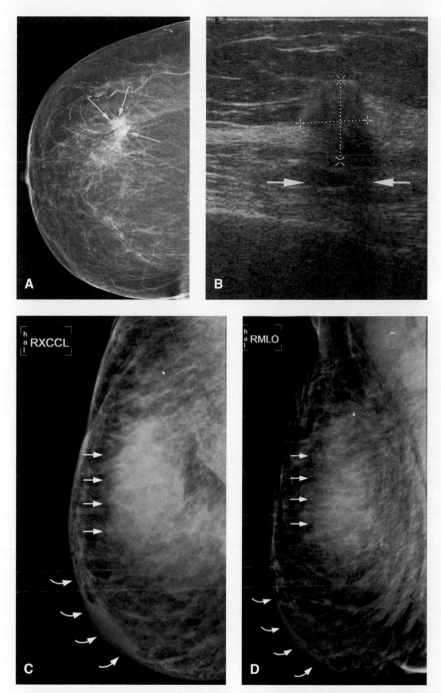

FIGURE 11.7. Carcinoma. A: Right breast CC digital mammogram shows an infiltrating ductal carcinoma in an 84-year-old woman. The high-density malignant mass lesion (*arrows*) has spiculated and poorly defined borders, which are in contrast to the sharp and well-defined border of the benign cyst in Figure 11.4A. **B:** Ultrasound image of the same patient shows an ill-defined hypoechoic mass, which is taller than wide. Note that there is posterior acoustic shadowing (*arrows*). The *X*s and *crosses* are electronic caliper marks that measure the dimensions of the mass. **C, D:** Inflammatory carcinoma. MLO **(C)** and XCCL **(D)** views of the left breast show a large ill-defined high-density mass (*straight arrows*) with surrounding thickened trabeculation. Note the markedly thickened skin (*curved arrows*).

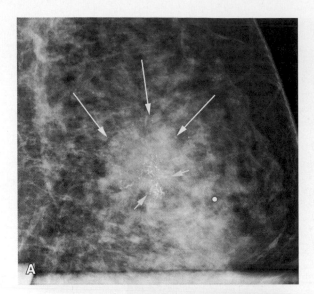

FIGURE 11.8. Carcinoma. A: A 38-year-old woman with an infiltrating ductal carcinoma. Left breast digital MLO magnification compression view demonstrates the classical appearance of malignant calcifications (*short arrows*) in the mass (*long arrows*). Note the difference between the coarse benign calcifications in Figure 11.3 and these pleomorphic malignant calcifications. Also, the high-density and poorly defined borders of the associated mass are more obvious in this magnification compression view. A skin marker (*white dot*) indicates that this mass is palpable. **B:** CC digital mammogram of the right breast shows scattered, diffuse calcifications that are round in shape. These calcification are benign and do not require biopsy.

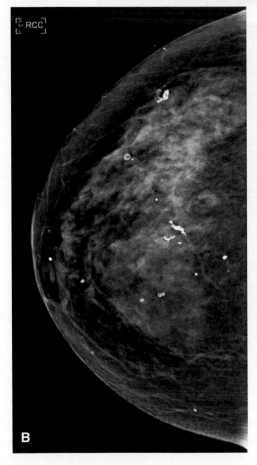

LIMITATIONS OF MAMMOGRAPHY

Overall, about 40% of women who have mammograms have dense breast tissue, which may mask small breast carcinomas. US can also find tumors that mammograms miss, but they produce even more false-positive examinations. If all women with dense breasts had US, more early cancers would be found, but thousands of unnecessary biopsies would also be performed.

Many limitations of conventional 2D mammography are overcome by digital breast tomosynthesis (DBT or 3D mammography), which provides radiologists with in-depth views (through a series of cross-sectional images) of the internal structure of the breast. DBT (3D mammography) is a modification of the standard two-dimensional (2D) digital mammography to yield a 3D image by using tomography, which allows better visualization/characterization of lesions by removing overlapping structures present in the planes other than the plane in which the lesion is located (Fig. 11.9).

Because DBT images remove overlapping dense breast tissue, breast cancers are more visible than on conventional 2D mammograms. DBT has shown to be a superior modality for early detection of breast cancer, with higher cancer detection rates and fewer patient recalls (false positives), thus improving the sensitivity and specificity of mammography. It is rapidly becoming the standard of care for breast cancer screening.

INDICATIONS FOR BREAST ULTRASOUND AND MAGNETIC RESONANCE

US is an essential imaging modality for breast diseases as it allows distinction between cystic and solid breast masses. Advances in technology now allow tissue characterization

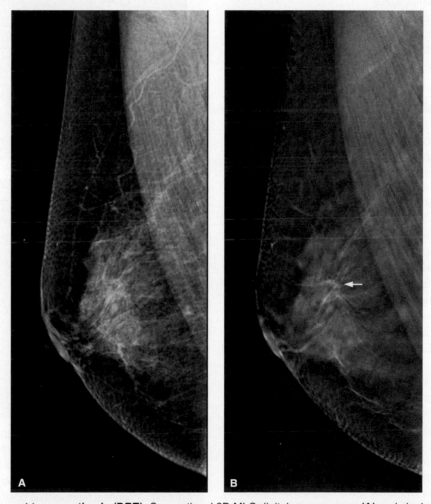

FIGURE 11.9. Digital breast tomosynthesis (DBT). Conventional 2D MLO digital mammogram **(A)** and single image from a 3D DBT scan **(B)** depicting a small irregular/spiculated mass (*arrow*) just above the nipple in the middle one-third of the breast. Note that the conspicuity of the mass is significantly better on the DBT image.

TABLE 11.7	**Indications for High-risk Screening Breast MR**

1. 20%–25% or greater lifetime risk of breast cancer, based on risk assessment models
2. BRCA1 or 2 gene mutation
3. First-degree relative with a BRCA1 or 2 gene mutation, have not had genetic testing themselves
4. Chest radiation therapy before age 30
5. Certain syndromes or have first-degree relatives with the syndromes, or other gene mutations (Li-Fraumeni, Cowden, and Bannayan–Riley–Ruvalcaba)

TABLE 11.8	**Indications for Diagnostic Breast MR**

1. Positive axillary lymph nodes with negative mammogram
2. Presurgical planning, extent of the disease
3. Monitor effect of chemotherapy
4. Evaluation of residual disease
5. Inconclusive mammogram and/or ultrasound
6. Silicone implant rupture

using harmonic imaging, compound imaging, elastography, and three-dimensional (3D) image acquisition. US is also used to guide percutaneous core biopsy, preoperative wire lesion localization and cyst/abscess drainage and has the advantage of real-time visualization while performing interventional breast procedures. The BI-RADS terms used to describe the ultrasonographic features of a mass include shape, orientation, margin, boundary with adjacent tissue, internal echo pattern, and posterior acoustic features. Characteristics suggesting benignity include circumscribed round/oval shape, parallel orientation with the ductal structures ("being wider than tall"), thin capsule, and gentle lobulation. Characteristics suggesting malignancy include an irregular shape, spiculated/angular/microlobulated border, antiparallel orientation to the ductal structures ("being taller than wide"), and surrounding architectural distortion (Fig. 11.7B).

MR is also increasingly used to evaluate the extent of disease in women diagnosed with breast cancer, especially those with dense breast tissue, which is not well imaged by mammography (Tables 11.7 and 11.8). For women at high risk for breast cancer, MR is used in addition to (not as a replacement for) screening mammography. Breast US has also been used as a supplemental screening test but has not been shown to be better than MR. Although US is less costly than MR, it has a higher false-positive rate. Advantages of MR include better evaluation of the 3D extent of the disease using intravenous contrast (Fig. 11.10A), diagnosis of

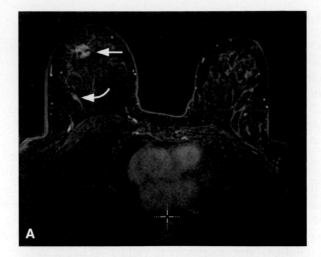

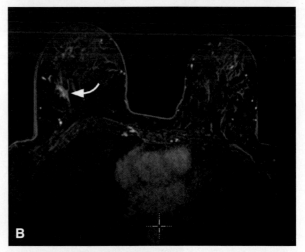

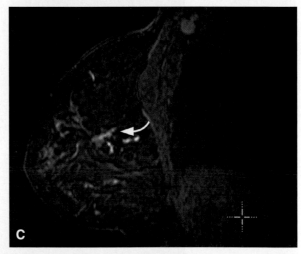

FIGURE 11.10. MRI of breast carcinoma. Postcontrast subtraction MRI demonstrate an irregular enhancing mass (*straight arrow* (**A**)) near 12-o'clock position of the right breast, which was a newly diagnosed invasive ductal carcinoma with internal nonenhancing component representing postbiopsy changes. **B, C:** A clumped linear nonmass enhancement in the upper outer right breast (*curved arrows*) was biopsied under MRI guidance, which confirmed ductal carcinoma in situ.

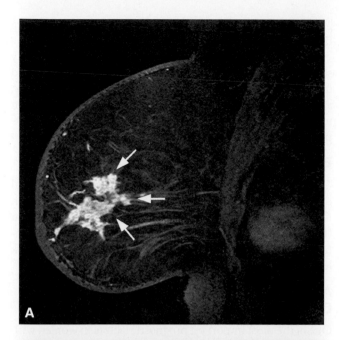

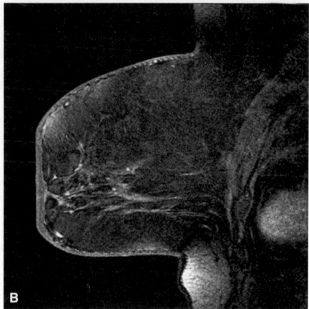

FIGURE 11.11. MRI posttreatment. Contrast-enhanced subtraction breast MR images before **(A)** and after **(B)** 3 months of neoadjuvant chemotherapy show a marked decrease in contrast uptake, indicating that the tumor (*arrows*) is responding to treatment.

additional, otherwise occult, malignancies in the same or opposite breast (Fig. 11.10B), differentiation between scar and recurrent cancer, presurgical planning in a known cancer patient (Fig. 11.10C), and evaluation of tumor response to chemotherapy (Fig. 11.11).

Breast MRI is also used to evaluate silicone implant rupture. It has much higher sensitivity to detect silicone leak

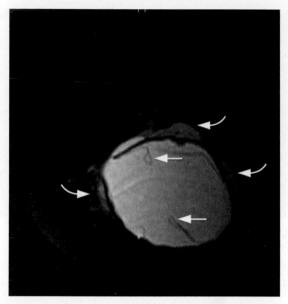

FIGURE 11.12. Silicone implant rupture. Noncontrast water saturation breast MR images demonstrate (1) silicone leak outside the capsule (*curved arrows*) consistent with extracapsular rupture and (2) a keyhole sign (*straight arrows*) consistent with intracapsular rupture.

both within or outside the fibrous capsule caused by the silicone implant. With MRI specific water saturation sequences, silicone that has leaked from the implant can be visualized clearly inside or outside of the implant envelope. When an implant rupture is contained by the fibrous capsule, it is termed intracapsular implant rupture and when silicone is detected outside the fibrous capsule, it is termed extracapsular implant rupture (Fig. 11.12).

BREAST BIOPSY

Biopsy and histopathology of a breast lesion are essential for diagnosis and treatment planning. Several options are available for image guidance of percutaneous breast biopsy (US, stereotactic, and MRI) and the type of biopsy needle used (fine needle, core needle, vacuum-assisted probe device). The choice of a biopsy technique used is based upon the clinical and radiographic features of the lesion. In general, more biopsy tissue is preferred so that additional testing (i.e., hormone receptors) can be performed, if indicated.

A fine-needle aspirate (FNA) biopsy is used to evaluate axillary lymph nodes when core biopsy of a suspicious breast lesion is performed and can also be used for aspiration of symptomatic (painful) or indeterminate cystic breast lesions. Analysis by an experienced cytologist is critical for accurate interpretation of FNA biopsy results. However, FNA biopsy does not distinguish between

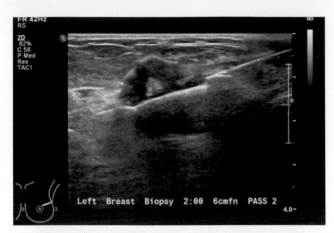

FIGURE 11.13. Ultrasound-guided core biopsy. A biopsy needle with parallel to chest wall orientation was inserted percutaneously into the suspicious lesion in the breast and the tissue sample was then obtained.

invasive and in situ breast cancer, and the false-negative rate for identifying breast malignancy is as high as 40%.

Core-needle biopsy uses a larger gauge needle (9G to 14G) to remove a narrow cylinder of tissue in contrast to a collection of cells obtained with FNA (Fig. 11.13). The larger sample permits more detailed pathologic analysis and determination of hormone receptor levels. Two types of core needles commonly used are spring-loaded (which requires separate needle insertions into the breast for each sample extracted), and vacuum-assisted biopsy needle, characterized by a single core needle insertion and acquisition of contiguous and larger tissue samples. Because most of the lesions detected during screening are impalpable, subsequent needle biopsy must be image guided. Ultrasonography-guided biopsy is usually the most straightforward approach, but some lesions, particularly microcalcifications, are better seen on mammography and require stereotactic needle biopsy.

Stereotactic biopsy is used primarily for calcifications and other lesions not visible on US. The stereotactic technique uses radiographic imaging performed in at least two planes to localize and guide the core biopsy needle to target a lesion in 3D space. To minimize sampling error, minimum of five to six samples are required when biopsying microcalcifications. Specimen radiography of the biopsy samples is also required to ensure that representative calcifications are contained within them. Once the biopsy is complete, an inert metallic clip is deployed into the biopsy site through the biopsy trocar as a marker for future reference (i.e., to guide subsequent surgical lumpectomy) in case the lesion can no longer be visualized after biopsy.

With the new development of a tomosynthesis-guided core biopsy device, breast lesion seen only on tomosynthesis can now be accurately biopsied using tomosynthesis

guidance with similar approaches as for stereotactic core biopsy.

If an enhancing mass or nonmass enhancement is only seen on breast MRI, core biopsy can also be performed under MRI guidance. During an MRI-guided breast biopsy, a vacuum-assisted biopsy needle is inserted to the lesion using MR imaging and 6 to 12 contiguous larger tissue samples obtained for histopathological evaluation.

Excisional Breast Biopsy

This biopsy is usually done surgically. A finding of atypical ductal hyperplasia on core-needle biopsy is an indication for open biopsy, which may reveal ductal carcinoma in situ (DCIS) in as many as 50% of patients. Radial scars diagnosed by core biopsy should also be regarded as high-risk lesions which may require excision biopsy.

Axillary Lymph Node Biopsy and Sentinel Node Biopsy

One of the most important prognostic factors in women with early stage breast cancer is the status of the axillary lymph nodes. The ipsilateral axillary region is often scanned at the same time when a suspicious breast lesion is seen on ultrasound to look for any suspicious axillary lymphadenopathy. If a suspicious lymph node is found, ultrasound-guided fine-needle aspiration or core biopsy will be performed to assist with cancer staging.

Traditional surgical axillary lymph node dissection (ALND) may be associated with postsurgical lymphedema and nerve injury in breast cancer patients. If a patient has clinically negative axillary nodes, sentinel lymph node biopsy (SLNB) is the preferred method of staging disease in the axilla because of less morbidity compared to ALND. Injection of a technetium-99m–labeled colloid and/or blue dye around the tumor or subareolar skin permits identification of a sentinel lymph node, which is then biopsied, usually at the time of lumpectomy. The false-positive rate for SLNB is less than 5%. Approximately 40% of patients with a positive sentinel lymph node will have residual disease in the axilla, which has been shown not to impact survival outcomes.

DISEASES OF THE MALE BREAST

All diseases that occur in the female breast can potentially occur in the male breast. The incidence of male breast carcinoma was approximately 2,190 cases in 2012 in the United States accounting for 1% of all breast cancers. Male breast cancers tend to be diagnosed at a more advanced stage and thus have a poorer survival. Because the overall incidence of breast cancer in males is low, mammography and clinical breast examination have no role for screening in males. The indications for male diagnostic mammography and the images obtained are similar to

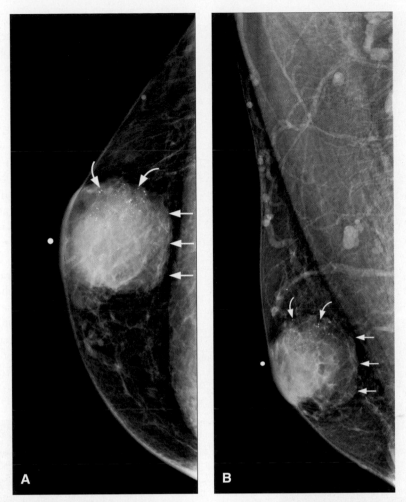

FIGURE 11.14. **Male breast carcinoma.** Left male breast CC **(A)** and MLO **(B)** digital mammograms. The *straight arrows* indicate the large round high-density mass with ill-defined margins and associated pleomorphic microcalcifications (*curved arrows*) in the subareolar left breast.

TABLE 11.9 Causes of Gynecomastia
Physiologic (neonatal, pubertal, elderly)
Adult men
• An increase in the ratio of estrogen to androgen (e.g., liver cirrhosis, testicular tumor, chronic renal disease)
• Drugs (spironolactone, digitalis, steroids)

those for females. Male breast carcinomas are similar in appearance to female breast carcinomas. They most commonly present as irregular or ill-defined solid masses (Fig. 11.14). Pathologically, invasive lobular carcinomas are less common in men than in women because of less developed lobular structures in men.

Gynecomastia is a benign enlargement of the male breast tissue due to proliferation of the glandular component and may be confused with breast cancer. The causes for gynecomastia are listed in Table 11.9. The presentation of gynecomastia is usually a tender subareolar breast mass, which may be unilateral or bilateral. On mammography, breast tissue is present in the subareolar zone and may contain calcifications (Fig. 11.15). The need for biopsy is determined by a combination of symptoms, physical, and mammographic or ultrasonographic findings. There is no association between gynecomastia and the subsequent development of breast carcinoma.

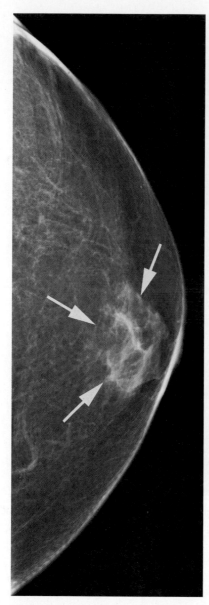

much more than normal cells do; therefore the areas with increased radioactivity will be detected by the gamma camera. MBI has been used as supplement screening test in some facilities; however, no large clinical trials have validated its efficacy for screening.

Whole-breast ultrasound is scanning of the entire breast either performed by a physician or ultrasound technologist using a handheld ultrasound probe or by automated whole-breast ultrasound machine with an ultrasound probe through an automated process. It can be used with mammography to screen the breast for breast cancers and is designed to improve the detection rate of breast cancer in women with dense breasts. If any abnormalities are found, a handheld ultrasound is then performed to further evaluate the findings noted from whole-breast ultrasound.

Galactography is a technique that opacifies the intraductal system by injecting contrast material to delineate abnormalities. Active nipple discharge must be present to perform this examination because the diseased duct must be identified prior to cannulation and contrast injection. An intraductal abnormality is seen as a "filling defect" in a contrast-filled duct or as abrupt cutoff of the visualized duct (Fig. 11.16). External compression by an extraductal

FIGURE 11.15. Gynecomastia. Left male breast CC digital mammogram. The *arrows* indicate the typically increased but normal appearing subareolar fibroglandular tissue without calcification. Normal male mammograms should not show any fibroglandular tissue.

OTHER IMAGING TECHNOLOGIES

PET scanning with fluorodeoxyglucose (FDG) is complementary to conventional staging procedures and should not be a replacement for either bone scintigraphy or diagnostic CT. PET and PET/CT have been shown to be particularly useful in the restaging of breast cancer and evaluating tumor response to therapy.

Molecular breast imaging (MBI) is a functional test that uses a radioactive tracer injected intravenously and gamma camera imaging to detect suspicious breast lesions. Breast cancer cells tend to take up the radioactive substance

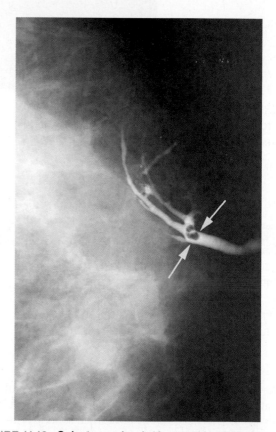

FIGURE 11.16. Galactography. A 48-year-old woman with intraductal papilloma in the left breast. Left CC view shows a small rounded filling defect (*arrows*) in the contrast-filled duct in left subareolar area.

abnormality may also be seen. Galactography has been largely replaced by improved US imaging techniques.

In summary, screening for breast cancer in the general and high-risk populations has resulted in reductions in breast cancer mortality. Breast imaging technologies continue to evolve, providing breast radiologists with improved tools to diagnose and manage benign and malignant breast abnormalities. The subspecialty of breast imaging is best practiced by specialty-trained breast radiologists in conjunction with their multidisciplinary colleagues, including breast surgeons, medical oncologists, radiation oncologists, and breast pathologists.

SUGGESTED WORKUP OF COMMON CLINICAL PROBLEMS

Suggested algorithms for the workup of two common clinical scenarios are shown in Figure 11.17.

FIGURE 11.17. Clinical algorithms. A: Screening for breast carcinoma. **B:** Workup of a palpable breast mass.

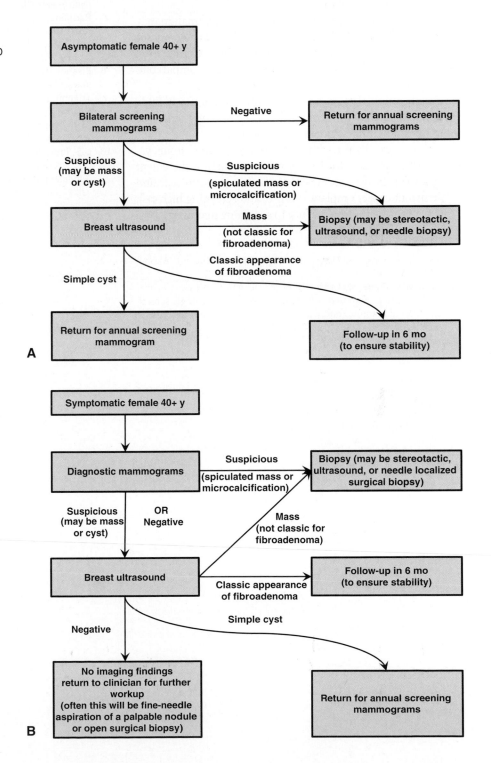

KEY POINTS

- Approximately one in eight females in the United States will develop carcinoma of the breast.
- Mammograms should be interpreted by qualified radiologists and high-quality mammography is imperative in the early detection of breast cancer.
- A screening mammogram consists of MLO and CC views.
- Screening mammography must be combined with regular breast examinations.
- Mammographic findings suspicious for malignancy include an irregularly shaped mass, pleomorphic microcalcifications, skin retraction or thickening, architectural distortion, or focal asymmetry (asymmetric compared to opposite breast).
- Calcifications that are suspicious for malignancy include new calcifications, pleomorphic calcifications, and fine linear branching/segmental calcifications.
- Ultrasonography is useful in differentiating solid from cystic breast masses. MRI is useful in evaluating the extent of known breast cancer, differentiating between scar and recurrent cancer, implant rupture, and screening high-risk patients as a supplemental test to screening mammography.

Further Readings

1. Berg WA, Yang TS. *Diagnostic Imaging: Breast*. 2nd ed. Altona: AMIRSYS; 2013.
2. Berg WA, Zhang Z, Lehrer D, et al. Detection of breast cancer with addition of annual screening ultrasound or a single screening MRI to mammography in women with elevated breast cancer risk. *J Am Med Assoc*. 2012;307(13):1394-1404.
3. Cardenosa G. *Breast Imaging Companion*. Philadelphia, PA: Lippincott Williams and Wilkins; 2007.
4. Lee CH, Dershaw DD, Kopans D, et al. Breast cancer screening with imaging: recommendations from the Society of Breast Imaging and the ACR on the use of mammography, breast MRI, breast ultrasound, and other technologies for the detection of clinically occult breast cancer. *J Am Coll Radiol*. 2010;7(1):18-27.
5. Conant E, Brennecke C. *Breast Imaging: Case Review Series (Case Review)*. Philadelphia, PA: Mosby; 2006.
6. D'Orsi CJ, Bassett LW, Berg WA, et al. Mammography. In: D'Orsi CJ, Mendelson EB, Ikeda DM, eds. *Breast Imaging Reporting and Data System (BI-RADS)*. 4th ed.. Reston, VA: American College of Radiology; 2003.
7. Independent UK Panel on Breast Cancer Screening. The benefits and harms of breast cancer screening: an independent review. *Lancet*;380(9855):1778-1786.
8. Pisano ED, Gatsonis C, Hendrick E, et al. Diagnostic performance of digital versus film mammography for breast-cancer screening. *N Engl J Med*. 2005;353(17):1773-1783.
9. Saslow D, Boetes C, Burke W, et al. American cancer society guidelines for breast screening with MRI as an adjunct to mammography. *CA Cancer J Clin*. 2007;57(2):75-89.
10. U.S. Preventive Services Task Force. Screening for breast cancer: U.S. Preventive services task force recommendation statement. *Ann Intern Med*. 2009;151(10):716-726.

Questions

1. Which is the best choice for the indications of screening mammogram?
   a. Asymptomatic women without high-risk factors starting at age 30 annually
   b. Asymptomatic women without high-risk factors starting at age 40 annually
   c. Asymptomatic women without high-risk factors starting at age 50 biannually
   d. Women with 1-week breast pain

2. The advantage of digital mammography compared with film-screen mammography includes the following except
   a. Use of computer-assisted diagnostic techniques (CAD) to aid in detecting abnormalities
   b. Better detection of breast cancer in pre- or perimenopausal women
   c. Rapid transmission of the imaging to another location and storage of the images electronically
   d. Better detection of breast cancer in women with fatty breast

3. Indications for diagnostic mammogram include the following except
   a. Recent lumpectomy to establish a new baseline
   b. 40-year-old women with bloody nipple discharge
   c. 50-year-old women with history of benign breast biopsy
   d. 50-year-old women with recent onset of unilateral skin indentation

4. Which one of the following calcifications is most suspicious for ductal carcinoma in situ?
   a. Round and punctate microcalcifications
   b. Dystrophic calcifications
   c. Amorphous microcalcifications
   d. Clustered pleomorphic microcalcifications

5. The differential diagnosis of the circumscribed solid mass on ultrasound is the following except
   a. Fibroadenoma
   b. Phyllodes tumor
   c. Simple cyst
   d. Medullary carcinoma

6. Which one of the following statement about male gynecomastia is true?
   a. It carries increased risk for malignancy
   b. It is always bilateral
   c. It can be due to certain medications, liver disease, or testicular tumor
   d. It occurs only in elderly

7. Indications for breast MRI are the following except
   a. Women with dense breast tissue
   b. Evaluation of extent of the disease with recently diagnosed breast cancer
   c. Silicone implant rupture
   d. BRCA mutations

8. Which one of the following is more suggestive malignancy?
   a. Circumscribed low-density oval mass on mammogram
   b. Circumscribed isoechoic oval mass on ultrasound
   c. Irregular high-density mass with spiculated borders on mammogram
   d. Lobulated anechoic mass with septations and posterior enhancement on ultrasound

9. The indications for high-risk screening mammogram prior to age 40 are the following except
   a. Mother was diagnosed with postmenopausal breast cancer
   b. BRCA mutations
   c. Mother diagnosed with premenopausal breast cancer
   d. History of lymphoma at young age of 8 years post chest radiation therapy

10. What is the best initial imaging modality to evaluate a 29-year-old women with a breast lump?
    a. Diagnostic mammogram
    b. Breast MRI
    c. Tomosynthesis
    d. Breast ultrasound

CHAPTER 12

Interventional Radiology

Thomas A. Farrell, MB, BCh

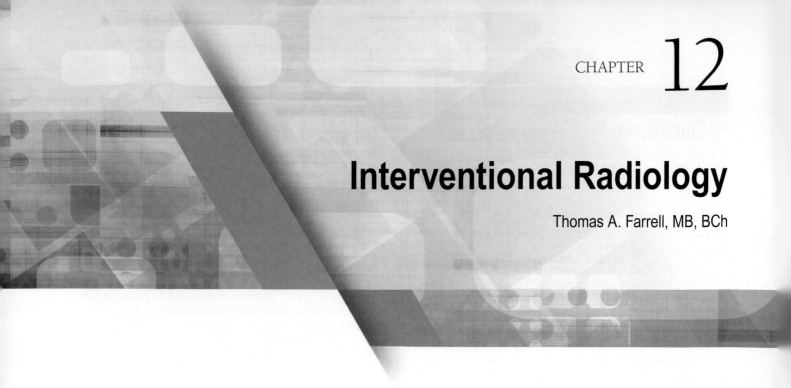

Interventional radiology (IR) is a diverse practice of patient care using minimally invasive image-guided procedures to diagnose and treat disease nonoperatively. Percutaneous diagnostic and therapeutic procedures are performed using fluoroscopy, ultrasound, computed tomography (CT), or magnetic resonance (MR) imaging for guidance. These procedures, which may be broadly categorized as vascular (i.e., arteriography, venography) and nonvascular (e.g., drainage of abscesses, obstructed kidneys, and bile ducts), are performed in a sterile IR suite under conscious sedation and are often done on an outpatient basis. Many procedures that were previously done surgically are now performed by an interventional radiologist with less morbidity and a shorter hospital stay.

Since 1953, when Dr Sven-Ivar Seldinger described a method of percutaneous arterial access using a hollow-core needle, guidewire, and catheter, IR has continued to evolve, as new techniques and devices are developed to enhance patient care. Technical advances have led to significant improvements in patient safety and procedural diversity. As these rapid changes in endovascular technologies continue to expand, so will the possibilities of image-guided, minimally invasive procedures.

Because IR is procedural, interventional radiologists are more involved in patient care than their colleagues in diagnostic radiology. Many IR practices offer a prompt consult service and employ specially trained nurse practitioners and physician's assistants as physician extenders. Patients are

TABLE 12.1	Interventional Radiology Preprocedure Checklist

Indication for procedure/question(s) to be answered from procedure
Contraindications for procedure
Review prior imaging and noninvasive studies
Check for contrast allergy
Written informed consent
Check coagulation parameters and serum creatinine
Need for prophylactic antibiotics
Patient should be fasting and well hydrated
Discontinue heparin infusion

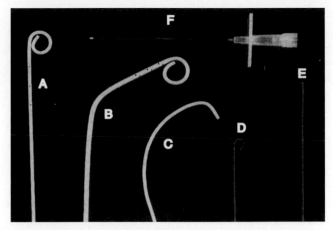

FIGURE 12.1. Tools of the trade. A: Pigtail catheter. **B:** Angled pigtail catheter. **C:** Cobra catheter. **D:** J-tipped guidewire. **E:** Straight (Bentson) guidewire. **F:** An 18G needle for vessel puncture.

routinely worked up by the IR service and are subsequently followed up postprocedure. The preprocedure workup consists of patient assessment as well as evaluation of previous imaging studies (Table 12.1).

Postprocedure follow-up is essential to determine whether the procedure has been successful and free of complications. This all-inclusive clinical service underscores that there is more to IR than simply doing procedures. Because procedures performed by interventional radiologists are invasive, the risk of complications should be discussed with the patient so that informed consent can be made by weighing the possible risks of a procedure against its potential benefits. A physician should never place a patient in a position of risk unless the risks, benefits, and alternatives of the planned procedure have been discussed, understood, and consented to before the procedure. It is in the physician's best interest to be honest and forthright when dealing with patients and their expectations about the outcomes of an IR procedure.

The aim of this chapter is to explain the background, indications, and basic techniques of the procedures commonly performed in IR so that the reader will gain an understanding of how this subspecialty contributes to and enhances patient care.

INSTRUMENTS AND TOOLS OF THE TRADE

IR procedures are performed in imaging suites with fluoroscopy and digital subtraction angiography (DSA). Ultrasound, CT, and MR imaging are also utilized by the interventional radiologist.

Endoluminal and endovascular procedures require administration of a contrast agent for improved visualization. Nonionic iodinated contrast is the most commonly used agent to visualize an artery, vein, bile duct, or the gastrointestinal (GI) or urinary tract. Alternatively, carbon dioxide gas can be used intravascularly in patients with renal insufficiency or who are allergic to iodinated contrast agents.

There is a variety of commercially available **angiographic catheters**, sheaths, guidewires, balloon angioplasty

catheters, vascular stents, and vena caval filters, and familiarity with them and their use requires training and experience. There are numerous preformed shapes and types of angiographic catheters, most of which are made from flexible plastic material such as polyethylene or polyurethane. Wire braiding may be incorporated into the catheter shaft to increase stiffness and improve its "torqueability." Catheter diameters are measured in French (F) size, where 3F = 1 mm (outside diameter). Most angiographic catheters are in the 4F to 7F range. Aortic angiography is performed with pigtail catheters that have several side holes proximal to the tip allowing rapid flow of a contrast bolus while the pigtail loop stabilizes the catheter preventing recoil (Fig. 12.1A,B). Selective angiography (renal, celiac, and superior mesenteric arteries) is performed with a curved end-hole catheter such as a Cobra C2 (Fig. 12.1C). A variety of catheters and guidewires may be necessary during a vascular procedure, and placement of a vascular sheath with a hemostatic valve at the site of access reduces vessel trauma and facilitates rapid catheter and guidewire exchange.

Percutaneous drainage catheters used for treatment of abscesses, obstructed kidneys (percutaneous nephrostomy), and bile ducts are usually made of polyurethane and are of greater diameter (8F to 22F) than angiographic catheters. These drainage catheters are usually placed using the Seldinger technique after which they are secured in position by deploying a locking pigtail mechanism formed by pulling on a suture that runs in the catheter shaft and is attached to its tip. The pigtail loop itself contains large side holes for drainage purposes. The smaller diameter catheters occlude more easily with debris and should be routinely changed over a guidewire every 6 to 8 weeks when long-term drainage is required.

Guidewires increase the ease and safety of catheter placement. The outer shell of a guidewire consists of a very tightly wound but flexible metal spring coil. A stiff central core provides rigidity over a variable length of the guidewire. The balance between the flexible and stiff components dictates the handling characteristics of the guidewire. For example, the distal 15 cm of a Bentson guidewire is floppy, allowing easy coiling (Fig. 12.1E), whereas a J-tipped guidewire reduces the risk of damaging the vessel wall because of its blunt tip (Fig. 12.1D). Guidewires usually range in diameter from 14 thousandths of an inch (0.014″) to 38 thousandths of an inch (0.038″). The standard length for most wires is 145 cm, while longer guidewires (260 cm) are available to facilitate catheter exchange.

Needles for vascular access vary in size from a 21G needle through which a 0.018-inch guidewire will pass to an 18G needle that accepts a 0.035-inch guidewire (Fig. 12.1F).

In order to perform procedures that are uncomfortable and sometimes painful, interventional radiologists use **moderate conscious sedation**, which is a drug-induced depression of consciousness during which patients respond purposefully to verbal commands, either alone or accompanied by light tactile stimulation. Typically this is achieved by administration of versed, a benzodiazepine in combination with fentanyl, a narcotic, both of which are titrated to effect. Monitoring of patient vital signs including end title CO_2, which is an earlier predictor of hypoxia than the arterial oxygen saturation level, is mandatory as is availability of trained personnel to administer these drugs and their reversal agents if necessary.

VASCULAR INTERVENTIONS

Angiography is a technique of imaging blood vessels, by injecting contrast material via an intraluminally placed catheter (catheter angiography) or noninvasively with CT angiography (CTA) and MR angiography (MRA).

Catheter angiography begins by accessing an artery (usually common femoral or radial) using the Seldinger technique (Fig. 12.2). After inserting a hollow-core needle into the artery, a guidewire is inserted through the needle and advanced into the artery. The needle is exchanged for a vascular catheter or sheath. Subsequent catheter movement and exchange is performed over a guidewire. Sonographic and fluoroscopic guidance is often necessary using this technique for needle and catheter placement, respectively. Large vessel arteriography is performed using flush catheters (pigtail). Smaller arteries are selectively cannulated using catheters of various shapes and sizes. Microcatheters (3F and smaller) are used for sub- or superselective arteriography.

After the catheter is safely positioned in the artery of choice, the guidewire is removed and contrast injected through the catheter during image acquisition usually with DSA, which involves the acquisition of several mask images before injection of contrast, allowing for subsequent subtraction of nonvascular structures from the next set of images, which are acquired as the contrast agent flows through the lumen of the vessel producing the arteriogram. The catheter can be exchanged or repositioned for additional imaging.

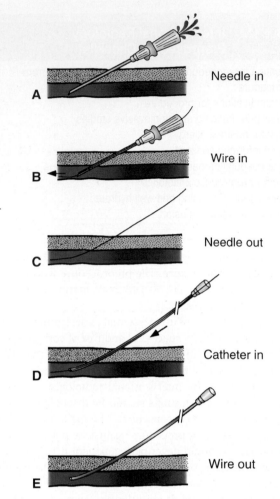

FIGURE 12.2. Seldinger technique. A: The vessel is punctured with the needle. **B:** A guidewire is advanced through the needle into the vessel. **C:** The needle is removed leaving the guidewire in place. **D:** A catheter is advanced over the guidewire into the vessel. **E:** The guidewire is removed and the catheter flushed.

After completion of the procedure, the catheter is removed from the artery and hemostasis obtained at the arteriotomy site using manual compression or a percutaneous closure device such as a nitinol clip or preformed suture, which closes the arterial wall externally in a purse-string fashion with minimal impact on the vessel diameter. Postprocedure recovery time for the patient is 2 to 6 hours.

Both CTA and MRA are widely used in the evaluation of arterial disease (Fig. 12.3) and have replaced diagnostic catheter angiography, except where intervention is planned or other examinations are inconclusive. Magnetic resonance angiography (MRA) takes advantage of the inherent contrast between flowing blood and stationary tissue with newer techniques not requiring the use of gadolinium.

Generally, the diagnosis of **peripheral arterial disease (PAD)** has already been made by the time an arteriogram is requested. The initial evaluation includes an assessment of the patient's symptoms (intermittent claudication, rest pain,

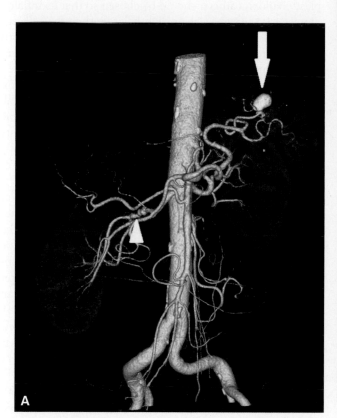
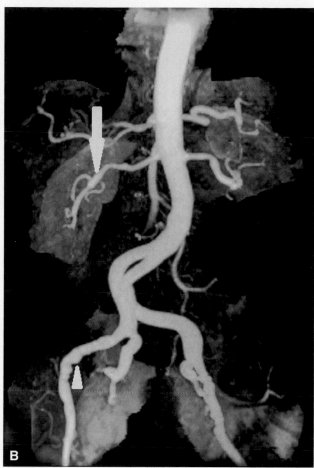

FIGURE 12.3. A: CTA of abdomen. Volume-rendered images of the abdomen show the abdominal aorta and its branches. There are multiple stenoses in the mid–right renal artery consistent with fibromuscular dysplasia (*arrowhead*). There is also a calcified splenic artery aneurysm (*arrow*). **B:** *MR angiography* of the abdomen and pelvis shows multiple stenoses of both renal (*arrow*) and external iliac arteries (*arrowhead*) consistent with fibromuscular dysplasia.

nonhealing ulcer), physical examination, and a review of the noninvasive imaging tests, such as Doppler US, CTA, MRA, and segmental limb pressures (Ankle Brachial Indices) before proceeding to angiography. Rather than being an end point, the angiogram helps formulate a comprehensive plan in the patient's subsequent management as it evaluates the extent and severity of disease and provides a road map for intervention (balloon angioplasty, stenting, surgery, etc.). Patients with diabetes may present with a more advanced stage of ischemia as they are prone to developing peripheral neuropathy that may mask the above symptoms. Diabetics also tend to have a greater prevalence of small vessel (infrageniculate) disease, which is more difficult to treat surgically and contributes to a less favorable long-term prognosis compared with other causes of PAD.

PAD is a marker of significant systemic atherosclerosis as over one-half of patients with PAD will have coronary artery disease, and up to one quarter of patients with PAD will have a significant stenosis in at least one carotid artery.

Arteriographic examination of patients with PAD may be divided into three anatomic regions: aortoiliac, femoropopliteal, and runoff (below the knee). Abdominal aortic aneurysms (AAA) occur most commonly below the level of the renal arteries. The number of renal arteries should also be noted, as should the presence of stenoses in these vessels. Bilateral oblique views of the pelvis should be obtained during arteriography, as hemodynamically significant stenoses can be missed if only a frontal view is performed. Patients with intermittent claudication typically have stenoses or occlusions of the iliac or femoral systems, most commonly the superficial femoral artery. Arterial collaterals fed by the profunda femoris develop in the thigh to bypass the superficial femoral artery occlusion, and flow may be reconstituted distal to the occlusion at the level of the popliteal artery. Ischemic rest pain or skin ulceration typically occurs with occlusive disease at or in the runoff vessels (anterior tibial, posterior tibial, and peroneal arteries) below the knee.

In general, **arterial stenoses** are not regarded as hemodynamically significant unless they reduce the lumen diameter by 50%. Measurement of a pressure gradient across it can more accurately assess the significance of an arterial stenosis, with a 10 mm Hg gradient or greater being regarded as significant and worthy of further treatment such as angioplasty or stenting. If the gradient is less than 10 mm Hg, a vasodilator such as nitroglycerin may be given intra-arterially to simulate exercise and possibly unmask a significant stenosis.

In the absence of satisfactory femoral pulses bilaterally, either the brachial or radial arteries can be used for percutaneous access.

Catheter-directed thrombolysis involves the dissolution of thrombus (blood clot) in order to reestablish patency of an occluded (thrombosed) vessel, using drugs such as urokinase and tissue plasminogen activator (t-PA). These drugs are infused directly into the thrombosed vessel (artery, vein, bypass, or hemodialysis grafts) via a catheter to ensure a very high local concentration of the thrombolytic drug. Contraindications to thrombolysis include internal bleeding, recent intracranial hemorrhage, or surgery (Table 12.2).

Complications of thrombolysis include bleeding and distal embolization of thrombus. The cumulative probability of bleeding increases with duration of infusion, rising from less than 10% after 16 hours to more than 30% at 40 hours. Routine monitoring of the patient's hemoglobin, hematocrit, and plasma fibrinogen is useful in diagnosing and avoiding this complication. Once thrombolysis is complete (which may take more than 24 hours), angioplasty, stenting, or surgery can be used to treat any underlying vessel stenoses that contributed to the occlusion. Treatment of an acute native arterial occlusion is better done mechanically, with either surgical embolectomy or catheter-directed aspiration.

Balloon Angioplasty

Percutaneous transluminal balloon angioplasty (PTA) results in a controlled vessel plaque and intimal fracture with localized dissection into the underlying media,

thereby increasing the intraluminal diameter. The plaque, intima, and media are subsequently remodeled to give a smoother endoluminal surface. The appropriate angioplasty balloon catheter should be chosen so that its inflated diameter is the same size or slightly larger than the adjacent nondiseased vessel. Initially, the stenosis is crossed with a guidewire that is left across the lesion until the procedure is finished. Heparin and nitroglycerin may be given intra-arterially to prevent thrombosis and vessel spasm, respectively. The angioplasty balloon is advanced across the stenosis, inflated, and deflated slowly under fluoroscopic guidance. Repeat angiography and pressure measurements should be obtained to evaluate the results of angioplasty. Suboptimal angioplasty results may require placement of an endovascular stent.

Iliac artery angioplasty improves inflow to the lower limbs and requires balloons that are 7 to 10 mm in diameter. Again, a guidewire is left across the stenosis during the procedure, the success of which is judged on angiographic and hemodynamic criteria. Stent placement should be considered if the postangioplasty pressure gradient is greater than 10 mm Hg, if there is residual stenosis of greater than 30%, or if a flow-limiting dissection is present (Fig. 12.4). Simultaneous PTA or stenting of both common iliac arteries, known as the kissing balloon or stenting technique, is effective in treating bilateral proximal common iliac artery stenoses.

Covered stents in the **femoropopliteal system** are associated with long-term patency similar to surgical bypass procedures. **Below-the-knee** angioplasty (anterior/posterior tibial and peroneal arteries) is usually performed for limb salvage or to reduce the extent of an impending leg or forefoot amputation for ischemia. This technique requires a narrow guidewire (0.014–0.018″) and angioplasty balloon (2–3 mm in diameter) because of the smaller vessel size.

Poorly controlled diabetes contributes to the development of peripheral neuropathy and arterial disease by complex metabolic pathways. Loss of sensation caused by peripheral neuropathy and ischemia due to peripheral arterial disease, or a combination of both may lead to foot ulcers, which may progress to amputation impacting long-term mobility and mortality. **Diabetic foot disease** tends to involve the small vessels of the leg and foot with progressive atherosclerosis and calcification. Measurement of the Ankle Brachial Index is unreliable as many of these lower extremity arteries are not compressible because of diffuse calcification. Management of patients with "diabetic foot" requires a multidisciplinary approach involving podiatrists, endocrinologists, vascular surgeons, and interventional radiologists. Regular physical examination and measurement of transcutaneous oxygen and doppler perfusion imaging are recommended as reliable tests. Balloon angioplasty using balloons 2 to 3 mm in diameter over 014 guidewires may be required to restore flow to both anterior and posterior tibial arteries into the pedal arches (Fig. 12.5A-C).

TABLE 12.2	Contraindications for Arterial Thrombolysis

Absolute

Active or recent (<10 d) gastrointestinal (GI) or genitourinary (GU) bleeding

Recent (<2 mo) cerebral hemorrhage/infarct/recent neurosurgery (<3 mo)

Irreversible limb ischemia

Relative

Recent thoracic/abdominal surgery (within last 10 d)

Recent trauma

Severe uncontrolled hypertension (SBP >180 mm Hg)

Renal artery angioplasty and stenting is usually performed with a 5- to 7-mm diameter balloon and stents, respectively. Atheromatous disease usually involves the proximal or ostial portion of the vessel in contrast to fibromuscular dysplasia that usually affects the midportion of the vessel (Fig. 12.6). Renal artery stenting is performed if there is a residual stenosis or significant dissection postangioplasty (Fig. 12.7). Ostial renal artery stenoses are often stented primarily, without balloon predilatation. It has been noted that improvement in hypertension and renal function is not universal postangioplasty/stent. In the CORAL Study (NEJM 2014), renal-artery stenting did not confer a significant benefit with respect to the prevention of major adverse renal and cardiovascular events when added to comprehensive, multifactorial medical therapy in people with atherosclerotic renal-artery stenosis and hypertension or chronic kidney disease.

Endovascular Stents

There are two main indications for endovascular stent placement: (1) A residual pressure gradient of more than 10 mm Hg postangioplasty, and (2) postangioplasty flow-limiting dissection, in which the goal of stent placement is to appose the dissected flap against the wall and improve flow. There are two general types of metallic endovascular stents, **balloon-expandable** and **self-expanding**. The balloon–stent combination is placed across the stenosis and the balloon is inflated, thus opening and deploying the stent. The balloon is then deflated and removed (Fig. 12.8). Deployment of the self-expanding stent, which does not require delivery on an angioplasty balloon, involves withdrawal of a covering sheath, after which the stent expands. Postdilatation with an angioplasty balloon may be necessary. Self-expanding stents

are usually more flexible than balloon-expanded stents, which is an advantage when stenting tortuous vessel. Covered (polytetrafluoroethylene [PTFE], Dacron) stents are available for treatment of vascular injury resulting in pseudoaneurysm, hemorrhage, or arteriovenous (AV) fistula (Fig. 12.9A and B).

Balloon angioplasty is limited by the elastic recoil and restenosis of the vessel. Stenting is limited by thrombosis and neointimal hyperplasia causing restenosis. Recent introduction of **drug-coated stents and balloons** that elute the drug paclitaxel significantly reduces the cellular response causing restenosis. These stents and balloons deposit paclitaxel on the endothelium. Sustained drug release (from a stent) may not be essential for the long-term antiproliferative action of paclitaxel as its uptake by vascular smooth muscle cells is rapid and can be retained for 1 week with a successful effect achieved by using drug-coated balloons (DCBs) instead of drug-eluting stents (DESs). The initial enthusiasm for the use of drug-coated technology has been tempered with a recent meta-analysis of randomized trials that suggests a possible increased mortality rate after two years in PAD patients treated with paclitaxel-coated balloons and paclitaxel-eluting stents compared to patients treated with control devices (noncoated balloons or bare metal stents).

Aortic stent grafts have revolutionized the treatment of aortic aneurysms including those occurring in the thoracic (TAA) and abdominal aorta (AAA), reducing the severity and duration of the operative procedure, morbidity, and hospital stay. The procedures, thoracic endovascular aneurysm repair (TEVAR) for TAA and endovascular aneurysm repair (EVAR) for AAA, are usually done in an OR or combined operative/fluoroscopy suite, under general or epidural anesthesia. A preprocedural CTA of the abdominal and pelvis is

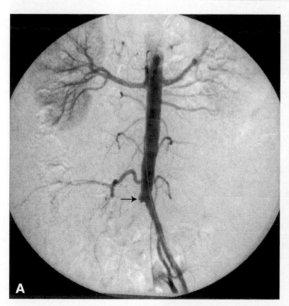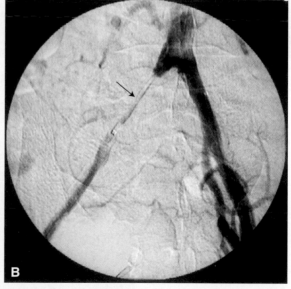

FIGURE 12.4. **Arterial thrombolysis, balloon angioplasty, and stenting of a common iliac artery occlusion. A:** Aortogram/pelvic angiogram shows occlusion of the right common iliac artery (*arrow*). **B:** Partial recanalization of the right common iliac artery following thrombolysis performed via an infusion catheter (*arrow*).

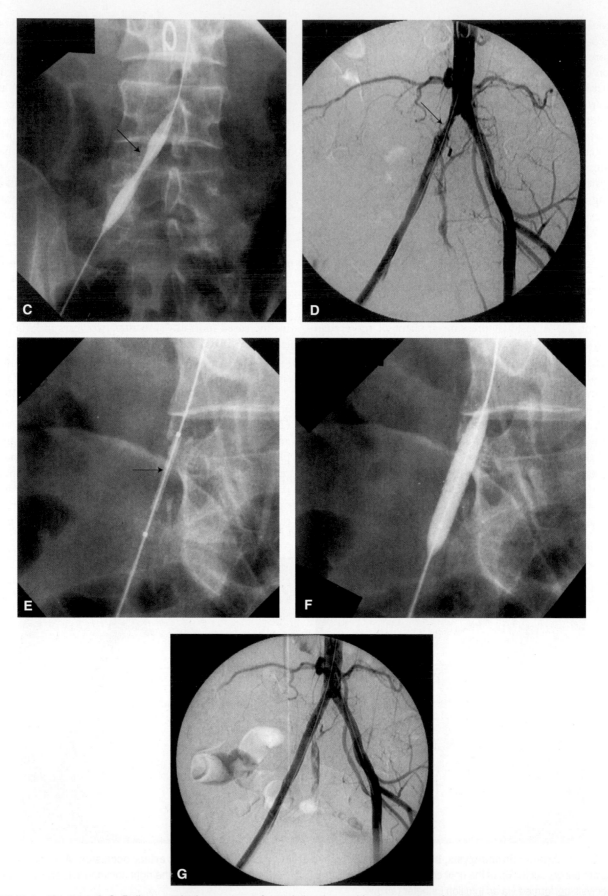

FIGURE 12.4. *(Continued)* **C:** Balloon angioplasty was performed showing residual narrowing of the balloon *(arrow)*. **D:** The common iliac stenosis persisted postangioplasty *(arrow)*. **E and F:** A balloon-expandable stent was deployed across the stenosis. The undeployed stent *(arrow)* can be seen on the distal portion of the angioplasty balloon. **G:** Poststenting, no residual stenosis is present.

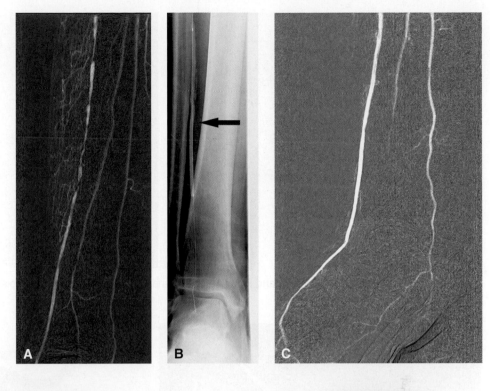

FIGURE 12.5. Anterior tibial angioplasty for a nonhealing ulcer of the big toe in a diabetic. A: Right lower extremity angiogram, demonstrating a diffusely diseased anterior tibial artery. **B:** Balloon angioplasty of the right anterior tibial artery with a 2.5 mm diameter angioplasty balloon. **C:** Follow-up angiography demonstrating improved flow in the right anterior tibial artery and dorsalis pedis.

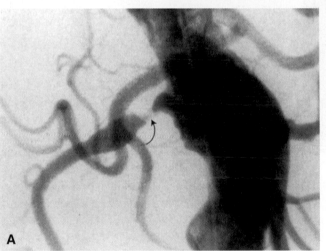
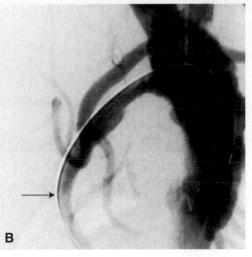

FIGURE 12.6. Renal artery angioplasty. A: Flush aortogram showing right renal artery stenosis (*curved arrow*). **B:** Residual stenosis persists post–balloon angioplasty. Note that the guidewire (*arrow*) is left across the stenosis.

essential for precise vessel measurement, aneurysm characterization, and localization of arterial branches. Through bilateral common femoral artery surgical cutdowns or percutaneous accesses, the modular components of the aortic stent graft are introduced and deployed at either end of the aneurysm, under fluoroscopic guidance. The device, which is composed of woven polyester covering on a wire exoskeleton frame, is deployed to exclude the aneurysm (Fig. 12.10). Post-EVAR follow-up with CT is important for the detection of complications such as endoleak, which is a leak into the aneurysm sac, which may cause the sac to enlarge. In the absence of such endoleak, the aneurysm sac should

reduce in size (Fig. 12.11). EVAR is associated with an early survival benefit because of an increased aneurysm such as aneurysm sac rupture, but the long-term survival is equivalent to open repair. Both TEVAR, and EVAR are also used to treat spontaneous aortic dissection, traumatic aortic transection, and acute rupture of AAA. Stent grafts have also been successfully used in the treatment of popliteal artery aneurysms.

Intravascular ultrasound (IVUS) is performed using a specially made catheter with a miniaturized ultrasound probe (20–40 Mhz) at its tip to visualize the lumen and endothelium (inner wall) of arteries and veins. IVUS is used

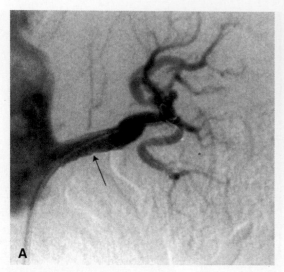

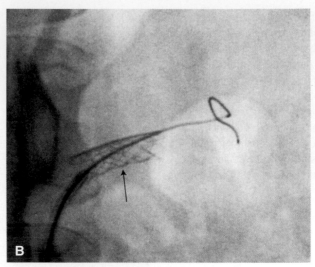

FIGURE 12.7. **Renal artery stenting. A and B:** A balloon-expandable stent (*arrow*) has been placed across a left renal artery stenosis.

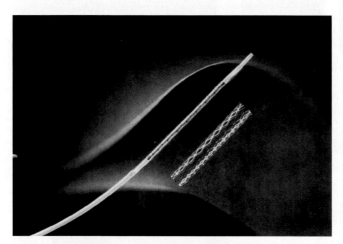

FIGURE 12.8. **Balloon-expandable stent** mounted on an angioplasty balloon and in its expanded form. (Courtesy of Cordis Corporation.)

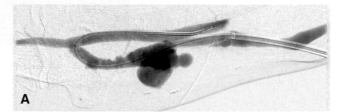

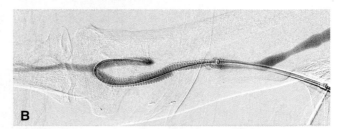

FIGURE 12.9. **A and B: Stenting of pseudoaneurysm. A:** Right arm dialysis fistulogram showing a large venous pseudoaneurysm in the antecubital fossa. **B:** The venous pseudoaneurysm has been excluded by placing a covered self-expanding stent.

in the coronary arteries to evaluate the amount of mural plaque, and in the venous system the technique is used for visualization of thrombus and stenosis in patients with chronic venous disease. IVUS does not require the use of contrast and this is advantageous when performing endovascular procedures such as EVAR or venous recanalization patients with renal failure.

Complications of Angiography

Complications of catheter angiography are rare and the main ones are listed in Table 12.3. Risk factors for these complications include hypertension and obesity and their prevention includes meticulous technique including common femoral artery puncture over the femoral head, and if a closure device is not being used, constant manual pressure directly over the puncture site after removal of the catheter until hemostasis is achieved. A postangiogram hematoma

may extend into the retroperitoneum when the puncture site is in the external iliac (above the inguinal ligament) rather than the common femoral artery (Fig. 12.12A). Incomplete or intermittent compression over the puncture site may also result in the formation of a pseudoaneurysm, which can be treated surgically or with ultrasound-guided injection of thrombin (Fig. 12.12B). Dissection of vessel wall may occur if the needle/wire or catheter is introduced subintimally (Fig. 12.12C), and distal embolization of mural plaque or thrombus is a risk following any endovascular manipulation (Fig. 12.12D). Complications following brachial or axillary arterial puncture are relatively more common than with femoral artery puncture because of the smaller vessel size and the close proximity of nerves in the arm. Radial

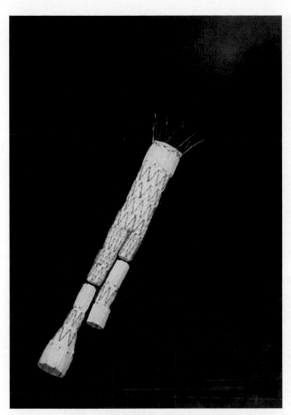

FIGURE 12.10. Aortic stent graft device is composed of three components—a main body and two iliac extensions—which can be custom-made to suit each patient. The components are placed through femoral artery cutdowns. (Courtesy of Cook Medical, Inc.)

artery access is now widely preferred if upper limb access is required. Dissection or thrombosis of the access artery may require endovascular intervention or surgical repair.

Contrast-induced nephropathy usually results in transient renal insufficiency, and occasionally, permanent renal failure. In most patients this complication is usually mild and self-limiting, with serum creatinine levels peaking by 3 to 5 days and returning to normal within 2 weeks. The pathophysiology of this complication is thought to be due to a combination of vasoconstriction and direct toxicity of iodinated contrast on the renal tubules. Patients with diabetes and patients with preexisting renal impairment (serum creatinine greater than 1.6 mg%) are at increased risk for developing contrast-induced renal failure. Clinical judgment, adequate hydration, iso-osmolar or low-osmolar iodinated contrast, should be used in high-risk patients (elderly, creatinine (Cr) >1.6, DM).

Systemic allergic or anaphylactoid reactions to iodinated contrast media are rare, with their severity depending on the type, dose, route, and rate of contrast delivery. Allergic reactions may be categorized as mild, moderate, or severe (Table 12.4). The prevalence of most allergic reactions to iodinated contrast is greater with the intravenous route. Many studies suggest a lower incidence of severe reactions

when nonionic iodinated contrast is used. The mortality rate is approximately 1 per 45,000 contrast exams and is equivalent for high and lower osmolar contrast agents. Moderately severe contrast reactions are characterized by hypertension, hypotension, wheezing, and laryngospasm and occur in 1% to 2% of contrast administrations. Mild allergic reactions—nausea, cough, hives, and flushing—are even more common and can be treated symptomatically. (Consult the ACR Contrast Media Manual for specific treatments.) The standard of care is premedication with steroids prior to contrast administration. (See Inside back cover for premedication of iodinated contrast reactions.) Allergy to seafood is not a predisposition to developing an allergic reaction to iodinated contrast.

Therapeutic Embolization

Gastrointestinal Hemorrhage

Selective angiography and therapeutic embolization are important techniques in the management of patients with acute nonvariceal upper and lower GI bleeding. Initially, a nuclear medicine study using radiolabeled red cells or a CTA of the abdomen may be helpful to confirm the presence and locations of bleeding. Selective angiography of the celiac, superior mesenteric, or inferior mesenteric arteries is then performed. Once a bleeding site has been identified, the catheter can be used to control bleeding by embolization with gelatin sponge pledgets or coils to mechanically occlude flow (Fig. 12.13).

Hemoptysis

Patients with massive hemoptysis may be successfully treated by embolizing the appropriate bronchial arteries, which arise directly from the thoracic aorta or from intercostal branches, using particles measuring 300 to 500 μm in diameter. Preprocedure CTA of the chest provides information on the site and nature of bleeding as well as the supplying bronchial arteries. Great care should be taken to avoid embolization of the arterial supply to the spinal cord, which may result in paralysis.

Uterine Fibroid Embolization

Fibroids are the most common benign gynecological tumors and may present as pain, menorrhagia, anemia, or pressure symptoms related to mass effect. Traditionally, patients were treated with hysterectomy or myomectomy. Uterine fibroid embolization (UFE) offers an effective and less invasive treatment option. After bilateral selective catheterization of the uterine arteries, particles up to 900 microns (0.9 mm) in size are injected, infarcting the fibroids, eventually reducing their size and improving patients' symptoms. The fibroid size typically reduces by 60% at 6 months after treatment and up to 90% of patients notice an improvement in their pain, menorrhagia, or pressure symptoms (Fig. 4.27). Preprocedure MRI is necessary to exclude other causes of menorrhagia including adenomyosis, which may not improve following embolization.

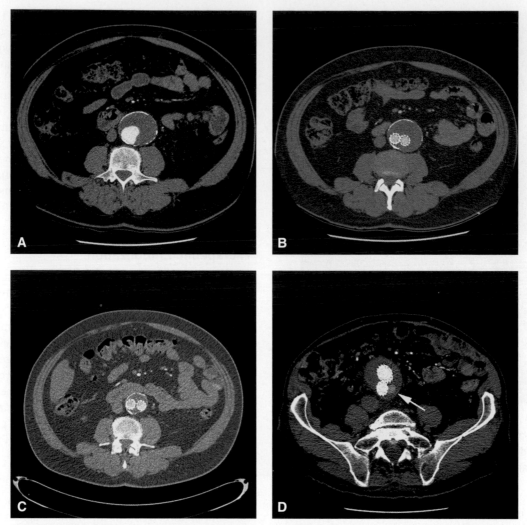

FIGURE 12.11. Aortic endograft follow-up. Serial CT studies show an infrarenal abdominal aortic aneurysm (AAA) measuring 4.5 cm in diameter **(A)**. Six months post–AAA endograft placement, the excluded aneurysm sac now measures 4 cm **(B)** and at 18 mo post-tendograft, it has further reduced to a diameter of 3.2 cm **(C)**. CT abdomen in a patient post–AAA endograft shows contrast within the aneurysm sac but outside the endograft (*arrow*) **(D)**. This is an endoleak (*arrow*) that occurs because of persistent blood flow into the aneurysm, which in this patient is due to retrograde flow from a lumbar artery.

TABLE 12.3	Complications of Angiography

Systemic
   Allergic contrast reaction
   Renal failure
Local
   Puncture site
     Hematoma
     Pseudoaneurysm
     Arteriovenous fistula
Intraluminal
   Subintimal dissection
   Thrombosis
   Distal embolization

Arterial embolization is performed to decrease arterial flow to a tumor, depriving it of nutrients. In the case of renal cell carcinoma, the kidney may be embolized prior to surgery to decrease intraoperative blood loss during nephrectomy or resection (Fig. 12.14).

The liver has a dual blood supply—hepatic arterial and portal venous—and liver tumors depend largely on the arterial supply for growth. **Chemoembolization** is performed in patients with primary or metastatic liver cancer, by subselectively embolizing the arterial supply of the tumor with a combination of chemotherapeutic drugs and inert particles. Chemoembolization has the advantage of prolonging the tumor exposure to a high concentration of drug(s) while also infarcting the tumor (Fig. 12.15). **Radioembolization** is another form of liver embolization in which numerous

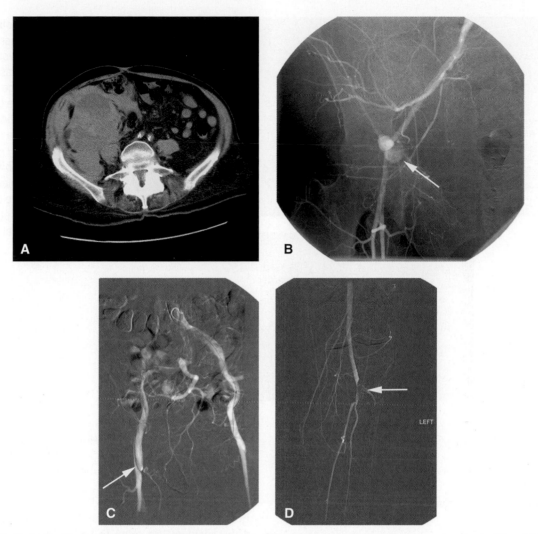

FIGURE 12.12. **Complications of arterial interventions. A:** This CT scan shows a hematoma occupying most of the right hemipelvis. The retroperitoneal hematoma could be traced down to the right external iliac artery where the physician performing an angiogram had made the initial arterial puncture. **B:** The well-defined focal bulge (*arrow*) is a pseudoaneurysm, which has formed at the site of a previous common femoral arterial puncture. **C:** The vertically oriented well-defined curvilinear filling defect (*arrow*) in the right external iliac is a dissection flap. **D:** The well-defined intraluminal filling defect in the distal popliteal artery (*arrow*) is an embolus, which migrated there after balloon angioplasty of a stenosis containing atherosclerotic plaque upstream in the superficial femoral artery.

TABLE 12.4	Allergic Contrast Reactions		
Type	**Mild**	**Moderate**	**Severe**
Incidence (%)	5–15	1–2	0.1
Clinical features	Nausea	Bronchospasm	Laryngospasm
	Vomiting	Dyspnea	Facial edema
	Urticaria	Vasovagal reaction	Cardiorespiratory arrest
		Hypertension	Seizures
Treatment	Monitor vital signs	Oxygen	Oxygen/IV fluids
	Observe for clinical deterioration	β2 agonist	Epinephrine SC or IV
			β2 agonist
			Diazepam
			ACR Contrast Media Manual 2018

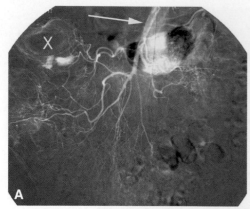

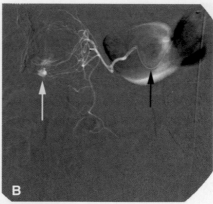

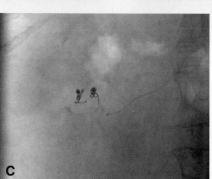

FIGURE 12.13. Embolization of a GI bleed. A: This superior mesenteric angiogram (*arrow*) shows extravasation of contrast, which represents hemorrhage into the colon at the hepatic flexure (*X*). **B:** This extravasation (*white arrow*) is confirmed on selective angiography of the right colic artery performed with a microcatheter (*black arrow*). **C:** Several stainless steel coils 2 to 3 mm in diameter were deployed through the microcatheter occluding the right colic branch at the bleeding site.

10 to 50 micron glass or resin beads, containing isotope yttrium-90, are injected intra-arterially, permitting a highly concentrated dose of radiation, which is confined to the liver. The maximum range of emission of Beta particles is 11 mm and 94% of the radiation dose is delivered over 11 days.

Trauma

The interventional radiologist has an important role in the management of trauma patients. Vessel injury with bleeding, intimal injury, pseudoaneurysm, or fistula can be diagnosed and immediately treated in the angiography suite, often using covered stents or embolization techniques (Figs. 12.16 and 12.17).

Prior to the introduction of external fixation devices, much of the early mortality associated with **pelvic fractures** was due to internal hemorrhage. Patients with pelvic fractures require angiography and embolization because laparotomy would decompress the pelvic hematoma, reduce the tamponade effect, and lead to further blood loss. The extent and nature of the pelvic fracture and associated hematoma are readily diagnosed on CT. A pelvic angiogram is performed with a pigtail catheter placed above the aortic bifurcation with acute hemorrhage being diagnosed by extravasation of contrast. The arterial branch may then be embolized with either a coil or gelfoam, both of which can be deployed through a selectively placed angiographic catheter. Gelfoam results in temporary vascular occlusion that recanalizes within

2 to 3 weeks, whereas a metallic coil usually results in a permanent occlusion. Pelvic ischemia following selective arterial embolization is rare because of the extensive collateral blood supply.

Eighty percent of those who sustain a laceration to the thoracic aorta following blunt trauma die at the scene of the accident, en route to the hospital, or shortly after arriving in hospital. The cause of death in most cases is exsanguination from **aortic transection**. The mechanism of injury is a sudden deceleration where the mobile descending aorta shears from the relatively fixed aortic arch, as the most common site for aortic transection is just distal to the origin of the left subclavian artery. As in all trauma patients, rapid clinical evaluation is important, but up to 50% of patients surviving accidents with blunt aortic injuries have no external physical signs of injury. CTA of the chest has replaced catheter aortography as the gold standard for diagnosing aortic arch injury (see Figure 2.105). One should be aware of a normal anatomic variant in the aortic arch that may be misdiagnosed as traumatic aortic injury—the so-called ductus bump, which lies proximally on the inferior surface of the aortic arch and represents the site of attachment of the ductus arteriosus (Fig. 12.18).

Venous Imaging and Interventions

Deep vein thrombosis (DVT) and acute pulmonary embolism (PE) are two manifestations of venous thromboembolism (VTE). Compression ultrasonography with

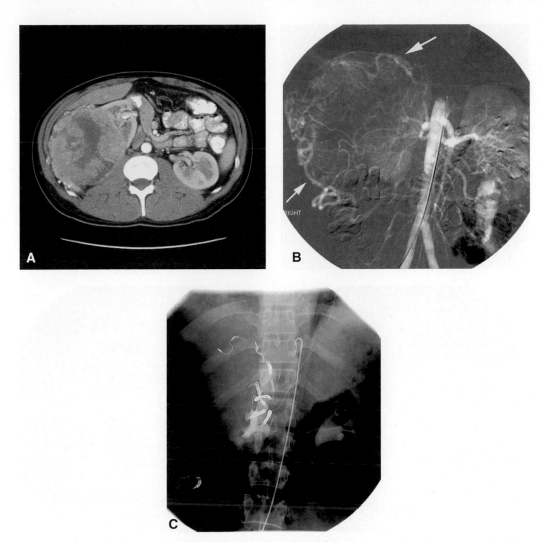

FIGURE 12.14. Preoperative embolization of a renal carcinoma. A: The CT scan shows a large hypervascular right renal carcinoma. **B:** Abdominal aortography confirms it hypervascular nature (*arrows*). **C:** Postembolization of the renal artery branches and nonrenal branches (lumbar and inferior phrenic arteries) with stainless steel coils. The prophylactic embolization reduced the operative morbidity and blood loss as the surgeon was operating in a "bloodless" field. (Courtesy of Dr D. Warner.)

Doppler is the diagnostic test of choice in patients with suspected DVT with an accuracy of over 95% for DVT in the thigh and lower accuracies for calf and pelvic DVT. DVT is diagnosed by demonstrating noncompressibility of the vein by the ultrasound probe. Anticoagulation is the standard treatment. If there is an underlying venous stenosis provoking the DVT, catheter-directed thrombolysis in which an infusion catheter is placed in the thrombus and thrombolytic infused may be indicated. Following resolution of the DVT, the underlying venous stenosis can be treated with either stent or surgery. Patients with **May-Thurner syndrome**, typically present with left lower extremity DVT. Anatomically, there is compression of the left common iliac vein by the overlying right common iliac artery. Following successful treatment of the DVT with catheter-directed thrombolysis, the left common iliac

vein stenosis is stented (Fig. 12.19). **Paget von Schroetter syndrome** describes the development of a upper extremity DVT in a patient with stenosis of the subclavian vein secondary to extrinsic compression by the first rib and associated ligaments. Following successful treatment of the DVT with catheter-directed thrombolysis, resection of the portion of the first rib is recommended to maintain long-term patency.

While catheter-directed thrombolysis has been widely used in the treatment of lower extremity DVT with variable success, the prospective **ATTRACT trial** showed that among patients with acute proximal lower limb deep-vein thrombosis, the addition of pharmacomechanical catheter-directed thrombolysis to anticoagulation did not result in a lower risk of the postthrombotic syndrome but did result in a higher risk of major bleeding.

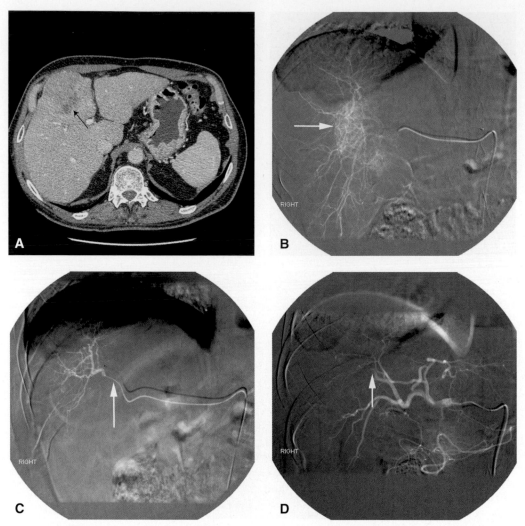

FIGURE 12.15. Chemoembolization of a hepatocellular carcinoma. A: CT shows a hypervascular hepatoma (*arrow*). **B and C:** Selective hepatic angiography confirms the tumor's hypervascularity (*arrow*) and more clearly defines its arterial supply. **D:** Angiography postchemoembolization of the hepatoma confirms occlusion (*arrow*) of its main hepatic arterial branch.

Venography is a commonly performed in interventional procedures such as placement of central venous catheters, caval filters, and adrenal vein sampling. **Primary hyperaldosteronism** is one of the most commonly treatable causes of hypertension and is due either to a unilateral adrenal adenoma (Conn disease) or bilateral adrenal hyperplasia. Adrenalectomy can be curative in patients with adenoma, whereas medication is effective in bilateral adrenal hyperplasia. **Adrenal vein sampling** distinguishes between these two forms of primary hyperaldosteronism, by measuring the secretion of aldosterone (corrected for cortisol) from both adrenal glands.

Central venous catheters are placed for a variety of indications including administration of antibiotics, chemotherapy, and hemodialysis (HD). There are essentially two types of catheters: **Tunneled and nontunneled**. Tunneling

refers to the creation of a subcutaneous tract in which the catheter lies before it enters the vein. The tunnel acts as a physical barrier reducing the incidence of catheter-related infection and also enhancing catheter security. A fibrous cuff on tunneled catheters causes a localized fibrotic reaction, stabilizing it within the subcutaneous tissues. The optimal **tip position** of all central lines is between the mid superior vena cava (SVC) and the mid right atrium. The right internal jugular vein is the preferred site for these catheters. Use of either subclavian vein as venous access site is **not** considered appropriate because of the risk of long-term venous stenosis and occlusion. Another type of tunneled venous access is a port device consisting of a subcutaneously implanted reservoir in the upper chest wall or upper arm to which the catheter is connected. Ports should only be accessed percutaneously with a noncoring needle (Fig. 12.20).

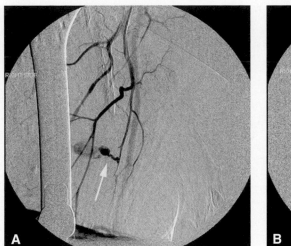
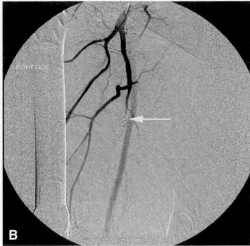

FIGURE 12.16. **Embolization of a leaking pseudoaneurysm.** This patient presented with a rapidly expanding thigh hematoma after hip replacement surgery. **A:** A thigh angiogram shows a pseudoaneurysm (*arrow*) in the distal profunda femoris artery. **B:** Several stainless steel coils were deployed through the angiographic catheter occluding the arterial branch proximal to the pseudo-aneurysm (*arrow*).

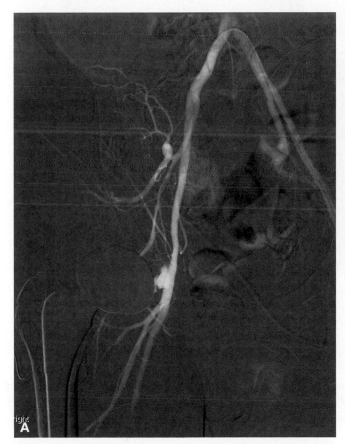
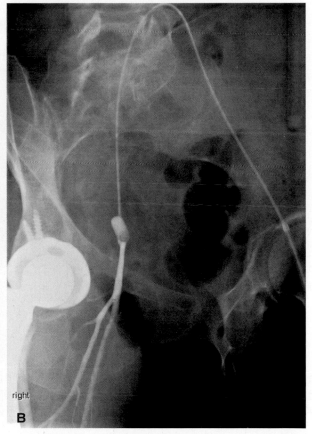

FIGURE 12.17. **Balloon tamponade above arterial tear. A:** Pelvic angiogram showing extravasation from the common femoral artery following inadvertent puncture during hip replacement. **B:** Balloon occlusion of external iliac artery proximal to common femoral laceration shows no extravasation. This allowed patient transfer to the OR for surgical repair of the laceration.

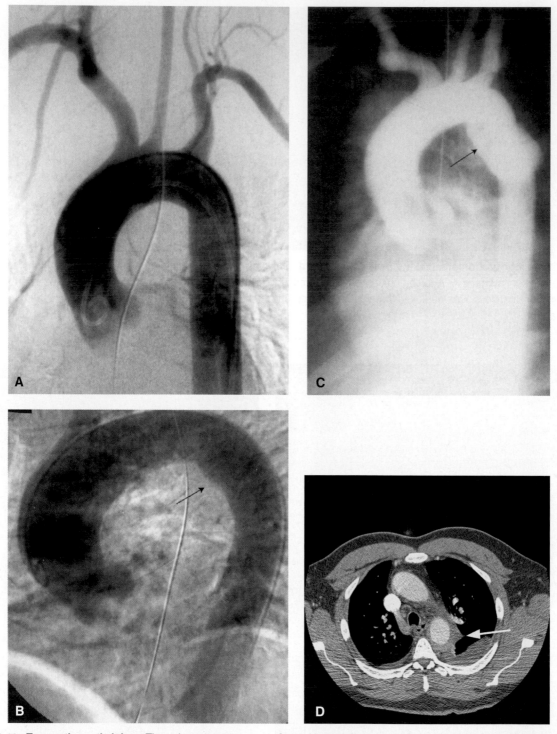

FIGURE 12.18. Traumatic aortic injury. Thoracic aortograms are performed in the left anterior oblique (LAO) view for optimal visualization of the aortic arch. **A:** Normal aortic arch. **B:** Ductus bump, normal variant (*arrow*). **C:** Aortic transection (*arrow*) distal to the origin of the left subclavian artery. **D:** CT scan of the chest shows a mediastinal hematoma (*arrow*) of the distal aortic arch consistent with aortic transection.

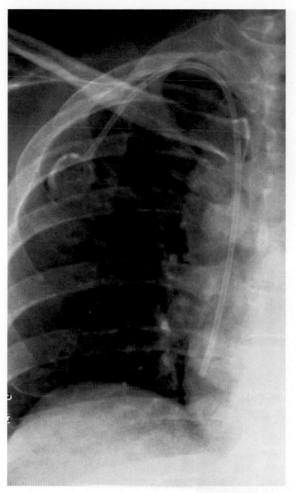

FIGURE 12.19. **Chest port** placement for chemotherapy. The port reservoir is in the infraclavicular subcutaneous tissue. The catheter passes subcutaneously to the right internal jugular vein on its way to the right atrium.

For short-term venous access (less than 90 days) a nontunneled catheter, such as a peripherally inserted central catheter (PICC) is appropriate. A PICC is inserted by direct percutaneous puncture of either arm or forearm veins and advanced under fluoroscopic guidance until the tip lies in the SVC.

The purpose of an **inferior vena cava (IVC) filter** is to prevent PE by trapping clot. Filter placement is indicated in patients in whom anticoagulation for DVT/PE is contraindicated or ineffective. Currently, there are several types of permanent filters available (Fig. 12.21), all of which are made from either stainless steel or nitinol, an alloy of nickel and titanium, and which are introduced percutaneously through the common femoral or internal jugular vein. The purposes of the filter legs are twofold: one to trap clot in the infrarenal IVC and secondly to attach to the IVC wall. **Retrievable** IVC filters may be placed in trauma patients or others at short-term risk of PE. They have a hook at the top to facilitate retrieval with a loop snare (Fig. 12.22). The design of retrievable filters differs from that of permanent filters in that their legs or struts are more likely to perforate the IVC wall. These filters should be retrieved from the IVC as soon as the risk of PE has lessened because of an increased risk of caval perforation and subsequent inability to retrieve them safely (Fig. 12.23).

Cirrhosis causes portal hypertension, which is manifested by esophageal varices, splenomegaly, and ascites. Massive hematemesis may occur from esophageal variceal bleeding, the initial treatment of which is endoscopic banding or injection of the sclerosant such as ethanolamine. If bleeding from esophageal varices due to portal hypertension persists, then creation of an intrahepatic shunt between hepatic and portal veins to decompress the

FIGURE 12.20. **Permanent inferior vena cava filters. A:** Greenfield filter. **B:** Braun Venatech filter (which has side struts to prevent tilt).

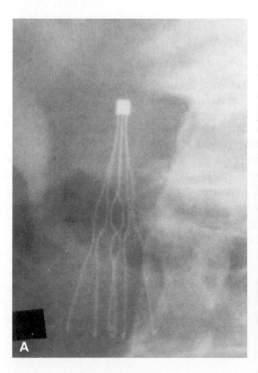

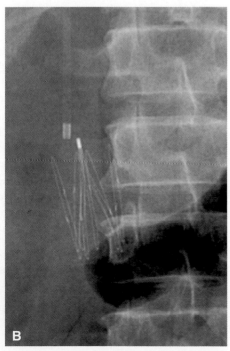

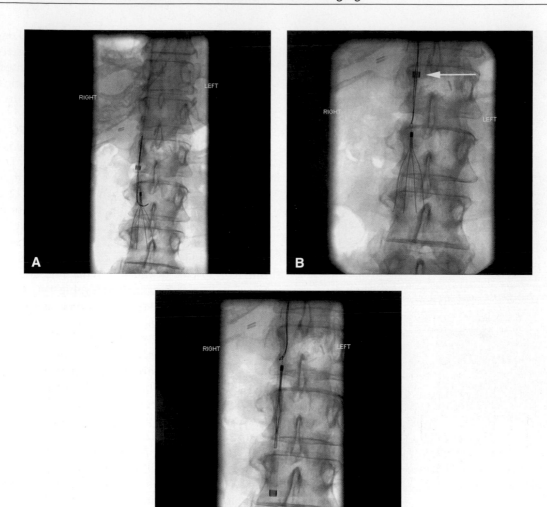

FIGURE 12.21. **Inferior vena cava (IVC) filter retrieval. A:** Under fluoroscopy a retrieval snare has been advanced from the right internal jugular vein to the retrievable IVC filter. **B:** The snare is then used to retrieve the filter by its hook and the filter is collapsed by advancing a sheath (*arrow at tip of sheath*) down over it. **C:** The snared filter and sheath are then removed from the internal jugular vein access site.

portal system is done. This shunt is called a **transjugular intrahepatic portosystemic shunt (TIPS)**. Typically, the right hepatic vein is accessed from a right internal jugular approach. A branch of the right portal vein is then accessed from the right hepatic vein, and this intrahepatic tract is stented decompressing the portal system by shunting blood to the systemic venous system (right hepatic vein and right atrium) (Fig. 12.24). The aim of the shunt is to reduce the pressure gradient between the portal and hepatic veins to less than 10 mm Hg. Depending on the patient's underlying liver status (Child Pugh classification or MELD score), up to 20% of patients may develop hepatic encephalopathy as a complication of this procedure.

Hemodialysis Access Interventions

At the end of 2013, almost 468,000 End Stage Renal Disease (ESRD) patients were being treated with some form of dialysis in the United States, the majority of whom were getting hemodialysis (HD) as opposed to peritoneal dialysis. Vascular access is a generic description where blood is removed from and returned to the body during HD. A vascular access may be an arteriovenous (AV) fistula (56% of patients on HD), an AV graft (36%), or a dialysis catheter (18%). **An AV fistula** is the preferred type of vascular access because it is associated with fewer complications such as infection and clotting. Catheters have the highest rate of infection compared with other access types. **The Fistula First Breakthrough Initiative** is dedicated to improving care for people with chronic kidney disease by increasing AV fistula placement and use in suitable HD patients. Surgically created AV fistulae should be 6 mm in diameter, should be less than 6-mm deep, and have flow rates of 600 mL/min at 6 weeks (**Rule of 6's**). However, as many as 25% of all AV fistulae fail to mature, mostly because of stenosis and competing accessory

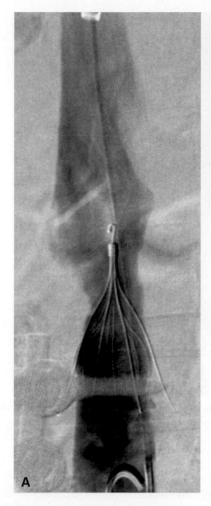

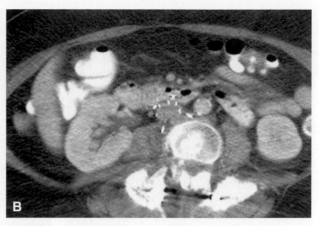

FIGURE 12.22. **Complication of temporary inferior vena cava (IVC) filter. A:** Inferior vena cavography shows perforation of the IVC wall by legs of a temporary IVC filter. **B:** CT abdomen confirms perforation of the IVC.

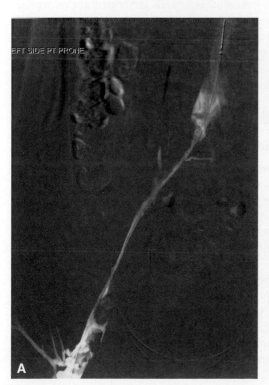

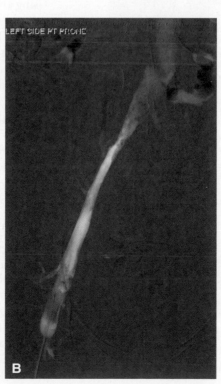

FIGURE 12.23. **Treatment of May–Thurner syndrome. A:** Pelvic venogram with the patient in the prone position shows extensive thrombosis of the left iliofemoral venous system across which an infusion catheter has been placed for thrombolysis. **B:** Follow-up venography after 24 h shows partial resolution of the clot.

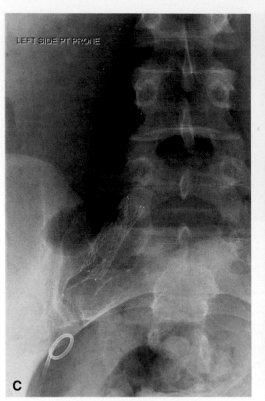

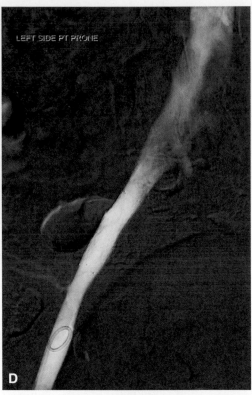

FIGURE 12.23. *(Continued)* **C and D:** At 48 h there is complete resolution of the iliofemoral clot, and a self-expanding stent has been placed to treat the underlying venous stenosis, which was due to external compression of the left common iliac vein by the left common iliac artery.

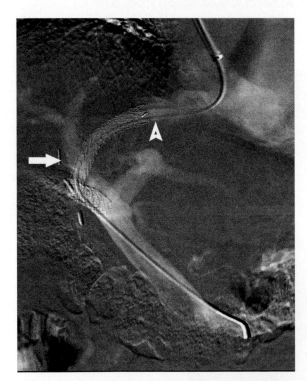

FIGURE 12.24. Transjugular intrahepatic portosystemic shunt (TIPS). A shunt has been created between the right portal vein (*arrow*) and the right hepatic vein (*arrowhead*), decompressing the portal venous system.

veins, which may be successfully treated with balloon angioplasty and coil embolization, respectively.

Using the percutaneous skills described above, including thrombolysis, angioplasty, and stent placement, HD access (AV) fistulae and grafts are declotted and maintained, preserving graft function and longevity. Proper graft or fistula maintenance can add many years to the life of an HD-dependent patient.

NONVASCULAR INTERVENTION

Image-Guided Biopsy

Biopsy allows the retrieval of cells or tissue for a pathologic diagnosis and usually involves the percutaneous introduction of a needle under image guidance (usually ultrasound or CT), which ensures a safe needle trajectory and sufficient material for analysis. As with all percutaneous interventions, bleeding is a risk, so the patient should discontinue their anticoagulants and have a platelet count above 50,000. There are two types of biopsy needles, Fine and Core. As its name suggests a fine needle has a narrow diameter (23G or 25G) and most often yields an aspirate of cells, suitable for cytology (Fig. 12.25A). Core needles are bigger and acquire their sample using a spring-loaded cutting mechanism yielding a core of tissue, for example, liver (Fig. 12.25B).

FIGURE 12.25. **Biopsy specimens.**
A: Cytology specimen obtained using a fine needle aspirate (FNA). Note details of the individual cells are visible. **B:** Core liver biopsy specimen shows tissue rather than individual cells.

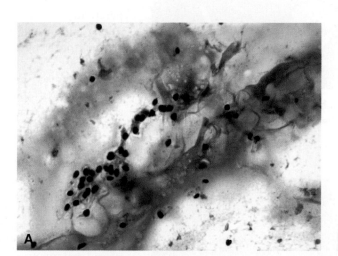
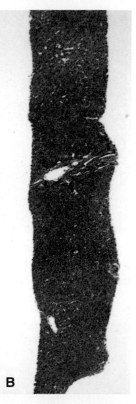

TABLE 12.5	Patients With a High Risk of Thyroid Carcinoma[a]
History of thyroid cancer in one or more first-degree Relatives
History of external beam radiation as a child
Exposure to ionizing radiation in childhood or adolescence
Prior hemithyroidectomy with discovery of thyroid cancer
[18]FDG avidity on PET scanning

[a]Biopsy is indicated in any patient with a 5-mm or greater thyroid nodule and a high-risk history (American Thyroid Association).

Thyroid

Thyroid nodules occur in almost 50% of adults and the majority of these nodules are benign, but this determination can only be made pathologically by reviewing cells aspirated using a fine needle (23G or 25G) inserted into the nodule under US guidance. Generally, US-guided biopsy is not indicated in nodules less than 10 mm unless the patient is at high risk of thyroid carcinoma (Table 12.5).

Lung

Biopsy may be done under CT or less commonly US guided if the lesion is adjacent to the pleura. There is a 10% to 15% risk of pneumothorax. A fine needle aspirate (FNA) is usually sufficient to distinguish small cell from non–small cell carcinoma (NSLC). However, with the advent of biologic chemotherapeutic agents such as tyrosine-kinase inhibitors,

measurement of biomarkers requires more tissue and this is best achieved with a core biopsy. **Transbronchial** biopsy is used to obtain random parenchymal tissue samples and is helpful in confirming the diagnosis of sarcoid.

Liver

The two main reasons for liver biopsy are diffuse parenchymal diseases such as hepatitis and cirrhosis and focal lesions such as malignancy, which may be primary (hepatoma) or secondary (metastases). A core biopsy is necessary for evaluation of the parenchyma and this is usually done percutaneously. The presence of ascites, low platelet count, or prolonged prothrombin time (which are all features of chronic liver disease) increases the risk of bleeding with percutaneous liver biopsy. An alternative biopsy technique involves advancing a long-core biopsy needle to the right hepatic vein from the right internal jugular vein, via the right atrium. After the liver tissue adjacent to the right hepatic vein is biopsied using this **transjugular technique**, any bleeding that occurs will be intravascular (hepatic vein) reducing the risk of significant complication.

Kidney

Similar to liver biopsies, core biopsies are necessary for the diagnosis of parenchymal renal diseases such as glomerulonephritis. FNA may be sufficient for lesions such as carcinoma or metastases. The main risk associated with core biopsy is bleeding (Fig. 12.26).

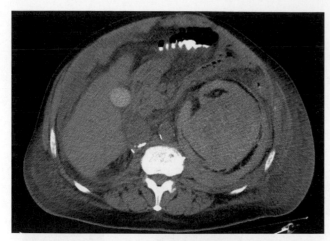

FIGURE 12.26. Post–renal biopsy complication. CT scan shows a large left perirenal hematoma following core needle renal biopsy.

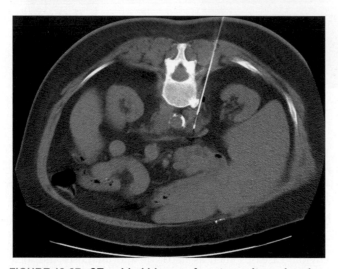

FIGURE 12.27. CT-guided biopsy of a retroperitoneal node. With the patient in the prone position, a right paraspinal approach is used to advance a core biopsy needle into a right para-aortic lymph node. The diagnosis was lymphoma.

Lymphoma or metastatic carcinoma may present as retroperitoneal adenopathy. CT-guided biopsy of these nodes is done with the patient in the prone position (Fig. 12.27). The technique is well tolerated and risk of bleeding is low.

Urologic Interventions

Percutaneous nephrostomy is a valuable tool in the treatment of urinary obstruction, which is most commonly caused by calculi, neoplasms, or benign strictures. With the patient in the prone position, the obstructed renal pelvis is accessed using the Seldinger technique during which an 8F or 10F pigtail drainage catheter is passed over a guidewire and the loop formed and secured in the

renal pelvis and connected to gravity drainage. Further intervention such as ureteral stenting or stone removal (nephrolithotomy) may be performed through this percutaneous renal access. Mild hematuria is not uncommon after percutaneous nephrostomy and usually resolves within 72 hours.

Percutaneous Biliary Drainage and Stenting

Obstructive jaundice may be diagnosed and treated by a percutaneous transhepatic cholangiogram (PTC) whereby a long 22G needle is advanced through the liver parenchyma from a site in the 11th intercostal space in the right midaxillary line or through the left lobe, using a subxiphoid approach and ultrasound guidance. The needle is then slowly withdrawn while injecting contrast to opacify any bile ducts that may have been traversed. Successful PTC is more likely if the ductal system is dilated. Once a bile duct is opacified, a larger (21G or 18G) needle is then used to percutaneously access one of the opacified ducts peripherally. The tract is dilated over a guidewire and an attempt to traverse the biliary obstruction is made, followed by placement of **an internal–external biliary drainage** catheter to decompress the ductal system. Permanent self-expanding metallic stents may be placed percutaneously or endoscopically when internalized biliary drainage is desired, as in the case of a malignant obstruction. Alternatively, temporary short plastic stents may be placed in the common duct when surgery is planned or in patients with benign strictures.

Percutaneous cholecystostomy (external gallbladder drainage) has become an accepted interim treatment for patients with acute cholecystitis. The gallbladder is accessed percutaneously and the tract dilated over a guidewire, over which a pigtail drainage tube is advanced into the gallbladder and connected to gravity drainage. A tube check is done after 5 to 7 days to confirm a patent cystic and common duct, at which time the tube is capped pending cholecystectomy. several weeks later.

Percutaneous Feeding Tubes

Radiologically guided placement of percutaneous gastrostomy and gastrojejunostomy tubes for enteral nutrition has gained widespread acceptance in the management of patients who cannot eat or swallow because of stroke, head injury, and head and neck tumors. The stomach is accessed percutaneously under fluoroscopic guidance using the Seldinger technique and the tract dilated over a guidewire. A 12F or 14F self-retaining pigtail feeding tube is placed over a guidewire and secured within the stomach (Fig. 12.28). If there is a risk of aspiration, delivery of liquid feeds directly into the small bowel rather than the stomach is preferred, and this is accomplished by a gastrojejunostomy tube, which is placed in a transgastric fashion as described above and the tip directed through the pylorus to the proximal jejunum.

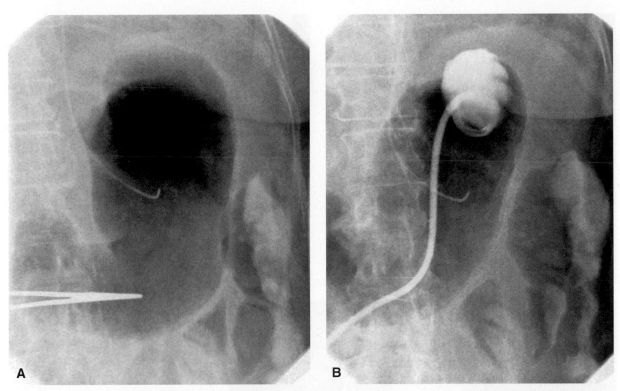

FIGURE 12.28. Fluoroscopic gastrostomy tube placement. A: The stomach is inflated and accessed percutaneously using a Seldinger technique. **B:** The tract is dilated over a guidewire and a 16F feeding tube placed.

Interventional Oncology

Ablation of Tumors

This minimally invasive technique is often used in the treatment of liver, lung, and bone tumors and results in a reduced hospital stay and complication rate. Under CT or ultrasound guidance, a radiofrequency ablation (RFA) needle is percutaneously inserted into the tumor. RFA involves the deposition of energy at 480 kHz, causing coagulation necrosis by heating the tissue to 60°C at which temperature cell death occurs (Fig. 12.29). More recently, microwave ablation has gained acceptance for solid tumor ablation because of its higher energy and more consistent ablation profile. Percutaneous cryoablation, which involves freezing, thawing, and refreezing a lesion, is preferred for renal masses as there is less risk of urine leak.

Vertebroplasty

In the United States, more than 1.5 million osteoporosis-related fractures occur every year, of which 700,000 are vertebral compression fractures. Vertebroplasty is the percutaneous injection of bone cement into a vertebral body fracture, thereby stabilizing it and rendering it less painful. With the patient in the prone position and under fluoroscopic guidance, an 11G or 13G needle is advanced percutaneously through each pedicle into the vertebral body, into which 3 to 5 mL of PMMA bone cement is then injected which hardens in 5 to 10 minutes (Fig. 12.30). Initial skepticism on the efficacy of the technique has been overcome

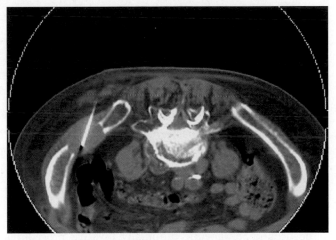

FIGURE 12.29. Radiofrequency ablation. CT pelvis shows a radiofrequency ablation needle in a bony metastasis in the right iliac bone, with the patient in the prone position. The heat generated locally will kill the pain fibers improving the patient's symptoms.

following publication of the **VAPOUR trial** (Lancet, 2016), which showed significant reduction in pain scores following vertebroplasty. A variant of this procedure is kyphoplasty where an attempt to augment the vertebral body height is made by temporarily inflating balloons. Following deflation and removal of the balloons, bone cement is then injected into the recently created cavity.

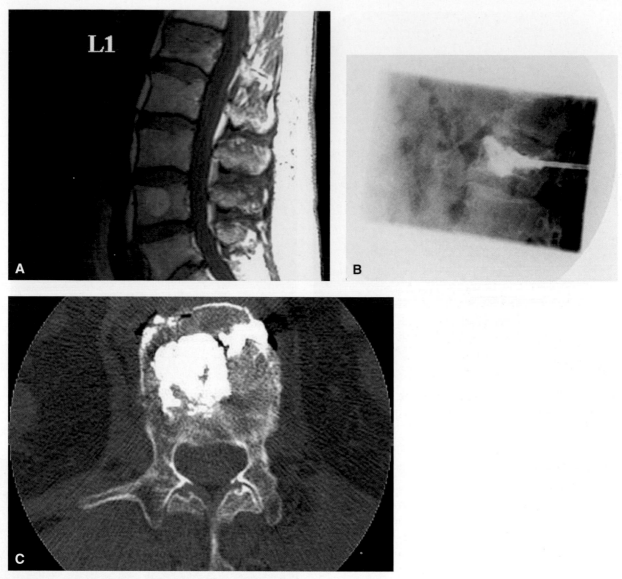

FIGURE 12.30. Vertebroplasty. A: MR of lumbar spine shows a compression fracture of L1. **B:** Bilateral transpedicular needle placement and injection of bone cement into the vertebral body. **C:** Postprocedure CT shows cement within the vertebral body.

KEY POINTS

- IR is a specialty of medicine that provides patients diagnostic and therapeutic minimally invasive procedures using imaging guidance.
- Written informed consent is necessary for most angiographic and interventional procedures. The benefits, risks, and possible complications must be discussed with the patient.
- The Seldinger technique describes a method for gaining vascular or visceral access using a needle, a guidewire, and a catheter.
- Most arteriograms are performed via the common femoral artery, which should be punctured over the femoral head.
- Iodinated contrast is nephrotoxic, particularly in patients with diabetes and patients with preexisting renal impairment.

- CT has superseded pulmonary angiography and ventilation–perfusion scintigraphy in the diagnosis of PE. CT is also essential in the diagnostic workup of AAA and their follow-up post–endograft placement.
- Some IVC filters are retrievable, ideally within 90 days of placement.
- A positive nuclear medicine scan is helpful in patients with GI bleeding because it not only confirms the diagnosis but also directs the angiographer to the site of bleeding.
- Arterial embolization is an important therapy for traumatic vascular injury, GI bleeding, uterine fibroids, and certain tumors.

References

1. *Contrast Manual Version 10.3.* 2018. www.acr.org.
2. Cooper CJ, Murphy TP, Matsumoto A, et al. Stent revascularization for the prevention of cardiovascular and renal events among patients with renal artery stenosis and systolic hypertension: rationale and design of the **CORAL trial**. *Circulation*. 2006;152:59-66.
3. Vedantham S, Goldhaber SZ, Julian JA, et al; **ATTRACT trial** Investigators. Pharmacomechanical catheter-directed thrombolysis for deep-vein thrombosis. *N Engl J Med*. 2017;377:2240-2252.
4. Clark W, Bird P, Gonski P, et al. Safety and efficacy of vertebroplasty for acute painful osteoporotic fractures (**VAPOUR**): a multicentre, randomised, double-blind, placebo-controlled trial. *Lancet*. 2016;388:1408-1416.
5. Harsha A, Trerotola S. Technical aspects of adrenal vein sampling. *J Vasc Interv Radiol*. 2015;26(2):239.

Questions

1. Which of the following types of endoleak is the most common post endovascular repair (EVAR) of abdominal aortic aneurysms (AAA)?
   a. Type 1
   b. Type 2
   c. Type 3
   d. Type 4

2. The most common endoleak post AAA EVAR arises most commonly from which combination of arteries?
   a. Lumbar and inferior mesenteric
   b. Lumbar and superior mesenteric
   c. Inferior mesenteric and median sacral
   d. Inferior mesenteric and internal iliac

Questions 3 to 5: A patient is admitted with acute onset right upper extremity pain and swelling. Venography demonstrates axillo-subclavian thrombosis with extensive collateral formation.

3. The most likely underlying cause for this is
   a. Pancoast tumor
   b. Trauma
   c. External venous compression due to a rib or muscle at the level of the first rib
   d. External compression due to lymph nodes

4. The initial treatment should include
   a. Anticoagulation alone
   b. Catheter-directed thrombolysis
   c. Surgical resection
   d. Thrombectomy
   e. SVC filter placement

5. The preferred definitive treatment is
   a. Surgical resection of the first rib
   b. Balloon angioplasty of the RT subclavian vein
   c. Stent placement in the RT subclavian vein
   d. Creation of an arteriovenous fistula

Questions 6 to 9: A patient's chest film shows a peripheral 2-cm solitary lung nodule.

6. Initial workup includes
   a. Review of previous imaging
   b. Bone (MDP) scan
   c. Wedge resection
   d. Transbronchial biopsy

7. Biopsy guidance of this lesion is best accomplished using
   a. PET
   b. CT
   c. MR
   d. Bronchoscopy

8. One hour after lung biopsy the patient complains of chest pain and dyspnea. A chest film is obtained and the most likely diagnosis is
   a. Flail chest
   b. Pneumothorax
   c. Hydropneumothorax
   d. Pneumopericardium

9. The patient's symptoms worsen and requires oxygen and IV analgesia. The next most appropriate treatment is:
   a. More oxygen and analgesia
   b. A chest tube in the second intercostal space, midclavicular line
   c. A chest tube in the fifth intercostal space, midaxillary line
   d. Bronchoscopy

10. A patient presents with back pain and weight loss. CT abdomen shows extensive retroperitoneal adenopathy. A biopsy is requested. This is best achieved by:
    a. CT guided using a posterior approach
    b. Transjugular route
    c. CT guided using an anterolateral approach
    d. Endoscopically

Answers

Answers to Chapter 2 Questions

1. b
2. a
3. a
4. d
5. False
6. False
7. True
8. True
9. True
10. False

Answers to Chapter 3 Questions

1. False
2. False
3. False
4. False
5. False
6. False
7. True
8. False
9. True
10. False

Answers to Chapter 4 Questions

1. False
2. False
3. False
4. True
5. d
6. False
7. False
8. True
9. True
10. True

Answers to Chapter 5 Questions

1. d
2. False
3. a
4. c
5. False
6. c
7. b
8. d
9. False
10. a

Answers to Chapter 6 Questions

1. b
2. c
3. a
4. c
5. a
6. b
7. d
8. c
9. d
10. a

Answers to Chapter 7 Questions

1. False
2. d
3. d
4. c
5. b
6. c
7. True
8. False
9. True
10. True

Answers to Chapter 8 Questions

1. c
2. c
3. e
4. b
5. a
6. False
7. c
8. True
9. b
10. a

Answers to Chapter 9 Questions

1. c
2. b
3. d
4. b
5. b
6. b
7. d
8. b
9. True
10. e

Answers to Chapter 10 Questions

1. d
2. b
3. d
4. a
5. b
6. a
7. d
8. True
9. False
10. False

Answers to Chapter 11 Questions

1. b
2. d
3. c
4. d
5. c
6. c
7. a
8. c
9. a
10. d

Answers to Chapter 12 Questions

1. b
2. a
3. c
4. b
5. a
6. a
7. b
8. b
9. b
10. a

Common Abbreviations and Acronyms

ABI	Ankle Brachial Index
ACR	American College of Radiology
ADC	Apparent diffusion coefficient
AMS	Altered mental status
ARDS	Acute respiratory distress syndrome
ARSA	Aberrant right subclavian artery
AVM	Arteriovenous malformation
BIRADS	Breast Imaging Reporting and Data System
BRCA	Breast cancer gene
CBCT	Cone beam CT
CBF	Cerebral blood flow
CBV	Cerebral blood volume
CC	Craniocaudal view
CDT	Catheter-directed thrombolysis
CECT	Contrast-enhanced CT
CGM	Cerebral glucose metabolism
CPPD	Calcium pyrophosphate deposition disease
CTA	CT angiography
CTC	CT colonography
CTE	CT enterography
CTU	CT urography
DAI	Diffuse axonal injury
DBT	Digital breast tomosynthesis
DCB	Drug-coated balloon
DES	Drug-eluting stent
DEXA	Dual energy x-ray absorptiometry
DISH	Diffuse idiopathic skeletal hyperostosis
DWI	Diffusion-weighted imaging
EVAR	Endovascular aneurysm repair
FAST	Focused assessment with sonography in trauma
FDG-PET	Fluorodeoxyglucose positron emission tomography
FLAIR	Fluid attenuation inversion recovery
GCS	Glasgow Coma Scale
GGO	Ground glass opacity
HAART	Highly active antiretroviral therapy
HCC	Hepatocellular carcinoma
HRCT	High-resolution CT
HSG	Hysterosalpingogram
HU	Hounsfield unit
IMH	Intramural hematoma
IPMN	Intraductal papillary mucinous neoplasm
KUB	Kidneys, ureters, bladder
LDCT	Low-dose CT
MDCT	Multidetector CT
MIP	Maximum intensity projection
MLO	Mediolateral oblique view
MPI	Myocardial perfusion imaging
MPR	Multiplanar reconstruction
MRA	Magnetic resonance imaging
MRCP	Magnetic resonance cholangio-pancreaticogram
MRE	MR enterography
mRECIST	Modified Response Evaluation Criteria in Solid Tumors
MRF	Mesorectal fascia
MUGA	Multigated acquisition scanning
NAFLD	Nonalcoholic fatty liver disease
NCCT	Noncontrast CT
NMO	Neuromyelitis optica
NSF	Nephrogenic systemic fibrosis
PAU	Penetrating atherosclerotic ulcer
PCOS	Polycystic ovary syndrome
PFA	Plain film of abdomen
PSMA	Prostate-specific membrane antigen
PTC	Percutaneous transhepatic cholangiogram
%RAIU	Radioactive iodine uptake by the thyroid
RIND	Residual ischemic neurological deficit
ROI	Region of interest
SAH	Subarachnoid hemorrhage
SBFT	Small bowel follow-through
SCIWORA	Spinal cord injury without radiographic abnormality
SES	Self-expanding stent
SLNB	Sentinel lymph node biopsy
SPECT	Single photon emission computed tomography
STIR	Short tau inversion recovery
SUV	Standardized uptake value
T1WI	T1-weighted image
T2WI	T2-weighted image
TACE	Transarterial chemoembolization
TAVR	Transvascular aortic valve replacement
TBI	Traumatic brain injury

TcO$_2$	Transcutaneous oxygen	TTN	Transient tachypnea of the newborn
TEVAR	Thoracic endovascular aneurysm repair	UFE	Uterine fibroid embolization
TIA	Transient ischemic attack	UIP	Usual interstitial pneumonitis
TIPS	Transjugular intrahepatic portosystemic shunt	USPSTF	US Preventive Service Task Force
TRALI	Transfusion-related acute lung injury	V/Q	Ventilation perfusion scan
TRO	Triple-rule-out (CT)	VATS	Video-assisted thoracoscopic surgery
TRUS	Trans rectal ultrasound	VRT	Volume rendering technique

Index

Note: Page numbers followed by "f" indicate figures, "t" indicate tables.